A Core Curriculum

PLASTIC SURGERY

A Core Curriculum

PLASTIC SURGERY

ROBERT L. RUBERG, M.D.
Professor and Director
Division of Plastic Surgery
Ohio State University
Columbus, Ohio

DAVID J. SMITH, JR., M.D.
Professor and Section Head
Section of Plastic Surgery
University of Michigan
Ann Arbor, Michigan

With 485 illustrations

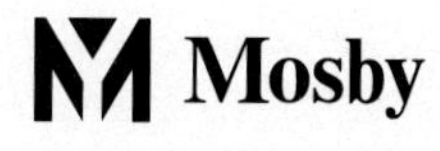

St. Louis Baltimore Boston Chicago London Madrid Philadelphia Sydney Toronto

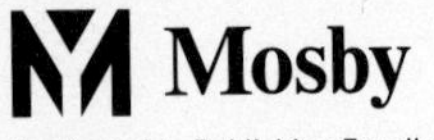

Dedicated to Publishing Excellence

Publisher: George Stamathis
Editor: Robert Hurley
Associate Developmental Editor: Lauranne Billus
Project Manager: Nancy C. Baker
Production Editor: Jerry Schwartz
Proofroom Manager: Barbara M. Kelly
Designer: Nancy C. Baker
Manufacturing Supervisor: Theresa Fuchs

Printed in the United States of America
Composition by Graphic World, Inc.
Printing/binding by Maple-Vail/York

Mosby–Year Book, Inc.
11830 Westline Industrial Drive
St. Louis, Missouri 63146

Library of Congress Cataloging in Publication Data
Plastic surgery : a core curriculum / [edited by] Robert L. Ruberg,
David J. Smith, Jr.
p. cm.
Includes bibliographical references and index.
ISBN 0-8016-6927-8
1. Surgery, Plastic. I. Ruberg, Robert L. II. Smith, David J.,
M.D.
[DNLM: 1. Surgery, Plastic. WO 600 P71455 1993]
RD118.P539 1993
617.9′5—dc20
DNLM/DLC 93-31210
for Library of Congress CIP
Rev

1 2 3 4 5 6 7 8 9 0 98 97 96 95 94

To Yetta and Norman Ruberg
For whom teaching was not just a profession, but a way of life

To my parents Carolyn and David Smith,
Who have taught by example

With love and admiration,
Bob and David

Contributors

Bruce M. Achauer, M.D.
Associate Adjunct Professor of Surgery
University of California, Irvine, College of Medicine
Active Staff
University of California, Irvine, Medical Center
St. Joseph Hospital
Children's Hospital of Orange County
Orange, California

Scott P. Bartlett, M.D.
Associate Professor of Plastic Surgery
University of Pennsylvania
Attending Surgeon
Children's Hospital of Philadelphia
Philadelphia, Pennsylvania

Fritz E. Barton, Jr., M.D.
Professor, Division of Plastic Surgery
University of Texas Southwestern Medical Center
Active Staff
Parkland Memorial Hospital
Baylor University Medical Center
Children's Medical Center
Presbyterian Hospital of Dallas
Dallas Veterans Administration Medical Center
Zale Lipshy University Hospital
Dallas, Texas

Joseph G. Bauer, M.D.
Clinical Instructor
Emory University
Plastic Surgery Associates of Atlanta, P.C.
Northside Hospital
Atlanta, Georgia

Ronald B. Berggren, M.D.
Professor Emeritus of Surgery
Ohio State University
Ohio State University Hospitals
Children's Hospital
Riverside Methodist Hospital
Columbus, Ohio

Arnold S. Breitbart, M.D.
Craniofacial Fellow
Clinical Instructor in Plastic Surgery
Institute of Reconstructive Plastic Surgery
New York University Medical Center
New York, New York

David B. Brothers, M.D.
Chief Resident, Division of Plastic and Reconstructive Surgery
University of North Carolina at Chapel Hill
Chapel Hill, North Carolina

Brently A. Buchele, M.D.
Assistant Professor of Clinical Surgery
Ohio State University
Ohio State University Hospital
Columbus, Ohio

Brian F. Burns, M.D.
Victoria Plastic Surgery Center
Victoria, Texas

Leland Chick, M.D.
Assistant Professor
University of Utah
Staff Surgeon
University Hospital
Shriners Hospital
Holy Cross Hospital
Salt Lake City, Utah

Steven R. Cohen, M.D.
Co-Director, Center for Craniofacial Surgery
Scottish Rite Children's Medical Center
Atlanta, Georgia

John J. Coleman III, M.D.
Professor of Surgery
Director, Division of Plastic Surgery
Indiana University School of Medicine
Indiana University Medical Center
Wishard Memorial Hospital
Veterans Administration Medical Center
Indianapolis, Indiana

Matthew J. Concannon, M.D.
Resident, Division of Plastic Surgery
University of Missouri Health Sciences Center
Columbia, Missouri

Gregory H. Croll, M.D.
Assistant Professor and Plastic Surgeon
Division of Plastic Surgery
University of Missouri Health Sciences Center
Columbia, Missouri

John W. Decorato, M.D.
Attending Plastic and Reconstructive Surgeon
Staten Island University Hospital
Staten Island, New York
New York Eye and Ear Infirmary
New York, New York

Earl J. Fleegler, M.D.
Adjunct Associate Professor, Department of Surgery
Head, Section of Hand Surgery
Department of Plastic and Reconstructive Surgery
Cleveland Clinic Foundation
Cleveland, Ohio

Warren Garner, M.D.
Assistant Professor of Plastic Surgery
University of Michigan
Attending Physician
University of Michigan Medical Center
Ann Arbor, Michigan

Mark Gorney, M.D.
Associate Clinical Professor
Stanford University School of Medicine
Former Director, Post-Graduate Training Program
St. Francis Memorial Hospital
San Francisco, California

Lawrence J. Gottlieb, M.D.
Associate Professor of Clinical Surgery
University of Chicago Pritzker School of Medicine
Co-Director, Genitourinary Reconstruction Team
University of Chicago Hospitals
Chicago, Illinois

Daniel P. Greenwald, M.D.
Assistant Professor
University of South Florida
Chief, Section of Hand Surgery
Division of Plastic Surgery
Tampa General Hospital
Moffitt Cancer Center
Tampa, Florida

Robert Hardesty, M.D.
Associate Professor and Chief, Division of Plastic and Reconstructive Surgery
Associate Professor of Pediatrics
Loma Linda University School of Medicine
Associate Professor, Department of Oral and Maxillofacial Surgery
Loma Linda University School of Dentistry
Section Head, Loma Linda University Medical Center and Children's Hospital
Loma Linda Community Hospital
Loma Linda, California
Riverside General Hospital, Riverside, California
San Bernardino County Medical Center, San Bernardino, California

Vincent R. Hentz, M.D.
Professor of Hand Surgery
Stanford University
Chief, Division of Hand Surgery
Stanford University Hospital
Stanford, California

Michael E. Hill, M.D., Ph.D.
Staff Plastic Surgeon
Wayne Memorial Hospital
Goldsboro, North Carolina

Charles E. Horton, Sr., M.D.
Professor of Plastic Surgery
Eastern Virginia Medical School
Norfolk, Virginia

Charles E. Horton, Jr., M.D.
Clinical Assistant Professor of Urology
Eastern Virginia Medical School
Norfolk, Virginia

David A. Janssen, M.D.
Attending Physician
Mercy Medical Center
Oshkosh, Wisconsin

Thomas J. Krizek, M.D. F.A.C.S.
Professor and Vice Chairman, Department of Surgery

Director, Division of Plastic and Reconstructive Surgery
University of South Florida
Tampa, Florida

John O. Kucan, M.D.
Professor of Surgery
Director, Regional Burn Center
Southern Illinois University School of Medicine
Memorial Medical Center
St. John's Hospital
Springfield, Illinois

J. Daniel Labs, M.D.
Assistant in Surgery
Harvard Medical School
Chief Resident in Plastic Surgery
Massachusetts General Hospital
Boston, Massachusetts

W. Thomas Lawrence, M.P.H., M.D., F.A.C.S.
Associate Professor and Chief, Division of Plastic and Reconstructive Surgery
University of North Carolina
UNC Hospitals
Chapel Hill, North Carolina

Laurence A. Levine, M.D.
Associate Professor of Surgery
Rush Medical College
Director of Reconstructive Urology
Rush Presbyterian-St. Luke's Medical Center
Chicago, Illinois

William Lineaweaver, M.D.
Associate Professor
Division of Plastic and Reconstructive Surgery
Division of Hand Surgery
Stanford University Medical Center
Stanford, California

Graham Lister, M.D.
Professor and Chairman
University of Utah
University Hospital
Primary Children's Medical Center
Shriners Hospital
Salt Lake City, Utah

Ramon Llull, M.D., Ph.D.
Fellow, Division of Plastic and Maxillofacial Surgery
University of Pittsburgh
Resident
University of Pittsburgh Medical Center
Pittsburgh, Pennsylvania

Ronald A. Lohner, M.D.
Clinical Instructor in Surgery
University of Pennsylvania School of Medicine
Resident in Plastic Surgery
Hospital of the University of Pennsylvania
Philadelphia, Pennsylvania

James W. May, Jr., M.D.
Associate Clinical Professor
Harvard Medical School
Chief of Plastic and Reconstructive Surgery and Hand Surgery Service
Department of Surgery
Massachusetts General Hospital
Boston, Massachusetts

Mary H. McGrath, M.D.
Professor of Surgery
Chief, Division of Plastic and Reconstructive Surgery
George Washington University Medical Center
Children's National Medical Center
Washington, District of Columbia

William D. Morain, M.D.
Professor of Plastic Surgery
Dartmouth Medical School
Staff Plastic Surgeon
Dartmouth-Hitchcock Medical Center
Lebanon, New Hampshire

Foad Nahai, M.D.
Professor of Plastic Surgery
Emory University
Attending Physician
Crawford W. Long Memorial Hospital
Emory University Hospital
Atlanta, Georgia

R. Barrett Noone, M.D.
Clinical Professor of Surgery
University of Pennsylvania School of Medicine
Director, Department of Surgery
Chief, Service of Plastic Surgery
Bryn Mawr Hospital, Bryn Mawr, Pennsylvania

Lankenau Hospital, Wynnewood, Pennsylvania
Pennsylvania Hospital
Children's Hospital of Philadelphia
Hospital of the University of Pennsylvania
Philadelphia, Pennsylvania

John A. Persing, M.D.
Professor and Chief of Plastic and Reconstructive Surgery
Yale University School of Medicine
Attending Plastic Surgeon
Yale-New Haven Hospital
New Haven, Connecticut

Linda G. Phillips, M.D.
Associate Professor of Plastic Surgery
Program Director, Residency in Plastic and Reconstructive Surgery
Chief ad interim, Division of Plastic Surgery
University of Texas Medical Branch
University of Texas Hospital Group
Shriners Burns Institute
Galveston, Texas

Carl I. Price, M.D.
Attending Physician, Plastic and Reconstructive and Maxillofacial Surgery
Cox Regional Medical Centers
St. John's Hospital
Springfield, Missouri

Charles L. Puckett, M.D.
Professor and Head, Division of Plastic Surgery
Plastic Surgeon
University of Missouri Medical Center
Columbia, Missouri

Riley S. Rees, M.D.
Associate Professor
University of Michigan Medical Center
Ann Arbor, Michigan

Edward Ricciardelli, M.D.
Assistant Professor of Plastic and Reconstructive Surgery
University of Iowa Hospitals and clinics
Iowa City, Iowa

Martin C. Robson, M.D.
Truman G. Blacker Distinguished Professor of Plastic Surgery
University of Texas Medical Branch
Galveston, Texas

Frank R. Rogers, M.D.
Assistant Professor of Surgery
Loma Linda University School of Medicine
Chief of Plastic Surgery
Riverside County General Hospital
Riverside, California

Robert C. Russell, M.D., F.R.A.C.S., F.A.C.S.
Professor of Surgery and Director of Microsurgery Unit
Southern Illinois University School of Medicine
Chairman, Department of Plastic Surgery
St. John's Hospital
Memorial Medical Center
Springfield, Illinois

Alan Seyfer, M.D.
Professor of Surgery and Chief, Division of Plastic and Reconstructive Surgery
Oregon Health and Science University
Veterans Administration Medical Center
Shriners Hospital
Portland, Oregon

Noel Tenenbaum, M.D.
Resident, Plastic Surgery
University of Michigan
Ann Arbor, Michigan

John W. Siebert, M.D.
Assistant Professor of Plastic Surgery
New York University School of Medicine
NYU Medical Center
Attending Surgeon
Bellevue Hospital
Manhattan Eye, Ear, and Throat Hospital
New York Eye and Ear Infirmary
New York, New York

Susan D. Vasko, M.D.
Clinical Instructor
Ohio State University Hospitals
Staff
Riverside Methodist Hospital
Columbus Children's Hospital
Columbus, Ohio

Jeffrey D. Wagner, M.D.
Assistant Professor of Surgery, Section of Plastic Surgery
Indiana University School of Medicine
Indiana University Hospital
Richard Roudebush's Veterans Hospital
Indianapolis, Indiana

Robert L. Walton, M.D.
Professor and Chairman, Section of Plastic Surgery
Department of Surgery
University of Chicago
Chicago, Illinois

John Woods, M.D.
Professor of Plastic Surgery
Stuart W. Harrington Professor of Surgery
Mayo Medical School, Mayo Foundation
Rochester, Minnesota

Jack Yu, M.D.
Fellow in Craniofacial Surgery, Division of Plastic Surgery
Hospital of the University of Pennsylvania
Children's Hospital of Philadelphia
Philadelphia, Pennsylvania

William A. Zamboni, M.D.
Assistant Professor, Division of Plastic and Reconstructive Surgery
Southern Illinois University School of Medicine
Springfield, Illinois

Elvin G. Zook, M.D.
Professor of Surgery
Southern Illinois University School of Medicine
Memorial Medical Center
St. John's Hospital
Springfield, Illinois

Preface

This textbook is designed principally for use by plastic surgery residents and residents in related specialties. It is the ultimate outcome of an effort which began almost 10 years ago to define the essential curriculum of the plastic surgery resident. The evolution of this work is described in the following:

In 1985 the Association of Academic Chairmen of Plastic Surgery was created as a distinct and separate organization; for the previous 10 years it had existed as a committee of the American Association of Plastic Surgeons, the Program Directors Committee. One of the very first efforts of the AACPS was to develop a comprehensive curriculum to define the scope of plastic surgery residency education and training. After several unsuccessful efforts to achieve consensus on the activities of residents, a Comprehensive Plastic Surgery Curriculum was produced.

The initial document included a long list of "learner objectives" and "clinical practice activities" which could comprise the full scope of plastic surgery residency training. Then an "evaluation panel" of 25 AACPS members was assembled. The panel consisted of program directors and non-program directors, older and younger members, university and private practice physicians. Based on the recommendations of this panel, each of the Learner Objectives and "Clinical Practice Activities" was classified as **essential**, desirable, or *optional*. The document thus produced was intended for use by program directors in structuring their training programs and residents in deciding their study patterns and selection of clinical activities.

This textbook is the natural outgrowth and extention of the Comprehensive Plastic Surgery Curriculum. The scope of each chapter in the text has been determined by the corresponding unit in the curriculum. The emphasis of each chapter has been guided by the designations of **essential**, desirable, and *optional* in the curriculum: each unit stresses principally the **essential** and desirable components, with minimal attention to the *optional* elements.

At the start of each chapter we have printed the appropriate section from The Comprehensive Plastic Surgery Cirriculum. The "Learner Objectives" and "Clinical Practice Activities" are classified by different type: **essential is represented by bold type**; desirable by text type; and *optional in italics*.

The goal of the text was to present the most important material ("A Core Curriculum") in a concise form, with uniform illustrations and multiple tables. In this way a thorough overview of all basic material might be mastered by a plastic surgery resident in 1 year of training. Similarly, the basics of plastic surgery would be easily accessible to residents and physicians in related specialties. And a concise reference to the most important plastic surgery topics would be available to all physicians.

The authors are deeply indebted to the Association of Academic Chairmen of Plastic Surgery for granting permission to publish the Comprehensive Plastic Surgery Curriculum and to utilize the curriculum as the basis for the text.

We wish to thank our Editor Jim Ryan and Associate Editor Karyn Fell Taeyaerts for their guidance and for their great help in keeping this project on track. We are delighted with the excellent work of our illustrator Jaye Schlesinger. We could not have completed this entire effort without the support of our hard-working secretaries, Jane Van Straten and Gretchen Lowry in Columbus and Jeanne Jeager and Donna Miller in Ann Arbor. And finally, we give special thanks to our families, who put up with the many late night and week-end hours spent putting this effort together.

Robert L. Ruberg, M.D.
David J. Smith, Jr., M.D.

Contents

PART I

Core of Knowledge: General Plastic Surgical Principles and Techniques

Chapter 1

Wound Repair: Principles and Applications

Martin C. Robson, M.D.
Brian F. Burns, M.D.
Linda G. Phillips, M.D.

■ CONTENTS

NOTE: The material in this chapter is frequently covered during the **prerequisite** training period of many plastic surgery residents. This chapter should serve as a valuable review of important material in such cases. For residents who have **not** mastered this material previously, this chapter is essential.

■ CHAPTER OBJECTIVE

At the end of this chapter the resident understands the physiology of wound healing and manages complex wounds by utilizing a variety of techniques to achieve complete healing and maximum aesthetic benefit.

■ LEARNER OBJECTIVES

On completion of this chapter the resident

1. **Is thoroughly familiar with the physiology and biochemistry of normal wound healing.**
2. **Understands the physiology and biochemistry of abnormal wound healing, including hypertrophic scars and keloids.**
3. **Is familiar with common agents and**

processes that result in abnormal wound healing.

4. **Is familiar with the pharmacologic agents and other nonsurgical methods for the treatment of abnormal healing of skin and subcutaneous tissue.**
5. **Is competent in the management of dressings, splints, and other devices and techniques utilized in wound management.**
6. **Understands the principles of healing of bone, tendon, cartilage, nerve, skin, and muscle.**
7. **Recognizes the differences in the healing of cortical and cancellous bone and membranous and endochondral bone.**
8. **Is thoroughly familiar with the principles and techniques for achieving optimal healing of bone, tendon, cartilage, nerve, skin, and muscle.**
9. **Is skilled in the application, planning, and surgical performance of techniques to alter scars (such as Z-plasty, W-plasty).**
10. **Recognizes the various lines of the skin (such as relaxed skin tension lines) and their importance in the placement of incisions for maximum aesthetic benefit.**
11. **Understands the role of nutrition in the wound healing process and is familiar with standard methods for diagnosis and treatment of nutritional deficiency.**
12. **Understands the pathologic processes involved in keloid formation and the methods available to treat keloids.**
13. Recognizes techniques for preservation of skin, bone, cartilage, tendon, and nerve.
14. Understands differences in suture materials and indications for the use of different materials.

CLINICAL PRACTICE ACTIVITIES

During the course of the training program, the resident

1. **Treats complex wound problems such as dehiscence, delayed healing, and multiple complex traumatic wounds.**
2. **Evaluates patients with scar problems and revises scars to achieve maximum functional and aesthetic benefit.**
3. **Performs surgical and pharmacologic treatment of hypertrophic scars and keloids.**
4. **Utilizes splints, casts, dressings, topical agents, etc., to optimize wound healing.**
5. **Places incisions for elective surgery in such a way as to achieve maximum aesthetic benefit.**
6. **Performs surgical procedures to repair tendon and nerve injuries.**
7. **Treats fractures with casting and open reduction techniques.**
8. Utilizes biological and artificial skin substitutes in wound management.

BASIC SCIENCE OF HEALING

Wound healing is the restoration of anatomic integrity and function of injured tissue. In humans, regeneration of normal cellular elements is limited to epithelium and liver; most wound healing and repair result in scarring. While this scar provides "healing," it may also severely limit the ultimate function of injured structures. Although wound healing was once considered a generic term, it is now recognized to be the summation of a number of complex processes including coagulation, inflammation, matrix synthesis and deposition, angiogenesis, fibroplasia, epithelialization, contraction, and remodeling (Fig 1–1). The degree to which any single process plays a part in the repair of a given wound is variable. A partial-thickness skin abrasion heals almost entirely by epithelialization, whereas a deep chronic pressure ulcer may require very little epithelialization and rely more on matrix synthesis, angiogenesis, fibroplasia, and contraction.

Wound healing activities begin almost simultaneously with the wounding event. There is local activation of phospholipase A at the injured cell membrane that causes the me-

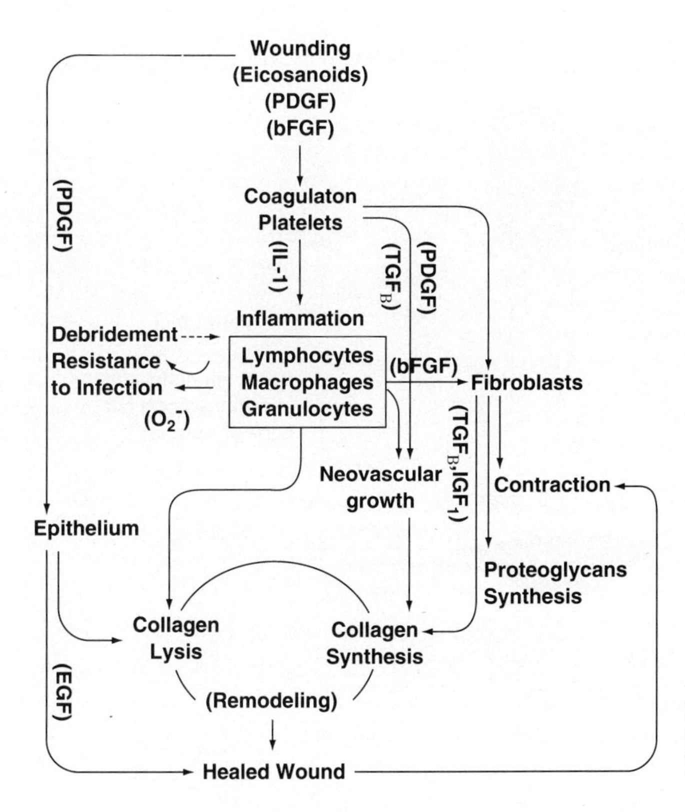

FIG 1–1.
Scheme of multiple processes of wound healing.

tabolism of arachidonic acid to the eicosanoid soluble mediators, especially the prostaglandins and leukotrienes. The bleeding that occurs following wounding activates the body's hemostatic mechanisms to terminate blood loss. These mechanisms include vascular constriction, platelet plug formation, fibrin formation, and fibrinolysis. As the coagulation cascade is activated, so are portions of the complement cascade. These events occur simultaneously to produce the primary messengers orchestrating the various processes of healing.

Physiology of Wound Healing: Phases of Healing and Cellular Sequence of Repair

Although artificial phases or stages of wound healing have been described, it is important to realize that these are both separate and distinct. The repair process proceeds in an orderly and timely manner, but with different tissues and in different circumstances, the phases of the process may be indistinct.

Inflammation is the basic physiologic process that is common to all wounds. Clinically, inflammation is identified by the cardinal signs of redness (rubor), heat (calor), swelling (tumor), pain (dolor), and loss of function (functio laesa). The physiology underlying these cardinal clinical signs is a complex amalgam of biochemical and cellular events. A variety of biochemical processes including the coagulation cascade, the complement system cascade, arachidonic acid metabolism, and histamine and kallikrein release are initiated immediately after wounding. While these biochemical events are occurring, leukocytes are marginating, sticking to vessel walls, and emigrating through the walls toward the site of injury. Simultaneously, venules are dilating, and lymphatics are blocked.

The inflammation that begins immediately after wounding is the first phase of healing. The main cells involved in this process are polymorphonuclear leukocytes (PMNs) and macrophages. Clots, foreign bodies, and bacteria are removed, and the substrates for extracellular matrix deposition and collagen synthesis are being arranged (Fig 1–2). In primary wound healing, this process of inflammation

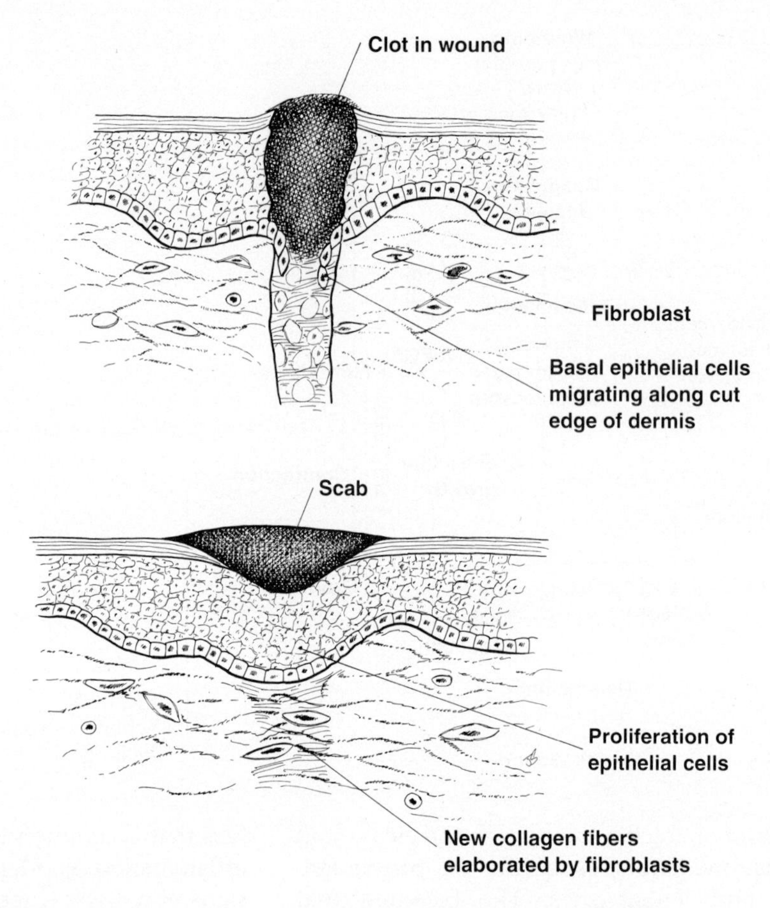

FIG 1–2.
Skin wound repair.

occurs in a brief 4- to 6-day period. During this time the wound appears erythematous and edematous because of the effect of various humoral mediators. In healing by secondary or tertiary intention, the inflammatory phase continues until the wound surface is closed by ectodermal or endodermal elements (epithelium for skin or gut and endothelium for blood vessels).

The second and third phases of wound healing are relatively constant and begin only when the wound is covered by epithelium. The proliferative (or collagen or regenerative) phase of healing is characterized by the production of collagen in the wound. The main cell present during this phase is the fibroblast, which produces the extracellular matrix and collagen. In a primarily approximated wound, production of collagen begins approximately 7 days after wounding, and net production continues over the next 6 weeks.

The third and final phase of wound healing is the remodeling (or maturation) phase. It is characterized by the maturation of collagen by cross-linking and continued turnover (synthesis and degradation) of collagen without a net gain or loss. This maturation may continue for as long as 2 years in adults and even longer in children.

The proliferative and maturation phases of healing may overlap to some extent. Since the process of collagen synthesis and degradation is dynamic, collagen laid down early is being remodeled as new collagen continues to be produced. These two phases of wound healing are separated in order to describe the predominant physiologic process occurring at a particular time.

After a wound is incurred, many different cell types become integrally involved in the process of healing. Their presence and interactions are determined by messengers that will be described in the section on biochemistry. These cells appear in an overlapping temporal sequence that begins with the formation of the aggregated platelet thrombus.

This is followed by the migration of various types of leukocytes into the wound and culminates in the appearance of fibroblasts and neocapillaries formed by endothelial cells.

Immediately after wounding, humoral and cellular elements of the clotting mechanism are activated to achieve early hemostasis. The platelet directs this response, and its granules contain substances necessary for wound repair to proceed. These substances include lysosomal enzymes, adenosine triphosphate (ATP), serotonin, and peptide growth factors. One such factor, platelet-derived growth factor (PDGF), is released only at sites of injury and has both chemotactic and mitogenic activity toward fibroblasts and smooth muscle cells. It appears to be primarily a wound hormone that results in early deposition of extracellular matrix, increased entry and proliferation of cells, and an increased rate of collagen deposition.

Shortly after the formation of a clot, PMNs appear and remain the predominant cell for approximately 48 hours. The activated PMN is the origin of many inflammatory mediators and bactericidal oxygen-derived free radicals. Since the neutrophil's absence does not prevent wound healing, it does not appear to be an essential cell. However, the macrophage is. Monocytes enter the wound after the PMNs and reach maximum numbers approximately 24 hours later. They quickly evolve into macrophages, which are the main cell involved in wound debridement. Macrophages persist for several weeks in wounds healing by primary intention and are numerous in chronic open wounds. Macrophages secrete substances such as basic fibroblast growth factor (bFGF) that are chemotactic and mitogenic for fibroblasts and endothelial cells and increase angiogenesis.

The fibroblast is the workhorse of the wound repair process. It is the cell responsible for the formation of all the connective tissue components in the healing wound, including collagen, glycosaminoglycans, and elastin fibers. As the collagen production reaches a maximum and remodeling of the collagen becomes the predominant process, the number of fibroblasts is gradually reduced, and the scar tissue becomes almost acellular.

Epithelialization is a prominent process in wound healing (Fig 1–3). The basal epithelial cell at the wound margin flattens and migrates into the open wound area. As the basal cells at the wound margin multiply in a horizontal direction, the basal cells behind this margin assume a vertical growth column characteristic of a normal epithelial barrier. Although this process is accomplished with relative ease in wounds healing by primary intention, in those healing by secondary intention or in partial-thickness burns the epithelium must often migrate over great distances, which requires a much longer time period. Migration of epithelial cells occurs only over viable tissue and only if the wound is not infected. An open wound remains in the inflammatory phase of healing with no effective collagen production until it has been covered with an epithelial element.

Epithelium in areas other than the skin may heal in a somewhat different fashion. Respiratory epithelial migration occurs in multiple planes, not just at the basal cell layer. Excessive scarring may lead to the loss of underlying mesenchymal structures necessary for differentiation of the epithelium into ciliated columnar cells. Intestinal epithelium is columnar except for the esophagus. The esophagus is stratified squamous epithelium and heals more like skin. Small-bowel mucosa is regenerated from the crypts of Lieberkühn,

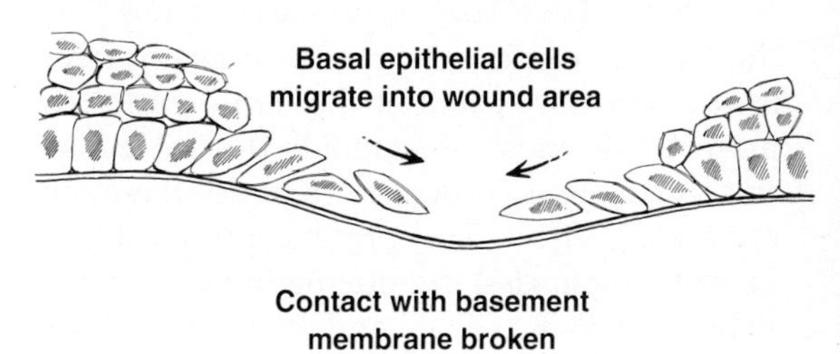

FIG 1–3.
Epithelial repair.

and turnover of mucosal cells is extremely fast and efficient. Colon epithelium migrates much more slowly. A defect that would be resurfaced in a few days in the small bowel may take up to 3 months to resurface in the colon. Regeneration of bladder epithelium is rapid and involves all layers of the stratified squamous cells.

Biochemistry of Wound Healing

Eicosanoids, Cytokines, Oxygen-derived Radicals—Primary Messengers of Repair

Just as there is a cellular sequence to healing, so also is there a humoral mediator, or messenger sequence. These substances carry the message for cell-cell and cell-matrix interaction. Initially, a number of substances collectively called "inflammatory mediators" modulate the wound healing process. Among the inflammatory mediators that contribute to the genesis of the signs and symptoms of the inflammatory process are the prostanoid derivatives of the arachidonic acid cascade (Fig 1–4). Rubor (redness) is caused by vasodilation. The most potent prostanoid vasodilator is prostacyclin (PGI_2). Others include prostaglandins A, D, and E (PGA, PGD, and PGE). While prostaglandins G_2 and H_2 (PGG_2 and PGH_2) initially evoke a vasoconstrictive activity, they are responsible for a secondary vasodilatory response.

Tumor (swelling) is primarily caused by the leakage of plasma proteins through gaps in the vascular spaces of the tissue endothelium. While most prostanoids do not evoke this edematous process, they do have an enhancing effect. The prostanoids most frequently implicated in potentiating edema are PGE_2 and $PGF_{2\alpha}$. PGI_2 and PGE_2 have little direct effect on vascular permeability, but they markedly enhance edema formation and leukocyte infiltration by promoting blood flow into the area of injured tissue.

The role of prostanoids as mediators of heat (calor) is less clear. Arachidonic acid, PGE, and PGE_2 have some potential for creating a febrile episode. The best evidence for this is the antipyretic effect of prostaglandin blocking agents such as aspirin.

Dolor (pain) is provoked by arachidonic acid in the experimental situation. The eicosanoid derivatives initiate or provoke varying degrees of hyperalgesia, especially PGI_2, PGE, and PGE_2.

The release of these prostanoids also triggers mobilization of the inflammatory cells, which interact with all known cells and cell structures. After release of the arachidonic acid cascade from the tissue membranes, the neutrophil is the first infiltrating cell present during the acute phase of inflammation. The activated neutrophil produces a wide variety of additional inflammatory mediators. Thromboxane A_2 (TxA_2) is present within 6 hours of trauma, possibly to help in hemostasis by its vasoconstrictive effect. The biosynthesis of prostaglandin F_2 (PGF_2) has a profound influence on the fibroblast function of the dermis after trauma to the skin. It has been reported that PGF_2 along with PGE_2 helps to initiate collagen biosynthesis. The concentration of hyaluronic acid in human skin and connective tissue increases in the presence of PGE_1. $PGF_{2\alpha}$ is also a potent stimulator of hexosamine-containing ground substance production by dermal fibroblasts.

Normal skin maturation and skin tissue function rely on maintenance of the permeability and integrity of all tissue membranes. It has been documented that prostaglandins (particularly the PGE_2–cyclic adenosine monophosphate [cAMP] relationship) are essential for normal skin maturation. Although PGE_2 is a vasodilator and PGF_2 a vasoconstrictor, they maintain a steady-state relationship through the effect of PGE_2 9-ketoreductase. When the host needs more PGE_2, $PGF_{2\alpha}$ is converted to PGE_2 by the enzyme and reduced nicotinamide adenine dinucleotide phosphate (NADPH). This reaction is reversible via NADPH and 9-ketoreductase to produce $PGF_{2\alpha}$. Concentrations of PGE_2 9-ketoreductase in normal skin are low, and their presence further supports the hypothesis of a steady-state relationship to maintain normal cell function and integrity. This steady-state relationship between PGE_2 and $PGF_{2\alpha}$ apparently maintains the flow and balance of intracellular and extracellular nutrients and waste fluids for cell and tissue viability and integrity. Through control of the

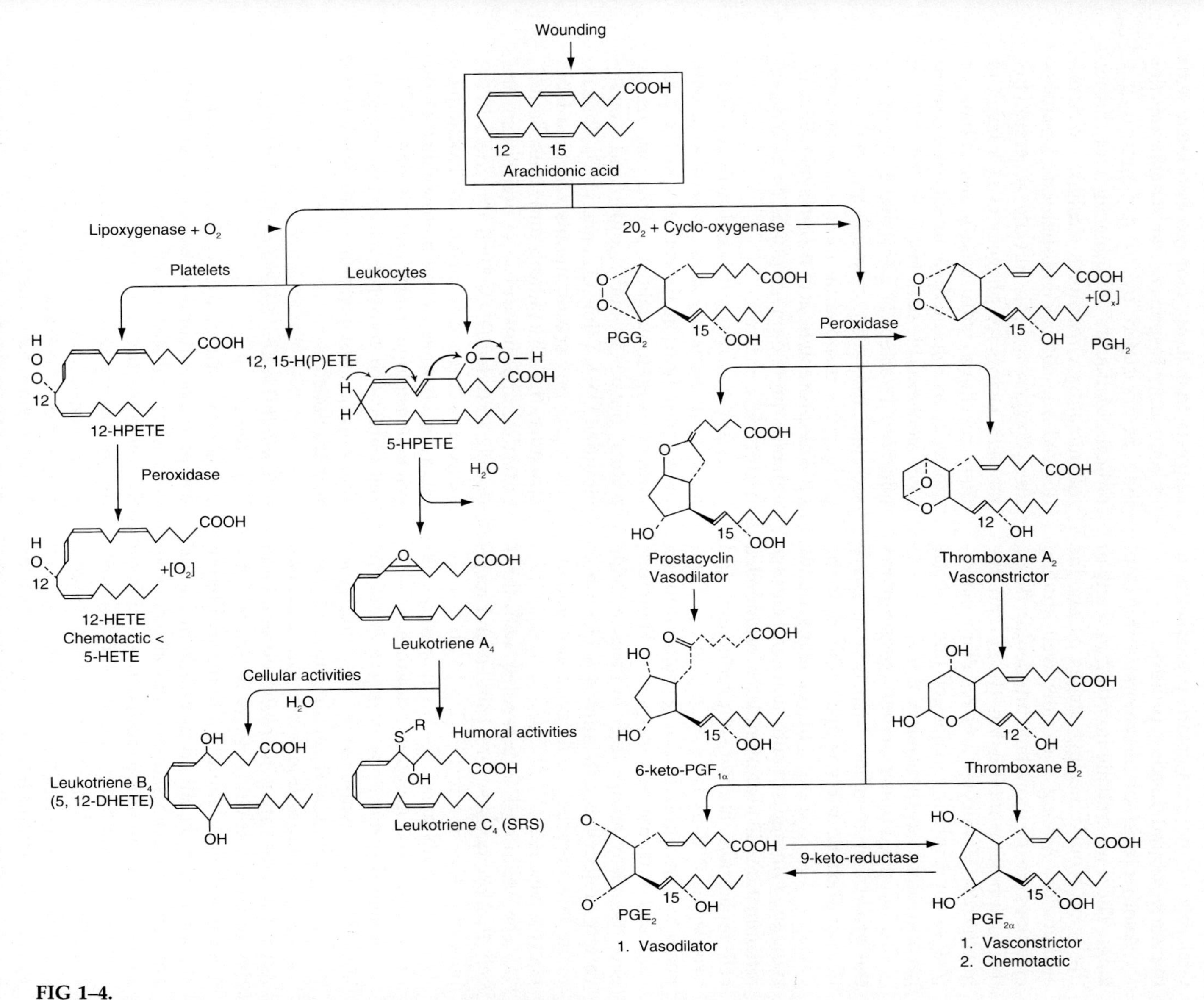

FIG 1–4.
Metabolism of arachidonic acid to various eicosanoid inflammatory mediators.

vasoactive and vasoconstrictive activities of these two prostanoids, cell viability and permeability and microvasculature patency are maintained. This mechanism points out the vital role of the inflammatory mediators in the early wound healing process.

Another class of mediators is the cytokines. These are initially involved in many of the same wound healing stages as are the eicosanoids. Among the most well studied cytokines are the monokine interleukin (IL-1), the lymphokine interleukin (IL-2), and the interferons. Monocytes and resultant macrophages constitute the major cell line that has been identified as the source of IL-1.

IL-1 derived from macrophages promotes the growth or metabolic function of every nonlymphocytic cell type that responds to the cytokine. IL-1 can account for many of the signs and symptoms of both acute and chronic inflammation. It also stimulates endothelial cell replication, fibrinogen production, and procoagulant activity. Consequently, it appears to play a role in clot formation during the early inflammatory response. Therefore, like the eicosanoids, IL-1 induces a wide variety of activities and functions like a hormone affecting both leukocytic and nonleukocytic cells.

The origin of IL-2 rests solely with the T cell. IL-2 promotes several cellular and metabolic functions in activated T cells prior to the onset of proliferation. IL-2–activated T cells can in turn produce other cytokines.

Just as IL-1 functions more as a monokine and IL-2 as a lymphokine, the interferons possess functions that mimic those of both classes of cytokines. Interferons can be defined as peptides that are genetically restricted and that promote antiviral activity in treated cells. They have been organized into three different classes (α, β, γ) based on physiochemical and antigenic differences. Interferons also have an influence on immune reactivity and inhibit cell proliferation but promote cell differentiation. The interleukins and interferons regulate the inflammatory response and the immune systems by controlling the cell responses. These responses alter cell proliferation and differentiation and can be either beneficial or detrimental to the process of wound healing.

During the metabolism of a variety of lipids, including arachidonate, oxygen-derived free radicals are produced. Current evidence suggests that tissue damage associated with inflammatory responses and ischemic injuries may be mediated by oxygen-derived free radicals. Mediators of both acute and chronic inflammatory reactions include oxygen-derived free radicals and subsequent metabolites. Oxygen radicals directly generate chemotactic factors for phagocytes as a result of their reactions with unsaturated lipids or indirectly as intermediate metabolites in normal biochemical pathways of the cell. In addition, a variety of lysosomal enzymes are secreted into the extracellular milieu by phagocytes responding to chemotactic stimuli. This proteolytic activity can synergistically enhance direct damage produced by oxygen-derived free radicals.

It appears that structural matrices of tissues at inflammatory sites can be altered with or without lysosomal proteases in the presence of oxygen metabolites. Free radicals can induce breaks in both single- and double-stranded DNA. While O_2^- and H_2O_2 alone do not create any significant alterations in DNA structure, the OH radicals and other peroxyradical compounds can sever both single- and double-stranded DNA. Such alterations in the DNA structure can result in biochemical changes, changes in the maintenance of the cell's physiologic state, and changes in the cell's ability to conserve its genetic constitution during subsequent division, thus leading to mutations.

Growth Factors: Secondary Messengers of Repair

Growth factors are peptides that promote cell proliferation and induce the migration of cells. These substances, which are chemotactic to inflammatory cells such as neutrophils and/or macrophages or mitogenic to cells such as fibroblasts and/or endothelial cells, play a major role in wound healing. Since wound healing is a well-orchestrated complex series of events involving cell-cell and cell-matrix interactions, the growth factors serve as messengers to regulate the various processes involved. If the inflammatory mediators are the "primary" messengers of repair, growth factors might be considered "secondary" messengers.

Although growth factors were thought to start acting following coagulation and the formation of a platelet plug, it now appears that they play a much earlier role. PDGF and bFGF are produced by the injured cell at the time of wounding. Once the platelet plug is in place, several growth factors are released that are chemotactic to and mitogenic for inflammatory cells. Transforming growth factor β (TGF-β) and PDGF are released from the platelet and mediate chemotaxis of neutrophils, monocytes, and macrophages into the wound. PDGF is the more important peptide during the period of inflammation and is responsible for the directed and sequential migration of neutrophils, macrophages, and fibroblasts into the wound over the first several days after wounding.

Following the introduction of monocytes and macrophages into the wound during inflammation, the extracellular matrix is laid down. Growth factors important during inflammation also have predominant roles during this stage. A single application of PDGF into experimental wounds increases the volume of granulation tissue dramatically. The extracellular matrix in these wounds has increased glycosaminoglycan deposition consisting largely of hyaluronic acid. TGF-β also causes an increase in the volume of granulation tissue.

Several growth factors are stimulatory for endothelial cells. These include PDGF, bFGF, and TGF-β. Factors that are chemoattractant and/or mitogenic for endothelial cells increase the rate of angiogenesis.

Fibroplasia and collagen synthesis appear to be regulated by various peptide messengers. bFGF is chemotactic and mitogenic for fibroblasts. PDGF and insulin-like growth factor 1 (IGF-1) act synergistically to promote mitogenesis of mesenchymal cells. PDGF is also chemotactic for fibroblasts, and IGF-1 stimulates collagen production. Although TGF-β works earlier in the wound healing scheme, evidence is now available that this growth factor can directly accelerate collagen synthesis and maturation in wounds. Tumor necrosis factor α (TNF-α) can also modulate wound healing in the fibroplasia phase by stimulating replication of fibroblasts. Recombinant TNF-α has been demonstrated to increase wound disruption strength in both normal and impaired healing situations.

Keratinocyte replication and epithelialization can be increased by epidermal growth factor (EGF), epidermal cell–derived growth factor (EDF), and PDGF. Not only is the rate of epithelialization increased, but there is also a greater degree of keratinocyte differentiation, especially with EGF. PDGF appears to affect only keratinocytes after wounding and is downregulated when epithelialization is complete. The role of bFGF in epithelialization is unclear at present, with some reports suggesting keratinocyte stimulation and others suggesting impairment of epithelialization.

As discussed previously, the primary cell responsible for wound contraction is the fibroblast. Therefore, growth factors chemotactic and/or mitogenic for fibroblasts would be expected to affect the rate of contraction. Experimentally, bFGF, PDGF, and granulocyte-macrophage colony-stimulating factor (GM-CSF) speed contraction. In human wounds such as pressure sores in which contraction is a major process in the healing scheme, PDGF and bFGF appear to be efficacious.

TGF-β, PDGF, and bFGF have many of the same roles in early fracture healing as they do in soft-tissue healing. In addition, acidic fibroblast growth factor (aFGF) appears to be an important intracellular growth factor in callus formation. In fracture healing bFGF is important because it is mitogenic to chondrocytes and osteoblasts, and TGF-β can differentiate mesenchymal cells into osteoblasts and chondrocytes.

Several clinical trials have reported success in using a platelet-derived wound healing formula (PDWHF). This is formulated from autologous or pooled homologous blood. The PDWHF contains PDGF, TGF-β, platelet-derived angiogenesis factors, platelet-derived EGF, and platelet factor 4. Stimulation of repair by such a compound underlines the importance of peptide growth factors in the wound healing scheme.

Collagen, Glycosaminoglycans, Elastin: Structural Components of Repair

Collagen is the principal structural protein of the body. It is a complex, three-dimensional structure, and there are several distinct types, depending on the component parts (Table 1–1). The process of collagen synthesis begins with the production of amino acid chains in the cytoplasm of the fibroblast. These α-chains are unique in that each third amino acid is glycine. Two amino acids, hydroxyproline and hydroxylysine, are found only in collagen and require hydroxylation (from proline or lysine) in their synthesis by specific enzymes, which require ferrous ion, α-ketoglutarate and ascorbic acid as cofactors.

The α-peptide chains are woven into a triple helix, and the entire structure is then twisted into a "super helix." Following attachment of a galactose unit, the molecule is excreted from the fibroblast as procollagen. Removal of several terminal amino acids from the α-chains produces tropocollagen. Tropocollagen aggregates to form collagen fibrils, and these aggregates are held together by cross-links created by the conversion of lysine to an aldehyde and then reaction with another aldehyde from an adjacent tropocollagen molecule (Fig 1–5).

TABLE 1-1.
Various Types of Collagen

Type	Distribution
I	Connective tissues and basement membranes
II	Hyaline cartilages and cartilage-like tissues
III	Distensible connective tissues
IV	Basement membranes
V	Essentially all tissues
VI	Essentially all tissues
VII	Dermal-epidermal junctions
VIII	Descemet's membrane, produced by endothelial cells
IX	Hyaline cartilage
X	Hypertrophic cartilage
XI	Hyaline cartilage
XII	May be similar to type I collagen
XIII	Synthesized by certain tumor cell lines

The deposition of collagen is a dynamic process that involves production and remodeling. Production of collagen begins between days 3 and 7 after the wound is closed. Making new collagen remains the dominant process in wound repair from day 7 to about day 42 after wound closure.

Remodeling of collagen is the process whereby randomly arranged collagen fibers and aggregates are gradually replaced by a more organized formation of fibers in response to local stress factors in the wound. Early in scar formation, type III collagen is also gradually replaced by type I collagen. Although there is no net collagen production after day 42, there is a dynamic turnover of collagen that results in continued gain in wound strength for up to 2 years after injury. This steady state of no net collagen production is the result of collagen synthesis equaling collagen lysis.

Another component of connective tissue and scar tissue is glycosaminoglycans, large polysaccharides of repeating disaccharide units. These glycosaminoglycans are usually connected to a protein moiety, the combination being designated a proteoglycan. Proteoglycans are the main component of "ground substance." Ground substance is the extracellular matrix that is felt to be responsible for directing and organizing collagen synthesis and deposition. Proteoglycans are divided into two major groups: sulfated and nonsulfated. Nonsulfated proteoglycans include hyaluronic acid, chondroitin, and fibronectin, whereas sulfated proteoglycans include chondroitin sulfate A, B, and C, heparan sulfate, and keratosulfate.

As wound repair proceeds, the particular proteoglycans involved likewise change. Early in the inflammatory phase the hyaluronic acid content rises rapidly. As collagen is laid down, hyaluronic acid levels decrease, and chondroitin sulfate levels increase. As the scar matures, the total proteoglycan levels are low, and only small amounts remain incorporated into collagen. This decrease in the proteoglycan level leads to a corresponding loss of water and the resultant tightly packed collagen scar.

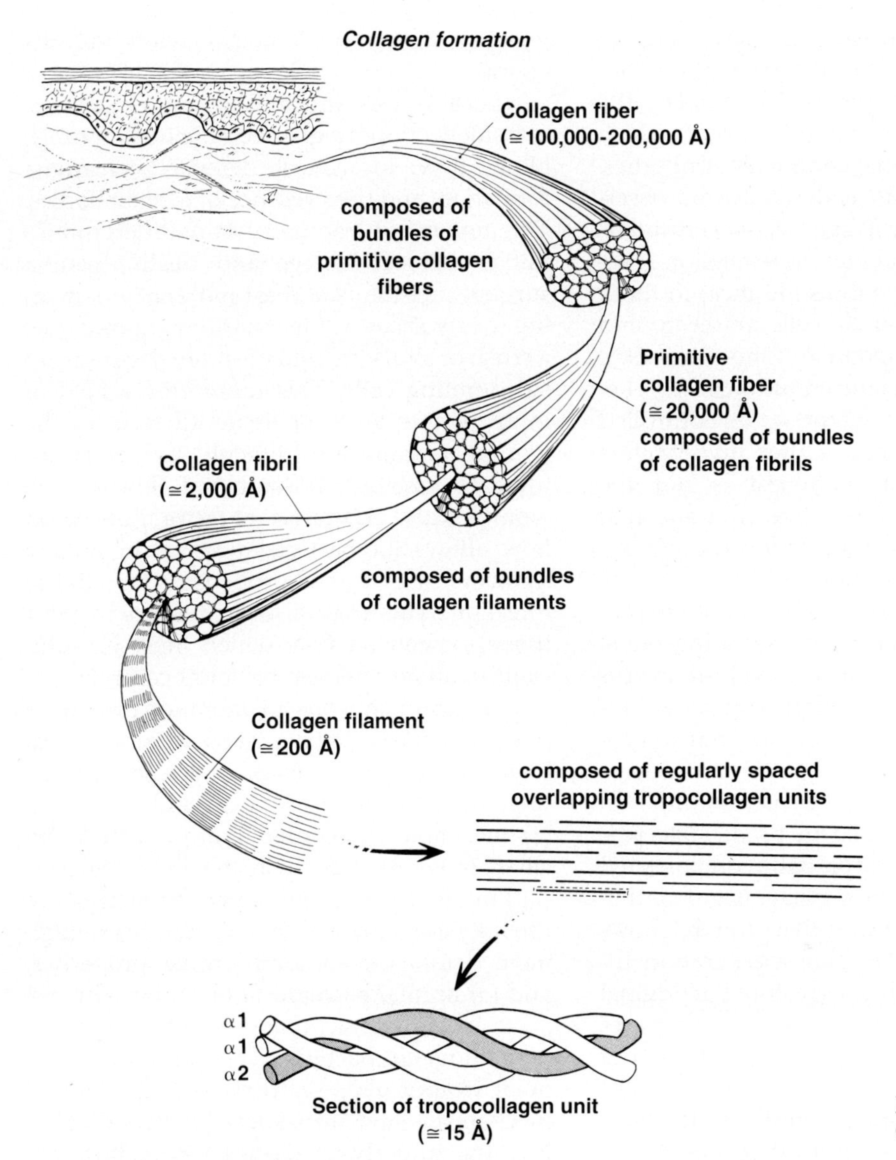

FIG 1–5.
Collagen formation.

Like collagen, elastin is a protein produced by the fibroblast. However, it is not readily replaced and is not an important component of wound repair. Elastic fibers are found in skin, arteries, ligaments, and certain fibrocartilaginous structures, all of which are subject to extreme, repetitive distortional forces. They act to restore the original shape and contour of the structures in which they are found. Specialized cross-links in the elastin molecule give it this remarkable property. The number of elastic fibers in tissue decreases with age.

Wound Contraction

The cellular physiology and humoral biochemistry just discussed can be applied to all healing wounds. However, one process of healing requires special attention when one considers healing of open wounds of the skin. Open wounds heal by the bimodal process of epithelial migration and contraction of the wound edges. Wound contraction is a pulling of the surrounding skin toward the center of an epithelial defect to make the defect smaller. Collagen formation is not essential for wound contraction, and even with vitamin C depletion, contraction proceeds normally. Most of the recent literature concerning wound contraction focuses on a specialized fibroblast, the myofibroblast, at the wound margin, which appears to have special contractile properties. The term *myofibroblast* is derived from observations concerning this specialized cell and its internal structure. Under transmission electron microscopy, myofibrils identical to those found in smooth muscle cells are seen, and these myofibrils respond to smooth muscle stimulants and relaxants. Contraction is believed by some investigators to be controlled by these myofibroblasts. Other investigators believe that the myofibroblast is not the functioning cell but only a skeleton and that actin and myosin in the wound margin are responsible for contraction.

A wound that is externally splinted to prevent advancement of the surrounding tissue does not contract. Thicker split-thickness grafts and full-thickness grafts can act as "internal splints" and will minimize but not totally inhibit the amount of wound contraction. As the wound contracts, the surrounding skin is stretched and thinned in predictable patterns. This is eventually partially compensated by the production of new collagen and epithelial cells. This "intussusceptive growth," however, does not represent skin regeneration. Intussusceptive growth does restore the original dermal thickness, but specialized structures such as hair follicles and sweat glands are not reproduced.

Contraction of open wounds is inevitable and somewhat predictable. It is not necessarily a detrimental process. The tension and deformity of surrounding tissues must be balanced against the successful coverage of the wound.

Microbiology and Immunology of Wound Healing

Every wound is to some degree contaminated with microorganisms. The result of this contamination on wound healing depends on a complex interaction among local tissue factors, host resistance, amount of bacterial inoculum, and preparation of the wound prior to closure. Before closing a wound, the surgeon must take these many factors into account.

Local factors affecting wound closure are extremely important and include trauma, blood flow, local host defense, hematoma formation, and the presence of foreign bodies. The amount of trauma sustained determines initial cellular damage and death. Even a surgical incision is at least minimally damaging to any tissue at the wound margins, while a crush or avulsion injury is more damaging to surrounding cells. This represents a field of injury where areas of tissue adjacent to the wound margin are difficult to assess for ultimate viability. Local blood flow to the wound is also an important factor. Low blood flow allows for bacterial survival in greater numbers and thus a propensity for clinical infection. This may also be related to poor tissue oxygen tension, which must be sufficient to allow effective bacterial control.

Skin and mucous membranes provide a structural barrier to bacterial invasion. Several biological decontamination processes are also ongoing deterrents to bacterial invasion: (1) mechanical decontamination such as by ciliary movement in the tracheobronchial tree, (2) chemical decontamination from tears or the fatty acids present on the skin surface that have demonstrated antibacterial properties, and (3) normal bacterial flora of the skin and gastrointestinal tract that prevent overgrowth of pathogenic bacteria. The presence of an open wound bypasses these natural defense mechanisms and introduces bacteria directly into the underlying tissues where host defenses must then be called upon for protection.

A hematoma interferes with normal wound healing because it provides a medium for bacterial proliferation and inhibits the orderly removal of foreign bodies from the wound. In addition, numerous studies have demonstrated various biochemical mechanisms whereby the components of the hematoma have been implicated in tissue destruction and potentiation of a bacterial inoculum.

Foreign bodies obviously impair healing and potentiate wound infection. One must recognize that sutures are foreign bodies and as such block local defense forces that kill bacteria. The presence of a silk suture can decrease the number of bacteria required to cause a wound infection by 10,000-fold in a clinical wound infection.

After bacterial contamination, neutrophils and monocytes are drawn to the area by chemotaxis. Opsonic fragments bind to the surface of microbes and interact with leukocyte receptors to accelerate ingestion of the bacteria. If chemotaxis and opsonization do not occur effectively, a wound is predisposed to infection. Following ingestion by leukocytes, bacteria are killed intracellularly by a burst of oxidative phosphorylation that produces hydrogen peroxide (H_2O_2) and superoxide radicals (O_2^-), both of which are highly toxic to the microbes through oxidation (Fig 1–6). Oxygen-independent killing mechanisms also exist in a variety of forms, including enzymatic digestion of cell wall and cationic binding proteins, which bind microbe walls and interfere with reproduction. However, oxygen is an essential substrate for effective bacterial killing.

Although leukocytes are necessary for efficient killing of most microbes, certain gram-negative organisms are lysed directly by an antibody and complement complex in serum. Another humoral mechanism is responsible for direct kill of gram-positive and gram-negative species. Wound fluid is not a medium for bacterial growth as hematoma is and in fact is actually independently bactericidal to a number of organisms.

The amount of bacterial inoculum introduced into a wound is critical for appropriate management of the wound. A dynamic equi-

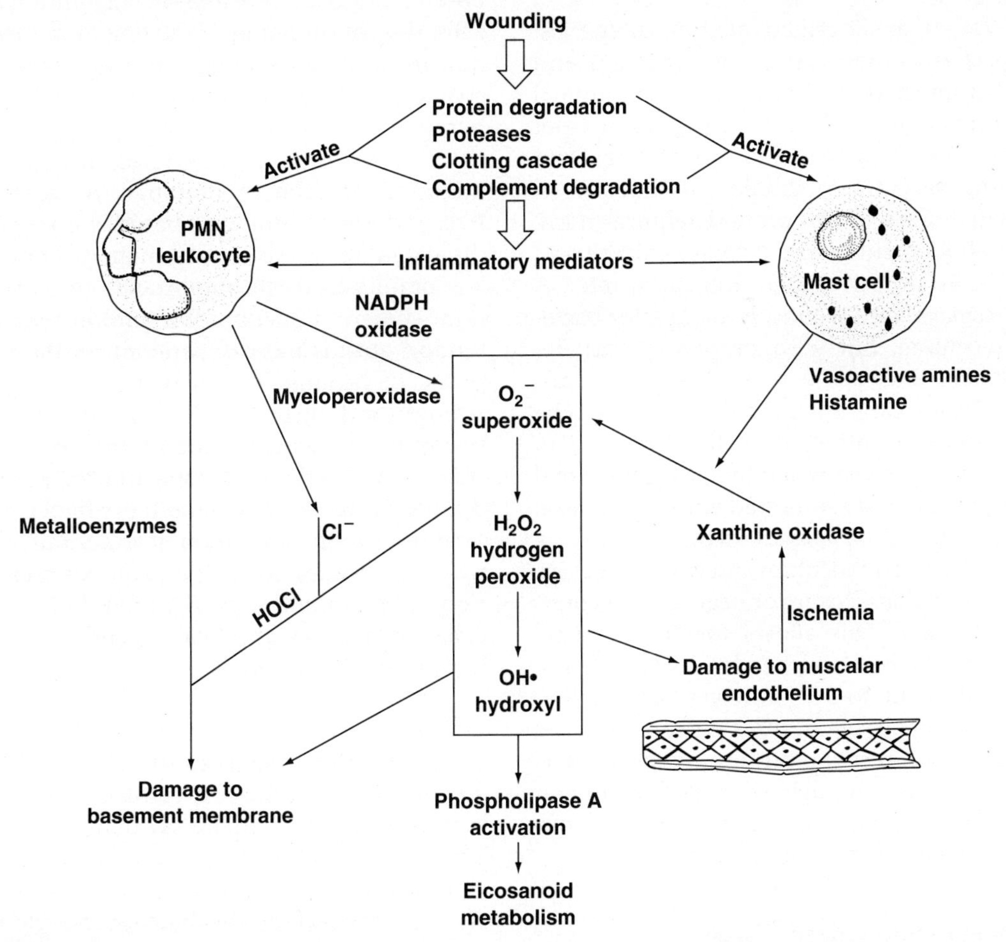

FIG 1–6.
Oxygen-derived radicals important in limiting microbial effect on healing.

librium exists between the bacteria in the wound and the host. This relationship is best described as a balance. With adequate wound host defenses and without interference by such factors as hematomas or foreign bodies, a wound can withstand a level of up to 100,000 (10^5) organisms per gram of tissue and still heal or be repaired successfully. If greater than 10^5 bacteria per gram are present, wound closure is likely to lead to clinical wound infection. The only exception to this occurs in the case of β-hemolytic streptococci, which can produce clinical wound infection if present in any number. Although the presence of bacterial balance in a wound can be surmised by a careful history and physical evaluation, it can only be confirmed by quantitative and qualitative bacteriology performed on a tissue biopsy specimen from the wound.

Wounds are classified into four categories: clean, clean-contaminated, contaminated, and dirty or infected. A *clean* wound has minimal contamination and is less than 12 hours from injury. The respiratory, gastrointestinal, and genitourinary tracts should not have been breached. Care of this wound requires minimal debridement before primary closure and results in a low (0.5%) infection rate. A *clean-contaminated* wound has a greater bacterial inoculum, but with proper wound debridement and saline lavage successful primary closure can be expected. This is the type of wound encountered in civilian trauma or in the operating room when the gastrointestinal or respiratory tract is entered with a minimum of spillage. *Contaminated* wounds have a greater bacterial inoculum and usually require delayed primary closure or healing by secondary intention. This allows for the bacterial balance to be reestablished by decreasing the bacterial count to 10^5 or fewer bacteria per gram of tissue by various means such as debridement and topical antimicrobial therapy. Examples of such wounds are human bites, gross spillage of gastrointestinal contents, or left-sided colon injuries.

Healing in Specialized Tissue

The discussion of the physiology, biochemistry, and microbiology of wound healing to this point has been directed at wounds involving the skin. Healing in wounds of other tissue involves the same series of orderly processes. However, each has some unique characteristics that will be detailed below.

Tendon

Tendon is composed of extracellular matrix, collagen, elastin, tenocytes, and associated blood vessels, lymphatics, and nerves. Tendons have the highest concentration of collagen of any tissue of the body. The extracellular matrix or ground substance in tendon is present in small amounts and is composed of glycosaminoglycans, glycoproteins, and noncollagenous protein. Three distinct cell populations have been identified: (1) epitenon cells, a thin cellular layer on the outer margin of the tendon; (2) endotenon cells, the continuation of the epitenon projection into tendon bundles; and (3) tenocytes, sparsely distributed cells within the tendon bundles.

Tendon healing progresses through the inflammatory, the proliferative or regenerative, and the maturation phases as previously discussed for soft tissue, although recent work has emphasized the importance of synovial nourishment. Function of a tendon repair or tendon graft is most dependent on the third phase of healing in which the repair gains strength and the peritendinous adhesions lose strength. In favorable conditions, the adhesions between the repair site and the peritendinous tissues are filmy and loose by 8 weeks. To minimize the formation of adhesions, early motion is indicated in the postoperative period. Nine months is required before the collagen fibers in the healing ends resemble normal tendon bundles.

Cartilage

Because of a sparsity of cell population and relative avascularity, cartilage has a low metabolic rate as compared with other tissues. The primary cell of cartilage is the chondrocyte. These cells metabolize sulfur to produce chondroitin sulfate, the mucopolysaccharide constituent of the protective cartilage matrix. In addition to production of extracellular matrix, the chondrocyte produces collagen.

Wounded cartilage can heal by neochondrogenesis and also by filling in surrounding connective tissue. Neochondrogenesis becomes less apparent and connective tissue replacement more prominent with aging. Since the long-term success of a cartilage graft depends on living chondrocytes to maintain the graft's bulk, adequate blood supply to the graft is paramount.

Bone

The healing process of bone is also divided into three phases of wound healing (Fig 1–7). In addition to these processes, however, bone also undergoes mineralization. Three cell types are present in bone: the osteoblast, the osteoclast, and the osteocyte. The osteoblast produces bone matrix, while the osteoclast functions to absorb bone material and matrix. Osteocytes constitute the majority of cells in mature bone and have matrix-producing as well as resorptive capacity in wound healing.

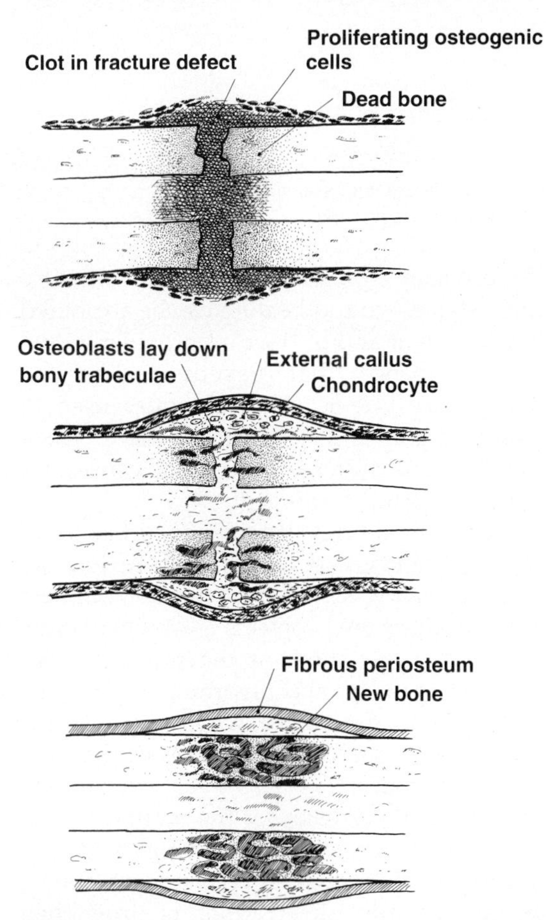

FIG 1–7.
Bone repair.

The inflammatory phase of bone healing lasts approximately 5 days and resembles the same phase in soft tissue, with monocytes and PMNs removing necrotic tissue and debris. The proliferative phase is characterized by mineralization and the formation of a fracture callus with transition to mature bone. Within the cells there is an orderly progression of endochondral ossification of cartilage, the formation of woven trabecular bone bridging the fracture site, and restoration of periosteal and endosteal blood supplies. The bone remodeling phase is the longest stage of fracture healing as the callus diminishes in size and angular deformities at the fracture site decrease. This occurs because of "strain-sensitive" cells that are able to perceive deformation forces and initiate adaptation. Bone remodeling follows Wolff's law, which states that bone adapts to functional forces acting upon it.

Cortical, or endochondral, bone provides weight-bearing functions and allows locomotion. Membranous bone serves to protect vital soft-tissue structures. Endochondral bone formation has a cartilage intermediate phase, while membranous bone is thought to form without a cartilaginous component stage. Endochondral bone contains an epiphyseal plate, while membranous bone has no identifiable epiphysis.

Nerve

Nerves do not heal the same as other tissue. The functional unit of the nervous system is the neuron, or cell body (soma). Usually, the axonal dendrite and not neuron itself is wounded. As a consequence of injury to a peripheral nerve there is a predictable sequence of distal (wallerian) and proximal axonal degeneration. Repair consists of coapting the nerve sheath so that regeneration can occur (Fig 1–8). Schwann cells, particularly those closest to the site of injury, respond vigorously to nerve wounding. They first swell and then proliferate. Proliferation is seen primarily in the distal nerve stump. Schwann cells become motile and form dense cords along the former line of the axon. The Schwann cell appears to be phagocytic and ingests portions of degenerating axon, frag-

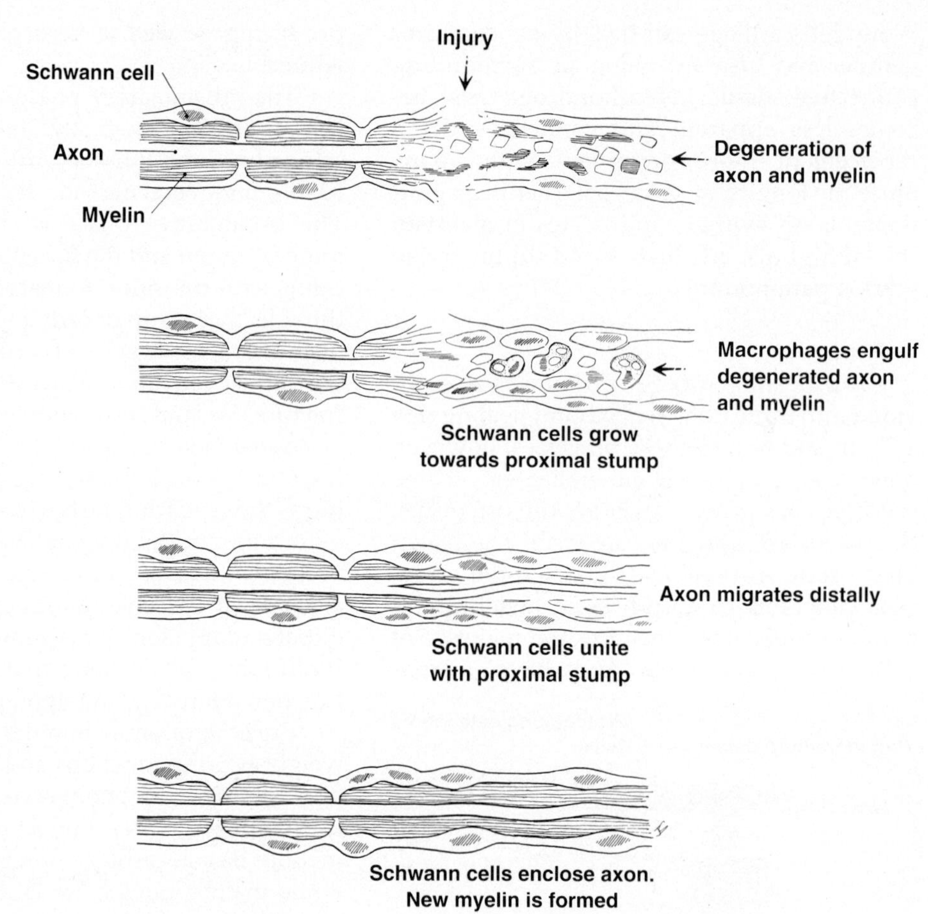

FIG 1–8.
Peripheral nerve repair.

ments of myelin, and other debris. If the injury does not lead to neuronal death, a sequence of regeneration proceeds. Myelin sheaths first make their appearance on the regenerating axon at about 6 to 7 days. Nodes of Ranvier appear some 2 weeks later. Myelin continues to be laid down for approximately a year.

ABNORMAL WOUND HEALING

Delayed Healing – Physiology and Treatment

Normally, the physiology of wound healing should progress as related previously. If the wound is debrided of nonviable tissue and repaired in a physiologic manner, the normal phases of wound healing should proceed without difficulty. When this does not happen, one must understand each component of the physiology, biochemistry, and microbiology of wound healing to successfully diagnose the problem and institute management. Disturbances of wound healing can be attributed to the patient and/or the care provider. Often the disturbances that prevent ideal wound healing are due to the techniques used in wound repair and not to the patient. There can be both systemic and local causes for delayed wound healing.

To evaluate the systemic disturbances of wound healing, it is necessary to review the wound healing scheme. One must evaluate whether there are problems with coagulation, systemic oxygenation, or the proteins. Also, the host (patient) and environment must be evaluated to determine whether a disease, condition, or medication is present that will affect healing.

Systemic perfusion of the wound is necessary to provide the oxygen necessary for healing. If the patient is receiving an anticoagulant or antiplatelet adhering drug, then wound healing may be delayed. Similarly, cancer chemotherapy may affect healing. In normal wound healing, the macrophages are the most important cells, more important than granulocytes. Corticosteroids can prevent macrophages from migrating and result in a wound healing disturbance. Just as an excess of a drug may delay wound healing, so might a deficiency such as occurs in scurvy and diabetes mellitus. Finally, if one cannot synthesize the proteins because of a lack of building blocks, there is no way to synthesize collagen, which is the *sine qua non* of wound healing.

Oxygen is important in wound healing for cell migration and multiplication and for protein and collagen synthesis because it facilitates hydroxylation of proline and lysine; the oxygen gradient also determines the rate of angiogenesis. Whatever decreases the level of oxygen delivered to the tissues—hypotension, hypovolemia, anemia, lung disease, low inspired oxygen concentration, hypothermia, or alkalosis—will interfere with wound healing. Hypovolemia is especially detrimental because it not only decreases oxygen delivery but also causes coagulation and sludging of the microcirculation, thus compounding the oxygen deficit.

Anti-inflammatory agents such as aspirin or indomethacin affect wound healing by interfering with the arachidonic acid cascade. Although aspirin in small doses can protect the microcirculation by preventing platelet adhesion, in larger doses it is detrimental.

Patients who receive cytotoxic drugs have little demonstrable impairment in their wound healing capacities. In patients who are severely debilitated by a cytotoxic regimen, nutritional status and wound healing are impaired. These effects are probably more directly related to the effect of the nutritional impairment than to the cytotoxic drug. Doxorubicin (Adriamycin), however, is one chemotherapeutic agent that has been demonstrated to delay healing.

The adverse effects of glucocorticoids on wound healing are observed principally when they are present in excess at the time of and in the early days after wounding. The inflammatory response to wounding is lessened dramatically, and there is a significant delay in angiogenesis, fibroblastic proliferation, and the synthesis of proteoglycans and collagen. Wound strength is impaired, as well as epithelialization and contraction of open wounds. These effects are seen in wounds of various tissues (e.g., skin, subcutaneous tissue, tendon, gut, bone) regardless of whether the glucocorticoids are given systemically or locally.

The specific mechanisms underlying these effects have not been fully elucidated. One possibility is that the steroid prevents release by the wounded tissue of chemical substances that are necessary for the initiation and completion of repair. Another is that there may be an inhibitory effect on cell proliferation and proteoglycan and collagen synthesis. The glucocorticoids may also act systemically by antagonizing insulin or growth hormone, or locally, perhaps by interfering with the production, secretion, or action of one or more growth-promoting cytokines or by retarding cell growth directly.

Supplemental vitamin A prevents or reverses the impaired healing resulting from excess cortisone. The specific mechanisms underlying the effects of vitamin A are not known, but its effects are believed to be due to an early increase in the inflammatory response. In culture, vitamin A increases the fibroblast receptors for EGF and increases fibroblast multiplication. Vitamin A appears to stabilize the lysosomal membrane (which is opposite to the effect of glucocorticoids).

Descriptions of markedly abnormal wound healing in sailors with scurvy appear in the writings of explorers and physicians as early as the 16th century and continue through much of the 18th century. This effect is the result of deficiency of vitamin C or ascorbic acid. The hydroxylation of proline and lysine requires molecular oxygen, α-ketoglutarate, iron, and ascorbic acid. It has been suggested that ascorbic acid may act as an electron transport substance between iron and oxygen in the hydroxylation reaction and in the activation of prolyl hydroxylase and lysyl hydroxylase, the enzymes catalyzing these reactions.

There are serious impairments of healing and decreased resistance to infection that occur in patients with diabetes mellitus. The mechanisms underlying the impairment in healing are multiple and not understood completely. The early inflammatory response after wounding is impaired, and fibroblast and endothelial cell proliferation is reduced, as is the accumulation of reparative collagen and gain in wound breaking strength. Some authors also report delayed epithelialization of open skin wounds. High levels of glucose interfere with cellular transport of ascorbic acid into various cells, including fibroblasts and leukocytes, and cause decreased leukocyte chemotaxis. Several reports have shown that some of the peptide growth factors and cytokines ameliorate the impaired healing in diabetic animals. Among these are PDGF, bFGF, EGF, GM-CSF, IL-1, and IL-4.

The indirect effects of a severe acute lack of insulin and hyperglycemia on wound healing are hyperosmolarity, dehydration, metabolic acidosis, and inadequate tissue perfusion, which may slow healing. If diabetes has been present for a long time, healing is impaired by the neuropathy and vascular abnormalities that have developed. Severe renal disease with its abundant metabolic and physiologic abnormalities, a common complication in such diabetics, and serious cardiac dysfunction also contribute to impaired healing. Finally, the decreased host resistance (local and systemic) of diabetic patients, especially those whose disease is inadequately controlled, may lead to serious wound infection.

Thyroid and parathyroid hormones affect the healing of several tissues. Clinical observations suggest that hypothyroidism is associated with impaired wound healing, especially in burn patients and in patients with enteric fistulas. Parathyroid hormone, a primary regulator of calcium metabolism, affects wound healing, particularly in skeletal tissue. Fracture healing is impaired in animals following parathyroidectomy.

Other abnormalities of wound healing are associated with genetic disorders of collagen synthesis. An example is Ehlers-Danlos syndrome, which results in integument that seems to have a great deal of elasticity. There are actually groups of variants of the syndrome (Table 1–2). It has been suggested that many more patients are afflicted with one of the variations of Ehlers-Danlos syndrome than previously thought. Marfan syndrome can also result in wound healing difficulties, as will osteogenesis imperfecta.

Despite these systemic causes of delayed wound healing, it is the local factors that most commonly cause delays in wound healing. These local disturbances may be secondary to iatrogenic causes or wound care technique and include temperature, ischemia, tissue trauma, denervation, and infection. Each can

TABLE 1-2.
Variants of Ehlers-Danlos Syndrome

Type		Clinical Features
I	Gravis	Soft, hyperextensible skin; thin, atrophic scars; hypermobile joints; easy bruisability; prematurity of affected newborns
II	Mitis	Similar to type I but less severe
III	Familial Hypermobility	Soft skin; large and small joint hypermobility
IV	Arterial	Thin, translucent skin with visible veins; easy bruisability; arterial, bowel, and uterine friability
V	X-linked	Similar to type II
VI		Muscle hypotonicity; scoliosis; joint laxity; hyperxextensible skin
VII	Arthrochalasis Multiplex Congenita	Congenital hip dislocation; severe joint hypermobility; soft skin with normal scarring
VIII	Periodontal	Generalized periodontitis; soft hyperextensible skin
XI		Soft, extensible, lax skin; bladder diverticulae and rupture; short arms, limited pronation and supination; broad clavicles
X		Similar to type II but with additional abnormal clotting studies

interfere with one or several of the processes of healing.

Excessive Healing (Hypertrophic Scars and Keloids)

In the integumentary system, even though the processes of wound healing have apparently progressed normally, proliferative scar formation (either a hypertrophic scar or keloid) may result. Hypertrophic scars are large masses of collagen that remain within the bounds of the original wound from which they arise. This differs from keloid formation, where the collagen mass extends beyond the original bounds of the wound. At the extremes, keloids and hypertrophic scars are easily distinguishable. However, in many cases, there is considerable overlap in features, which may blur this distinction. Since hypertrophic scars remain within the boundaries of the original injury, it appears that the normal wound healing process begins and seems to continue without a signal to shut off or downregulate. Normal wound contraction ends up with a hypertrophic scar. One way to reduce hypertrophic scar formation is to minimize the time in which normal wound contraction takes place. The duration and the intensity of the inflammation can also be reduced. It is desirable to reduce this time because it has been demonstrated that hypertrophic scars are related to the amount of time that the wound is allowed to remain in the inflammatory phase before it moves into the proliferative phase. The inflammatory phase should be reduced not only in wounds healing by secondary or tertiary intention but also in those healing by primary intention.

Grossly, a keloid appears raised and firm, with overlying epithelium that is often darker than normal. Microscopically, there are thick, homogeneous bands of collagen and a paucity of cellular elements. Hypertrophic scars are histologically similar to keloids, although the collagen tends to whorl about clusters of macrophages, fibroblasts, and vessels.

Keloids are not the result of wound healing out of control because they do not occur in every wound. For instance, they rarely occur distal to the wrist or knee. They have a predilection to form over the butterfly area of the sternum and in the mandible and deltoid areas. The rate of collagen synthesis is increased in fibroblasts derived from keloids. The water content of the collagen of keloidal tissue seems to be higher than collagen from either normally healing wounds or hypertrophic scars. Similarly, the amount of acid-soluble collagen appears to be more. The amount of glycocaminoglycans produced by the keloid fibroblasts is abnormally high. There is also a redistribution of the synthetic patterns of the proteoglycans, with chondroitin-4-sulfate being produced disproportionately.

Treatment of Hypertrophic Scars and Keloids

Hypertrophic scars are not the result of disturbance of the normal physiology of wound healing. Rather, they occur basically as a problem resulting from the degree and time of inflammation as well as the tension resulting from either tissue deficiency or misdirection of a wound that produces uncontrolled wound contraction. Surgery can be used to improve these scars because there is a normal healing mechanism. Changing the direction of the scar to lie within relaxed skin tension lines with techniques such as Z-plasty or W-plasty can bring additional tissue into the scarred area and reduce the amount of tension acting on the scar.

One very effective nonoperative treatment of hypertrophic scarring is the application of direct pressure. The mechanism of this modulation of collagen deposition is not certain. It may be related to a relative hypoperfusion of the area inasmuch as the external pressure required must exceed capillary blood pressure in order to be effective. The results of long-term treatment with graded pressure garments have been particularly rewarding in treating hypertrophic scars in burn patients, although the concept is generally applicable to other types of injury as well. Ultrasound, positive-polarity electrotherapy and topical application of silicone gel sheeting are additional physical modalities reported to decrease scar thickness.

The treatment of a keloid requires understanding the disturbance in the normal healing pathway and attempting to correct it. Current treatment uses triamcinolone injections rather than surgery. If triamcinolone is injected into the wound every 3 to 4 weeks, the collagen can be manipulated, and the amount of cross-linking in the collagen and the amount of collagenase present can be modulated. If injections are continued until there is no excess abnormal collagen, then the lesion can be excised. If abnormal collagen buildup can be prevented during this wound healing phase, then a normal scar may result rather than another keloid. There are other experimental ways that the collagen can be manipulated. Both the intracellular and extracellular synthesis of collagen can be controlled by the use of compounds such as the lysyl oxidase inhibitors β-aminoproprionitrile fumarate (BAPN) and penicillamine to change the cross-linking or by the use of colchicine to accelerate collagenase kinetics. Vitamin A, especially in the form of a retinoic acid, can reduce collagen production, as can the interferons α and γ. Keloid tissue grown in culture following treatment with interferon-α_{2B} reveals normalization of collagen, glycosaminoglycans, and collagenase production by the fibroblasts. Currently, these pharmacologic manipulations hold greater hope for the management of keloids than does surgery.

Unattractive scars can occur without a true disturbance in wound healing. The most common reasons for this are a lack of orientation of the original wound or incision in the normal lines of skin tension, failure of proper dermal approximation, and a pathologic extension of normal wound contraction. The simplest revision for these scars consists of scar excision and reapproximation of the wound edges. If the excessive scarring is due to an improper direction of the original wound, the wound direction can be realigned so that the new scar falls in the lines of minimum tension or relaxed skin tension. Occasionally an unacceptable scar is due to a true deficiency of tissue in which case skin may need to be added in the form of a graft or a flap.

Camouflage techniques may also be useful for unacceptable scarring. These can be both operative and nonoperative. Dermabrasion (which does not actually change the dermal portion of the scar) can be considered operative camouflage. By removing the epidermis and superficial dermis, it allows the reepithelialization process of healing to result in a more uniform flattened surface. It is more successful for depressed than for elevated scars. Another camouflage technique is tattooing. This can allow semipermanent matching of pigments to decrease color mismatch. Cosmetics and dress can provide final camouflage techniques. These should all be considered when normal wound healing has left a less-than-desirable result.

NUTRITION AS RELATED TO WOUND HEALING

Diagnosis of Deficiency

Many patients are malnourished because of other disease, loss of appetite, depression, or social circumstances. This affects wound healing by decreasing the rates of neovascularization, fibroblastic proliferation, cell synthesis, and wound remodeling. Malnourished patients are at greater risk while the wound is closing because both humoral and cellular immunity is impaired. Phagocytic activity and lymphocyte function are impaired after only 4 weeks of malnutrition. The alterations in the immune response can be tested with delayed hypersensitivity skin testing in which an antigen is injected intradermally. In a competent host, this antigen combines with sensitized lymphocytes, which release lymphokines that attack macrophages and unsensitized lymphocytes to clear the antigen and cellular debris. As cells and protein accumulate over a period of 24 to 48 hours after the injection, a skin wheal forms, which indicates a positive result. In the event that this sequence fails, the skin test result will be negative. When five common antigens are used as a test, a patient is considered immunocompetent with two or more positive results, relatively anergic with one positive response, and anergic with no positive responses.

Deficiencies in vitamins and minerals result in poor wound healing. Ferrous ion, oxygen, vitamin C, and α-ketoglutarate are all coenzyme factors required for hydroxylation of lysine and proline in the formation of collagen. Calcium is required in the conversion of procollagen to fibrillar collagen. In addition, calcium is an important coenzyme factor with granulocyte collagenase, tissue collagenase, and synovial collagenase types A and B. Cuprous ion (Cu^{2+}) along with oxygen and tropocollagen is required to deaminate and oxidize lysine. Manganese glycosylates OH-lysines and attaches glucose to O-lysyl galactose.

Wounds in severely protein-deficient patients cannot heal. Methionine, available in the diet, is converted to cystine. Cystine now appears to be required for the formation of disulfide bonds, which allows alignment of the amino acid chains in the formation of the triple helix of collagen. A lack of cystine inhibits all phases of collagen deposition. For this reason, patients who are in a severe state of malnutrition have an impaired ability to maintain skin integrity and to heal even minor breaks in the integument.

Protein synthesis must be increased at the wound site during the repair process if normal healing is to occur. A deficiency or imbalance of some amino acids has singular effects on protein synthesis and healing, just as it does on growth. The effects of specific amino acids vary quantitatively and qualitatively. All amino acids are essential physiologically, whether or not there is a dietary requirement for them. For example, glycine makes up about one third of the collagen molecule. When there is a dietary requirement for amino acids (the so-called dietary essential amino acids), this is generally not because the body cannot synthesize them but rather because they are synthesized too slowly to meet the body's needs. After injury the requirement for certain amino acids that are normally synthesized at adequate rates for maintenance of the adult steady state (e.g., arginine) may increase, so a dietary supply must be provided.

Disturbances in carbohydrate and fat metabolism have both direct and indirect effects on wound healing. The indirect effects are the result of excessive oxidation of amino acids for caloric needs when inadequate amounts of carbohydrate and fat are available. The role of fats in wound healing has not been studied as extensively as that of carbohydrates or proteins. Certain key unsaturated fatty acids must be supplied exogenously (that is, they are dietary essentials). Linoleic acid cannot be synthesized by mammals, and evidence suggests that the biosynthesis of linolenic acid and arachidonic acid from linoleic acid does not proceed at a rate adequate for the growing animal. These fatty acids are critical constituents of the triglycerides and phospholipids that are part of subcellular membranes. The unsaturated fatty acids are also essential building blocks for the prostaglandins that regulate many aspects of cellular metabolism and inflammation. Essential fatty acid deficiency causes impaired wound healing in skin and fascial incisions, small- and large-bowel anastomoses, and burn wounds.

Although vitamin C deficiency results in the delayed healing of scurvy, there is no evidence that wound healing can be accelerated by the administration of more vitamin C than is required to maintain normal tissue levels. However, since vitamin C is not stored to any great extent in the body, physiologically significant deficiency may rapidly develop in seriously ill and injured patients unless ascorbic acid supplementation is given.

There are few data regarding the specific influences of the B-complex vitamins on wound healing. It is to be expected, however, that serious deficiencies of some of these vitamins will interfere with healing since the B vitamins serve as cofactors in a wide variety of enzyme systems and in their absence disturbances in protein, carbohydrate, and fat metabolism occur. Deficiencies of the B-complex vitamins, notably pyridoxine, pantothenic acid, and folic acid, decrease resistance to infection, in part because antibody formation and some white blood cell functions are impaired.

Vitamin K is involved in the synthesis of prothrombin, clotting factors VII, IX, and X, and calcium-binding protein. When vitamin K deficiency exists, there is excessive bleeding in wounds, impairing healing, and a predisposition to infection. Parenteral vitamin K is indicated for obstructive jaundice, severe chronic pancreatitis, and other disorders of fat digestion and absorption. Patients with serious liver disease may not be able to synthesize adequate amounts of prothrombin even when vitamin K is absorbed and available.

There is no clear-cut evidence for a special role for vitamin E in normal wound healing, although an excess of vitamin E can result in delayed healing. It is possible that vitamin E deficiency may occur in patients with severe prolonged impairment of fat absorption. Also, because fatty acid deficiency has been reported in patients receiving long-term parenteral nutrition without lipids, vitamin E deficiency may develop in seriously ill and injured patients if parenteral vitamin E is not given during a prolonged illness requiring such nutritional therapy.

The body stores of most trace minerals are not large, but the economy of trace minerals in healthy individuals is high. Recognition of trace mineral deficiency has become more frequent with long-term parenteral feeding of highly purified nutrients. Also, chronic conditions may induce trace mineral deficiencies when dietary intake of these minerals is marginal. Associating a specific deficit in wound healing with a deficiency of a specific trace mineral is complicated by the fact that metabolic and nutritional deficiencies in patients are almost always multiple. Zinc is an important coenzyme for cell replication because both DNA polymerase and reverse transcriptase are zinc-dependent. If zinc stores are depleted, neither epithelium nor fibroblasts will proliferate since mitosis is inhibited. Iron is necessary for the hydroxylation of lysine and proline. It is only when iron deficiency anemia is severe and acute that it may have an adverse effect on oxygen transport and thus secondarily on wound healing. Copper is essential for normal erythropoiesis. As in the case of zinc deficiency, clinicians became more aware of copper deficiency when it developed in patients who received long-term total parenteral nutrition (TPN) without the inclusion of copper in the solutions. Copper is a component of a number of metalloenzymes of direct importance in wound healing, specifically lysyl oxidase, the enzyme catalyzing collagen cross-link formation, and Zn-Cu superoxide dismutase.

Treatment of Nutritional Deficiency

If wound healing impairment resulting from malnutrition is suspected and diagnosed, the patient's daily caloric requirements can be estimated and supplied. A negative nitrogen balance may require increased caloric intake and nutritional supplements. The calories may be delivered by mouth, enteral feedings, or in certain circumstances, intravenous alimentation.

Once the proper caloric, protein, carbohydrate, and fat intake is ensured, proper vitamin and mineral supplementation requires direct attention. Many severely debilitated patients have vitamin or mineral deficiencies that prevent wound healing. Although nutritional supplements slowly correct these, the specific administration of a multivitamin preparation with the addition of specific vitamin supplements may be required. If necessary, trace elements in the serum can be measured and replaced. The copper, iron, magnesium, and calcium can be restored to normal levels. Zinc levels must be carefully monitored to avoid overdosing. Ascorbic acid levels are quickly depleted, and this requires the administration of daily doses of vitamin C. Patients who have a history of significant alcohol intake require replacement of vitamin B_6. Patients receiving chronic high doses of steroids benefit from the systemic administration of vitamin A to allow collagen formation within the healing wound.

Finally, if the patient has a specific metabolic problem such as diabetes, malabsorption, or hepatic insufficiency, these conditions have to be corrected as much as possible to allow nutritional improvement. As long as the patient is malnourished, collagen deposition or epithelialization of the wound is delayed, the immune status is impaired, and the proper balance between catabolism and anabolism is disrupted, allowing further breakdown.

SURGICAL INCISIONS

Selection in Relation to Skin Lines

Any elective incision should be placed in Kraissel's lines of minimum tension or resting skin tension lines as opposed to Langer's lines

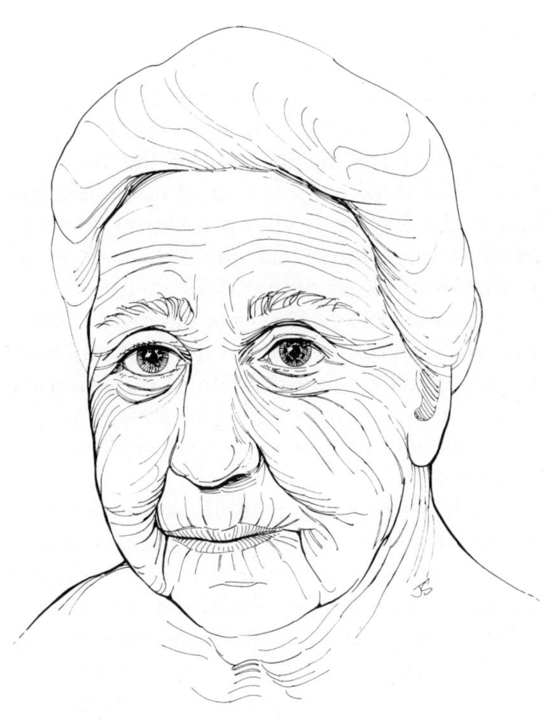

FIG 1–9.
Skin tension lines of the face and neck in a relaxed state.

of tension. Kraissel's lines, those lines perpendicular to the underlying muscular pull, minimize the tension in the incision even when the muscle contracts (Fig 1–9). Wounds perpendicular to Kraissel's lines are under constant tension and therefore have a high propensity for hypertrophic scar formation. Incisions in between these extremes have an increasing chance of normal healing the closer they mimic Kraissel's lines. In the nonelective (traumatic) situation, selection of wound direction is obviously not an option.

Technique for Incisional Closure

The best technique for wound closure will be as atraumatic as possible. Wound edges should be coapted to permit healing without a step-off and yet not so tightly approximated that the edema causes further ischemia in the coapted edges of the wound. The major strength in the skin is in the dermis. The collagen fibers in the dermis will give the wound its tensile strength. Good approximation of the dermis will minimize the step-off between the two edges and minimize the width of the resultant scar. Sutures placed in fat will cause necrosis of this tissue and serve as a foreign body and a nidus for infection.

While fascia has sufficient collagen to permit approximation with sutures and promote collagen formation in the scar, the underlying muscle will not support sutures and may even undergo necrosis if the edges are tightly approximated. For this reason, the best closure of a wound extending through muscle includes good apposition of the fascia and dermis. A buried dermal closure with an inverted suture will place the knot in the depth of the wound and minimize the likelihood of its erosion to the surface of the skin or the formation of a stitch abscess (Fig 1–10).

The epidermis can then be approximated with a nonabsorbable suture such as nylon, which will best approximate the wound and give a polished effect to the eventual scar. These sutures should be removed prior to invasion of collagen bundles into the suture holes. The density of the dermal appendages in the area will determine the timing of the suture removal. Areas such as the face, which has a high density of dermal appendages, should have the epidermal sutures placed only through the depth of the epidermis. If the dermis is included in the suture, suture tracks may occur when these stitches are left in place for as short as 4 days. Areas such as the palmar or plantar surfaces have such a low density of dermal appendages that these sutures may be left in place through both the dermis and epidermis for as long as 3 weeks without suture track formation. A truly epidermal

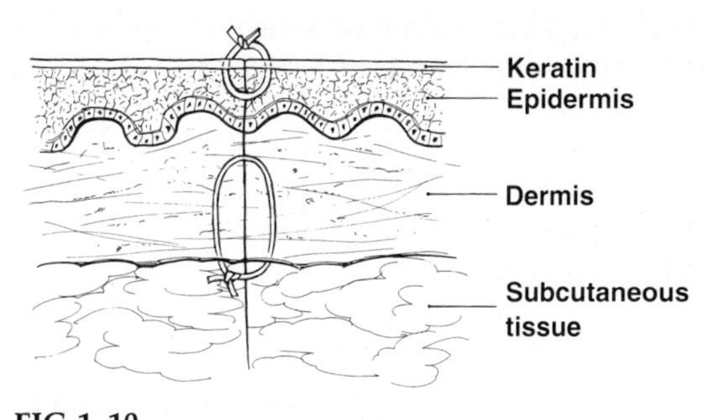

FIG 1–10.
Technique of inverted dermal suture and continuous fine epidermal suture for primary wound repair.

suture will be sloughed as the epidermal cells are sloughed and will fall out in 7 to 8 days.

When the sutures are removed, if desired, the surface of the wound may be further covered for a period of time with plastic bandages. Adhesive tape used to primarily close the epidermis will not approximate the epidermal edges as well as the nylon suture will and may result in inversion of the migrating epidermis.

Suture Materials—Types and Uses

Buried dermal sutures most commonly consist of an absorbable material that will be less likely to eventually erode or serve as a continuous foreign body. Chromic or plain gut sutures are rapidly degraded by hydrolysis and do not remain in the wound long enough to allow adequate tensile strength to occur in the scar. The use of these sutures not only increases inflammation but may also lead to widening of the scar as the dermis is no longer tightly approximated. Polyglycolic or polygalactic sutures are enzymatically degraded. These tend to be degraded on an average of 14 to 40 days after placement. Therefore, these sutures remain in place long enough to allow a greater tensile strength to occur in the wound and minimize the widening, which will occur as these sutures are degraded. The use of a braided suture leaves more interstices for bacterial adherence and proliferation with a higher incidence of wound infection. Therefore, a monofilament suture or a coated suture that mimics a monofilament suture is a better choice. As previously stated, a fine monofilament suture such as nylon or Prolene is usually chosen for the epidermis. These are less reactive than silk or cotton.

PRINCIPLES OF WOUND MANAGEMENT

Debridement

As mentioned before, any wound considered for closure should be evaluated for the level of necrotic tissue, debris, and bacterial contamination. Necrotic tissue requires sharp debridement. Fluorescein can help determine tissue viability. Irrigation will aid in removal of foreign bodies and debris. Once a bacterial imbalance has been accurately diagnosed, the principle is reestablishment of the bacterial balance. Sharp debridement of nonviable tissue is the key to reaching bacterial balance. Wound irrigation as usually delivered, even with voluminous amounts of solutions, removes little but surface contamination. Pulsating jet lavage is an improved modification. A further practical modification of pulsating jet lavage uses a syringe with a 19-gauge needle. This has been shown to be quite effective in small wounds.

Closure of acute wounds is divided into three categories: primary, secondary, and tertiary. In primary healing, the wound is usually closed by direct approximation of the wound edges as discussed above. Larger defects may be closed by flaps or skin grafts, but this still represents healing by primary intention since immediate closure of the wound is obtained. In traumatic injuries, if at all possible the wound should be closed primarily. Those wounds that appear unfavorable at the time of injury may eventually heal well. Any method to revise the scar at the time of the acute injury may be more than eventually needed. In addition, the use of "Z"-plasties or other complicated closures in the acute setting may prevent the use of these when reconstruction is necessary at a later date. If there is a true lack of tissue, occasionally the edges may be coapted simply by undermining the adjacent edges of the dermis. When this is insufficient, acute placement of a graft or flap may be necessary to achieve closure.

In secondary healing, the wound is left open and allowed to heal spontaneously. Spontaneous wound closure is a bimodal process of wound contraction and epithelialization. In the open, central areas of a wound healing by secondary intention, the inflammatory phase continues unabated. The product of this prolonged inflammatory process is granulation tissue consisting of inflammatory cells, bacteria, and a proliferation of capillaries. There are a number of options for closure of "granulating" wounds. The surgeon may elect to excise all of the granulating wound and perform tertiary closure, to skin-graft the wound, or simply to allow healing by secondary intention to continue.

Tertiary wound healing is closure of a wound by active intervention after a delay of days to weeks. This process is characterized by the intentional interruption of healing by secondary intention either by wound approximation or by a skin graft or flap. Tertiary wound closure can be performed at any time after wounding. However, closure should be performed only on wounds that are in bacterial balance.

Chronic wounds do not proceed with the orderliness or timeliness of acute wounds. However, management is similar to the acute wound. The wound must first be cleansed of all necrotic debris. The bacterial load should be assessed as previously discussed. If infected, the wound should then be treated with topical antimicrobials to decrease the bacterial count and allow for wound healing. These topical creams, such as silver sulfadiazine or mafenide acetate, decrease the bacterial count. Systemic antibiotics will not penetrate the chronic scarring in this relatively ischemic open wound. Surrounding wound cellulitis, however, should be treated with systemic antibiotics. Once the chronic wound is in bacterial balance, it can be modulated by wound healing agents such as growth factors or undergo delayed closure by wound edge approximation, a skin graft, or a pedicled flap.

Use of Topical Agents, Dressings, Splints, and Casts

Topical agents such as antimicrobial or anti-inflammatory creams or ointments are often placed over wounds. From a wound healing perspective, this is difficult to justify. Primarily approximated wounds need no such topical agents, and indeed application of them may be detrimental. The fibrin seal in the wound cleft is often dissolved by such agents. An open contaminated wound may benefit from an antimicrobial cream, but the use of these should be discontinued once the wound is in bacterial balance since most inhibit fibroblast and keratinocyte proliferation.

A dressing serves several important functions for the wound. Acutely, it protects the wound from additional bacterial contamination and from further injury. A dressing of absorptive gauze will allow exudate to be trapped in the gauze away from the skin. A grease-containing gauze such as Xeroform, Xeroflow, or Scarlet Red will not stick to the wound when it is removed. However, these gauzes also contain an excess amount of grease and must have most of this removed prior to use to prevent the dressing from becoming occlusive. Occlusive dressings such as hydrocolloids trap the exudate between the dressing and the wound and provide a moist wound healing environment. Although this raises concerns about increased infection, to date there is no evidence to support this concern and at least some evidence to support enhanced epithelialization.

A wound that is likely to create a great deal of edema either because of a dependent position or the force of the injury can be gently compressed with gauze wrappings to minimize the edema and the pain. The edema in the wound can, by diluting the sebum, make the wound more prone to infections.

Some wounds, especially over joints or in highly mobile areas, may benefit from a period of immobilization by a stiff dressing or even a splint or cast. Limiting mobility will minimize pain and edema formation as well as allow fragile structures to remain coapted during the healing period. A well-executed dressing will be more aesthetic to the patient and observers.

PRESERVATION OF SKIN, BONE, TENDON, CARTILAGE, AND NERVE

Principles and Techniques

Tissues used in wound repair and for reconstruction can be obtained from stored sources, if necessary. Techniques for storage need to allow preservation of the tissue in a usable state. The stored tissue can originate from an autogenous or allogeneic source. Allogeneic donors for tissue donation must be free from malignancy and transmissible diseases. If the tissue source is a cadaver, tissues should be retrieved within 12 hours if the body has remained at room temperature and 24 hours if the body has been refrigerated. Preservation can be short-term if the tissue will be used in the near future or long-term if the usage date is not predictable.

Short-term storage of skin can be done by placing the skin in sealed containers and storing at a temperature of 4°C (2 to 8°C) for up to 14 days. The addition of antibiotics and other agents such as nutrient media to the hypothermic storage is optional. This technique is used for delayed application of autografts and when fresh allograft skin is desired. Long-term preservation of skin involves cryopreservation at −70 to −196°C. Storage solutions should minimize osmotic damage to the skin by containing physiologic levels of salts as well as a cryoprotectant such as glycerol or dimethyl sulfoxide (DMSO). Skin allograft should be frozen at a slow rate of −1 to −5°C/min with minimizing of the exothermic plateaus. When frozen skin is to be used, it should be thawed by placing its packet in 20 to 37°C water. Unused thawed skin can be refrigerated at 4°C in an appropriate hypothermic storage medium for an additional 7 days. If thawed skin that has been rerefrigerated is not used after 7 days, it should be discarded.

Bone preservation consists primarily of preserving cadaver allograft bone in a frozen state. This freezing probably does not preserve living osteocytes but leaves only the organic collagen matrix and associated inorganic salts. Bone can be freeze-dried, dehydrated, lyophilized, or cryopreserved. The simplest technique is dehydration (evaporation) by placing the bone in a dehydrator and maintaining the temperature at less than 60°C until the residual water content is less than 5% of initial weight by gravimetric analysis and 8% by nuclear magnetic resonance (NMR) spectroscopy. The more common technique is cryopreservation using a solution of DMSO or glycerol and a liquid nitrogen freezing device to keep the specimen at or below −70°C. Once frozen, the bone can be stored at −40°C or colder. If large skeletal segments are required to provide allograft structural support, the donor should be free of any osteogenic disorders. Women donors should preferably be under 50 years of age and men under 55 years of age. The donor should have closed epiphyses and thus should be over 15 years of age.

Tendons and cartilage can be stored short-term and transplanted within days by maintaining them in an isotonic solution or nutrient media at 2 to 10°C. Antibiotics such as cephalosporin and gentamicin are usually added to the storage solution. They can be preserved for longer periods in a fresh frozen or freeze-dried state.

Nerves have been less successful as allografts. They are most frequently preserved fresh for brief durations in a hypothermic solution containing a nutrient medium similar to skin and connective tissue. Data on long-term preservation have not shown survival of the Schwann cell, and as will be discussed below, the axons are not useful as a graft.

Biological Substitutes

When autogenous tissue necessary for wound reconstruction is either unavailable or the price of sacrificing it from a functioning donor site is too high, a substitute must be sought. When possible, biological substitutes are preferable to alloplastic material. Various biological substitutes are available for skin, bone, tendon, cartilage, and nerve.

Of all the tissues attempted for allograft substitution, skin has been the least successful because of its marked antigenicity. The only successful permanent coverage with allograft skin has been with the use of immunosuppression with agents such as azathioprine (Imuran) or cyclosporine. Imuran depresses the host defenses to such a great degree that overwhelming sepsis often follows the allotransplantations. Temporary coverage with allograft skin as a "biological dressing" is common and can be lifesaving. When used in this manner, the skin is regularly changed at intervals calculated to precede any evidence of tissue rejection. Amniotic membranes, which embryologically and histologically simulate skin, have also been successfully used as temporary biological dressings. The problems with both of these substitutes for autogenous tissue is their human source and the risk of viral disease transmission (e.g. hepatitis or acquired immunodeficiency syndrome [AIDS]).

Cultured epithelial cells, although fairly successful when from autogenous sources, have been less successful when used as a skin substitute from allogeneic sources. The rate of growth of the keratinocytes in culture depends on the age of the donor, with cells from neonatal sources growing faster. Cultured epithelial allografts are of most functional value in structurally intact tissue such as partial-thickness wounds. Persistence of cultured epithelium from allogenic sources has not been well documented in humans.

Xenogeneic tissue has also been used as a temporary biological dressing. Commercially available pigskin has been utilized and must be changed every few days. This commercially available xenograft is nonviable, and a true graft take does not occur with this material. Fresh, viable xenograft functions better, but logistics make this substitute quite difficult to use.

There have been several attempts to engineer a skin substitute from biological sources. One consists of a "dermal" layer of enzymatically digested bovine collagen cross-linked with chondroitin-6-sulfate. This "dermal framework" is covered by a thin adherent Silastic sheet. This xenogeneic substitute is nonviable, and the bovine collagen framework is replaced by host collagen. To achieve permanent closure of the wound, the Silastic layer must be removed after vascularization of the dermal component and a thin epithelial autograft applied. This extremely thin autograft offers the practical advantage of more frequent harvesting of autologous donor sites since the healing time for the donor site is related to the depth of the split-thickness graft taken.

Another concept is that of a living skin equivalent composed of allogeneic cultured fibroblasts and a collagen matrix with an overlying lattice of autogenous keratinocytes. Preliminary studies with such substitutes suggest that allograft fibroblasts do not provoke a rejection response.

Finally, it is thought that allograft dermis may be less antigenic than epidermis, and attempts are being made to use frozen or irradiated allograft dermis, devoid of epidermis, as a skin substitute to be later covered by cultured epithelial autografts.

Biological substitutes for bone are also available. Bone allograft that has been rendered nonviable has enjoyed popularity for large tissue defects secondary to surgical tumor ablation or trauma. In these cases, the donor site is inadequate for autogenous bone reconstruction. Since this bone is nonliving, it is replaced by creeping substitution by host cells over a prolonged period of time. Periodic contamination of bone banks has resulted in patient infection with both bacteria and viruses (AIDS). Vascularized live bone allograft transplanted across strong histocompatibility barriers results in rapid rejection. The clinical use of vascularized allograft remains highly experimental but may be feasible with immunosuppression by cyclosporine.

Although whole-bone allografts have problems, allogeneic, lyophilized decalcified transplants can induce the formation of new bone by host osteogenic precursor cells. This bone induction factor appears to be a glycoprotein that stimulates new bone formation from cells migrating from the perivascular connective tissue. Bone morphogenic protein and decalcified, freeze-dried, allogeneic cortical bone grafts can be substituted for autogenous grafts.

Fresh xenograft bone has been unsuccessful because it elicits a strong immune response. It is possible that freeze-dried xenogeneic bone could produce a lesser response, but with the availability of allograft bone, this attempt has not gained popularity.

Substitutes for autogenous tissue are available. Freeze-dried tendon allografts have little antigenicity because of their relative paucity of cells. These grafts remain intact and are repopulated by host fibroblasts. Mechanical strength studies reveal the allografts to be similar in strength to tendon autografts. Fascia allografts have also been used as tendon substitutes with limited success. There are experimental data that glutaraldehyde-treated bovine xenografts may be useful substitutes. The problem with them is a problem of adequate attachment of the xenograft to the donor tendon.

Cartilage substitution is usually performed with allogeneic material. Because of its relative acellularity as compared with its matrix structure, cartilage tends to lose bulk when grafted. This is more significant with allograft cartilage than with autograft cartilage. Calcification and fracture of allograft cartilage is a frequent complication not seen with autografts. Xenograft cartilage has proved less successful than the allogeneic material.

Nerve substitution has been sought for over 100 years. Although originally it was thought that a whole-nerve allograft would be useful, it is now recognized that only the nerve sheath is desirable to form a conduit for axonal regeneration. Allograft nerve sheaths contain Schwann cells, which are very antigenic. However, with immunosuppression, the rejection can be delayed long enough to allow axonal growth to proceed through the allograft conduit. Substances with less antigenicity than allograft nerve sheaths have been studied to produce a substitute conduit. Blood vessels such as umbilical veins and skin or amniotic membranes formulated into tubes have been tried. Although all of these techniques have had initial success in animal trials, none has become routinely clinically useful.

The ultimate in biological substitutes for wound healing is the composite tissue allograft. What better way to solve the amputation wound of an extremity than to replace it with an allograft limb? Experimentation to reach this goal continues with each new immunosuppressive agent discovered. As mentioned under the skin substitutes, the greatest immune stimulation from composite allografts will come from the skin.

SUGGESTED READING

Cohen IK, Diegelmann RF, Lindblad WJ: *Wound Healing, Biochemical and Clinical Aspects.* Philadelphia, WB Saunders, 1992.

Heggers JP, Robson MC: *Quantitative Bacteriology: Its Role in the Armamentarium of the Surgeon.* Boca Raton, Fla, CRC Press, 1991.

Peacock EE: *Wound Repair,* ed 3. Philadelphia, WB Saunders, 1987.

Robson MC: Growth factors as wound healing agents. *Curr Opin Biotech* 1991; 2:863.

Robson MC, Raine TJ, Smith DJ, et al: Principles of wound healing and repair, in James E, Corry RJ, Perry JF (eds): *Principles of Basic Surgical Practice.* Philadelphia, Hanley & Belfus, 1987, pp 61–72.

Robson MC, Stenberg BD, Heggers JP: Wound healing alterations caused by infection. *Clin Plast Surg* 1990; 17:485.

Technical Manual for Tissue Banking, revised. American Association of Tissue Banks, 1992.

Chapter 2

Grafts and Flaps

Thomas J. Krizek, M.D., F.A.C.S.

CONTENTS

CHAPTER OBJECTIVE

At the end of this chapter the resident understands the physiology of flaps and grafts, is thoroughly familiar with surgery in all types of flaps and grafts, and utilizes flaps effectively for reconstruction in the full spectrum of plastic surgical practice.

LEARNER OBJECTIVES

On completion of this chapter the resident

1. **Understands the terminology of flap movement including advancement flap, rotation flap, transposition of flap, etc.**
2. **Understands the terminology of flap vascular supply including random flap, axial flap, island flap, free flap, etc.**
3. **Understands the variations in flap anatomy including cutaneous flap, fasciocutaneous flap, musculocutaneous flap, etc.**
4. **Recognizes the physiology of normal flaps, ischemic flaps, and the "delay" phenomenon.**
5. **Knows the physiology and microbiology of acute, intermediate, and chronic wounds, and the impact this has for the timing and techniques of wound closure surgery; is thoroughly familiar with the factors influencing the choice of flap vs. graft for wound closure.**
6. **Understands in detail the specific physiology of split- and full-thickness skin grafts, dermal grafts, cartilage grafts, bone grafts, tendon grafts, nerve grafts, fascial grafts, and composite grafts.**
7. **Knows specific grafting techniques including the operation of various types of dermatomes, management of graft donor sites, and care of graft recipient sites.**
8. **Understands the principles and applications of special grafting techniques including dermabrasion and over-grafting, the crane principle, xenografts, and cadaver grafts.**
9. Understands technological, pharmacological, and physiological monitoring techniques including fluorescence, capillary refill, thermal monitoring, laser flow probes, oxygen saturation, pH monitoring, etc.

CLINICAL PRACTICE ACTIVITIES

During the course of the training program, the resident

1. **Performs operations incorporating the full spectrum of flaps and grafts including skin grafts, local flaps, fascial and musculocutaneous flaps, free tissue transfers, bone grafts, composite grafts, etc.**
2. **Treats patients who have complications of flaps and grafts including skin graft loss, flap necrosis, wound dehiscence, wound infection, etc.**

Reconstructive surgeons are the managers of the most difficult and complex of wound problems. Our ability to mobilize, shift, transpose, transfer, and otherwise move tissue from one place to another is our special contribution to the art and science of surgery—and it is in part science and in large measure art. All complex tissue transfers can be divided into the major categories of "grafts" and "flaps."

In choosing any individual technique to close a wound, the surgeon employs what has been referred to as the "reconstructive ladder," the bottom rung of which is the most simple approach. As one climbs the ladder, the steps become more complex; therefore, it is a ladder of complexity. The choice of technique is based on three factors: the wound, the donor site, and the patient. The needs of all three must be matched; avoid the accusation that your work is the triumph of technology over reason. In the wound healing process the critical step most under control of the surgeon is successful closure of the wound. It is *only* when the wound edges cannot be approximated as in an incised wound (primary closure) or when spontaneous closure by contraction/epithelialization (secondary closure) is not desirable that one ever considers the use of flaps and grafts.

GRAFTS

Skin

A skin graft is defined as the transfer of a segment of skin by totally separating the tissue from its original blood supply (from the "donor site") and transferring the skin to a different part of the body (to a "recipient site") from which the skin must derive its new blood supply. All skin grafts initially adhere to the recipient bed by the formation of fibrin, which "glues" the graft to the bed. Skin grafts initially derive the oxygen and nutrients necessary for survival by diffusion from the underlying recipient bed ("plasmatic diffusion" or "imbibition") through this fibrin glue. The thinner the graft, the less nutrition it requires and the more likely it is to be successfully transplanted (to "take"). The thicker the graft, the more complex its metabolic needs; permanent take depends not on diffusion alone but the actual establishment of a new blood supply to the grafted skin. The intrinsic blood supply of skin is complex but basically includes deeper dermal vessels that course horizontally in the reticular dermis in parallel with the skin surface and send vertical vessels up toward the papillary dermis where they arborize into smaller nourishing twigs. In thicker skin grafts there is a rapid matching up of the cut vessels between the raw undersurface of the graft and the surface of the recipient wound, a process known as "inosculation." The graft's vessels then form the framework for the spread of a new endothelial lining from the vessels in the bed, thus establishing a permanent neovasculature.

Split-Thickness Skin Grafts

Any skin graft in which less than the full thickness of the skin is transferred is known as a split- or partial-thickness skin graft. Split grafts may be subdivided into epidermal, thin, intermediate, and thick, but the distinction is always based on its thickness relative to the full thickness of the skin from which it was removed and not as an absolute number. The skin of the body varies in thickness from 2 to 3 thousandths of an inch in the eyelid to 30 to 40 thousandths of an inch over the back. Since dermatomes are calibrated in thousandths of an inch, it is tempting to want to employ some universal guideline that, for instance, 10 thousandths of an inch would be a nice figure for moderate thickness grafts. Unfortunately, that thickness removed from the back of an adult produces a graft that is actually rather "thin" relative to the total thickness of the skin: skin of 10 thousandths of an inch taken from the medial aspect of the thigh of an infant or from an older patient might well be the total thickness of the skin and some fat for good measure.

Whereas the transfer of "flaps" (in which the tissue remains attached during the transfer) dates to antiquity, the use of grafts is a relatively modern development. Although certainly others must have tried the technique, even successfully, credit must go to the one who truly gave it to the world. In this case Jacques Louis Reverdin in 1869 described the first grafting of human skin to an open wound.

Epidermal Grafts. Some of these earliest grafts were shavings of the epidermis only (Fig 2–1, A). Since the epidermis lacks most of the structural integrity and complexity of skin, it provides only the most primitive coverage. Lacking structure, these grafts do little to retard wound contraction. They lack the dermal appendages and are devoid of pigmentation. They were almost abandoned until interest was renewed for the possibilities of removing skin and culturing the epidermis, i.e., allowing small amounts of tissue to be spatially multiplied and then reapplied to cover large areas. The application of cultured epidermis, because of the disadvantages of such thin grafts, is limited to use as a potential lifesaving technique in major burns.

Thin Grafts. Grafts that include some but not all of the basal cell layer of the epidermis and some of the papillary dermis are described as thin (Fig 2–1, B). They have considerably more structural integrity than epidermal grafts and, because they are thin, require only

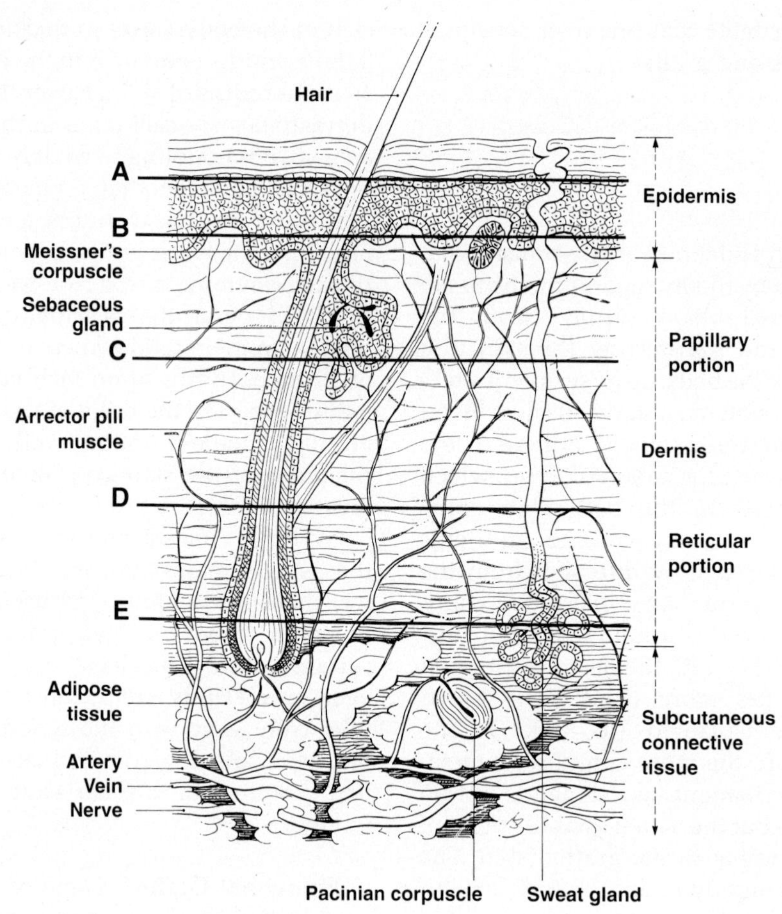

FIG 2–1.
Cross section of the skin and subcutaneous tissue. **A,** epidermal grafts remove only the thin layer of epidermis. **B,** thin split-thickness grafts remove some of the basal cell layer. **C,** moderately thick split-thickness grafts most commonly have a range of thickness from just below the papillary dermis through about three fourths of the thickness of the skin. **D,** thick split-thickness grafts remove more than three fourths of the thickness of the skin. **E,** full-thickness skin grafts by definition remove the entire thickness of skin but not the subcutaneous tissue.

modest nourishment to survive. Vascular ingrowth is over short distances, and such grafts can "take" quickly. They are thin and lack some of the aesthetic niceties of skin, are without hair follicles and glands, and do not inhibit wound contraction in the bed as well as thicker grafts do. Because they require less nourishment, their use in less vascular recipient sites or in burned patients may be desirable. The donor sites of these thin grafts have most of the skin elements left behind and heal more rapidly (thus permitting reharvesting if needed) than those from which thicker skin has been removed.

Moderately Thick Grafts. To obtain a moderately thick graft the surgeon removes the epidermis, including the basal cell layer and most if not all of the papillary dermis (Fig 2–1, C). The lining of the remaining hair follicles, sebaceous glands, and eccrine glands provides the residual epithelial elements necessary for the donor site to epithelialize and repair itself. The moderately thick graft has some real substance and provides durable and functional coverage. Since only portions of the glands and hair follicles are transplanted, the grafts are hairless, tend to be dry, and are often pruritic, as are most grafts. Whether from increased activity of the melanocytes or from their compression during wound contraction, the grafts tend to be more heavily pigmented than the original donor site. The final color is not predictable, and this lack of color match is one of the major aesthetic impediments to truly successful skin transplantation.

Thick Grafts. Thick grafts are those in which more than 75% to 80% of the thickness of the skin is removed, which leaves a rather tenuous donor site of reticular dermis through which the underlying subcutaneous tissue may occasionally be seen (Fig 2–1, D). These grafts contain most of the elements of skin. The recipient wound conditions must be truly favorable for the surgeon to anticipate "take" of these grafts. They are the most aesthetically pleasing, pliable, and durable of split-thickness grafts and are most valuable on the face, hands, and feet. The donor sites must be managed with meticulous care since dehydration, infection, or further injury could convert these wounds into full-thickness tissue loss.

Full-Thickness Skin Grafts

A full-thickness skin graft contains all of the skin elements and none of the underlying fat (Fig 2–1, E). Full-thickness skin grafts, particularly when the donor and recipient sites are very similar in color and texture, may provide a very acceptable functional and aesthetic result. A prime example of a clinical situation is the removal of the full thickness of the skin of the upper eyelid to serve as the cover for a denuded lower eyelid. Historically, many of the grafting techniques (Wolfe grafts for example) were developed to solve problems around the eye, particularly ectropion of the lower lid.

Since the entire skin thickness is transferred, the donor site obviously results in a wound the same size and shape as the graft that was removed. This is truly the situation where the surgeon cannot "borrow from Peter to pay Paul unless Peter can afford it." In the eyelid example, many if not most adults have a surplus of skin in the upper lid that allows removal of enough skin to cover the lower lid and still allows closure of the donor site without difficulty, usually with a very pleasing result. On the other hand, it is almost never possible to remove sufficient tissue from a lower lid to be of any use without serious risk of ectropion. Only under the most unusual circumstances would a surgeon remove a full-thickness graft so large, from any area, that the donor site could not be easily closed by primary intention. Traditional donor sites are the postauricular skin, the inguinal region, and the medial aspect of the upper part of the arm, all sites that tend to be inconspicuous when healed. Other sites used often are the neck, the antecubital fossa, and dreadfully, the volar aspect of the wrist. (Although this site may be temptingly nearby when skin is required for the hand, the resulting scar has social consequences that are unacceptable.)

The full thickness of the skin requires substantial nourishment to survive, nourishment that is by definition parasitic until inosculation and reendothelialization can occur. A full-thickness graft should therefore be used only when the recipient bed is most receptive (e.g., well vascularized and without excessive contamination).

Composite Grafts

Composite grafts include skin *and* another tissue such as fat or cartilage. The term is also used to describe such grafts as a combination of mucous membrane and cartilage. Although most complex tissue transfers are now accomplished by microvascular techniques, composite grafts are still occasionally of value. Since vascularity of thick tissue is predictably tenuous at best, such grafts are usually both small and limited to use in highly vascular recipient areas such as the ears, nose, and nipple/areolar complex. An example is the use of a portion of the earlobe or helical rim (with cartilage included) as a donor site for tissue to reconstruct defects in the alar rim. Another common type of composite graft is a "nipple-sharing" approach to reconstruct a nipple with the opposite side as a donor. Careful approximation of the graft to the wound bed is paramount. Rapid inosculation and prompt capillary refill of the graft after blanching has occasionally been observed within hours of transfer. Replantation of amputated fingertips of skin and fat are occasionally successful without microvascular techniques, particularly in children. As with full-thickness grafts, the donor site from composite grafts leaves an open wound that must be closed or allowed to contract.

Hair Transplants. The most common form of composite grafting is probably the hair transplant. Since the hair follicles extend for variable distances into the subcutaneous tissue, plugs of tissue with hair follicles are most safely transplanted as skin-fat composite grafts. The usual technique involves removing a plug of tissue containing a number of hair follicles with a dermal punch and placing the plug in a defect in a hairless area (using a slightly smaller punch in the recipient site allows the size discrepancy to facilitate the graft fitting snugly). The individual donor sites contract and close by secondary intention. Strips of hair-bearing scalp may also be transferred as larger units, particularly to recreate a hairline.

"Pinch Grafts"

It is of historical importance and current practice to first define and then condemn the use of pinch grafts. Some of the earliest efforts at skin grafting utilized a technique whereby the operator lifted a portion of skin with a hypodermic needle or other sharply pointed instrument and shaved off the tented tissue. The divot thus created tended to be full thickness in the center and then gradually thinned toward the margin where it was very thin. The graft was therefore composite in the center and then graded through thick to thin and epidermal at the margin. This simple technique of skin harvesting persisted in the hands of the less skilled; unfortunately, these grafts heal with a telltale cobblestone appearance. They were usually applied in regular rather than artistic patterns, often resembling a checkerboard (with the checkers in place). The donor sites (unfortunately often the anterior aspect of the thigh) were equally unsightly. The development of modern techniques and instruments for harvesting skin has made pinch grafting obsolete.

Dermal (Dermal/Fat) Grafts

Completing the possible types of skin grafts is the use of dermis from which the epidermis has been removed, with or without underlying fat. The removal of the epidermis allows the dermis to be buried at the recipient site. The use of such grafts has almost exclusively been for the correction of contour defects, particularly of the face. The fat all too often liquefied and could rarely be identified at reexploration. The dermis also shrinks variably, sometimes as much as 50% since presumably it does not completely vascularize. Even though the epidermis has been removed, there is a tendency for the dermal elements of hair follicles or glands to become cystic, although atrophy of these elements is more likely.

Skin Graft Transfer

The major elements in preparing for skin grafting for wound repair involve both diagnostic and technical aspects. The diagnosis is directed to the needs of the patient and the characteristics of the recipient site, including the opportunities, limitations, and constraints. The technical aspects refer to the means of obtaining the graft, transferring and affixing it, and managing the donor site.

The Patient

Wounds are attached to people who are unique, each with special needs. One patient may wish to exchange some scarring for the opportunity to return quickly to work; for another the aesthetic appearance may in actuality outweigh the functional result in importance. No patient should be subjected to an operation more complex and dangerous than the situation requires. Many wounds allowed to close secondarily will, in actuality, provide a result the quality of which matches a more complex operative closure. The ultimate aesthetic result at the donor site is too often ignored; discolored scarring of the anterior aspect of the thighs of a young girl may be a handicap long after the site to which the skin was transferred is forgotten. Reconstructive surgery is truly a scientific art form and not a mere repertoire of techniques. It truly must be reiterated that "if your only tool is a hammer, all the world begins to look like a nail." It is incumbent on the reconstructive surgeon to be knowledgeable and facile with all the reconstructive techniques, able to recognize the pros and cons of various options, and be in a position to offer each patient the best approach to the individual problem.

Wounds

There are certain characteristics of a wound that either promote or inhibit the "take" of a skin graft. Since the graft must derive its new vascularity from the recipient bed, wounds that are avascular, such as bone denuded of its periosteum, are poor candidates for supporting the graft. Some general observations regarding skin graft transfer may be made:

1. Skin grafts do nicely on well-vascularized wound beds, either clean granulating beds or those created by the excision of tissue. Regular surfaces such as provided by the reticular dermis (as in the tangential excision of a burn wound), by fascia, or by intact peritenon are examples of "good" wound beds. Irregular, less vascularized surfaces such as fat are less desirable.
2. Cooperative patients do better since the grafts must be immobilized and the donor sites tended. It is best when the patient can help.
3. The best results are accomplished when the donor tissue matches the recipient bed in texture and color (e.g., upper eyelid-to-lower eyelid graft).
4. The avascular wound is not suitable for nourishing a graft. Such wounds include bone without its vascular periosteal cover, tendon without peritenon, and denuded cartilage.
5. Wounds may be rendered marginally suitable by the presence of peripheral vascular disease or other factors such as radiation that compromise local wound healing ability.
6. Contamination by microorganisms is an important cause of graft loss. Surface contamination can often be eliminated by topical preparation. More important are organisms that are in the depth of the wound; they can be identified with great precision as to both their type and quantity either preoperatively or rapidly intraoperatively. Bacterial presence in quantities exceeding 100,000 organisms per gram of tissue is accompanied by frequent graft loss, possibly by eliciting products that activate plasmin, which in turn dissolves the fibrin glue holding the graft. Streptococci may be a significant cause of graft loss at levels even below 10^5 organisms per gram. Such contamination should be managed by excision/debridement or topical antibacterials. Systemic antibacterials have little effect on the bacterial levels in the depths of the granulation tissue.
7. Granulation tissue that has fewer than 10^5 microorganisms per gram is usually a healthy recipient of grafts and should *not* be scraped away. Such maneuvers tend to cause bleeding, which may interfere with graft take.
8. Grafts can survive on plasma through which oxygen and nutrients can diffuse. Grafts *cannot* survive on blood clots.
9. Grafts must remain adherent to the bed until such time as they revascularize; wound beds that are subject to motion, particularly shear forces, are not easy to cover with grafts. The periscapular region is notoriously difficult to graft since it is most difficult to immobilize.
10. If the patient has been chosen well, if the wound is appropriate for a graft, if the wound has been properly prepared, if the grafting is performed accurately, and if the postoperative management is conducted well, then skin grafts *always* take!

Techniques of Grafting

Donor Sites

The choice of the donor site is critical and is a decision with lifetime consequences. A relatively thin graft removed accurately from a donor site that reepithelializes promptly may leave no scarring and only a small amount of discoloration (almost always lighter than before). A thicker graft produces a deeper donor wound that may heal with difficulty and, in younger patients (particularly deeply pigmented patients), may leave very unsightly scars or even keloids. Although the anterior aspect of the thigh is a readily accessible donor site from which even the least talented technician can obtain skin, it is also a highly visible body part in both younger men and women. The use of the thigh and the subsequent development of scarring are unconscionable when less visible sites such as the buttock could be used instead. A rather challenging but highly suitable donor site for split-thickness grafts is the scalp, which when shaved and ballooned with saline makes removal of a graft technically simple. The healed wound (since all the hair follicles were deep to the level at which the graft is usually removed) is a wound totally hidden by the regrown hair.

It is obviously desirable to match the color and texture of the donor site and recipient site. Would that it were even remotely possible to accomplish this with any consistency. The donor site almost always winds up lighter than before, and the transferred skin is usually not only darker than it was originally but rarely matches the neighboring tissue at its new site. The Nobel prize awaits the inventive and imaginative investigator who can predictably enable the reconstructive surgeon to control and manage color match. No particular "truism" is as predictably false as the idea that removing skin from a so-called blush area of the upper part of the chest or neck gives a better aesthetic result when placed on the face.

Dermatomes

Skin grafts were originally removed with the free knife blade, the size and accuracy of the depth and uniformity of the graft being directly and proximately dependent on the skill of the surgeon. The initial modifications were to extend the width of the blade to enable the surgeon to obtain grafts perhaps 3 to 4 in. in width and as long as the donor site allowed; grafts 2 to 3 ft long could be obtained, although it was hard to imagine where to put them. An important modification was the placement of a guard on the blade that enabled the depth to be controlled and required substantially less skill in use. These freehand knives have a variety of names such as Braithwaite, Humby, Weck, and a small one developed by Goulian that employs a narrower width and fixed shims to control the depth. These instruments are now used more often to tangentially excise burn wounds than to obtain skin grafts.

The drum dermatomes were developed in the 1930s and 1940s by Padgett and Reese. The Padgett dermatome has a semicircular drum 4 in. in width and 8 in. in length. A blade fixed in the movable handle can be adjusted to determine the thickness of the skin graft to be obtained. Glue or, more commonly now, sticky tape applied to both the drum and skin forms a bond between the skin and the drum; the blade neatly incises the skin at thicknesses varying from thin to thick that can be altered during the course of removing the graft. The Reese dermatome is essentially identical to the Padgett one in concept except that the thickness of the skin graft is controlled by shims of varying thickness. Both of these dermatomes should remain in the reconstructive surgeon's armamentarium since they provide very uniform grafts, they are suitable for even difficult donor sites, and the 4-in. width is occasionally of real value.

The "motorized" dermatomes, first developed by Brown, made it possible for even the minimally trained to obtain nice skin grafts. The dermatomes, driven by electricity or air pressure, cut the graft with a rapidly oscillating blade. Fairly uniform grafts of almost unlimited length can be obtained. It has been observed that the motorized dermatome is perhaps the greatest advance in burn care in the last century; it made it possible for any surgeon to rapidly learn and then obtain skin grafts.

Donor sites are easier to use when the surface is smooth; irregular surfaces can be bulked out by injecting fluid such as saline into the subcutaneous tissues. A donor site of 150 to 200 cm^2 for a moderately thick graft can be anticipated to lose 60 to 75 mL of blood. This can be reduced by injecting vasoconstrictors in limited amounts under careful monitoring or by the topical application of vasoconstrictors or thrombin.

A variety of devices is now available to perforate the graft in a regular, grid-like pattern that allows the skin to be expanded.

The "mesh" grafts originally were tedious to use since each piece of skin had to be stretched on a plastic carrier to insert into the mesher; new models eliminate this step.

Donor Site Management

The donor site is a raw wound with all nerve endings exposed. The donor site is therefore almost always substantially more painful than the recipient site where the graft is placed (Moriarity's law). The donor site, as any partial-thickness wound, heals only when closure is accomplished by reepithelialization from the margins or from the dermal elements in the glands and hair follicles. This process proceeds most efficiently in a moist environment. The formation of a crust (scab) is the body's way of holding moisture against the wound and should be promoted. Any dressing placed against the raw wound should remain until epithelialization allows it to separate without pain. Various impregnated gauzes are traditional. Xeroform is fine-mesh gauze impregnated with Vaseline and preservatives; it is often packaged in a 5 × 9-in. size (since the original drum dermatomes removed a 4 × 8-in. graft, the nice fit and overlap are not an accident). Gauze impregnated with scarlet red ointment has a scientific legitimacy since the agent is a known epithelial stimulator. There are now a variety of "veil-like" materials that can be placed between the gauze adherent to the wound and the bulky absorbent dressing usually applied in the operating room. This intervening layer enables the outer dressing to be removed with less discomfort. Exposing the wound to the air or sometimes a warming lamp will "dry" it out. Actually this maneuver promotes the formation of a protective scab and thus preserves the moisture at the wound interface. The hydrocolloid and other dressings that preserve moisture at the wound surface but also protect from injury or bacterial invasion are fundamentally sound approaches to donor site management. In actuality there is a "Hawthorne effect" in managing donor sites: any technique that leads to care givers being interested in and tending to the wound will promote healing, and changing the technique occasionally will heighten and renew this interest.

Dermabrasion

The technique of dermabrasion is presented here since management of a dermabraded wound most nearly represents the care of a donor site. The concept of dermabrasion evolved from efforts to "smooth" skin that suffered from contour irregularity within the superficial layers of the skin. Scalpels are used to shave, and wire brushes or abrasive wheels are used to abrade or scrape the outer layer of the skin to remove irregularities. The tissue remaining is thus very much like a donor site: raw, weeping, and in need of protection from dehydration and bacteria. When healed, the "new" skin will tend to be smoother, pinker, and then lighter than the surrounding tissue and may have a more prominent pattern of pores. It usefully smoothes the finest of rhytids, acne rosacea, and the more superficial craters from healed acne vulgaris. What dermabrasion cannot do is eliminate the "ice pick" scars or other problems that involve the full thickness of the skin; sufficient regenerative tissue must be left behind to allow healing, or the result will be a scar. (For additional discussion of dermabrasion, see Chapter 5.)

Graft Application

The *sine qua non* of all graft application is careful approximation of the undersurface of the graft to the raw surface of the wound. The graft must be kept in position until adherence has occurred, with or without complete revascularization. This requires roughly a week and varies, of course, with the location and vascularity of the recipient site and the thickness of the skin graft. In all cases the junction between the graft and the neighboring normal skin (or an additional adjacent graft) is comparable to the closure of an incised wound. Particularly in full-thickness or thicker split-thickness grafts, this seam will form a scar that should be managed with the same care as for any other wound closure. No pressure or even compression over and above atmospheric pressure is necessary to promote graft take. When the wound bed is irregularly contoured, it may be desirable to use a bolus dressing. Some of the marginal sutures between the graft and adjacent skin are left long, and when the graft is in place, a conforming dressing that may be moist cotton, gauze, dental compound, or any other conforming material is tied in place by using the long ends of the sutures. This is often referred to as a "stent." Conformation to irregular surfaces can also be promoted by perforating the graft at regular intervals, the result of which is the "mesh" graft; when skin is in short supply, such as in major burns, the meshed skin may be expanded in ratios of 2:1 on up to 9:1.

"Postage stamp" graft was a term used to describe the result of taking larger pieces of skin graft of any thickness and cutting them in stamp size, which then allows them to conform to and cover a larger area. The meshed graft has largely replaced this more cumbersome maneuver. The interstices of the meshed graft *must* fill with epithelium from the edge of the graft; the more the skin is expanded, the larger the interstices and the more space that must fill and heal with scar epithelium. Meshed grafts have been referred to as *"puka"* grafts (*puka* meaning "air"), pointing out that *puka* heals with scar. Albeit acceptable, no mesh graft ever looks as good as a uniform nonperforated graft.

"Pie crusting" is a useful technique for decompressing the crusty surface of fruit pies; since pies predictably expand and do so uniformly, small cuts in the surface allow liquid to egress. It is nonsense to believe that this culinary technique is transferrable to the operating room. In the first place, the wound bed is not fruit, and it is unpredictable where plasma will accumulate beneath the graft. It is difficult to know in advance where to perforate. Additionally the pie-crusting perforations seal with fibrin within minutes, as do the interstices of the meshed graft. Mesh grafts are successful in allowing the grafts to conform to the wound and minimize plasma collections, and not because the interstices allow drainage. Additionally, if fluid does accumulate, accurate aspiration with a fine needle and syringe is kinder to the graft than a series of random cuts. Finally, the fluid should also *not* be "milked" to the margin; why convert that small area where the graft is not adherent to an entire track where, by milking, you have lifted the already adherent graft from its bed.

Long-Term Management

After the initial "take," grafts must still be protected during the early maturation stages. Particularly for grafts in dependent areas, compression and external support are desirable. Grafts and donor sites are dry and often pruritic. Soothing lotions and compression will help. Although full-thickness and some other thicker grafts may present an acceptable, even pleasing appearance rather early in the healing process (weeks to months), more often the graft is rather ugly in the eyes of the patient and family. Meshed grafts in particular may develop a cobblestone appearance and look worse at 2 months than they did at 2 weeks. The surgeon must be sensitive to the difference between a result that may be exciting to the surgeon but shocking and disappointing to a patient who, not quite knowing what to expect from a graft, may not share the surgeon's enthusiasm. Fortunately, grafts like other wounds will improve with time.

Overgrafting

Overgrafting is a technique designed to thicken a thin graft to allow it to become a sturdier, more protective cover. Most commonly used on leg ulcers, the healed split-thickness graft is dermabraded and, instead of allowing the bed to heal like a donor site, is subsequently covered with another skin graft. This process can be repeated several times, at the risk, however, of ultimately producing a thick scar rather than a pliable graft.

Reinnervation

All grafts are initially without sensation. Thicker, more complex grafts may preserve some of the sensory endings during the transfer, and ingrowth of nerve fibers from the bed of the wound may result in acceptable sensibility. Again, donor and recipient graft sites should be matched when possible for their relative sensibility. A denuded fingertip should not be covered with a piece of skin from the back; the back's skin has only mediocre intrinsic sensibility and a paucity of specialized sensory endings. It is implausible that this tissue would ever provide the same sensation as tissue removed from another place on the hand such as the hypothenar skin.

Other Types of Tissue Transfer

Although almost all tissue transfer is from one part of a single patient to another place on the same person, there are other forms of transfer. The terminology and concepts are reviewed below.

Autograft

An autograft (to the geneticist this is referred to as a *syngeneic* graft) refers to tissue transferred from one place on the patient to another location on the *same* patient.

Isograft

An isograft (the geneticist term is *isogeneic*) is tissue transferred from a donor to a recipient who is *genetically identical.* The first successful renal transplant by Joseph Murray was between identical twins. Successful skin transfers from an unburned twin to a burned twin have been reported as well. There are also isogeneic animals bred with identical immune systems.

Allograft

An allograft (the geneticist term is *allogeneic,* and the old, all-but-obsolete term is "homograft") is tissue transferred to and from members of the *same species.* Most solid-tissue transfers (kidney, liver, heart, etc.) are of this category. The immune response, which is known to be cell mediated, can be suppressed, and the long-term survival of such grafts of solid organs is known. Patients and families are often surprised to learn that no such long-term successful skin allografts have occurred.

George David Pollock, who performed the first skin autograft on a burned patient in 1870, subsequently used his own arm as a donor site for the first allograft on the same patient all within a few weeks' period. He watched his own skin seem to take, in the same manner as the patient's own skin, and then 10 to 14 days later it began to dissolve—the fate of skin allografts even now. Medawar, in rabbits, observed that if an allograft from the same donor was used a second time on the same patient (animal), rejection was accelerated ("second-set phenomenon").

Removed from cadavers up to 12 hours after death, skin can be stored for up to 30 days in culture media under refrigeration or frozen and used many months later. The skin must be tested for bacterial or viral contamination to prevent transfer of infectious diseases, including acquired immunodeficiency syndrome (AIDS). Survival of allografts on burned patients, who are immunocompromised from the injury, is prolonged, and longer survival has also been shown investigationally when immunosuppression is used. However, immunosuppression risks infection in any patient whose wounds are not closed and should not be considered as a routine.

Other terms applied to solid-organ transfer include "orthotopic," which refers to organs that are transferred to the same anatomic position in the recipient as was the original organ; the term "heterotopic" is used when the organ is placed in a site anatomically foreign to the graft.

Amnion

The placental membranes have been used on occasion over the last 60 years or so as a temporary cover for burns and other wounds. The unseparated amnion/chorion, when applied with the chorion against the wound, seems to "take" and provides serviceable cover temporarily. The thin, transparent amnion is also a tidy dressing for partial-thickness wounds. Although amnion comes in large sizes and is readily available at essentially no cost ("except for the labor"), its use runs a risk of transfer of infective agents, which decreases its clinical value. Moreover, the availability of preserved (frozen) skin allograft has decreased the need for amnion.

Xenograft

A xenograft (the geneticist term is *xenogeneic,* and the old term is "heterograft") is tissue transferred from a member of one species to a recipient of a *different species.* The lay press is endlessly fascinated by the occasional transfers of baboon kidneys or hearts, which have been uniformly unsuccessful. Almost ignored is the use of bovine valves and vessels, which have been employed successfully for years. The reconstructive surgeon may use porcine skin xenografts for temporary wound cover in burned and other patients with open wounds. Pigskin stores well and is readily available commercially. It does not "take" and may not provide the same degree of wound control from bacteria that allograft provides.

FLAPS

It is curious that descriptions of flap transfer date to antiquity whereas grafting is relatively modern. Almost all would agree that flap transfer is substantially more complex and the technology more sophisticated than for grafts. A graft is totally separated from its blood supply both during and after transfer and must derive its nourishment and ultimate survival from the underlying bed to which it is applied. In contrast, a flap remains attached to its original blood supply during the entire transfer process, thereby accounting for its terminology. The "flap" is likened to fabric raised on three sides from the surface but attached along one margin, as the flap over a pocket. The term "pedicle," often redundantly used with flap as in "pedicle flap," refers to the vascular "pedicle" derived from the word for "foothold." Although Alexis Carrel described the anastomosis of small blood vessels in 1905 and transferred kidneys in rodents by reattaching the vascular pedicle, use of the vascular pedicles of muscle, skin, or composite tissue was not developed until the 1960s. The ponderous terminology used previously, "transplantation of composite tissue by microsurgical vascular anastomoses," has been shortened to "free flap." Some incorrectly refer to all flaps as "pedicle grafts"; I believe that this term would only be applicable if tissue normally considered to be a flap were transferred by microvascular techniques, and a preferable term is free tissue transfer or free flap.

The breakthrough that allowed this to happen was a new understanding of the blood supply to the skin. The intrinsic reticular and papillary dermal vascularity was described in the section on grafts. How the blood gets to the skin forms the basis for rational flap transfer. At its most fundamental, all skin is supplied by variations of three patterns of vascular distribution. These patterns form the basis for dividing "flaps" into three kinds, random, axial, and musculocutaneous/fasciocutaneous. It is clear that there is substantial overlap, but the divisions, although arbitrary, are very useful.

Random Flaps

It is almost disingenuous to suggest that none of the blood supply to the skin is truly random since ultimately the vascularity is always, at its origin, precisely determined and identifiable. Functionally, however, much tissue transfer is accomplished without sophisticated identification of the specific vascularity. A random or random-pattern flap is one in which the specific blood supply is not identified but is rather derived from nonspecific dermal and subdermal vessels (Fig 2–2). Such flaps are the most commonly used and are the dominant form of *locally* transferred flaps, either from immediately adjacent or nearby tissue. It is the random flap that was described by Sushruta in the *Samhita* in about 600 B.C. whereby tissue was advanced from the cheek to correct defects of the nose (perhaps the real origin of our specialty). These flaps have a number of commonly used descriptions and configurations.

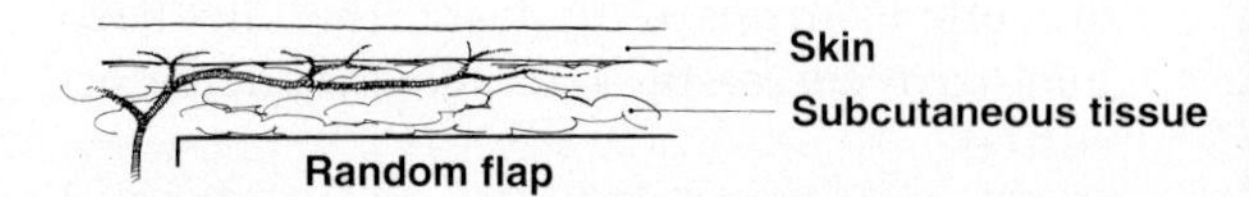

FIG 2–2.
Cross section of the skin and subcutaneous tissue with functional divisions of vascular supply. Random flap vascularity is derived from subcutaneous plexuses.

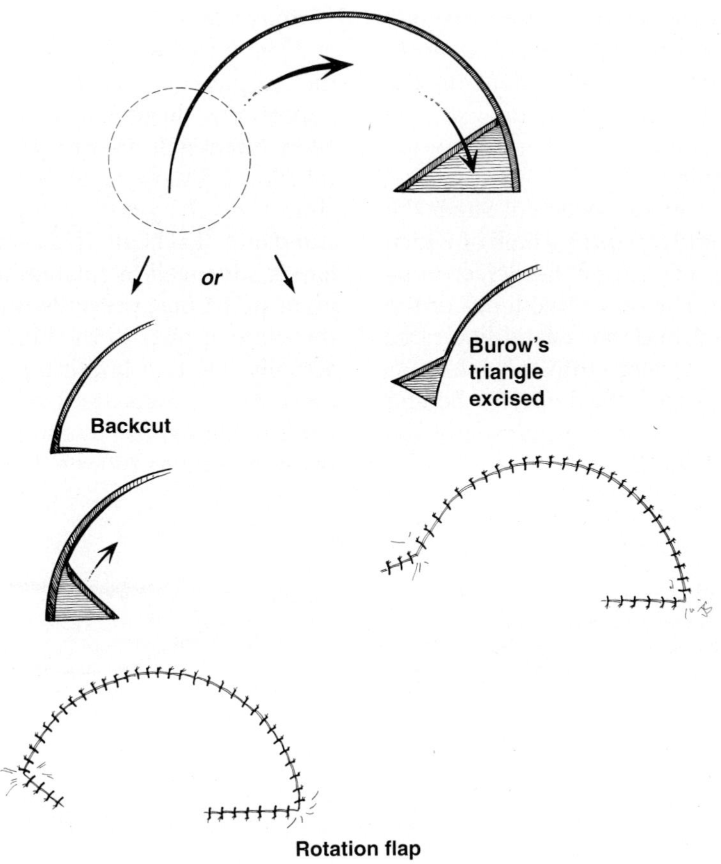

FIG 2–3.
Rotation flaps are based adjacent to the defect and turned into the defect. There is often an opportunity to "backcut" the base of flap to lengthen it (Burow's triangle).

Rotation

The base or the pedicle of a rotation flap is usually located as immediately adjacent to the defect to be filled as is possible. The tissue is incised on three sides, undermined, and transferred ("rotated") into the defect (Fig 2–3). If such a maneuver were attempted with rigid material, the defect produced at the site from which the material was moved would be of the same size and approximate shape as the material moved, and nothing would be gained. Fortunately, human tissue is elastic and expansive, and when the neighboring tissues are undermined, it is usually possible to close the donor defect. When this is not possible, a skin graft or another somewhat smaller flap may be rotated into the defect to be closed. When the flap is truly rotated, it is inevitable that the tissue most adjacent to the defect must fold on itself and cause a raised fold known as a "dog-ear." It is tempting to obliterate this fold by excising it; the peril is hidden in the fact that this fold contains a variable, sometimes critical portion of the blood supply to the flap.

Advancement

Whereas a rotation flap is designed adjacent to the defect, an advancement flap is designed such that the defect lays beyond the tip or distal portion of the flap. The flap is raised, undermined, and then pulled or pushed into the defect. As in the rotation flap, folds of tissue, now one at each side of the base of the flap, will be created. To avoid these small folds, a triangle of tissue at the base may be excised (Burow's triangle). Such advancement flaps are obviously dependent on the forgiving elasticity of human tissue.

V-Y Advancement

An example of an advancement flap is the creation of a triangular flap, one limb of which forms part of the margin of the defect to be filled (Fig 2–4, B). The other two limbs of the triangle are incised, and the "island-like" area of tissue is shifted forward into the defect. As the triangle is advanced, the defect left behind is closed primarily; the resulting closure has the configuration of a Y.

Bipedicle

The bipedicle flap is perhaps the flap in the surgical repertoire that is most often improperly designed. The non–plastic surgeon often will attempt this maneuver and trivialize it by referring to it as a "backcut"; it almost never works when designed and executed as a "backcut" (Fig 2–4, A). Whenever a flap is advanced or rotated, there is a limiting pivot point that prevents further movement; the same applies to the bipedicle flap, which actually has two limiting pivot points. Since these pivot points are fixed, if the "relaxing" cut is made parallel to and the same length as the edge adjacent to the defect, any advance-

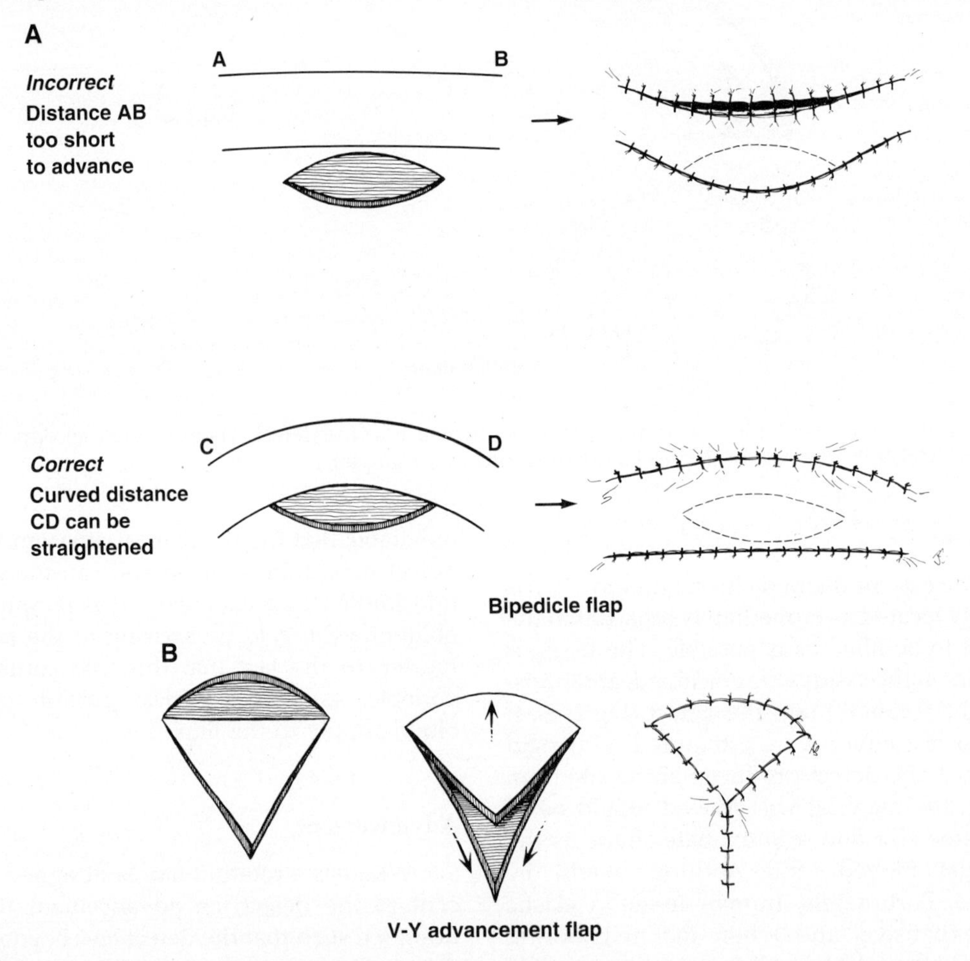

FIG 2–4.
Advancement flaps. **A,** bipedicle. The bipedicle flap has two attachments, one at either end. If the incisions are parallel, the tissue simply does not have enough length to advance (sometimes it is sufficiently elastic). It is better to design curved parallel lines so that as they straighten they allow the tissue to advance. **B,** V-Y-plasty. The flap is created adjacent to the defect and fashioned into a triangular shape by cutting on two sides (the V). The subcutaneous tissue is then teased and stretched, not cut, and the triangle advanced. As the defect behind is closed, the configuration is that of a Y.

ment is impossible, even with elastic tissue. The limbs *must* be curved, with one of the limbs longer. Only then, as the limbs are straightened, can the tissue be advanced. Try this with a piece of cloth and the principles become very apparent.

Transposition

The transposition flap refers to the technique of moving tissue either over or under intervening normal tissue. Alternatively, the transposed tissue can be exchanged with tissue nearby; it is then called an *interposition* flap. The classic examples of these flaps are the *rhomboid,* the *Z-plasty* (zed plasty), and the *W-plasty.*

Rhomboid

The rhomboid, a geometric phenomenon looking like a tilted square, has lent itself to the transposition of either a single or opposing rhomboid-shaped flaps into the defect (Fig 2–5). Since the maneuver is so aesthetically elegant and satisfying to the surgeon, it deserves its own category. It also heals particularly well since it is not circular. Many lesions grow in a centrifugal fashion and are largely circular in shape, and the defect created by surgery also tends to be circular. Unfortunately, few of the normal expression lines or aesthetic units are circular; so too, since wounds contract end to end, when a wound is circular it contracts toward the center. Any flap or graft that is circular in shape and fitted into the circular defect will contract toward the center, and the tissue in the middle will be "trapped" and will often become raised above the surface and look like a hamburger bun. Since grafts and many if not most flaps are fairly uniformly vascularized, there is little purpose in making them circular other than the fact that the defect is circular. The creation of a rhomboid defect avoids the circular contraction, the flap does not contract the way a circular flap tip would, and the result is therefore fairly uniformly pleasing.

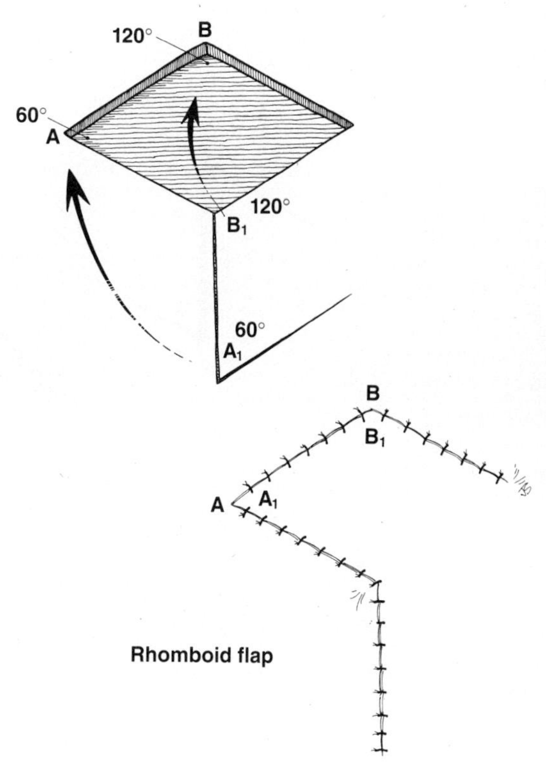

FIG 2–5.
Rhomboid flap. The defect resembles a tilted square, and the flap is designed to match the rhomboidal shape. The tissue is rotated, advanced, transposed, and since the normal tissue adjacent to the flap is used to close defect, also interposed.

Z-Plasty

An understanding of the principles and applications of the Z-plasty is fundamental to and an intellectual milestone in the learning of reconstructive surgery. The Z-plasty involves the interposition of two flaps that are triangular in shape (Fig 2–6, A). The original design and the resulting closure both have the configuration of the letter Z. The Z-plasty has a number of characteristics that are of substantial value in reconstruction.

It Lengthens. The Z-plasty, since it moves triangles of tissue from the sides of the wound and places them in the center of a linear defect, gains length at the expense of width. The amount of length gained is related to the angle of the tips of the triangles; the greater the angles, the more length gained (more gain from 45-degree angles than 30-degree angles, up to a maximum of about 60 to 70 degrees, beyond which the tissue cannot be interposed easily). With 60-degree angles, a Z-plasty gains 75% in length.

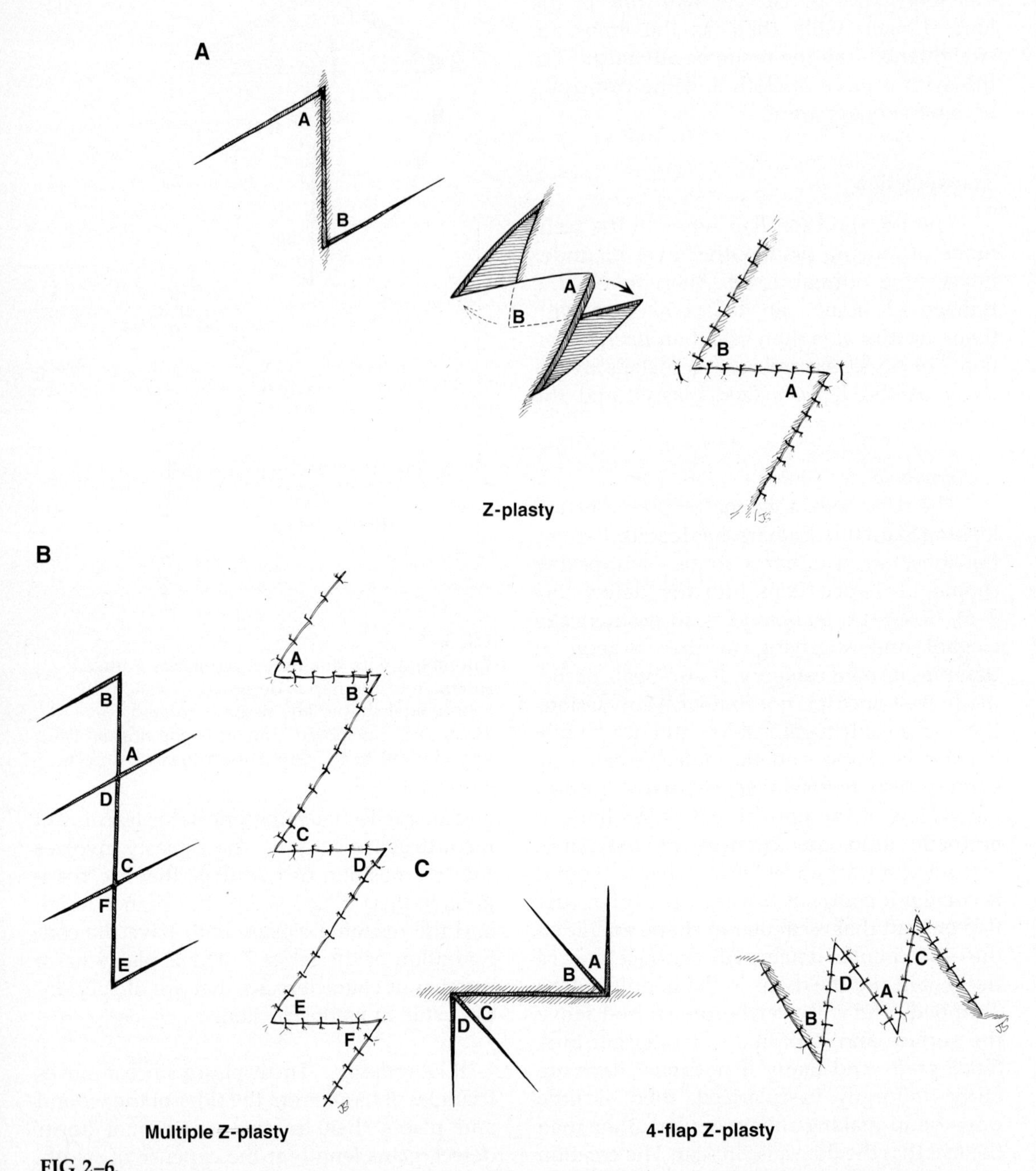

FIG 2–6.
Transposition flaps. **A,** Z-plasty. There are several steps involved: (1) the wound is incised along the scar, (2) two flaps (*A* and *B*) are raised with angles of 60 degrees, and (3) the flaps are then interposed. **B,** double or serial Z-plasty. The same steps as used in the Z-plasty are carried in series along the wound. Each pair of flaps is interposed. **C,** four-flap Z-plasty. The four-flap Z-plasty involves several steps: (1) opposing flaps of about 90 to 100 degrees are raised, and then each is bisected into two flaps with angles half the original flap, and (2) each pair of flaps is interdigitated (interposed) as depicted.

It Changes the Direction. Although the orientation and direction of a scar cannot be completely changed, the overall appearance of the scar can be altered sufficiently to suggest that the scar lays in a different direction. This is often functionally critical since the forces that tend to contract a wound always act along the long axis of the wound; the interposed Z-plasty breaks up these forces of contraction. Additionally, the resulting closed wound (thus the scar) can often be placed in a more aesthetically acceptable position.

It Changes the Appearance. A single long scar is often more noticeable and therefore less visually desirable than a series of shorter scars. This is, of course, most dramatic when the original scar was hypertrophic; the resulting scars are smaller and shorter and, since they are subject to different stresses, may heal more kindly.

Variations of the Z-Plasty

Serial Z-plasties A number of Z-plasties may be constructed along a single wound or scar. If these are two in number, they are called double Z-plasties (Fig 2–6, B). In such areas as a contracted web space between digits, a series of small Z-plasties accomplishes the lengthening as well as a single large Z-plasty and yet keeps the scarring from extending onto the dorsum or palm of the hand.

The Four-flap Z-plasty. To construct a four-flap Z-plasty, two opposing incisions are made at about right angles to the original scar or wound, and then each of these wide flaps is divided into narrower-degree angle flaps that are then interposed along the wound (Fig 2–6, C). This increases the length beyond what could be produced from a single flap.

The Single-limb Z-plasty. The Z-plasty principle can be used in circumstances in which there may be a relative surplus of tissue on one side of the wound (such as from a dog-ear) and a deficiency on the other. A single limb is created and fitted into a defect on the opposite side of the wound. It should be clear that these distinctions of the various flaps and Z-plasties are a bit artificial and each of these maneuvers could also be called a form of transposition or advancement flap.

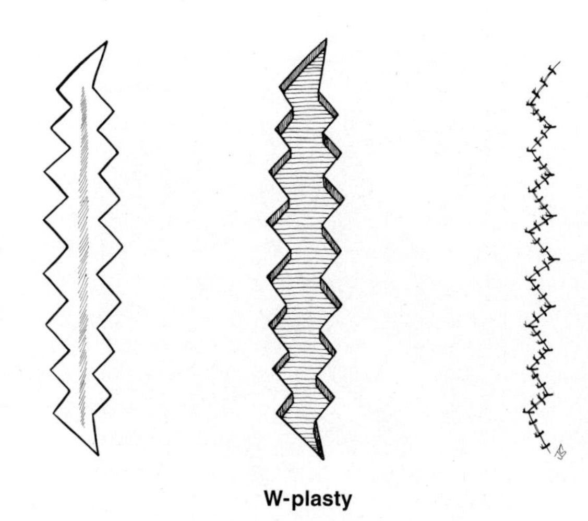

FIG 2–7.
W-plasty. The W-plasty involves the sacrifice of a series of small triangular excisions on either side of the wound. The remaining, jagged edges are then interposed or interdigitated along the length of the wound.

W-Plasty

The W-plasty describes a series of triangular flaps fashioned on either side of a wound and then interdigitated in the closure (Fig 2–7). The W-plasty may elongate the overall length of the wound but substantially less than what is accomplished with a Z-plasty. Its greatest value is in changing the orientation of the wound along better lines of stress so that the appearance is better than that of a single incision.

Other Flaps

There are many other flaps with specific designations that in actuality are variations on the random flaps listed above.

Tubed Pedicle Flap. A "tubed pedicle flap" is nothing more than a bipedicle flap in which the two lateral edges are rolled around the subcutaneous tissue and sutured to each other to result in the appearance of a tube. If one raises an identical area of tissue and then does not suture the margins, the forces of wound contraction will roll the tissue into a tubular shape; the tube pedicle does this

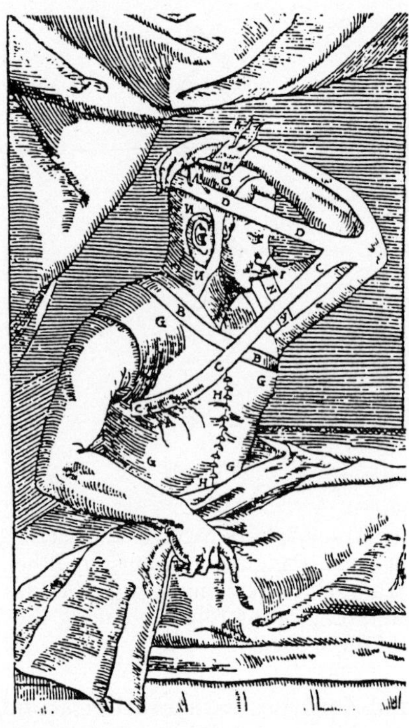

FIG 2–8.
G. Tagliacozzi's arm-to-nose transfer with the pedicle contracted on itself to form a tube. This most famous drawing in all of plastic surgery is the basis for the logo of the American Association of Plastic Surgeons. (From Tagliacozzi G: *De Curtorum Chirurgia per Insitionem.* Venice, Gaspare Bindoni, 1597.)

surgically. Gaspar Tagliacozzi in his treatise of 1597 described a technique of fashioning a flap from the inner aspect of the upper part of the arm by making two parallel incisions and placing a fabric beneath the flap to prevent it from adhering to the original bed. When he came to transfer the flap by cutting one end of the flap, his diagrams clearly show that the flap has rolled itself into a tube (Fig 2–8). Tubed flaps were the ultimate in the sophistication of flap transfer for many generations; the flap was raised and tubed and then one end cut and either transferred to its new, permanent location or attached to a carrier such as the forearm, which would in turn carry the flap to a new location. The tubed flap was a closed wound that prevented distortion, contraction, or infection of the flap.

The Lined Flap. To prevent the raw undersurface of a flap from contracting or becoming infected and particularly to give the flap two epithelial surfaces, the undersurface of a flap can be exposed at a preliminary stage and a skin graft (usually split thickness) applied to the undersurface. The lined flap can then be transferred to a site where two surfaces are normal such as to correct a full-thickness defect of the side of the nose, the cheek, or the neck. The lined flap can also be tubed on itself to form an epithelialized channel of value, for instance, in replacing a lost segment of esophagus.

The "Crane" Principle. On occasion a flap may be placed on a wound for a short period of time (e.g., to cover exposed tendons on the dorsum of the hand) and then returned to its original location while leaving behind a layer of tissue at the recipient site to be skin-grafted. In this circumstance the flap serves as a carrier for the covering tissue, i.e., it is a "crane."

Flap Physiology

The use of random flaps is constrained by the blood supply of the tissue. Sir Harold Gillies, the 20th century "father of reconstructive surgery," referred to it as the ongoing and endless "battle between beauty and blood supply." From Tagliacozzi to Gillies to the present transitional generation, this was a battle of imagination, technology, and an immense body of information about the physiology and technical manipulation of the random flap. Much of this science was incorrect, what was not incorrect was largely inaccurate, and finally, what was neither incorrect nor inaccurate has proved to be irrelevant in the light of our new understanding of axial and musculocutaneous/fasciocutaneous circulation. All tissue requires adequate oxygenation and nutrition. In the axial and other flaps to be described, the blood supply is now readily identifiable with predictable anatomic position either from named and consistent vessels or through underlying fascia/muscle units that are also predictable. The problem with the random flaps is that the blood supply is not readily identifiable or measurable. To improve consistency a number of factors became axiomatic in flap transfer: "length-to-width ratio," "delay," and the many techniques to measure some of these phenomena.

Length-to-Width Ratio

It always seemed intuitively correct that if the surgeon designed the base or pedicle of the flap as wide as possible, the length of the flap and the area of tissue that could be transferred would thereby be larger, and there would be greater security. Within well-confined limits, this is true. Unfortunately some of the presumptions were implausible and incorrect.

For example, if the base of a basically square flap that is 1 cm on each side were to be doubled to 2 cm, the length of the flap *cannot* also be doubled, even though the theoretical amount of blood supply was doubled. The reason is obvious; the surface area and volume of tissue were not merely doubled but actually increased *four-fold* from 1 cm^2 to 4 cm^2 (2 cm × 2 cm). In actuality, Milton showed that unless another "feeding" vessel were randomly encountered in the now-widened base of the flap, the blood supply was not really increased other than in small increments.

Since the randomly distributed skin on the body has a tremendously variable blood supply, generalities about length-to-width ratios really do not make any useful sense. In some areas of the face, for instance, a flap that is twice as long as it is wide will survive transfer quite nicely, while a comparable flap on the leg with its lesser blood supply will die every time. Experience with random flaps dictates that, in general, the width of the base of a flap should be at least equal to the length of the flap to be transferred, except where experience has shown that a longer flap will survive. That is not very scientific, which is why flap transfer is an art.

Delay

One of the wonders of our specialty is the body of information collected on the subject of "delay" of flaps. It was presumed, correctly, that if the randomly oriented blood supply of the flap were "shocked" in some way (surgically, pharmacologically, or mechanically), the tissue could be taught to survive in circumstances where, without such a "delay" maneuver, tissue death would be predictable.

Other biological phenomena confirm that such effects are common in the body; the person in whom peripheral vascular disease develops over a period of time will have an extremity accommodate to and survive on a degree of blood supply that if occlusion were to occur suddenly, would be totally inadequate and the extremity would die. This development of "collateral" blood flow may be part of what happens in a "delay" of the flap. The flow may also be reoriented and actually can be made to reverse its direction. For instance, when one end of a pedicle flap, such as a tube pedicle, is implanted, within days to weeks the flap will begin to gain a blood supply from the implanted end, sufficient eventually that the original pedicle can be divided and the flap now survives from perfusion from the opposite direction.

One intriguing theory of the "delay" mechanism relates to the activity of arteriovenous shunting in the flap; when the flap is challenged, under the control of the sympathetic nervous system the shunts open, and blood is diverted from the smaller vessels. As the tissue in the distal end of the flap recovers, the shunts close, and perfusion is reestablished. This theory would be far more attractive if arteriovenous shunts could be consistently demonstrated in human tissue other than in the glomus mechanism in the nail bed. The delay phenomenon may also work by having the tissue accommodate to a lesser degree of vascularity. "Delay" is usually accomplished surgically by incising the proposed flap margins at a preliminary stage and resuturing the wound. The process requires some experience since inadequate division of the distal blood supply fails to set the accommodation process in motion but too aggressive division of the distal blood supply may kill the flap. Other techniques include the pharmacologic use of vasoactive drugs, a technique that is of most interest in experimental animals. There is no totally satisfactory experimental model that mimics human skin. The panniculus carnosus of the rat makes most of the standard rodent flaps musculocutaneous flaps rather than skin-only flaps. In some circumstances vasoconstrictor drugs designed to close down the presumed arteriovenous shunts are of varying success; in other models vasodilators have been used and thought successful. The literature, although vast, has shed little consistent light of clinical value.

The axial and musculocutaneous/fasciocutaneous flaps described below are based on known, identifiable, consistent vascular systems, and the entire subject of flap "delay" is clinically less important than it was a generation ago.

Flap Monitoring

Since the blood supply of a random flap is usually not well known, it is desirable to be able to monitor the vascularity of the tissue during preparation and after transfer. The use of the "capillary refill" time after the tissue is blanched by compression is beneficial. However, there can be substantial variation in how the tissue is compressed (the sturdy pressure of an entire fingertip produces a rather different refill time from that resulting from the light stroking with an instrument such as a fine hemostat). The technique is also of little value in darkly pigmented skin. Suffice it to say that the capillary refill time in a flap *should* be the same as uninvolved tissue in the region that is compressed in a comparable fashion.

Far more accurate is the intravenous instillation of fluorescein. Fluorescein will actually perfuse to the capillary level and can often be visualized easily with the naked eye, but even more accurately with a Wood's lamp, which is usually readily available. A wait of 5 to 10 minutes is appropriate after injection; tissue that fails to perfuse will rarely survive, and failure to remove the tissue that does not perfuse is usually the triumph of hope over experience. If the surgeon is unwilling to act on the findings, the use of the technique can be eliminated.

Most other techniques are mechanically cumbersome or are representative of vascular patency in larger vessels rather than perfusion at the tissue level. The Doppler image of any type is usually reflective of flow in larger vessels and only indirectly the adequacy of tissue perfusion. Clinically, a diabetic with bounding pulses in a foot with ischemic toes is an example of good flow but limited perfusion.

Indirect Flaps and Flap Division

Most flaps are moved into position to cover the defect for which they were intended, and no division or alteration of the base of the flaps at a secondary procedure is either planned or necessary. There are circumstances in which the flap must be moved to an intermediate position as part of its transfer, or for other reasons the original base of the flap must be divided. The most common example of this circumstance is that in which a "carrier" is used to move the tissue from its original position to the defect. An example might be the creation of a tubed pedicle flap based on the abdomen, transferred first to the wrist or forearm, and then when suitably vascularized to the wrist, divided from its original bed. The cut end is then carried by the extremity to a new position such as in the head and neck. Variations on this theme include reattaching the two ends alternately until the flap can be finally positioned in a new site ("waltzing" or "caterpillar" technique). These maneuvers have become technical and historical curiosities in our era of microvascular flap transfer.

We have learned from clinical experience with these flap maneuvers that a flap does in fact derive a new blood supply from its new site. Experimental studies in which impervious material is placed either in the bed or at the margins of the flap to prevent vascular growth indicate that it is the margins rather than the bed of the wound that are the primary source of the new blood supply. A flap with a larger margin proportionate to its area will develop a secure blood supply more rapidly. Studies of perfusion of flaps from their new position indicate that flaps may be adequately vascularized, sufficient to allow division of the base, as early as 6 days after transfer. More classically an interval of 2 to 3 weeks was widely accepted as the appropriate time before flap division. No less than Tagliacozzi himself specified that the flap should initially be delayed ("It is not well to implant the flap in its age of infancy because then it is not strong enough") and further specified that this period should be 14 days. Certainly the surgeon's judgment is critical in determining when, between 1 and 3 weeks, it is safe to separate the flap from its original attachment. This judgment might also include "delaying" the flap before division, just as one might do in the preparatory stage.

A curious "given" of flap design is that flaps should never be based on a scar. Despite the fact that flaps are regularly divided and survive on the new blood supply that crossed the incised wound, there seems to be a time beyond which this neovasculature is no longer rich. Tagliacozzi described the phenomenon of waiting too long: "Nor yet should one await its old age for by then it has become too wrinkled, blanched, pallid, and juiceless," an unsavory description, but in actuality, the blood supply across healed scars is not dependable, and the "given" should probably be taken.

Why Flaps Fail

There are a number of reasons why flaps fail; these may be conceptual, technical, mechanical, and occasionally acts of the patient. The most common underlying factor is inadequate blood supply, either on the arterial side or, more infrequently, from venous congestion.

Conceptual

The fundamental decision making in the design of the flap is the size and shape of the flap necessary to fill the defect for which the operation is being undertaken. The flap may be too long, occupy too large an area, or be based on a blood supply that is fundamentally inadequate for any flap (a scar, for instance). The idea that a wider base *automatically* allows for a longer flap is conceptually incorrect.

Technical/Mechanical

Excessive tension on the flap may be a factor in tissue with a marginal blood supply (such as the tightened skin flap on a face-lift). This can be aggravated seriously by a hematoma under the flap that compresses the flap from underneath or from too tight a dressing that does the damage from outside. Bacterial contamination of a hematoma or of a marginal flap can cause necrosis, and some suggest treating compromised flap surfaces with topical antibacterial agents such as silver sulfadiazine. Flaps that are twisted, kinked, or otherwise mistreated will also fail.

Patient Factors

There are actually circumstances not really under the surgeon's control. The elderly, the cachectic, and the florid (high hematocrit, such as in polycythemia vera) are not good candidates; the anemic may actually have better flow (less chance for blood cells to sludge).

Smoking

Smoking is such a hazard to successful flap transfer that it deserves its own section. Cigarette smoking results in vasoactivity, either directly or by stimulating epinephrine release. It is also a danger because of the diminished oxygen carrying capacity of blood, with a 4 to 6% carboxyhemoglobin level seen in smokers. The clinical observation of increased flap necrosis in smokers is so real that the failure of experimental data to confirm or validate mechanisms is not relevant. A wise surgeon will recognize the risks and counsel the patient. Then whether to accept the risk on a face-lift or abdominoplasty "flap" becomes a shared responsibility—one that even then some surgeons will not accept. The "recovery" time after cessation of smoking is not well defined; perhaps the accepted time of 3 to 4 weeks is factual but not completely validated scientifically. It should be recognized that in our society smoking has "gone into the closet" and many patients are unable to quit and might well exaggerate or falsify their history to gain access to a desired aesthetic operation.

Axial Flaps

The concept of axial flaps is derived from the observation that certain tissue territories have an identifiable vascular system with an artery and vein capable of supporting the tissue. An obvious example is a finger or toe in which a single digital artery and vein can

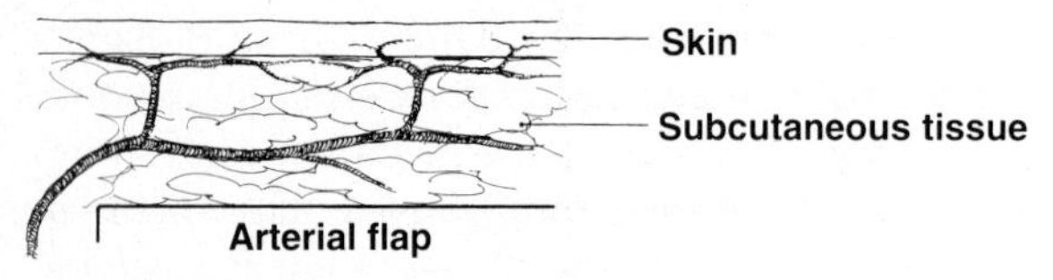

FIG 2–9.
Cross section of the skin and subcutaneous tissue with functional divisions of vascular supply. Axial flap vascularity is derived from the arterial flow, identifiable in the subcutaneous tissue.

support the digit. There are a number of skin territories with an axial blood supply, such as a portion of the forehead supplied by the supraorbital vessels, the entire forehead on the temporal vessels, and other areas such as the dorsum of the foot (dorsalis pedis), the groin (superficial circumflex iliac artery), and the deltopectoral area (perforating vessels of the internal mammary artery). Each "axial" area has a vascularity that is independent of the underlying fascia or musculature; rather, the vessels tend to course through the subcutaneous and subdermal areas (Fig 2–9). Each of the axial flap areas can be raised as an island of skin and subcutaneous tissue and transferred *en bloc* to a new site either on its intact pedicle or by division and reattachment at a new site by microvascular techniques.

The pure axial flap represented an important transition in the development of reconstructive surgery. It became clear that any tissue with an identifiable blood supply had the potential for being transferred over great anatomic distances in a single super bound. The specific anatomic territory could often be enlarged to also support a "random" flap at the distal end of the axial flap. Unfortunately, many of these axial flaps leave truly unacceptable donor sites, and other available flaps can be used at less expense.

The most commonly considered axial flaps are outlined in Table 2–1. The full *forehead flap* served for years as a flap to line the inside of the oral cavity after cancer surgery. Supplied by the superficial temporal vessels, the flap can be raised as an "island" (i.e., the skin bridge is divided) and then turned either inside or outside the zygomatic arch into the oral cavity. The donor defect requires a skin graft with an aesthetic result that while tolerable, fails the test of acceptability when alternatives are available (and they usually are).

The *median forehead flap* has great historical significance. It was the flap that Carpue brought back from India in the early 19th century; it replaced the Tagliacozzi arm flap as the flap of choice to restore a lost nose (and noses were often lost; nasal amputation was the penalty for many crimes for many centuries in many different cultures). Based on the supraorbital vessels, this flap is often sufficient in area to resurface the entire nose or any of its anatomic subunits. The defect can usually be acceptably closed primarily. Burget has used this flap to define a new level of elegance in reconstructive nasal surgery. It has probably been rarely if ever used as a free flap.

The *temporoparietalis flap* is not strictly an axial flap since it does not involve skin but is

TABLE 2–1.
Commonly Considered Axial Flaps

Axial Flaps	Use/Advantage	Disadvantage
Forehead Flap	Intraoral reconstruction, readily available in area	Bad donor site defect
Medial Forehead Flap	Nasal reconstruction, wonderful texture	Limited size
Temporoparietalis fascia	Ear reconstruction, free flap	Fragile, not always available
Deltopectoral	Head and neck reconstruction	Poor donor site defect
Lateral arm	Quite thin, use only as free flap	Poor donor site defect
Forearm	Thin, hairless, used as free flap	Poor donor site defect
Scapular	Skin thick, can include bone	Need to turn patient
Groin	Free flap for anywhere	May be thick, dissection also as direct flap variable
Dorsalis pedis	Very thin, free flap	Often hairy, often bad donor site defect, dissection tough

included here since it is otherwise comparable. The temporoparietalis is a loose, semiareolar tissue beneath the subcutaneous tissue and external to the temporal fascia. Its vasculature from the superficial temporal system supports it as an island flap. Brent has demonstrated its use as a thin, filmy, but very vascular cover for denuded or newly reconstructed ears and, like Burget for the nose, has set standards for the ear against which any reconstruction must be measured. The temporoparietalis is used occasionally as a free flap, for example, for the dorsum of the hand.

The *deltopectoral flap* was popularized by Bakamjian in the 1960s and became the workhorse for reconstruction of the head and neck for the next two decades. The flap is based on the perforating vessels of the internal mammary artery and vein, which course subcutaneously in an "axial" fashion toward the shoulder. When a random portion is extended from the end of the axial flap, the flap will then include a portion of the relatively thin tissue over the shoulder. This flap is used as a rotation flap.

The *lateral arm flap* includes a territory on the lateral portion of the arm, is relatively thin, and has a constant blood supply through the posterior radial collateral artery off the brachial artery. The disadvantage to this flap is that it can only be used as a microvascular flap transfer.

The *forearm flap* was introduced and popularized in China, primarily for reconstructing the penis. The flap is based on the radial artery and branches of forearm veins and has variable sensation through cutaneous branches from any of the forearm/hand nerves. It can be used as a turnover island to cover the hand but is usually considered for a free flap.

The *scapular* flap is supplied by the branches of the circumflex scapular artery, a branch of the scapular artery, and has an advantage as a free flap in that it can also carry a portion of vascularized bone for complex reconstructions.

The *groin flap* is the clinical application of the original dog flap used experimentally. It was also one of the flaps that McGregor used to define the difference between axial and random flaps. The vessels are reasonably constant through the superficial circumflex iliac artery and accompanying veins, which supply an area of the groin that can be used either as a direct or a free flap.

The *dorsalis pedis flap* is supplied as the descriptive implies and is a territory of very thin, varying hairy to hairless skin from the dorsum of the foot with good potential as a sensate flap. It is a superb flap with a very troublesome donor defect that may be slow to heal, and meticulous attention to the grafted donor site is mandatory.

The *scalp* may also serve as a donor site for island flaps or free flaps based on the superficial temporal vessels. It has the obvious potential for moving hair-bearing tissue to reconstruct the eyebrow, for instance.

There certainly are other potential axial flaps, but except as described, they have largely been superseded by myocutaneous and fasciocutaneous flaps.

Microvascular Flaps and Techniques

In 1905, Alexis Carrel transplanted solid organs in animals and performed microvascular anastomoses in humans (he attached the radial artery of a father to the popliteal vein of an infant to accomplish a direct transfusion; it was reported as being successful). In the early 1960s an axial flap on a dog's abdominal wall was described and survived as an island of tissue, and Krizek used microvascular techniques to transfer the flap to the dog's neck. Within the decade, microsurgery had reached clinical fruition through the relentless dedication of Bernard O'Brien and Harry Buncke.

An important surgical principle that I learned early was when in trouble, "make the incision longer." The point of this was, of course, that most surgical problems can be solved by being able to see better; the operating microscope has functionally enlarged our incisions. All who have operated under the microscope are in awe of the exquisitely fine movements of which our hands are capable when we can see. It must be emphasized that microsurgery represents a technique and its body of knowledge a "technology." It is not, however, a surgical specialty, and its applications must be fitted into the broader category of "reconstructive surgery."

Although presented under axial skin flaps, the technology of microsurgery has been successfully applied to more complex skin-muscle and skin-fascia combinations, nerves, bones, and the intestine. Many complex tissues (such as the intestine) can only be transferred by such techniques, unable as they are to tolerate the period of relative ischemia that accompanies all grafting maneuvers.

The factors leading to success in microsurgery are very similar to the success factors in other reconstructive surgery: precise diagnosis of the problem to be solved, careful planning, and technically accurate surgery. (For a complete discussion of microsurgery, see Chapter 3.)

Myocutaneous and Fasciocutaneous Flaps

For more than a century before Tagliacozzi described a skin-only flap from the medial aspect of the arm to reconstruct lost noses in 1597, the Branca family of Sicily held within their family the "secret" of a technique for reconstructing noses with muscle and skin-muscle flaps. Their secret remained hidden, and their technique of using muscle was "undiscovered" for more than 400 years. Jurkiewicz, McCraw, and Dibbell are just three of the prominent names in the modern era of flap transfer whose fundamental contribution was based on the recognition that the blood supply to much of the skin of the body, rather than being totally random, is quite orderly and based with remarkable consistency on the vascular pattern of the underlying muscle or fascia. Theirs was as truly a "eureka" observation as our specialty has ever encountered. They identified that vessels course into the muscles from "named" vessels and form regular patterns of distribution in the muscle or fascia (Fig 2–10). The muscle or fascial vessels then branch from the muscle and then, oriented vertically, supply the overlying skin. It is clear in the light of this fact that the many efforts to raise random flaps, to tube them, to rotate them, or to "delay" them were in actuality dividing these vessels and potentially devascularizing the skin at each step. It is somewhat amazing that it worked at all and even more amazing that generations of surgeons knowingly divided these vessels without recognizing the significance of what was happening.

A skin territory, matching in size and shape the underlying muscle or fascial territory, represents one of the most secure units of tissue available for transfer that we have ever encountered. Flaps based on the pectoralis major, latissimus dorsi, and rectus abdominis muscles have been transferred with almost uniform success in very large series.

The recognition that the blood supply of much of the body skin is derived from the underlying musculature has resulted in a detailed reexamination of the blood supply of muscles.

Mathes and others have detailed with exquisite reproducibility the significant, clinically relevant blood supply of muscles; it can be divided into five types (I to V), depending on where the vasculature enters the muscle and how it is distributed (Fig 2–11).

- *Type I.*—The muscle derives its major blood supply from a *single dominant pedicle.* This configuration is particularly advantageous since the vasculature is usually proximal and allows the muscle, when elevated with or without the

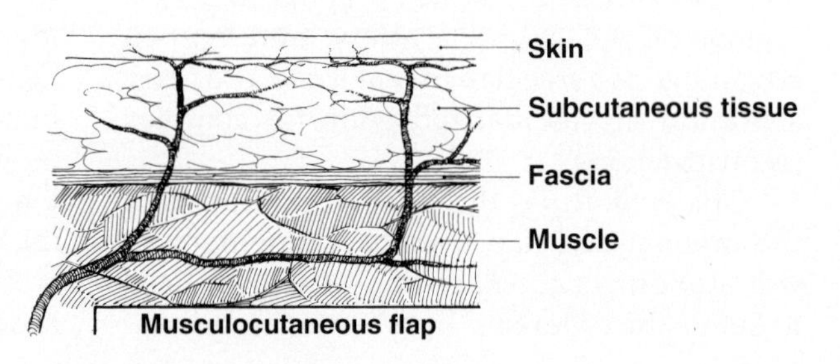

FIG 2–10.
Cross section of the skin, subcutaneous tissue, fascia, and muscle with functional divisions of vascular supply. Musculocutaneous flap vascularity is derived from muscles, with vertical supply to the skin.

overlying skin, to have a good arc of rotation. Examples are the gastrocnemius and tensor fasciae latae muscles.

- *Type II.*—The muscle has a dual blood supply, of which there is *a dominant and a minor vasculature.* The muscle and its overlying skin will survive on the dominant vasculature after the minor blood supply is divided. Even though there is a dual blood supply, the muscle is functionally as effective a flap as the type I. This is the *most common* type of blood supply for muscles; examples are the gracilis, soleus, and trapezius muscles.
- *Type III.*—The muscles of this group have *two major pedicles* that may enter the muscle either in parallel or from opposite ends of the muscle, such as the blood supply to the rectus abdominis. The great value of this blood supply is that the muscle may survive on either vascular pedicle.
- *Type IV.*—These muscles have *multiple pedicles,* each of which tends to supply a segment of the muscle. Unfortunately, the division of a pedicle tends to devascularize that portion of the muscle. Many of the extremity muscles, such as the sartorius, are of this type and are of rather limited value for flap transfer.
- *Type V.*—The type V muscles have *one major and a number of secondary vascular pedicles* that tend to be segmental. Both sets of pedicles provide important vasculature. The latissimus dorsi and pectoralis major are of this category and are among the most important of the muscular flaps.

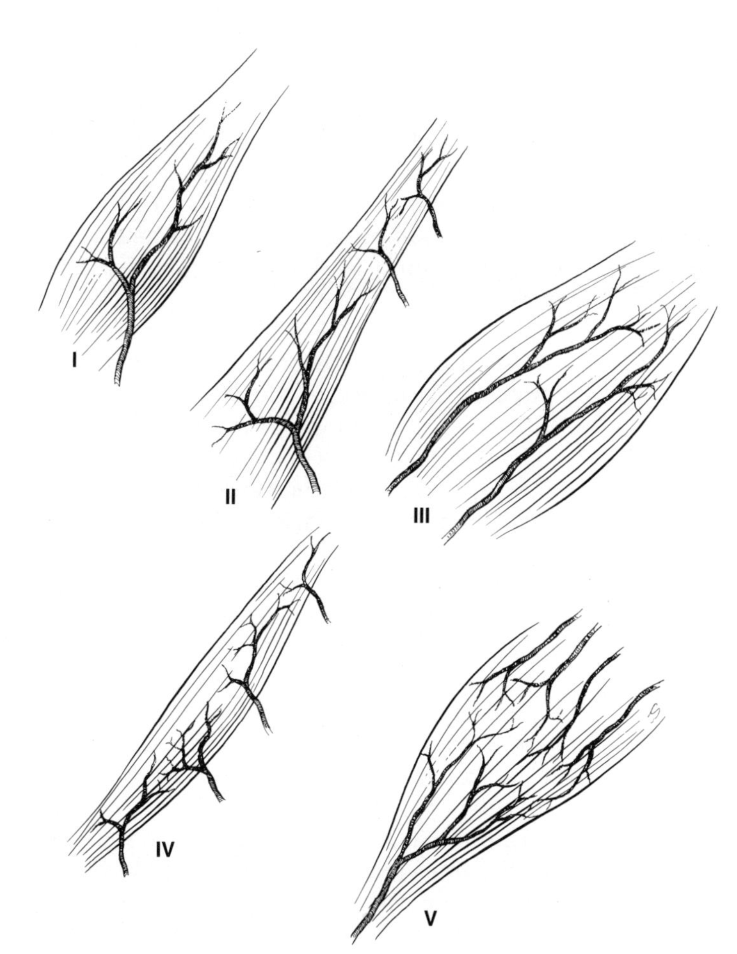

FIG 2–11.
Muscle categories based on blood supply (Mathes and Nahai). *Type I,* single major pedicle. *Type II,* dominant pedicle and minor pedicles. *Type III,* two dominant pedicles either in parallel or from opposite ends. *Type IV,* multiple minor pedicles (not much overlap to vascularity). *Type V,* dominant pedicle and many minor pedicles (similar to type II but with richer minor pedicles).

Principles of Muscular Flaps

1. The flap transfer is dependent on the muscle surviving on the remaining vascular pedicle. Each of the types, except type IV, has a blood supply that will support rotation, transposition, or when appropriate, free microvascular transfer. Types I and II can be rotated or transferred on the dominant pedicle and type III on either pedicle, and type V may be moved on either the single major or the multiple segmental vessels (the latissimus dorsi muscle may be transferred on its dominant vasculature from the thoracodorsal proximally or moved on its distal segmental vasculature).
2. Function is usually lost. When the muscle flap is transferred, it will no longer serve its original function and will leave a functional or aesthetic defect. The latissimus dorsi, pectoralis major, rectus abdominis, and the medial head of the gastrocnemius are examples of muscles whose use is accompanied by acceptable functional and aesthetic consequences.
3. These flaps can be transferred with or without the overlying skin. In many cases the wound is better covered by transferring the muscle without the skin and then applying a skin graft to the muscle. When muscle is used to cover defects, particularly of the lower extremities, the bulk of the muscle and the immobility of the skin at the margins of the original defect make it hard to obtain closure with any skin paddle transferred with the muscle, and a skin graft works much better.
4. Muscle and skin/muscle flaps have several potential advantages over skin-only flaps:
   a. The vascularity of the muscle is often more vigorous and dependable than that of the skin islands.
   b. The muscle will often dress into irregular defects and obliterate dead space better than skin flaps will. This is of particular value in contaminated wounds.
   c. Muscle flaps are more resistant to bacterial invasion and tolerate transfer into contaminated wounds better than skin-only flaps.
   d. The blood vessels to the muscles are usually larger and more easily dissected than the vessels to the skin pedicles, which makes microvascular transfer easier.
   e. The defect left when the muscle flap is moved (particularly when it is not a skin/muscle flap) is aesthetically more pleasing than that left from a skin flap.
   f. The muscle and its overlying fat and skin provide more bulk than any skin-only flap does. This is critical for reconstructive procedures designed rather specifically to add bulk such as breast reconstruction.
   g. Muscle and tendon transfers, when the nerve supply is preserved, add functional restoration to paralyzed or otherwise diminished functional areas, particularly in the upper extremity.

Important Muscle Flaps

There was an effulgence of descriptions of methods for turning almost any muscle and its adjacent skin into the "flap of the month" until the possibilities were exhausted. From these, experience has identified a half dozen or so that form the essential core of useful flaps.

Platysma. This flap is mostly of historic interest since its use was described in the 1950s without recognizing its musculocutaneous characteristics. History again must credit not those who may have been the first but rather those who gave it to the world.

Latissimus Dorsi. This flap was described in the early part of the 1900s by Tansini, but its value was unrecognized until Bostwick popularized its use for breast reconstruction. A type V flap, its proximal dominant vasculature is from the thoracodorsal vessels, and it may easily rotate through a wide arc from its insertion on the humerus. It may also be transferred as a free flap and may be split into smaller units that can be transferred independently. The vascular supply from near the origin through the posterior intercostal and lumbar perforators allows the insertion and the dominant vascular pedicle to be divided and the flap to be folded and turned to cover posterior midline defects. The skin paddles are supplied by vertically oriented vessels.

Pectoralis Major. The pectoralis major muscle (another type V flap) is supplied by the vessels through the dominant pedicle from the thoracoacromial vessels and the perforating vessels of the intercostal and internal mammary vessels. Ariyan demonstrated that when based on its dominant vessel and the insertion on the humerus, the flap may be rotated through an arc that carries the distal end of the flap and an accompanying skin paddle to almost any site on the head and neck including the oropharyngeal cavity. The flap is often used by advancement or turnover, unilaterally or bilaterally, to cover sternal wounds and defects following cardiac surgery.

Rectus Abdominis. The most exciting flap of the 1980s, the rectus abdominis has become the workhorse of reconstructive surgery for chest and sternal defects, for the pelvis when turned internally, and for breast reconstruction. Hartrampf and others clearly delineated the vascular territories that could be supported by the rectus abdominis muscle (a type III flap). The transversely oriented skin paddles have led to the acronym TRAM (the *t*ransverse *r*ectus *a*bdominis *m*usculocutaneous flap). The rectus is supplied from either end by the superior and inferior epigastric vessels respectively and may survive on either pedicle: the superior when the flap is turned cephalad to reconstruct the chest wall or breast and the inferior when the flap is used for microvascular transfer. Elegance in conception and refinement in technique have evolved to allow this muscle to serve as a "carrier" of tissue while preserving most of its fascial encasement, thus allowing closure of the defect with only an occasional hernia. Bilateral muscles may be used when the skin territory needed is large or when two flaps are used—for instance, one to each side for bilateral breast reconstruction. The final nuance is to occasionally "supercharge" the flap by an anastomosis at the recipient site on the chest wall to the cut end of the epigastric vessel.

Gracilis. The gracilis, a long muscle along the medial aspect of the thigh, has a dandy type II vasculature; the dominant vessel, entering proximally, will carry this long flap after the distal minor pedicle is divided. The skin paddle can be generous and can be brought to the perineum and vaginal areas and is most useful in genital surgery. The gracilis without skin is useful as an innervated, functioning muscle that can mimic a sphincter around the anal area. Unfortunately, its bulk is rather puny, which limits its value in larger perineal defects.

Gastrocnemius. The medial and the lateral heads and bellies of the gastrocnemius provide double flaps, each with a type I vasculature. This flap has been of inestimable value in proximal leg/knee defects.

Tensor Fasciae Latae. The tensor fasciae latae is a muscle with type I vasculature through the proximal lateral femoral circumflex artery and accompanying vein. There is a large skin paddle involving much of the lateral aspect of the leg.

Gluteus Maximus. The gluteus maximus is really two muscles, each with its own blood supply. The superior portion of the muscle is supplied by the superior gluteal artery, and the inferior portion is supplied by the inferior gluteal artery. Either or both are valuable as muscle or skin muscle flaps for the sacral region and have been used, particularly in breast reconstruction, as a free microvascular flap transfer.

Fasciocutaneous Flaps

The fascia is obviously interposed in any given musculocutaneous flap. The fascia, without the underlying muscle, has been included in some skin flaps to augment the vasculature to the skin (Fig 2–12). This has been used most often in the forearm and the scapular flaps. The fundamental difference in fasciocutaneous flaps is that even in circumstances in which there is no true "axial" skin

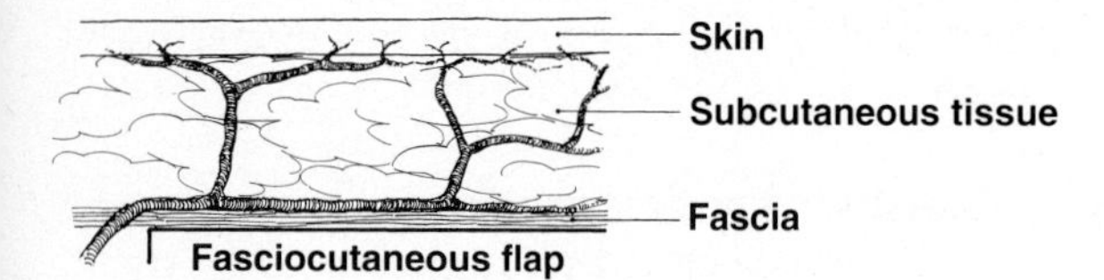

FIG 2–12.
Cross section of the skin, subcutaneous tissue, and fascia with functional divisions of vascular supply. The fasciocutaneous flap vascular supply may serve an axial-type function.

flow, the fascial territory beneath the skin may serve the same purpose and can be transferred as a transposition or a free fasciocutaneous flap based on the fascial vessels.

OTHER TISSUES

In addition to skin and muscle, other tissues are valuable to the reconstructive surgeon and may be transplanted to another site, either for structure, for improved function, or for restoration or augmentation of contour. Some of these tissues may be available only as graft tissue, while others may lend themselves to vascularized transfer, either by transposition or by free transfer using microsurgical techniques.

Bone

It would be most economical and convenient for the patient if some substitute for the patient's own living bone were to be identified. Unfortunately, as an ideal for skeletal reconstruction, replacement, or augmentation, only the patient's own bone provides the durability and permanence and is therefore the choice for reconstruction whenever available.

Osteoconduction

The healing of normal bone requires bone to be in contact with bone. There is serially in the healing phase the formation of granulation/vascular tissue, a fibrous callus, osteoclast degradation of bone, and finally osteoblastic deposition of new bone. The process of healing of transplanted bone is similar. When bone is transplanted into an area where it is not in contact with other bone, such as into skeletal muscle, there occurs neovasculature and the appearance of "osteoprogenitor" cells that are derived from stem cells from skeletal muscle or migrating mesenchymal cells; these cells differentiate into osteoblasts to form new bone. The transplanted bone resorbs and induces bone to be formed from the osteoblasts—a process called *osteoinduction.* This process is far more effective when bone is placed in contact with other bone and the supply of osteoblasts is present in greater quantity from the recipient bone. Bone not placed in contact with other bone is largely dissolved. Although bone is the usual bone-inducing substance clinically, there is a biological curiosity that the most effective bone-inducing substance is uroepithelium derived from the bladder or renal pelvis. Identified by Huggins and thoroughly investigated by Urist, the exact substance responsible and the clinical implications of this remain elusive.

Incorporation

The process whereby donor bone is accepted at its new site and new bone gradually replaces the graft is called incorporation; this requires vascularization. These processes are comparable to those described for skin flaps and grafts; the best vascularization is from tissue transplanted by microvascular techniques. Vascularization of grafted bone, as for thick skin grafts, occurs from both the random matching of vessels from donor and recipient bone as well as the new growth of vessels, primarily along vascular channels in the donor bone. The vascularization, as for skin, is dependent on the nature of the donor tissue, and faster revascularization and faster resorption and replacement will occur in cancellous bone as compared with compact bone. The nature and degree of the bone contact also influence the "take," and faster and more complete vascularization occurs when the surface interface is large in relation to the volume of bone transplanted. Finally, the relationship of the donor to the recipient is critical; there is more vascularization, resorption, and final replacement in an autograft than there is in allograft or xenograft bone. (For additional discussion of bone healing and bone grafting, see Chapters 1 and 4.)

Advances in internal rigid fixation and external fixators have revolutionized the technology of handling bone. This technology and the approach to craniofacial surgery by Tessier have had a quantum influence on improved survival of grafts and the healing of bone in general—far more than any understanding of underlying physiology.

Autograft

Autografts again refer to transfers in which the patient serves as both donor and recipient. Such grafts have the highest degree of short-term success as well as long-term survival and durability. There are a variety of circumstances in which bone grafts are desirable, and for each circumstance there are donor sites that more nearly meet the needs than others.

Donor Sites

Cranial. Since the advent of craniofacial surgery, the cranium itself has become the donor site of choice for most facial reconstruction. This membranous bone has predictable survival, and particularly in children, the donor site has tremendous regenerative capacity. The donor site is less uncomfortable than other donor sites and has less morbidity in healing. In general, except for small children, the full thickness of the cranium is removed and the layers split; the outer table becomes the graft, and the inner table is replaced in the donor defect. Depending on the curvature of the donor site, the graft can be nicely matched to the needs of the recipient site for appropriate contour.

Iliac Crest. The iliac crest, more particularly the ilium just below the crest, provides a large volume of cancellous bone. The nice curve and large size have made this tissue the desirable bone for reconstructing an absent hemimandible. The crest is transected and folded back to allow access to the wing of the ilium. When the graft is removed, the crest is rewired in place to prevent an unsightly defect in the pelvis. The inner or outer table of the bone (or both) can be used, and the bone may also serve as a donor for a free microvascular transfer. There is more morbidity in this site, including hematoma, considerable discomfort, and occasionally some weakness in gait resulting from stripping of muscle. When smaller amounts of cancellous bone are needed (e.g., for a maxillary alveolar cleft), a window can be cut in the ilium to permit access without disturbing the iliac crest.

Rib. The rib has been used for many different purposes, both as a sturdy replacement (such as for the mandible) or when split longitudinally. It serves as an excellent onlay for the facial skeleton and skull either as a graft or as a free microvascular transfer. The subperiosteal stripping of bone for the donor site may allow the rib to regenerate and to be used again in the future.

Extremities. When used as donor sites, the extremities provide a combination of compact and cancellous bone. The tibia was used by many as a donor for clefts of the alveolus or palate. The distal end of the radius and proximal third of the ulna have served as readily available bone for use in hand surgery, and the fibula is the traditional donor bone for bridging defects in the long bones.

Vascularized Bone Grafts. Large segments of bone may be transferred with the security of substantial survival by using microvascular techniques. For small gaps between bone ends, for smaller defects, and for augmentation purposes, the use of standard bone grafts is appropriate. When the defect exceeds 5 to 6 cm, the reported failure of traditional bone grafts is more than 30% and increases when longer defects must be bridged. In these circumstances, free vascularized bone is indicated, and very successful results (more than 90% take) have been reported. Suitable bones for transfer include the fibula, the iliac crest, the cranial bone (on a temporal vessel supply), and the rib.

Allograft

The use of cadaver bone is one of the more successful uses of allograft in reconstructive surgery. Although skin allograft is useful, it is only as a temporary coverage; bone, however, forms the structural framework for long-term survival.

Bone allograft is subject to the same histocompatibility reactions as among any genetically disparate tissues. Long-term survival is not possible, and the immunosuppression that might prolong survival is not appropriate in the less-than-lifesaving situations in which bone grafts are used. Rather, the antigenicity of the allograft bone is usually purposely altered to destroy the donor cells and render the graft tolerable to the recipient. The methods of freezing or freeze-drying alter the strength of the graft but allow for long-term storage of bone allograft and the later matching of size and shape. Sterilization by radiation or chemical means reduces or eliminates any osteoinductive capability of the allograft. Allograft is most useful in bridging defects from removal of large segments of long bones. It is in these circumstances that the external rigid fixation, compression, and distraction maneuvers have made the difference, and truly, "a difference to be a difference must make a difference," and here it made a difference. The incorporation of the allograft is a framework into which the recipient bone grows, ultimately replacing the allograft with living tissue.

Xenograft

The use of tissue from other species (xenograft) has found some popularity for augmenting contours of bony structures. The most popular was the use of bovine grafts. The bovine preparation is prepared in such a fashion as to eliminate any antigenicity, also thus eliminating any possibility of osteoinduction. Most often the bovine implant served as a foreign body that was usually isolated and then dissolved.

Bone Substitutes

Bone is a tissue more easily mimicked structurally than other tissues, and the search for inorganic, nonbiological substitutes is tempting. The characteristics sought are those of a compound with some structural similarity to bone and porous enough to allow vascular ingrowth. Such a substance found in nature is the apatite found in coral, which has similarities to the haversian system of bone. Coral and hydroxyapatites have been extensively studied experimentally and are of some use clinically in non–load-bearing circumstances, such as for contour irregularities.

Cartilage

Cartilage has an elasticity and a "spring" to it that is most difficult to reproduce when lost, except with other cartilage. Fortunately, cartilage can be successfully transferred from one area to another and, unlike bone, does not have to be in intimate contact with other cartilage to survive. Cartilage transplanted into the subcutaneous tissue will survive as cartilage. The elasticity of cartilage is also its "weakness" in that it has a tendency to "warp" and alter its shape after transfer. Gibson demonstrated beautifully that when the surface of the cartilage was altered by scoring, abrading or crushing, the cartilage would curve to the opposite direction; scoring the concave surface would tend to make the cartilage straighten. Preparation may include scoring, morselizing, or crushing to overcome these tendencies. (For additional discussion of bone and cartilage grafting, see Chapter 4.)

Donor Sites

Cartilage is not available in large quantities. On the other hand, the needs, except for total ear reconstruction, are also not for great volumes of tissue. The following are the available sources for cartilage:

Costochondral (fibrous cartilage). The seventh to ninth ribs form the richest source of cartilage in any volume. This cartilage is the most useful for volume replacement or for structuring large areas such as an ear. Subperichondrial harvesting allows the cartilage to regrow and be harvested again.

Septal (hyaline cartilage). Septal cartilage is most useful in augmenting and contouring areas of the nose during reconstructive nasal surgery. Readily available in the operative field, it can be harvested from its position with or without its overlying mucosa. The cartilage has also been used with mucosa to reconstruct the trachea.

Auricular (elastic cartilage). The elastic conchal cartilage is most useful for reconstruction of the tarsus (eyelid), the nose, and the malar areas and has been diced to form the appearance of Montgomery glands in areolar reconstruction.

Cartilage requires some imagination and skill to use effectively. The tendency for it to assume shape, as if it had a mind of its own, requires that it be purposely altered in advance. It may be useful to cover it with dermal grafts or temporalis fascia to soften the tendency to form sharp edges in the ear or on the nasal dorsum.

Tendon

In many ways, tendons are far more complex "grafting" materials than bone, cartilage, or even skin. The normal tendon has an exquisite structure designed to fulfill its specialized function of movement. The tendon itself is not particularly complex, a bundle of longitudinally oriented collagen fibers and groups of fibers. Its vascularity, however, is very special. The gliding of tendons through tissue, particularly through the confining sheaths of the hand, required the evolution of a vascularity that could alternately curl and then unfurl as the tendon moved to and fro, likened most closely to the mesentery of the intestines. It is easy to graft a tendon, but it is another matter to graft a tendon that will then glide.

Tendon repair is almost always preferable to tendon grafting. When the injury is complex and the tendon destroyed or when the tendon sheath is destroyed, particularly when infection is involved, it may be necessary to graft and place the proximal and distal junctions of tendon and graft outside the worst of the injured site. The bed into which the graft is placed should be as favorable as possible; a preparatory period in which a silicone rod is laid in the bed may help prepare the bed.

Tendon grafts heal by diffusion of nutrients initially and subsequently by the neovasculature of ingrowing vessels, either joining the cut ends of the vessels to the graft (exceedingly unlikely) or from new growth into tendon. The inflammatory response necessary to healing disposes to scar formation, which destroys any possibility of motion. Scar must be minimized, which requires ideal circumstances; ideal circumstances mean no bleeding, no infection.

Unlike most other grafts, the tendon graft must be *forced* to move before it is biologically "ready"; it is a battle between technology and biology. The tendon must be encouraged (actively and then passively) to move through its normal excursion and stretch the new blood vessels so that they will mimic the original coiled vessels. A tendon graft "healed" but encased in unyielding scar is of no value.

The donor sites for tendon grafts require the availability of "spare" tendons that fortunately are provided. The *palmaris longus* tendon is present in some 80% of patients, and its size and shape mimic the upper extremity tendons; its loss has negligible functional consequences. The *plantaris* tendon is also present in about 80% of persons and, although not in the operative field in upper extremity surgery, is readily accessible and is long enough to often supply several grafts, if necessary. The toe extensors also serve as possible graft material.

There are no allograft, xenograft, or artificial materials readily available as a substitute. Kangaroo tendon was formerly available but was used more as a suture material than a tendon substitute.

Nerve

The functional element of the nerve is the axon, the extension of the central nervous system. The axons and their accompanying Schwann cells with their myelin sheath are surrounded by protective layers that encase the nerve into fascicles. The protective covering is much like the tendon sheath; it provides vascularity and allows the nerve to glide with joint motion.

When the nerve is cut, the critically altered structure is the axon, and unlike most other tissues, the damage extends far out of the original field of injury. All axons distal to the site of injury degenerate (wallerian); they also degenerate proximally for varying distances. Successful repair is dependent on the proximal, regenerating axon finding a suitable distal passageway, a passageway that will lead to an appropriate distal nerve ending. A motor nerve should desirably find a motor end point, and similarly, a sensory nerve should find some sort of sensory end organ; otherwise the regenerative trip is wasted. It is no biological surprise that a pure motor nerve (for example, facial nerve VII) when cut has an excellent chance for recovery; all the fibers are motor fibers, and all will find some sort of motor end plate. Similarly, a purely sensory nerve (for example, a digital nerve) will also recover well. The mixed nerves such the median and the ulnar fare less well.

A major mechanical impediment to successful nerve regeneration is the formation of scar at the site of the nerve injury and at the site of any repair. The chance of scar is greatest when there has been a complex injury, when there has been infection, or particularly when the nerve ends were repaired under tension. Within the technical constraints, the best results for nerve regeneration occur when there is an accurate repair of the individual fascicle to the matching cut end and particularly when repaired without tension. There are many techniques, such as transposing the nerve to a new position to relieve tension. When these cannot be accomplished, it is better to bridge the gap with a nerve graft or other conduit.

Autografts

As with tendon, autografts are the most desirable, clinically applicable material for nerve grafts. When a nerve is grafted, the graft, like all other grafts, must initially derive its blood supply by diffusion of nutrients while awaiting neovasculature. The axons of the graft also undergo wallerian degeneration, and the proximal regenerating axons will grow down this vacated space. The argument for nerve itself being the ideal replacement and "bridging" material is based on the survival of grafted Schwann cells and the myelinated sheath for the new axon. If revascularization is delayed or prolonged, the Schwann cells will also fail to survive, and the argument for nerve as the conduit is less persuasive. There is little clinical evidence that vascularized nerve grafts transferred by microvascular techniques are ultimately superior to free grafts.

It is assumed that proximal motor fibers, when directly sutured to a distal fascicle that previously contained motor fibers, are the theoretical ideal. There have been a variety of techniques, anatomic and physiologic, for identifying motor and sensory fibers and fascicles. Histochemically, the presence of acetylcholinesterase and choline acetyltransferase indicates motor fibers, and carbonic anhydrase indicates sensory fibers. Unfortunately, these tests are not clinically available; moreover, the fascicular pattern follows a course best described as a twisting and turning one.

Donor Sites

Donor nerves are in obvious short supply; the sural nerve is the most commonly used. Also available are the saphenous nerve, the lateral femoral cutaneous nerve, the medial and lateral antebrachial cutaneous nerves, and the intercostal and cervical nerves.

Nerve Conduits

The nerve graft may be the ideal, but there are other materials that may serve as conduits through which nerve fibers may grow.

Although a nerve is an extraordinarily complex extension of the central nervous system, bridging of the gaps between nerve ends serves not much purpose other than as a conduit. There clearly exists some signal sent by the distal cut end of the nerve (neurotropic factor) that indicates to the nerve that it should regenerate. In the absence of this signal the nerve does not regenerate. It has been further described by Brushart that the distal end sends *different* signals for motor and sensory fibers. Experimentally, if a mixed nerve regenerates through a Y-shaped conduit, the motor nerves will seek out the limb of the Y that leads to motor fibers, and the sensory fibers will seek out the sensory ends. There may therefore be a real question as to whether ultimately the coaptation of nerve ends is, in actuality, the best management. It may turn out that a conduit should always be placed and the proximal fibers be given the opportunity to find the proper distal channel.

Types of Conduits

Veins. Chiu and Krizek used autologous vein to bridge the gap between nerve ends experimentally and demonstrated that over short distances (2 cm) the nerve would grow through the lumen of the vein and connect with the distal cut nerve end. Clinically, this has been used successfully in digital nerves.

Nonbiologicals. There have been as many tubular conduits developed as there are materials: silicone, polyglycolate copolymers, polyvinylidene fluoride, etc. Each has been experimentally successful. The tubes seem to exclude much of the inflammatory wound-healing and scar-forming materials and to create an internal wound-healing environment that allows the nerves to regenerate. Since all cause some foreign-body response, an entirely satisfactory material has not yet been identified. The ideal substance, when developed, will possess the characteristics of any perfect biological substitute. It will be biodegradable, nontoxic, nonantigenic, noncarcinogenic, and flexible and will disappear at a time coincident with the formation of new axons. Since all empty tubular materials must first fill with fibrin or other biological material, new studies are concentrating on filling the tubes with the best milieu for nerve growth (laminin, type IV collagen, etc).

Fascia

Fascia is perhaps less important than other grafting material since it is less frequently used. This may be unfortunate since it is exceedingly valuable both for function and for contour.

The functional uses of fascia have been as strips laid along the face to mimic the pull of the muscles of facial animation. When the facial nerve is irretrievably lost and cross-facial nerve grafting is not possible, the use of fascial strips can maintain the tone of the face. The fascia is laid along the lip, the cheeks, and the eyelids at a first stage. The fascia becomes vascularized by the diffusion and ingrowth of vessels. Several months later, the proximal portion of the strips can be drawn upward and backward to hold the face in a position of symmetry with the opposite side, particularly when the face is in repose. When possible the proximal ends may be made dynamic by attaching to the masseter or temporal muscles, which are often functional even when the seventh nerve–innervated muscles are absent. Fascial survival as a graft is predictable.

Fascia for coverage of other grafted tissue or material is underused. Cartilage grafts to the nose, for instance, tend to develop sharp edges that are visible or palpable. The draping of fascia (temporal fascia, for example) over the graft softens the contour.

Although any fascia may serve as a donor site, the fascia lata and the temporal fascia are most commonly used.

Temporoparietalis Fascia Flap

The thin, almost areolar temporoparietalis covering of the actual temporal fascia has its own blood supply and can be raised as a vascularized covering material, particularly for a reconstructed ear.

AFTERTHOUGHT

After reviewing almost all of what used to be considered reconstructive surgery—and in a single chapter—it may be useful to reflect on the three "eureka" phenomena of recent years. These three have altered our approach to reconstructive surgery more than any comparable events in the 2,600 years of our specialty.

Microsurgery

Microsurgery, beginning in the 1960s, altered our concepts of tissue transfer and expanded our technology to a degree of sophistication and elegance. It literally rendered meaningless many of our concepts of flap transfer and exchanged them for a new body of knowledge.

Musculocutaneous Flaps

The musculocutaneous flap changed not only our approach to flaps but the entire way in which we thought of them. The blood supply of the muscle/skin system has been rewritten in the last 20 years.

Craniofacial Surgery

The concepts of craniofacial surgery and the technology of bone grafting and rigid fixation devices altered much of our thinking about not only congenital disease but traumatic and aesthetic deformity as well.

What's Next?

The prediction of a "eureka" phenomenon is difficult since the finding may represent a new way of looking at old problems and "seeing" for the first time as it was for musculocutaneous flaps. It may also, as did microsurgery and craniofacial surgery, be the culmination of a number of related observations building toward a solution being assiduously sought. I shall bet on the latter and predict the next breakthrough to be the overcoming of the allograft rejection phenomenon. When it becomes possible to transplant living tissue successfully from one to another, our specialty will be uniquely poised to apply the principles in this chapter.

SUGGESTED READING

Georgiade GS, Georgiade NG, Riefkohl R, et al: *Textbook of Plastic, Maxillofacial and Reconstructive Surgery,* ed 2. Baltimore, Williams & Wilkins, 1992.

Gillies HAD, Millard DR: *The Principles and Art of Plastic Surgery.* Boston, Little, Brown, 1957.

Jurkiewicz MJ, Krizek TJ, Mathes SJ, et al: *Plastic Surgery, Principles and Practice.* St. Louis, Mosby–Year Book, 1990.

Mathes SJ, Nahai F: *Clinical Applications for Muscle and Musculocutaneous Flaps.* St Louis, Mosby–Year Book, 1982.

McCarthy JG: *Plastic Surgery.* Philadelphia, WB Saunders, 1990.

Smith JW, Aston SJ: *Grabb and Smith's Plastic Surgery,* ed 4. Boston, Little, Brown, 1991.

Urist M: *Fundamental and Clinical Physiology of Bone.* Philadelphia, JB Lippincott, 1980.

Chapter 3

Microsurgery

William Lineaweaver, M.D.

CONTENTS

CHAPTER OBJECTIVE

At the end of this chapter the resident is familiar with the principles of microsurgery and has mastered basic microsurgery techniques including microneural repair and microsurgical anastomosis.

LEARNER OBJECTIVES

On completion of this chapter the resident

1. **Is familiar with the use of the operating microscope and the technical aspects of microvascular anastomosis (artery and vein) and microneural repair.**
2. **Understands the indications for, the contraindication to, and the techniques for accomplishing replantation of amputated parts; recognizes the common methods of monitoring the success of replantation.**
3. **Understands the varying types of blood supply to discrete units of tissue (including arterialized flap, musculocutaneous flap, fasciocutaneous flap).**
4. **Is familiar with the terms and types of free tissue flaps—skin, skin/muscle, skin/muscle/bone, skin/tendon, muscle alone.**
5. **Knows in detail the anatomy for harvesting the most common free flaps, including the latissimus dorsi and rectus abdominis.**
6. **Recognizes the indications for harvesting various flaps and matching specific donor sites to specific recipient site needs.**
7. **Is familiar with radiologic techniques for evaluation of both donor and recipient sites.**
8. **Recognizes the mechanisms and consequences of the no-reflow phenomenon; knows how to treat a failing flap.**
9. **Understands the technological, pharmacologic, and physiologic principles of postoperative monitoring of free flaps.**
10. **Knows the basic physiology of nerve injury (axonotmesis, neurotmesis, neuropraxia, wallerian degeneration) and nerve healing.**
11. **Understand intraneural anatomy and anatomic relationships to surrounding structures of the major peripheral nerves.**
12. **Understands the principles of repair of nerve injury, including the need**

for nerve grafting, the anatomy of nerve graft donor sites, and the physiology, timing, and techniques of primary, delayed primary, and late nerve repair.

13. Understands the principles and techniques of hematologic manipulation of normal and abnormal vascular flow characteristics.

CLINICAL PRACTICE

During the course of the training program, the resident

1. **Learns how to use the operating microscope and performs microvascular anastomosis and microneural repair in the laboratory (experimental animal) and clinical settings.**
2. **Participates in surgical procedures for free tissue transfer; harvests flaps and manages donor sites; when competent, performs vascular anastomosis for free tissue transfer.**
3. **Diagnoses and treats a variety of nerve injuries by using microsurgery and nerve grafts where appropriate.**
4. **Conducts preoperative evaluation and postoperative management of patients undergoing free tissue transfer.**
5. **Manages long-term aspects, including donor site problems, of patients who have undergone free tissue transfers.**
6. Participates in surgical procedures for replantation of amputated parts; when competent, performs vascular anastomosis and nerve repairs during replantation procedures.
7. Conducts preoperative evaluation and postoperative management of patients undergoing replantation of amputated parts and revascularization procedures.
8. Manages long-term aspects, including rehabilitation, of patients who have undergone replantation and revascularization procedures.

EQUIPMENT

A modern microsurgeon should be sufficiently familiar with microsurgical equipment to make decisions regarding its purchase, upkeep, and replacement. The tools of microsurgery include loupes, operating microscopes, surgical instruments, and sutures.

Loupes are mounted on spectacle frames, the flat lenses of which must be made to correct any visual abnormality of the surgeon. Loupe magnification of 3× to 4× is most practical, and a maximally wide magnified field is desirable. Although expensive, a backup pair of loupes is a wise investment.

The microscope itself must meet certain critical specifications. Its stand must be stable but easily repositioned. "XY" maneuverability (the ability of the microscope to move back and forth, to and fro) should be easy and precise, whether done manually or by foot control. Foot controls for focusing and magnification should be sturdy and easy to use. The fiber-optic light source should be reliable and easy to service and have a variable intensity control. Magnification should range from 6× to 40×, and the focal length lenses should be easily interchangeable. Two operating ocular sets should be oriented so that the surgeon and assistant may sit face to face and share the same field of focus. Each ocular set should have an adjustable intraocular distance and vertical adjustment. Video and photographic adjuncts can be added as desired.

The basic microsurgical instrument set consists of fine forceps for tissue handling, a forceps-type vessel dilator, curved scissors for dissection, straight scissors for vessel transection, and a needle holder. The hinged instruments should be nonlocking.

Vessel clamps are critical pieces of equipment, and individual clamp types should be tested in the laboratory. Low clamp pressures will not provide hemostasis, while pressures greater than 30 g/mm^2 can cause vessel necrosis. Clinically, any clamp that has rough edges or a faulty clamping mechanism should be discarded immediately. Selections of straight and curved clamps allow optimal exposure and vessel stabilization within different wound configurations. Different-sized clamps should be available for vessels of different calibers. Two clamps fixed parallel to each other on a connecting bar offer a stable framework for vessel repair in ideal circumstances. Individual clamps allow more maneuverability and fine adjustment in actual clinical circumstances.

Nylon is the most commonly used microsurgical suture material. The sutures are available in gauges of 8-0, 9-0, 10-0, and 11-0, and the surgeon's experience must match these sizes with vessel caliber and wall thickness. Tapered, curved needles no greater than 100/μm in diameter should be used to minimize vessel trauma.

INTRODUCTORY MICROSURGICAL TRAINING AND BASIC OPERATIVE TECHNIQUES

Laboratory training should be the technical foundation of every practicing microsurgeon. In a training program, the microsurgical laboratory should have a director skilled in basic techniques and teaching. The trainee should be systematically introduced to posture, field organization, microscope adjustment, instrument use, and suture handling. Following these basic steps, the trainee is introduced to the basic elements of microsurgery: vessel and nerve dissection, vessel transection, end-to-end vessel repair, end-to-side vessel repair, and nerve repair (Fig 3–1). These procedures are usually performed in rats by using the femoral vessels and sciatic nerve.

Skeletonization of vessels and nerves gives the trainee the experience needed to develop coordination and instrument handling ability under the microscope. End-to-end vessel repair should be performed in arteries and veins. The surgeon learns vessel transection and clamp placement prior to suture placement. Suturing techniques such as the backwall first, 180-degree suture placement, and triangulated suture placement are necessary exercises with roles in clinical surgery. The use of irrigating catheters and background material is also learned. End-to-end anastomoses of superficial epigastric vessels to femoral vessels offer a greater challenge to microsurgical technique. Nerve repairs should include epineural and fascicular repair.

More sophisticated exercises include vein grafting, nerve grafting, limb replantation, and microvascular flap and organ transplants. All these procedures can be performed in rat models, and they teach not only technical facility but also organization of complex procedures.

CLINICAL MICROSURGERY: ANATOMY, PHYSIOLOGY, AND HEMATOLOGY

Clinical microsurgery is primarily based on the anatomic concept that many body parts and regions have identifiable and reliable axial blood supplies (pedicle vessels) on which the tissue can survive with no other vascular attachments. Replantation is based on the knowledge that amputated parts can survive following repair of axial arteries and veins. This concept also provides the foundation for toe transplantation. Early pedicled flaps of omentum and skin flaps designed around axial vessels were the precursors for actual transplantation of omentum and such flaps as the groin flap and the dorsalis pedis flap. Clinical applications of regional vascular anatomy have led to the design and use of a great variety of transplants of skin, muscle, and bone.

The two broad areas of physiologic study in microsurgery consist of the response of tissue to ischemia and hematologic processes that lead to thrombosis at anastomotic sites in small vessels and capillary beds.

Primary ischemia time is the period for which a tissue can tolerate interruption of circulation prior to reperfusion. Secondary ischemia time is the period for which a tissue can tolerate a second interruption of circulation prior to a second reperfusion. Generally, secondary ischemia time is less well tolerated than primary ischemia time. Clinical observation of the characteristic critical ischemia time

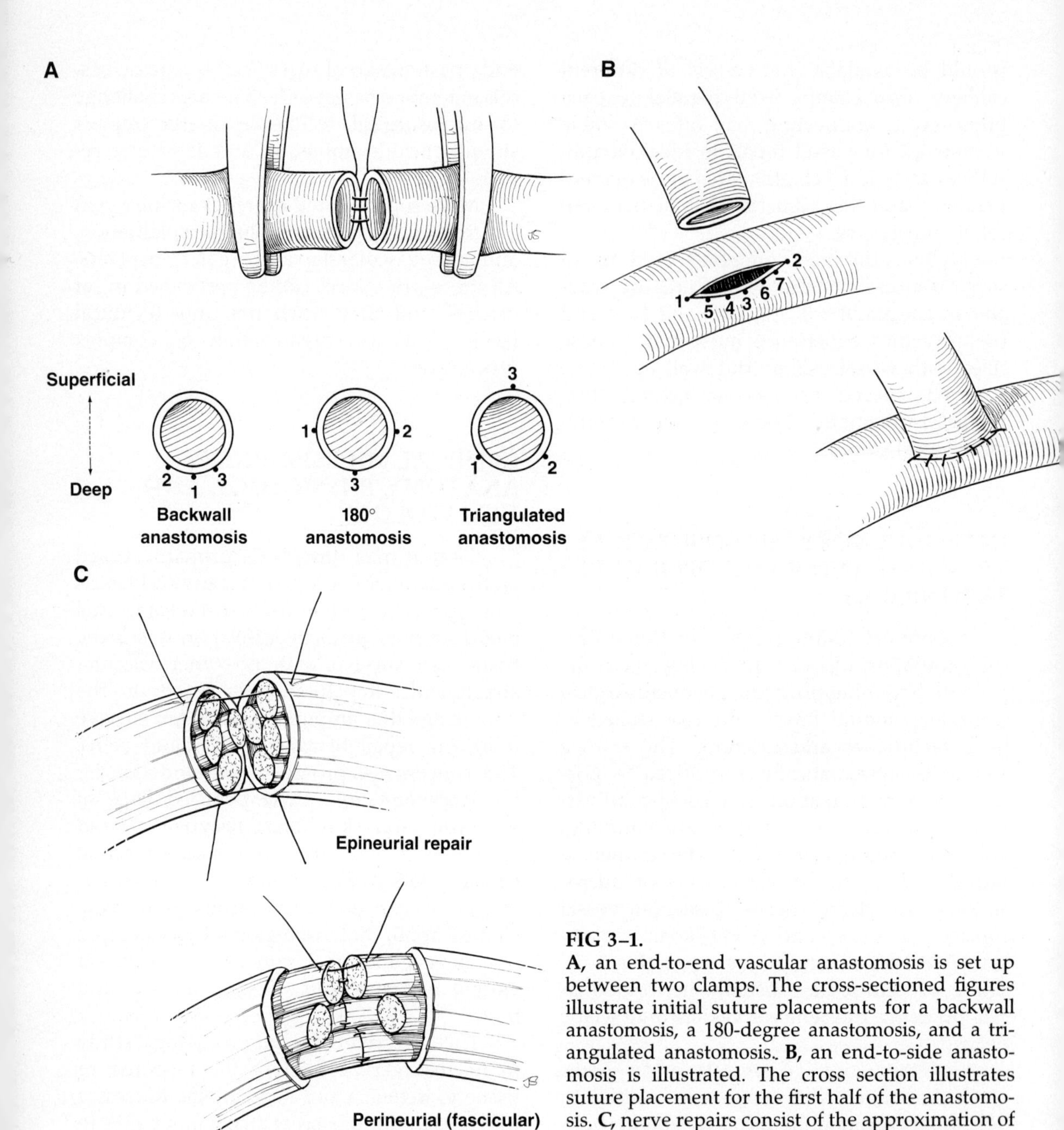

FIG 3–1.
A, an end-to-end vascular anastomosis is set up between two clamps. The cross-sectioned figures illustrate initial suture placements for a backwall anastomosis, a 180-degree anastomosis, and a triangulated anastomosis. **B,** an end-to-side anastomosis is illustrated. The cross section illustrates suture placement for the first half of the anastomosis. **C,** nerve repairs consist of the approximation of the epineurium or individual fascicular repairs.

of fingers, hands, limbs, and muscle have led to clinical strategies to minimize ischemia electively by operative organization and, in cases of amputation, by cooling.

Study of the end point of tissue response to ischemia, the "no-reflow phenomenon," has led to sophisticated investigations of tissue response to and recovery from ischemia. First described in organ transplant failure, the "no-reflow phenomenon" is more than a euphemism for death. The physiologic consequences of ischemia and reperfusion mount with time until injury is so great that despite reestablished blood flow in pedicle vessels, the capillary beds of the tissue do not perfuse, and the tissue dies. The mechanisms of this state are numerous and still being defined. Ischemia causes derangements of oxygen and glucose metabolism, capillary stasis, decreased red cell deformability, hypothermia, and hypoxanthine release. Reperfusion is implicated in the formation of toxic superoxide and hydroxyl free radicals, as well as the introduction of activated neutrophils and other cells that produce a destructive acute inflammatory response.

The cumulative results of these processes include capillary stasis, endothelial swelling, and diffuse cellular damage throughout the tissue. Investigation of these processes raises possibilities of intervention for tissue preservation. Possible routes for such intervention may include perfusion of tissues with metabolic substrates or anticoagulants, as well as systemic metabolic and hematologic manipulation. For example, allopurinol may, as a xanthine oxidase inhibitor, block xanthine oxidase–related aspects of ischemic and reperfusion injuries, thereby promoting tissue viability.

The study of thrombosis of microvascular anastomoses has led to detailed investigation of the roles of platelets and fibrin. Platelets can initially adhere to areas of vessel injury at the anastomotic site. The level of platelet adherence may be related to undefined factors of tissue damage and systemic factors. Once initiated, platelet adherence can progress to platelet emboli, which may complicate distal anastomoses (e.g., vein grafts) and disrupt capillary bed circulation. Platelets may also proceed to convert fibrinogen to fibrin at the anastomotic site and lead to the development of a stable, occlusive fibrin clot. Microvascular thrombosis therefore appears to have anastomotic and postanastomotic components. Investigation of these interactions may lead to more rational uses of antiplatelet and antifibrin adjuncts.

CLINICAL MICROSURGERY: REPLANTATION

Following a significant amputation, replantation offers the possibility of a one-stage reconstruction that usually surpasses any secondary reconstruction. Replantation is most often attempted following amputation of fingers, but hands, upper extremities, lower extremities, ears, scalp, and genitalia can be replanted under favorable circumstances.

The selection of patients for replantation requires a thorough assessment of the patient and the amputated part. The patient must be carefully examined to make certain that significant coexisting injuries are not overlooked in the excitement of addressing the amputation. Problems such as compartment syndromes, intra-abdominal injuries, and cervical spine injuries must be satisfactorily managed before replantation can be considered.

Significant preexisting illness such as a recent stroke or myocardial infarction may make replantation unfeasible. Acute psychosis, especially if the patient has committed an autoamputation, is a controversial factor, but in several cases replantation has been successful, and with intensive acute and long-term psychiatric care, the patients have gone on to a functional recovery. Age is no contraindication, nor are stable chronic diseases such as diabetes or hypertension.

The amputated parts must then be considered. Certain amputations, including thumbs, ears, scalp, genitalia, and amputation in children, should always, if possible, be examined by a microsurgeon to determine whether replantation is feasible. Other injuries given a high priority for replantation include multiple-digit amputations and sharp amputations at the hand, wrist, or forearm. Sharp digit amputations distal to the superficialis insertion are worthwhile replantations, even if only a single digit is involved. Any complex extremity injury that could reasonably be helped by revascularization and/or early flap transplantation should also be examined by a microsurgeon.

Single-digit amputations proximal to the superficialis insertion, avulsion and crush injuries, and multiple-level injuries are relatively unfavorable circumstances and may not merit referral for microsurgical evaluation. Major limb amputations should be considered for replantation only if the injuries are favorable (i.e., reasonably sharp without significant crush, avulsion, or multiple-level components); associated injuries are not significant, and referral can be prompt.

Transportation to a replantation center is arranged following the initial conference between the referring doctor and the microsurgeon. Transportation should be based on the tolerance of the amputated part to ischemia time. For example, the critical ischemia time of an amputated finger is approximately 8 hours at room temperature. If the finger is properly cooled by placing it in a plastic bag on ice, the finger's ability to recover from ischemia is extended to 20 to 24 hours. Ground transport is therefore sufficient for properly cooled amputated fingers within a range of about 200 miles. Major hand and limb amputations that contain skeletal muscle and that have a critical ischemia time of only 6 to 10 hours, even when cooled, should be transported as rapidly as possible.

When the patient arrives at the replantation hospital, the patient and microsurgeon should discuss replantation in detail before proceeding. The discussion should include blood transfusion, hospitalization time, chances for success, rehabilitation time, and the possibilities of secondary surgery.

The replantation procedure is ideally started by two surgeons (or two teams). One surgeon takes the amputated parts to the operating room for exploration and tagging. An amputated finger, for example, should have all its important structures identified through two midlateral incisions. The bone is debrided of loose fragments, tendons debrided of shredded ends, and the profundus tendon tagged by placing a modified Kessler tendon repair suture. Under loupe magnification, each digital artery, each digital nerve, and one or two dorsal veins should be tagged with fine silk (Fig 3–2).

The other surgeon completes the emergency room workup, including reviewing radiographs of the amputated parts and the injured extremity, and brings the patient to the operating table. Tourniquets are placed on the injured extremity and also on an uninjured lower extremity if vein grafts are anticipated. Following induction of anesthesia and draping, the second surgeon irrigates and explores the proximal amputation injury and debrides and tags significant structures.

For fingers and hands, replantation generally proceeds from parts requiring rougher manipulation to parts requiring microsurgical maneuvers. For the hands and fingers, the usual replantation sequence consists of skeletal fixation (using K-wires, interosseous wires, or plates), flexor tendon repair on the volar side, arterial repairs, and digital nerve repair. Following volar skin closure, the finger is turned, and the extensor tendon is approximated. One or more dorsal veins are repaired and the dorsal skin closed. Usually the replantation of one finger is completed before starting on another finger, and fingers are replanted in order of functional importance (thumb, little, ring, middle, index). In cases of multiple amputation, if a critical digit such as the thumb is not replantable, one can consider replanting a relatively noncritical digit (e.g., the index) into the critical position.

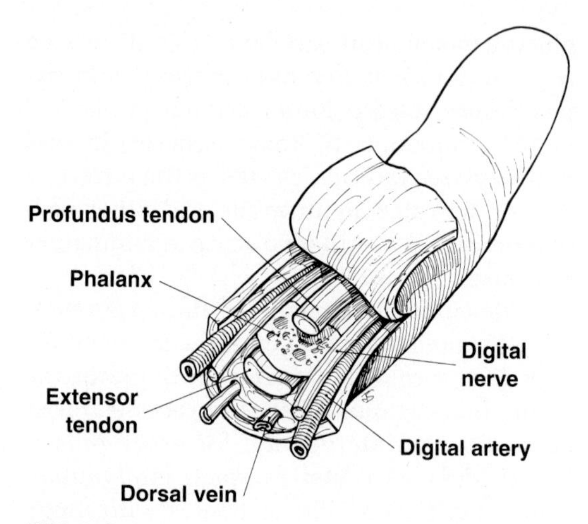

FIG 3–2.
An amputated finger is prepared for replantation by identification and tagging of important structures.

In extremity replantation, the initial operative step reestablishes arterial circulation with a dialysis shunt to minimize ischemia time. Skeletal fixation is then performed, followed by radical debridement of skeletal muscle and compartment releases. Microscopic vascular and nerve repairs are then completed. Muscle, tendon, and skin approximation follows.

Postoperatively, patients are monitored in an intensive care unit. In our unit, circulation is assessed by quantitative fluorometry. Arterial compromise is usually reexplored operatively, while venous obstruction in fingers is increasingly being treated by leech application with results comparable to operative reexploration. Patients with uncomplicated finger replantation receive dextran, aspirin, and antibiotics for a week and are discharged between 8 and 10 days after surgery. Postoperative hand therapy is initiated in the hospital.

Replanted limbs should be reexplored operatively for venous or arterial obstruction. These patients often require serial debridements and skin grafts or flap closures during the initial hospitalization.

CLINICAL MICROSURGERY: FLAPS

Microsurgical technique allows the surgeon to reconstruct complicated defects with tissue transplanted from sites distant from the defect. The preparation for a microsurgical transplant should include a thorough resection of the defect, be it an acute wound, a chronic wound, or a neoplasm. This ablation should define the requirements for reconstruction, either at the time of resection or at a second stage. For example, acutely, the amputation stump of a thumb is resected to skeletonize the remaining bone and the stumps of necessary tendon and digital nerves and to explore local vessels. This procedure gives measurements for the components of the great toe transplant harvested simultaneously. A complex scalp tumor, however, might be best handled by resection and temporary dressings while the specimen is thoroughly studied to determine adequacy of resection. Once the tumor is judged to be excised, a flap can be transplanted.

Arteriography should be considered preoperatively to delineate the anatomy of recipient vessels in areas altered by trauma or previous surgery. Preoperative planning should include banked blood since many of these procedures require transfusion. In totally elective cases, the patient may wish to donate autologous blood.

A microsurgical transplant procedure requires meticulous placement of the patient on the operating room table. The defect and the flap donor site should be positioned in such a way as to permit one team to prepare the recipient site while another team harvests the flap. Fields for vein grafts and skin grafts should be anticipated.

Postoperatively, patients with flaps are placed in an intensive care unit. Most flaps can be monitored in some way for circulatory competence, and any persistent sign of arterial or venous obstruction should prompt operative reexploration. There is no place for nonoperative management of a flap with compromised circulation if the patient's condition permits surgery. Most patients with uncomplicated flap placement leave the intensive care unit in 1 to 2 days and the hospital in 7 to 14 days.

An enormous number of flaps, composite flaps, and specialized tissue components have been successfully transplanted. The following catalog outlines transplants that have been widely used.

Skin Flaps

The *lateral arm flap* consists of skin, subcutaneous tissue, and fascia (see Fig 3–3). The flap territory extends in length from the insertion of the deltoid to the lateral epicondyle of the humerus. In an adult, the flap can be up to 6 cm in width and still permit primary closure of the recipient site. Wider flaps require a skin graft to the donor site. The posterior radial collateral artery (a terminal branch of the profunda brachii artery) and its accompanying vein are the flap's vascular pedicle, and these vessels are dissected from the fascial layer between the biceps and triceps muscles. The pedicle vessels can be up to 8 cm in length and 1 to 1.5 mm in width. The lower lateral cutaneous nerve of the arm can be taken with the flap for sensory reinnervation.

The *radial forearm flap* is a very thin unit of skin, subcutaneous tissue, and fascia based on the underlying radial artery, its accompanying veins, or subcutaneous veins. The flap can be designed to include all the skin of the distal volar forearm. Its thinness makes it ideal for intraoral defects. A segment of radius can be taken with the flap as a vascularized bone graft. The donor site usually requires a skin

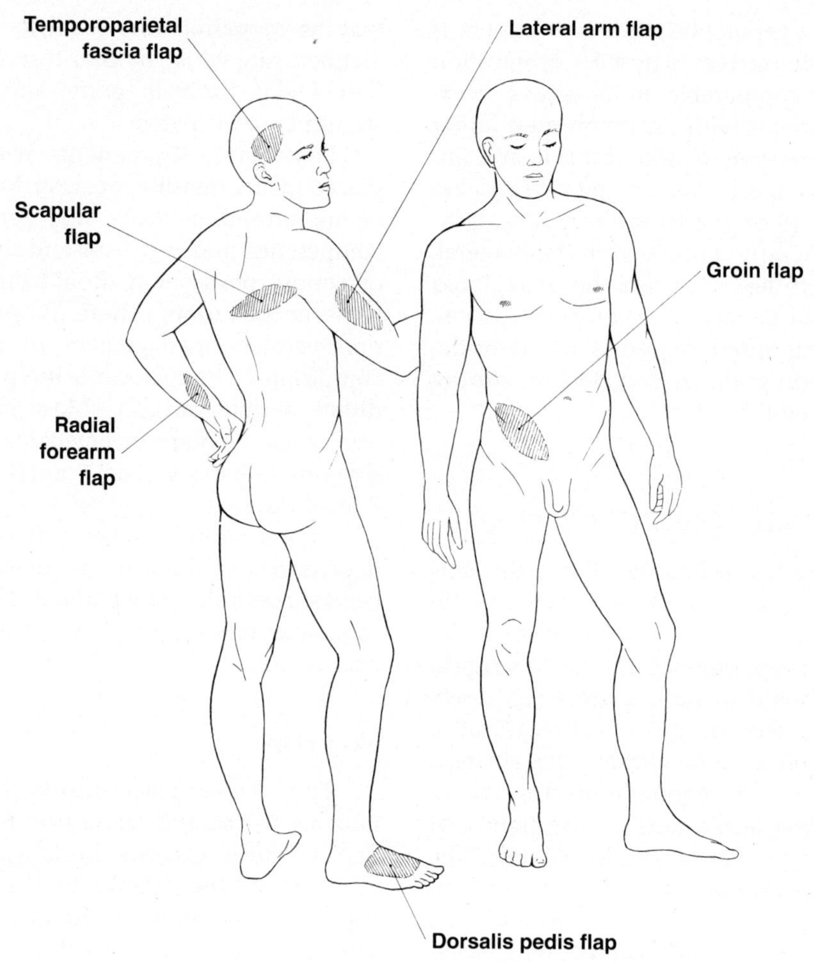

FIG 3–3.
Donor sites for skin and temporoparietal fascia flaps.

graft. Prior to using this flap, it is necessary to ensure that the patient has intact and sufficient ulnar circulation to the hand by either an Allen test or, if the extremity is traumatized, by arteriography.

The *groin flap* is a bulky unit of skin and fat based on the superficial circumflex iliac vessels. These vessels, which are dissected to the femoral vessels along the medial border of the sartorius muscle, are small and variable, and their suitability as a flap pedicle should be determined before the flap is completely mobilized. A branch of T12 can be incorporated into the flap for sensation. The flap can be designed as a large unit (8 × 20 cm in adults) parallel to the groin crease, and the donor site can be closed primarily and inconspicuously. Besides filling large cutaneous defects, the flap can be deepithelialized for subcutaneous contour reconstruction.

The *scapular flap* can be taken as a large (10 × 20 cm) cutaneous unit oriented transversely over the central portion of the scapula. The circumflex scapular vessels coming through the triangular space from their origins on the subscapular vessels serve as the vascular pedicle. The lateral border of the scapula can be taken with the flap as vascularized bone. The origin of the circumflex scapular vessels allows the flap to be raised as a unit with other tissue based on the thoracodorsal vessels, i.e., the latissimus dorsi and serratus flaps. This flap has played a major role in head and neck reconstruction, and it can be deepithelialized for subcutaneous placement to correct contour defects.

The *dorsalis pedis flap* is a thin cutaneous unit that can be innervated by the deep superficial peroneal nerves. The flap is based on the dorsalis pedis artery, which can be harvested in continuity with the anterior tibial artery to provide a long pedicle. Venous drainage is obtained by including a subcutaneous vein in the flap. The vein can usually be taken in continuity with the saphenous vein. The underlying second metatarsal can be included as vascularized bone. The long pedicle of this flap makes it useful in difficult defects of the face and hands that would otherwise require vein grafts for flap insertion. The donor site requires a skin graft, and chronic donor site breakdown is a recognized complication.

Temporoparietal Fascia

The temporoparietal fascia is a thin layer of the scalp deep to the fat and superficial to the temporalis muscle and its fascia. The flap is harvested after raising the overlying scalp layers as anterior and posterior flaps. The temporoparietal fascia is transplanted with the superficial temporal vessels. Above the temporalis muscle, the temporoparietal fascia has extensive vascular connections to the underlying skull, and split-thickness and full-thickness cranial bone segments can be incorporated with the flap. This flap has been used for thin coverage of facial defects and hand defects. The donor site is closed primarily by reapproximating the scalp flaps. The temporoparietal fascia must be covered by a skin graft.

Muscle and Myocutaneous Flaps

The *latissimus dorsi* is a large fan-shaped muscle that originates in the posterior layer of the lumbodorsal fascia and inserts on the humerus (see Fig 3–4). Its large, reliable pedicle consists of the thoracodorsal vessels,

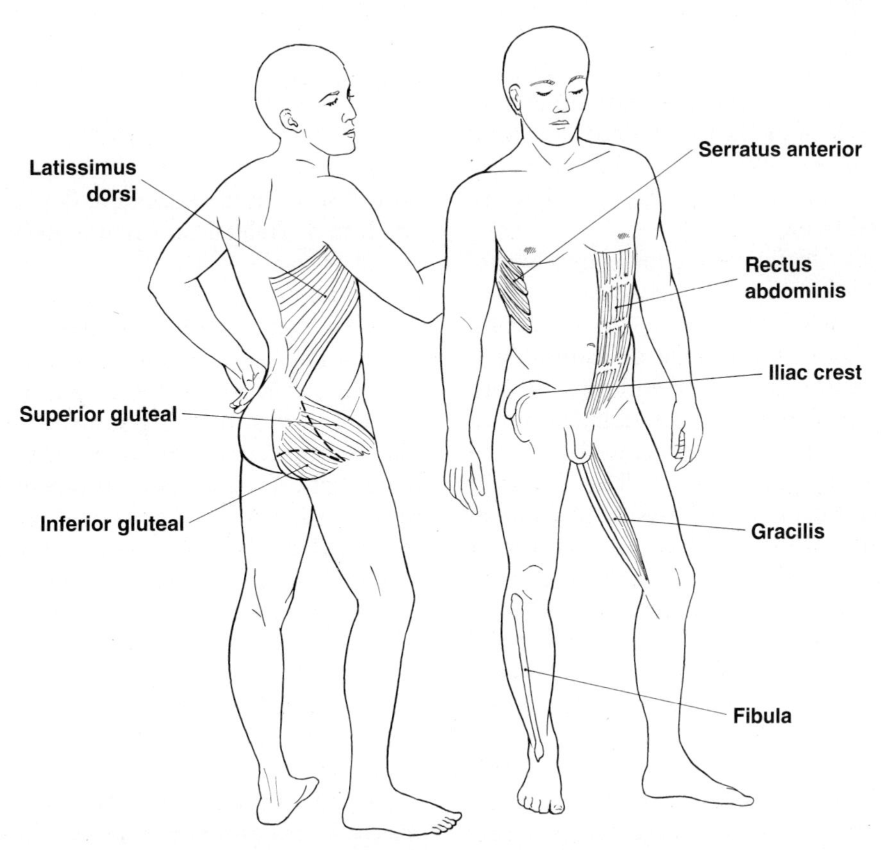

FIG 3–4.
Donor sites for muscle and bone flaps.

which when taken in continuity with the subscapular vessels, yield a long pedicle with vessel diameters of up to 4 mm. The thoracodorsal nerve travels with the vascular pedicle and can be used for reinnervation. The overlying skin can be reliably taken with the muscle, and the muscle will reliably support a skin graft. The donor site is closed primarily, over suction drains. This large muscle is a reliable flap for complex defects of the extremities and scalp.

The *serratus anterior* muscle lies beneath the latissimus dorsi. It arises from the first nine ribs and anchors the scapula. The most caudal four slips of muscle can be transplanted on vessels continuous with the thoracodorsal vessels, which themselves can be incorporated into the pedicle for extra length. The distal portion of the long thoracic nerve is taken with the flap and can be used for reinnervation. The proximal portion of the nerve must be protected to maintain innervation to the upper serratus slips and prevent scapular winging. The serratus is a malleable piece of tissue that can be molded into irregular defects, and it has been used for functional reconstruction of the face and hand. The long vascular pedicle makes flap positioning very flexible. Underlying ribs can be taken as vascularized bone.

The *rectus abdominis* is a long muscle that can cover defects with dimensions of up to 10×25 cm. Overlying skin can be taken, either parallel to the muscle or transversely oriented over the distal third and extending to the iliac crest. The muscle is mobilized out of the rectus sheath and transplanted with the deep inferior epigastric vessels. The myocutaneous variant using the transverse abdominal skin is being increasingly utilized for breast reconstruction. The muscle flap is a very reliable cover for appropriately sized defects of the extremities and head. Careful closure of the rectus sheath is necessary to prevent herniation or diffuse bulging at the donor site.

The *gracilis* muscle originates at the pubic tubercle and inserts on the tibia below the condyle. This long, narrow muscle was originally used for general coverage, but it is now being used less frequently because the rectus and serratus have been applied to moderate-sized defects. The gracilis, however, continues to be useful as a functional muscle in facial and extremity reconstruction. The muscle is harvested through a medial thigh incision. The primary vascular pedicle is composed of terminal branches of the medial femoral circumflex vessels. The terminal obturator nerve is taken with the gracilis for reinnervation. A cutaneous component can be reliably taken with the proximal third of the muscle.

The *gluteus maximus* muscle can be segmentally used as a myocutaneous flap, and these flaps are used in breast reconstruction. The superior gluteal flap is a transverse myocutaneous unit based on the superior gluteal vessels, which enter the gluteus muscle after passing between the piriformis and gluteus medius muscles. The inferior gluteal flap is a transverse myocutaneous unit based on the inferior gluteal vessels, which exit the pelvis between the piriformis and coccygeus muscles. Both flaps take only a portion of the gluteus muscle around the vascular pedicle.

Bone

Several of the flaps described above can be designed to carry components of vascularized bone. These multicomponent flaps can solve a combined skeletal–soft-tissue defect with a single transplant. The most commonly used combination flaps are temporoparietal fascia/calvarial bone, radial forearm flap/radius, scapula flap/scapula, and serratus/rib.

The *fibula* is a tubular bone that can be transplanted with the peroneal vessels. The fibula can provide over 20 cm of vascularized bone that can be shaped with osteotomies to replace such multidimensional structures as mandibular segments. Careful preservation of septocutaneous perforators allows an island of overlying skin to be transplanted with the bone.

The *iliac crest* can be transplanted with the deep circumflex iliac vessels. Flap elevation may involve division of the inguinal ligament if the pedicle vessels originate from the iliac vessel, and careful donor site reconstruction is necessary to prevent herniation. The iliac crest yields a thick flap of bicortical bone that can be 14 cm long in adults. Osteotomes can be safely used to shape this bone flap also. A skin component based on periosteal perforators can be included with the flap.

Toes

Toe transplantation offers a single-stage reconstruction for a missing digit. Most often applied to thumb reconstruction, toe transplantation can also provide multiple opposable digits for a severely injured or maldeveloped hand.

Great toe transplantation can be used to replace a missing thumb if at least a third of the metacarpal shaft remains. Thumb amputation at the metacarpophalangeal or proximal phalangeal level can be reconstructed with great toes amputated at the appropriate level. The dorsal radial vessels in the snuff box are preferred as recipient vessels, and if doubt exists about their availability, the recipient area should be studied by angiography.

The terminal segment of the dorsalis pedis artery (the first dorsal metatarsal artery) is the preferred arterial supply for the toe, and a dorsal subcutaneous vein provides venous return. If doubt exists that the dorsalis pedis supplies the great toe either because of trauma or the existence of a dominant plantar arterial system, then the foot should be studied by arteriography. Dissection of the recipient site should provide measurements for the toe transplant, including skeletal, tendon, vessel, and nerve length (Fig 3–5). The donor defect of the foot requires careful closure, guided mobilization, and occasional secondary revision for soft-tissue problems or neuroma, but eventually most patients recover with minimal or no functional defect.

The *second toe* has been used for thumb reconstruction, but it seems best suited as a replacement for an ulnar digit to provide pinch. Two second toes can provide ulnar grip as well as pinch. Hands requiring such recon-

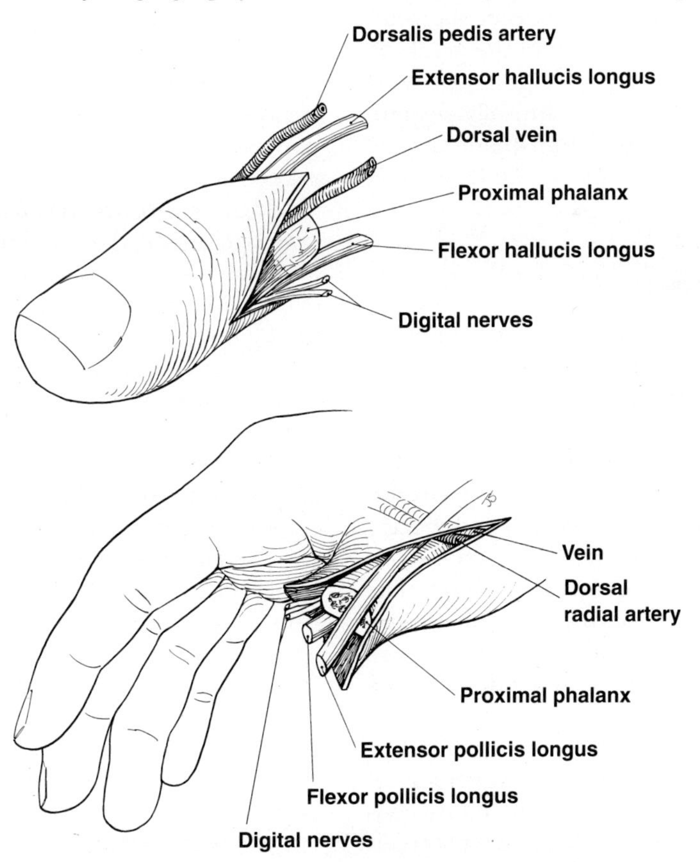

FIG 3–5.
Complementary dissections for a great toe transplant for thumb reconstruction.

struction generally have suffered severe injuries, and arteriography is recommended to delineate recipient site vessels in the palm. The second toe may receive a dominant blood supply from either the dorsal first metatarsal artery or from plantar arteries, and the largest pedicle vessel must be chosen after carefully dissecting both options. The donor site is closed as a ray amputation with negligible morbidity.

Combined second and third toe transplants can provide two digits in a single unit. These units are suitable for replacing fingers that have been amputated proximal to the web space. This transplant is also based on either the first dorsal metatarsal artery or plantar vessels.

Subtotal toe transplants, or "wrap-arounds," take only a portion of the great or second toe. For example, a partial thumb amputation can be reconstructed by taking only part of the donor toe, e.g., the distal phalanx, nail bed, and a portion of the pulp from the great toe. The stump of the great toe can then be covered by skin grafts or local flaps. These operations are technically elegant, but resorption of the small transplanted bone and chronic breakdown of the toe stump can occur.

Visceral Transplants

The *jejunum,* first transplanted in humans in 1957, has become a widely used flap for the repair of defects of the pharynx and cervical portion of the esophagus. The jejunum segment is harvested 60 to 80 cm distal to the ligament of Treitz. The mesentery is transilluminated to identify pedicle vessels to a specific bowel segment, and the jejunal segment and its vessels are then harvested as a unit. The jejunum is closed primarily, as is the mesenteric defect. The jejunal segment can be used as a tube or a patch, depending on the defect.

Omentum, first clinically transplanted in 1971, was originally used for coverage of soft-tissue defects. More recently, its use has been concentrated in areas of subcutaneous contour reconstruction such as Romberg's disease. The omentum is usually taken with the right gastroepiploic vessels as a pedicle, and careful division of arcade vessels can produce an elongated flap.

CLINICAL MICROSURGERY: PHARMACOLOGY AND LEECHES

There are many metabolic, neurovascular, and hematologic factors that could be theoretically manipulated pharmacologically to enhance microsurgical success. In practice, however, few pharmacologic agents are widely or consistently used in microsurgery, and these pharmacologic adjuncts are used empirically with inconclusive experimental and clinical evidence to support such practice. Agents used clinically are hematologic or vasodilating agents. No metabolic or anti-inflammatory agents currently play roles in clinical microsurgery, although future research may make such agents useful.

Intraoperatively, heparin in saline (100 units/cc) is used to irrigate vessels and to keep sutures and instruments from becoming sticky. Lidocaine (1%), bupivacaine (2%), and papaverine (0.3%) are applied to vessels to relieve spasm.

Most microsurgeons use some adjunctive systemic medication following replantation and transplantation procedures. Acetylsalicylic acid may be given perioperatively (3 mg/kg/day) for its antiplatelet effect. Low–molecular-weight dextran 40, a plasma expander, may interfere with some aspects of platelet adherence and may act as a fibrinolytic agent in capillary beds. Dextran is administered at a rate of 7 to 8 cc/kg/day for 6 to 7 days postoperatively.

Systemic heparinization is not used routinely, but its antithrombin activity is called upon for complicated cases, including vein grafts and anastomotic revisions. Local infusion and systemic administration of fibrinolytics such as streptokinase are sometimes used in complicated cases, especially if thrombosis has propagated into a flap pedicle.

Medicinal leeches have been used in microsurgery for over a decade. Their role is best defined in digit and ear replantations. If a replanted part has intact arterial circulation but obstructed or unreconstructible veins, the part will usually die. The application of leeches, usually one every 4 to 6 hours, can produce survival rates of up to 60% in such "artery-only" replants. The leeches evacuate blood and inject anticoagulant and vasodilating substances that promote bleeding from the leech site for up to 4 to 6 hours. This bleeding can substitute for venous return and sustains capillary circulation until venous capillary return is reestablished across the wound. *Aeromonas hydrophila,* a leech enteric organism, can complicate leech application with clinically significant infection. This complication may be eliminated by giving the patients systemic antibiotics effective against *A. hydrophila* prior to leech application.

CLINICAL MICROSURGERY: MONITORING

The ability of tissue to survive a second ischemia-reperfusion cycle is less than its ability to survive a first such episode. Vascular occlusion following initially successful transplantation produces a secondary ischemia time episode. Postoperative monitoring, by promptly detecting circulatory interruption, could shorten secondary ischemia time and improve the salvage rate of complicated flaps, currently reported to be about 50%.

Except for clinical observation, no monitoring method has gained wide use. Monitors attempt to measure some parameters associated with intact flap circulation. The parameter can be pedicle vessel patency (as measured by Doppler probes, either surface or implanted), capillary circulation (as measured by quantitative fluorometry, laser Doppler, or pulse oximetry), or metabolic measurements associated with perfusion (as measured by temperature probes or pH monitors). Convincing studies supporting the use of any monitoring system must include data documenting the monitor's sensitivity, specificity, and the effect of monitor use on the salvage of complicated flaps. Such studies are beginning to appear and may soon provide an objective basis for monitor selection.

NERVE REPAIR

The major nonvascular application of microsurgery is nerve repair. The basic techniques of microsurgical nerve repair were described previously. The application of these techniques is extensive and expanding. Repair of nerves, large and small, is more reliably successful when magnification and microsurgical instruments are used. Nerve grafting has become an established microsurgical technique. Vascularized nerve grafts may have a role in nerve reconstruction in extensively scarred or irradiated beds. These innovations have found applications in primary nerve repair, nerve grafting of traumatic or surgical defects, facial palsy reconstruction, brachial plexus reconstruction, and functional muscle transplantation.

Current concepts of the mechanisms of nerve regeneration across a gap include contact guidance (by which proximal axons grow through a tube or along a framework bridging the gap to the distal nerve or end organ); neurotropism, or factors influencing the direction of nerve regrowth; and neurotrophism, or factors influencing the maturation of regenerated nerve fibers and their appropriate functional reconnection to distal motor and sensory organs. Neurotropism and neurotrophism may be functions of the distal nerve end or end organ, and the structure that provides contact guidance serves as a bridge by which the proximal nerve end can respond to the distal stimulations. Microsurgeons have applied these concepts to the development of alternatives to nerve grafts for the bridging of nerve defects. Denervated muscle tissue, vein grafts, collagen bridges, and synthetic tubes (e.g., polyglycolic acid) have been used for nerve bridging, and successful clinical application of vein grafts for short defects of small nerves and polyglycolic acid tubes for defects in small and large nerves has been reported.

SUGGESTED READING

Buncke HJ (ed): *Microsurgery: Transplantation—Replantation.* Philadelphia, Lea & Febiger, 1991.

Foucher G, Braun FM, Smith DJ: Custom-made free vascularized compound toe transfer for traumatic loss of the thumb. *Plast Reconstr Surg* 1991; 87:310.

Johnson PC: Platelet-mediated thrombosis in microvascular surgery: New knowledge and new strategies. *Plast Reconstr Surg* 1990; 86:359.

Kerrigan CL, Zelt RG, Daniel RK: Secondary critical ischemia time of experimental skin flaps. *Plast Reconstr Surg* 1984; 74:522.

Khouri RK, Cooley BR, Kenna DM, et al: Thrombosis of microvascular anastomoses in traumatized vessels: Fibrin versus platelets. *Plast Reconstr Surg* 1990; 86:110.

Lineaweaver W, Buncke GM, Alpert BS, et al: Pitfalls in replantation surgery, in Vistnes L (ed): *Procedures in Plastic and Reconstructive Surgery*. Boston, Little, Brown, 1991, p 699.

MacKinnon SF, Dellon AL: *Surgery of the Peripheral Nerve*. New York, Thieme Medical, 1988.

O'Brien BM, Morrison WA, Gumley GJ: Principles and techniques of microvascular surgery, in McCarthy J (ed): *Plastic Surgery*. Philadelphia, WB Saunders, 1990, p 413.

Raine T: Microvascular techniques, in Jurkiewicz MJ, et al (eds): *Plastic Surgery: Principles and Practice*. St Louis, Mosby–Year Book, 1990, p 1573.

Wei F, Colony LH, Chen H, et al: Combined second and third toe transfer. *Plast Reconstr Surg* 1989; 84:651.

Chapter 4

Implants/Biomaterials

Robert L. Walton, M.D.

CONTENTS

CHAPTER OBJECTIVE

At the end of this chapter the resident is familiar with both the biology and the surgical use of the various implant materials including bone, cartilage, and alloplasts.

LEARNER OBJECTIVES

On completion of this chapter the resident

1. **Knows the local wound factors that have an influence on bone graft survival.**
2. **Recognizes the biological differences between vascularized and nonvascularized bone grafts.**
3. **Understands the influence of perichondrium and a "balanced cross-sectional area" on the warping of cartilage grafts.**
4. **Recognizes the various types of breast implants and the factors involved in implant choice.**
5. **Recognizes the various injectable materials for subcutaneous filling and the principles of their use.**
6. Understands the processes of bone repair: incorporation, osteoconduction, and osteoinduction.
7. Recognizes the difference in incorporation between cortical and cancellous bone grafts and membranous and endochondral autografts.
8. Is familiar with the immunology of bone and cartilage transplantation.
9. Understands the comparative characteristics of bone and cartilage autografts, allografts, and xenografts.

10. Knows the chemistry and biocompatibility of the commonly implanted biomaterials including silicone, methyl methacrylate, hydroxyapatite, tricalcium phosphate, and Proplast.
11. Understands the factors involved in the choice of implant materials for varying reconstructive problems.

CLINICAL PRACTICE ACTIVITIES

During the course of the training program, the resident

1. Prepares methyl methacrylate prostheses.
2. Performs surgical procedures using solid implant materials, including
   a. Cranioplasty
   b. Silicone implantation to breasts, orbital floor, malar area, chin, or joints
   c. Bone substitution for small defects, such as orthognathic advancements
   d. Nonvascularized bone grafts for a variety of defects:
      (1) Cancellous (iliac)
      (2) Cortical-cancellous (iliac, rib, scapula)
      (3) Cortical (cranial, radius, ilia)
   e. Vascularized bone grafts
   f. Carving procedures (nasal grafts, ear reconstruction) using rib cartilage or other alloplastic materials
3. Performs soft-tissue augmentation by using injectable material.

BONE

Bone grafts are employed for the reconstruction of acquired or congenital defects of the bony skeleton. The two major types of bone, membranous and endochondral, may be used for bone grafts and are defined by their embryologic development. All bones are derived from mesenchyme by two different processes depending on anatomic location. The flat bones of the face and calvarium and the ribs develop by the direct deposition of bone in areas of vascularized mesenchyme by the process of *intramembranous ossification* and hence are termed membranous bones. The long bones and the iliac crest develop from a cartilage precursor by the process of *endochondral ossification* and are thus termed endochondral bones.

Membranous and endochondral bones are composed of a cortical outer layer and a spongy, cancellous inner layer (in membranous bone this is termed the *diploë*). Both components of bone, cortical and cancellous, may be used for bone grafts either individually or together depending on the requirements for reconstruction. The relative amount of cortical and cancellous components in each type of bone varies according to body location, but in general endochondral bone contains a greater amount of cancellous material than does membranous bone. The anatomic configuration of the cortical and cancellous components of bone has an influence on their healing as bone grafts (Fig 4–1). Cortical bone is characterized by a very dense or compact arrangement of the organic matrix and the predominantly hydroxyapatite (HA) inorganic mineral component. The cortical layer is traversed by microtubules termed *haversian canals* that contain capillaries that connect with each other and with larger tubules termed *nutritive canals.* Osteocytes occupy lacunae within cortical bone and derive their nourishment through communication with the haversian system. Bone is deposited in concentric layers around the haversian canals to create the microscopic unit, the osteon.

Cancellous bone is composed of loosely woven trabeculae of organic and inorganic bone separated by large spaces filled with blood and marrow cells and osteoprogenitor (mesenchymal) cells. Cancellous bone does not contain haversian systems.

The most common source of bone graft is *autogenous,* and this represents the "gold standard." Bone *allografts* are derived from living or cadaver donors of the same species. These grafts generally elicit an immunologic response in the recipient and, like other allografts, are at risk for the transfer of certain diseases. Bone allografts are occasionally employed in situations where the need for bone graft material exceeds the availability and

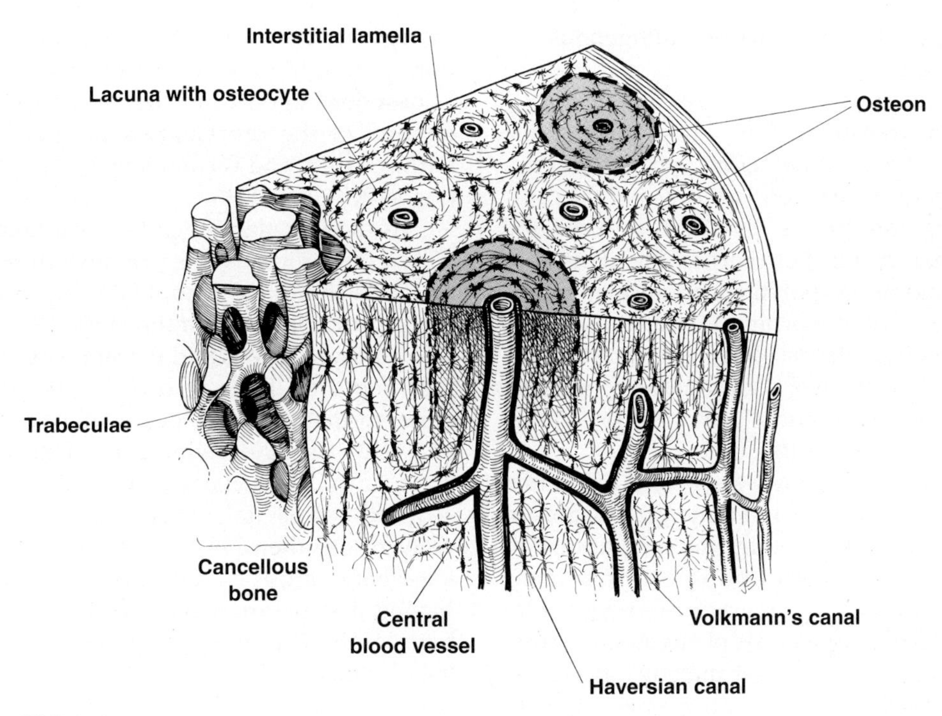

FIG 4–1.
Morphology of bone.

practicality of autogenous donor sites (i.e., whole femur or humerus grafts). Bone *xenografts* are derived from different species (usually bovine or porcine) and are infrequently used because of their immunogenicity and high rate of resorption.

Autogenous bone graft repair occurs by the processes of *incorporation, osteoconduction, osteoinduction,* and *osteogenesis.*

Incorporation is the process of adherence of the host tissues to the bone graft and the envelopment and admixture of necrotic and viable new bone. Incorporation ideally requires immobilization of the bone graft, close contact of the surrounding soft tissues and bone to the bone graft, and a viable and well-vascularized recipient bed. The incorporation of cortical and cancellous bone is similar but is variably influenced by the age and physiologic skeletal metabolism of the recipient as well as the proliferative activities of local and regional osteoprogenitor cells and the biomechanical properties of the repair site.

Osteoconduction is the predominant mechanism by which free, nonvascularized bone grafts "take" and is characterized by capillary and osteoprogenitor cellular ingrowth from the recipient bed into the bone graft, usually along the vascular channels and spaces previously occupied by the graft's cells. A bone graft therefore serves as a scaffold or stable template for cellular ingrowth and the deposition of new bone as the old bone is resorbed. This process is known as "creeping substitution."

Osteoinduction is the process by which local mesenchymal cells in contact with the matrix of the bone graft differentiate into osteoprogenitor cells and form new bone. This process is thought to be regulated by bone morphogenic protein (a component of the organic matrix) and specific enzymes and enzyme inhibitors.

Osteogenesis is the formation of new bone by surviving cells within the bone graft. It is the predominant mechanism for new bone growth in vascularized bone grafts. Osteogenesis occurs to a much lesser extent in nonvascularized bone grafts and especially in cortical bone grafts where the density of the bone impairs early revascularization; survival of graft surface cells and osteocytes is limited to a maximum depth of 0.3 mm.

Healing of Nonvascularized Autogenous Bone Grafts

Primary Stage

After transplantation, the graft is surrounded by a blood clot, and an intense inflammatory reaction ensues in the surrounding soft tissues. By the first week the inflammatory reaction bathes the graft in a fluid exudate of polynuclear and mononuclear cells (polymorphonuclear leukocytes, lymphocytes, plasma cells, osteoclasts) suspended in a lattice of scant fibrous connective tissue. Capillary buds begin to proliferate around the graft at this time.

During the second week, the inflammatory reaction around the bone graft begins to subside and is replaced by fibrous granulation tissue and giant cells having osteoclastic activity. Within the bone graft, osteocytic autolysis proceeds to necrosis of the tissue within the haversian canals and marrow spaces. As the granulation response progresses, capillary buds infiltrate the graft through these anatomic portals, and the necrotic cellular debris is phagocytized by invading macrophages. Coincident with the ingrowth of capillaries, the now empty lacunae, haversian canals, and trabeculae are repopulated with primitive mesenchymal cells.

This primary stage of autogenous bone graft repair lasts for approximately 2 weeks and is similar in cortical and cancellous grafts. Following the primary stage of bone graft repair, cortical and cancellous bone grafts diverge with respect to their rate, mechanism, and completeness of repair.

Secondary Repair

Cancellous Bone Grafts. Following the primary period of repair, cancellous bone grafts are usually completely revascularized owing to the larger channels available for capillary penetration and the facilitated access of phagocytes and osteoclasts. The rate of revascularization and repair of cancellous bone is related to its density (i.e., its number of trabeculae). Under certain circumstances, revascularization of cancellous bone may occur within several hours of transplantation by the process of inosculation (end-to-end alignment of the transplant and recipient vessels), although the primary method of revascularization is thought to occur by capillary ingrowth as described above. In general, capillary penetration of the cancellous bone graft occurs within 4 days and is complete by 2 to 4 weeks (Fig 4–2).

As the vascular integration of a cancellous bone graft proceeds, the primitive mesenchymal cells that have repopulated the edges of the vacant trebeculae of the graft differentiate into osteogenic cells and then into osteoblasts that deposit a layer of osteoid (appositional bone formation) that eventually surrounds and seals the underlying core of devitalized bone graft. Osteoclasts attack these isolated sequestra of devitalized bone graft and gradually resorb them. In time, the entire cancellous bone graft is replaced by new bone having a structure similar to that of the old bone graft. The marrow spaces of the renovated cancellous bone graft eventually refill with hematopoietic marrow cells.

Since the mechanical strength of a cancellous bone graft is not appreciably affected by necrosis, the initial deposition of new bone onto its necrotic bony surfaces tends to increase the mechanical strength and radiodensity of the graft. Over time, as the necrotic bone is gradually resorbed, the mechanical strength of a cancellous bone graft returns to normal.

Cortical Bone Grafts. The vascular integration of a cortical bone graft occurs through the preexisting haversian canals, starting first at the periphery and then proceeding to the interior of the graft. Because these channels are smaller and more widely dispersed than the vascular spaces of cancellous bone, the rate of revascularization and repair in a cortical bone graft is substantially decreased. Generally, the capillary penetration of a cortical bone graft does not occur until the sixth day, and complete vascular integration takes 1 to 2 months (Fig 4–3).

Capillary ingrowth into a cortical bone graft is facilitated by increased osteoclastic activity, which results in resorption and widening of the haversian canals. By the fourth week, the osteoclastic activity of the periphery of the graft and its interior is quantitatively

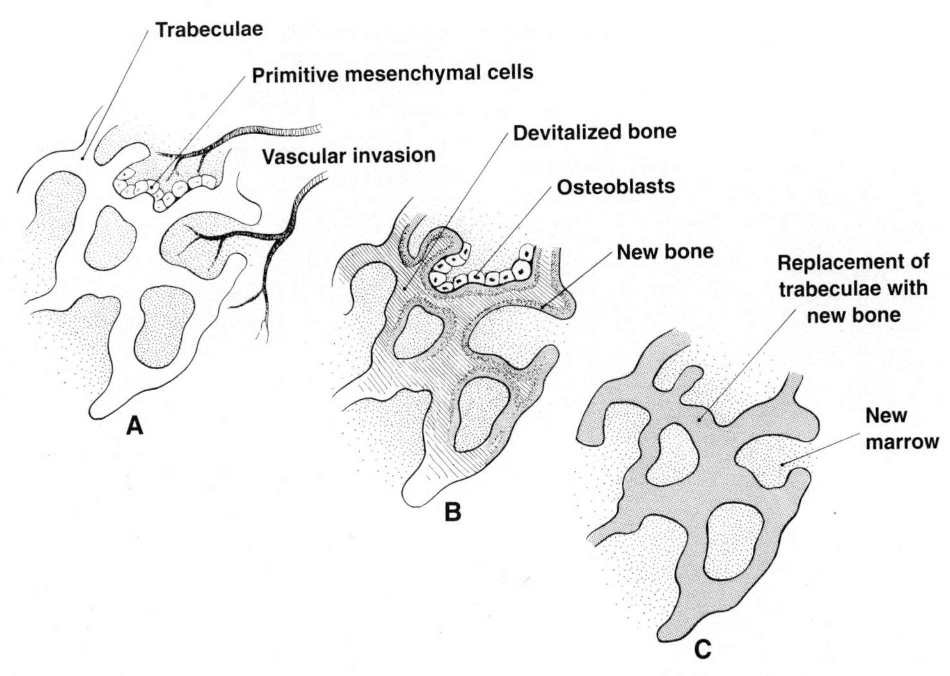

FIG 4–2.
Healing of cancellous bone grafts.

equivalent. The increased osteoclastic activity in a cortical bone graft persists for over a year following grafting. Although increased, this osteoclastic activity is directed primarily toward widening of the haversion canals with very little resorption of the remaining interstitial bone. After the haversian canals are widened to an appropriate size, the osteoclastic activity ceases. Mesenchymal cells then line the canals, differentiate into osteoblasts, and begin to form new appositional bone approximately 12 weeks following grafting. The new bone effectively seals the necrotic bone from further osteoclastic activity. The result is an admixture of new and necrotic bone that persists over time. The proportion of viable new bone to necrotic bone in cortical bone grafts increases for up to 6 months following transplantation and remains unchanged thereafter.

Owing to the fact that a cortical bone graft is initially repaired by osteoclastic activity, the mechanical strength of the graft decreases as a direct function of the graft's porosity. These grafts are approximately 40% to 50% weaker than normal bone at 6 weeks to 6 months following transplantation. As new bone is formed to create a permanent admixture of new and necrotic bone in a cortical bone graft, its mechanical strength and radiodensity gradually increase over time and by 1 to 2 years are nearly normal.

Local Wound Factors in Bone Graft Repair

The repair of cortical and cancellous bone grafts is characterized by the appearance of osteocytes, osteoblasts, and osteoclasts in and around the graft site. These cells exert their respective activities on the repair process, which differs according to the type of graft. The observation of these cells in the bone soon after grafting suggests that some osteogenic elements survive the transplantation process. It is thought that the three basic cell types of bone (osteocytes, osteoblasts, and osteoclasts) are incapable of mitosis and therefore the production of new bone cells resides in a primitive mesenchymal or osteoprogenitor cell. The periosteum, endosteum, intracortical elements, and marrow elements represent the four main sources from which surviving osteoprogenitor cells in the bone graft may be derived. Endosteal lining cells and marrow

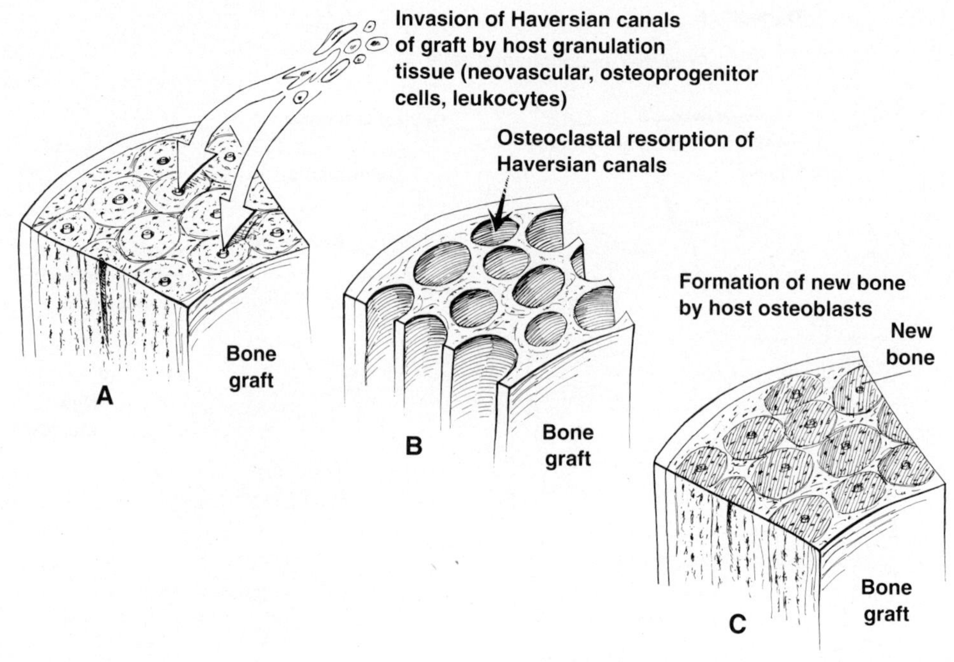

FIG 4–3.
Cortical bone grafts.

stroma cells together are responsible for the production of more than half of the new bone in the graft.

The remaining new bone is derived from the recipient site osteoprogenitor cells. The most likely sources for these cells are the capillary endothelial cells, circulating monocytes, reticuloendothelial cells, and fibroblasts; all of these are components of the granulation tissue ingrowth that characterize cortical and cancellous bone grafts. The inducement of osteoprogenitor cells to differentiate into bone repair cells is thought to be the result of their contact with substances released from the necrotizing bone and marrow tissue within the graft. Studies have shown that a non–species-specific glycoprotein component of bone matrix, bone morphogenic protein, is the active moiety in bone induction. With respect to endochondral bone induction, the recipient site mesenchymal cells that produce type II collagen serve as the progenitors of chondroblasts. These cells lay down a cartilage precursor that induces the attachment of osteoprogenitor cells and ultimately leads to new bone formation. In membranous bone grafts, the target cell for bone morphogenic protein is the perivascular connective tissue cell, or "pericyte," in the recipient bed. The membraneous bone graft provides a supplementary supply of marrow mesenchymal cells and a requisite structural framework upon which new bone formation may occur.

Local nutritional and electromechanical forces can exert a profound effect on the differentiation of primitive mesenchymal cells into osteogenic, chondrogenic, or fibrogenic cell lines and thus have an influence on the repair of transplanted bone. Conditions of high oxygenation and compression lead to osteoblast formation, as opposed to conditions of low oxygenation and compression, which favor chondrocyte formation. Compression forces and concave surfaces tend to generate electronegative potentials that favor osteoblastic activity and the production of new bone. Tensile forces and convex surfaces tend to generate electropositive potentials that promote osteoclastic activity and bone resorption. These forces collectively act on a surviving bone graft and influence its remodeling to achieve a state of electrical neutrality.

The site of bone graft placement can have an influence on its ultimate fate. For example, a bone graft that is transplanted to reconstruct a defect normally occupied by bone *(orthotop-*

ically transplanted) favors new bone formation and retention. Bone grafts placed into sites not normally occupied by bone *(heterotopically transplanted)* are usually resorbed, and this is unrelated to the vascularity of the recipient tissues. Exceptions to the latter are seen in the transplantation of vomer, nasal bone, and the perpendicular plate of the ethmoid, which demonstrate very little resorption regardless of their site of transplantation.

The survival of bone grafts is also influenced by the presence or absence of attached periosteum. Bone grafts transplanted with intact periosteum undergo less resorption and demonstrate improved survival over comparable bone grafts without periosteum. Survival is enhanced when the periosteal surface is placed in direct contact with the surrounding soft tissues. Bone grafts without periosteum undergo less resorption when their cancellous surfaces are placed in direct contact with recipient bone and their cortical surfaces are in contact with the surrounding soft tissues.

When used as an onlay bone graft to the facial skeleton, membranous bone demonstrates less resorption, earlier vascularization, and more new bone formation as compared with an endochondral bone graft.

The recipient site can be characterized as either bone resorptive or depository depending on its location. In a growing child, bone grafts transplanted to periosteal depository sites (i.e., zygoma or mandible) maintain significantly more volume than those transplanted to periosteal resorptive sites (i.e., orbital vault or nose).

Other local factors that may have an influence on the healing and ultimate survival of a bone graft include the quality of the recipient bed (irradiation, scarring, contracture, or infection), the age of the patient, the type of fixation or lack of fixation of the graft, the size of the graft, and the positioning of the graft with respect to local mechanical forces (i.e., inlay, onlay, bridging).

Common Sources of Nonvascularized Bone Autografts

Iliac Bone Grafts

The ilium is an excellent source of cortical, cancellous, or combined cortical-cancellous bone grafts. It is the most commonly used donor site for autologous bone graft material and is employed for the reconstruction of a wide variety of bony defects throughout the body. Iliac bone has a tough, dense cortical layer that lends itself well to the reconstruction of high-stress areas such as in defects of the long bones and hand. Its dense cortical component also facilitates anchorage by pins and screws for rigid fixation. These desirable qualities are offset by the relative rigidity and brittleness of the cortical component, which makes shaping and bending quite difficult. The inner table of the ilium is preferably harvested because of its decreased points of muscle attachment. A large volume of cortical and cancellous bone can be harvested from the ilium. The iliac crest is especially applicable in situations requiring a large amount of cancellous "filler" bone in reconstructions such as in the treatment of bony nonunions, alveolar cleft defects, and arthrodeses. In children, the iliac crest is covered by a cartilaginous apophysis that must be preserved for normal growth and development of the ilium. The primary disadvantage of the iliac crest donor site is its postoperative morbidity, which is related to the amount of bone harvested. Patients frequently experience prolonged pain and may require crutches to support ambulation. Care must be taken to avoid injury to the lateral femoral cutaneous nerve during bone graft harvest because this may result in meralgia paresthetica—severe pain in the distribution of the nerve.

Rib Grafts

Autologous rib grafts are cortical-cancellous, membranous bone grafts that are used primarily in the reconstruction of cranial defects and as onlay bone grafts of the facial skeleton to correct acquired and congenital deformities. Rib grafts are quite soft and flexible, particularly in younger patients, and are therefore less desirable for the reconstruction of defects subjected to high stresses. Rib grafts provide an extraordinarily large volume of bone graft material for reconstruction, and they are relatively easy to harvest. If the rib periosteal envelope is left in situ at the donor site, the rib will regenerate in both children and adults. As with any bone graft, the "take" of a rib graft is enhanced if its periosteum is left intact.

The primary disadvantage of rib grafts is their resorption when used as onlay grafts. This is perhaps due to the greater cancellous component of rib as compared with calvarial bone. The harvest of a rib graft carries the risk of pneumothorax and postoperative atelectasis as a result of splinting. Split-rib grafts provide an excellent material for cranioplasty, and when compared with alloplastic materials, the incidence of infection is reduced with their use.

Calvarial Bone Grafts

The calvarium is composed of membranous bone with a predominantly cortical component represented by the inner and outer tables. The cancellous component of calvarial bone is the diploë, which varies in thickness and is poorly developed in children. Calvarial bone can be used as a source of bone graft material for a wide variety of reconstructive problems in the facial skeleton. Because of its proximity to the face and ease of inclusion into one operating field, the calvarium is a preferred donor site for bone grafts to the face and calvarium. It is usually harvested as a split graft to preserve the inner table of cortical bone for protection of the brain and meninges. When large amounts of bone are required for reconstruction, the calvarium is harvested as a full-thickness graft and then split ex vivo into its inner and outer tables with one of the tables returned to the donor defect. Split calvarial bone grafts are excellent as onlay, inlay, or bridging grafts of the facial skeleton and calvarium since they retain their volume much better than endochondral bone grafts. In children, split calvarial bone is quite flexible and can be easily contoured. In adults, calvarial bone becomes rigid and brittle and does not lend itself well to bending. As with other bone grafts having a cortical component, calvarial bone can be rigidly fixed with wires, plates and screws, or pins. In older children and adults, the well-developed diploë can be harvested as a cancellous bone graft for closure of alveolar clefts and smaller spaces in the facial skeleton. The harvest of calvarial bone is technically difficult and carries a risk of injury to the brain and meninges. While the volume of bone that can be harvested is limited, the area of bone available is considerable; an entire hemicalvarium can be reconstructed with local split calvarial bone grafts.

Vascularized Bone Autografts

The transplantation of vascularized bone for reconstruction has many advantages over nonvascularized bone autografts, namely, earlier bony union, hypertrophy, and greater mechanical strength. Preservation of the nutrient blood supply in vascularized bone grafts allows survival of the vast majority of the cells, thereby preempting the need for healing by "creeping substitution." The method of repair of vascularized bone is similar to that of fracture repair, with the formation of callus and subsequent remodeling. The indications for vascularized bone grafts over conventional bone grafts are in the treatment of large defects in long bones (i.e., greater than 6 to 8 cm), in composite defects (bone, mucosa, skin), in the treatment of difficult nonunions, and for bone grafting in scarred, poorly vascularized, or irradiated fields.

Vascularized bone grafts derive their blood supply from either the endosteal or periosteal route or both. The primary blood supply to endochondral bone is through nutrient vessels that penetrate the cortex through identifiable foramina to supply the medullary or endosteal system. The contribution of the periosteum to cortical blood supply in endochondral bone is relatively minor. In most long bones, a dominant nutritive vascular pedicle is present and allows for isolation and transfer of the bone as a vascularized pedicled graft. Common donor sites for vascularized endochondral bone grafts include the ilium based upon the deep circumflex iliac system, the fibula based upon the peroneal system, and the spine of the scapula based upon the circumflex scapular system (Fig 4–4).

In membranous bone, the predominant blood supply is also by the endosteal route, which for calvarial bone is derived from the meninges, thus making it impractical to harvest with an endosteal supply. Calvarial bone will survive to a variable degree on its periosteal attachments and has been successfully transferred as a vascularized bone graft based

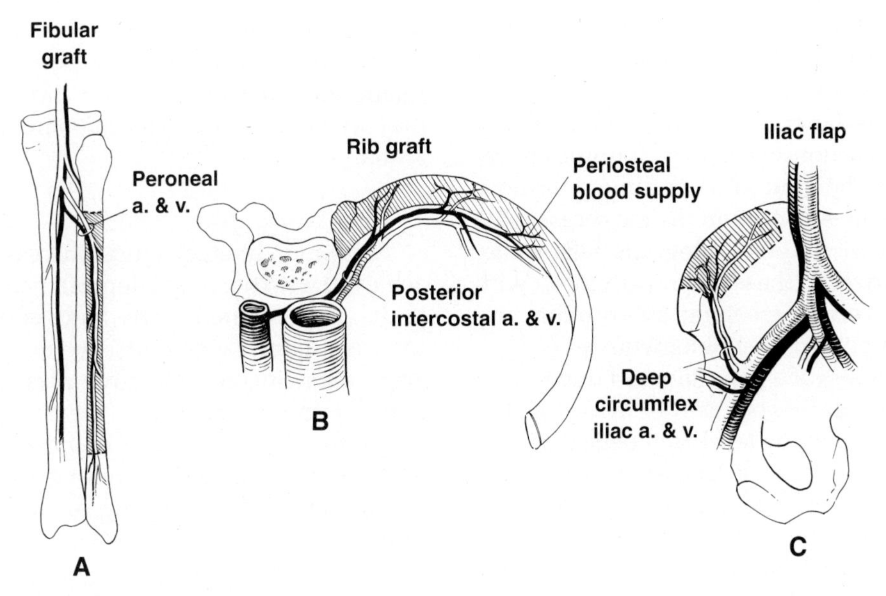

FIG 4–4.
Common donor sites for vascularized bone grafts.

upon the superficial temporal system or through attachments of the temporalis muscle to reconstruct defects of the mandible, orbit, and maxilla. Rib will also survive on its periosteum nourished by the internal mammary system or by attachments to the pectoralis major muscle. The dominant blood supply to the rib and its periosteum, however, is through the posterior nutrient artery, a branch of the posterior intercostal system. Vascularized rib grafts based on the posterior system have improved survival and healing characteristics. Owing to the curved shape of the rib, vascularized rib grafts have been employed extensively in mandibular reconstruction. In the few successful cases in which vascularized rib grafts have been transferred for reconstruction of tibial defects, hypertrophy of the graft has been observed (a remodeling response to the forces imposed by weight bearing). Because these grafts have limited weight-bearing capabilities, their use in reconstruction of the long bones is not recommended.

Immunology and Antigenicity of Bone

The use of bone allografts for reconstruction is appealing from many perspectives: their use obviates donor site morbidity and the additional operative time required for graft harvest, and there are no practical limitations on the quantity of graft material available for reconstruction. The shortcomings of bone allografts lie principally in the immunogenicity resulting from the genetic disparity between the host and recipient and the adverse effects that the host immune response has on graft incorporation and healing.

Immunogenicity in bone allografts is derived primarily from the cells of the graft and to a lesser extent the organic matrix. The cell surface transplantation antigens found on the heterogeneous cells of skeletal tissue are the most potent sources of sensitization. Fresh bone allografts will elicit from the host a cell-mediated immunologic reaction. Antibodies to the major histocompatibility antigens in the graft develop in proportion to the level of genetic disparity between graft and host. Removal of the marrow has little effect on stifling the immunologic reaction. Freezing will remove the antibody response but has little effect on cell-mediated immunity. Freeze-drying of the bone graft will decrease both types of immune response but will not completely eliminate them.

Bone Allografts

The host response to bone allografts is similar to that of other tissue allografts and varies from complete acceptance and repair of the graft to frank rejection based on the level of genetic disparity between the graft and host. In the former scenario, the graft heals in much the same fashion as an autogenous bone graft. In the latter, an intense inflammatory rejection reaction results in continuous resorption of the graft at its periphery without any creeping substitution. In most cases, the host response to bone allografts falls somewhere between these two extremes, with variable levels of creeping substitution and resorption occurring simultaneously.

The success of a bone allograft depends in large part on its rate of incorporation, which is dependent upon the level of genetic disparity between graft and host. The primary phase of healing in a bone allograft is similar to bone autografts with the formation of an inflammatory granulation tissue response. By the end of the first week the host capillaries invading the graft occlude, depending on the level of immunologic response. Both host and graft osteoprogenitor cells within and around the graft selectively die in response to this vascular shutdown, and the graft undergoes regional or complete necrosis. A secondary osteogenic response may be initiated by the host 4 to 6 weeks following bone transplantation and persist until final healing is concluded.

Bone allografts generally progress to a satisfactory result, although their healing rate may be substantially delayed. Union of the graft to the host bone occurs gradually by callus formed both periosteally and endosteally. The replacement of necrotic bone by creeping substitution of new bone to create the typical admixture of new and necrotic bone (as seen in bone autografts) is limited or absent in bone allografts. This, combined with the selective resorption of the graft, substantially reduces its structural ability to withstand stress and results in an increased incidence of fractures. Periosteal new bone formation around the bone allograft serves as the interface for attachment of the soft tissues, which is rather tenuous when compared with bone autografts.

Because of the superiority of autogenous bone for graft material and the variable immunogenicity of allogeneic bone, the clinical use of bone allograft in plastic surgery remains limited. Demineralized freeze-dried bone allografts have been shown experimentally to retain the capacity for bone induction and may well find future application in the clinical arena.

Bone Xenografts

Although limited clinical success has been achieved with the use of deproteinated bovine grafts impregnated with autogenous bone marrow, bone xenografts have very little application in reconstructive plastic surgery and are poor substitutes for autografts or allografts. The major pitfall of bone xenografts lies in their marked immunogenicity even when subjected to freezing or deproteinization.

Technical Considerations

The successful clinical application of bone grafts for reconstruction depends on numerous technical factors intrinsic to procurement, preservation, placement, and fixation of the graft material. Bone grafts should be harvested and tailored with the least amount of surgical trauma to minimize injury to the resident cells and periosteal attachments. This is preferably accomplished by the use of sharp osteotomes, bone cutters, rongeurs, and curets. The use of high-speed saws and burrs should be kept to a minimum because these instruments generate high temperatures (temperatures in excess of 42°C will kill bone cells) and result in significant local mechanical trauma to the bone. Prolonged irrigation or bathing of the graft with physiologic saline should be avoided because this may be toxic to the viable cells on and within the graft. Similarly, the bathing or irrigation of bone grafts in antibiotic solutions such as neomycin and bacitracin may be deleterious to graft survival. Accidental contamination of a bone graft in the operating room should be managed by sterilizing the graft in 70% alcohol followed by washing in 0.6N hydrogen chloride solution for 1 hour. As an alternative to this, the graft may be sterilized in ethylene oxide for 30 minutes. Both of these methods kill the viable cells within the graft but preserve its bone induction properties. Autoclaving or irradiation of the graft (in sufficient doses to sterilize it) destroys both the cellular and matrix components of the graft, thereby diminishing its usefulness. Of note is the adverse effect that freezing has on autologous bone graft take, commonly resulting in aseptic necrosis of the graft.

For optimum survival, bone should be transplanted immediately following harvest. If this is not practical, the graft should be placed in a moistened, blood-soaked sponge and stored in a container covered by moist sponges. In this manner, the graft will remain viable for up to 4 to 6 hours. When placed into the recipient site, the graft should be in intimate contact with bone and the surrounding soft tissues. Dead space around the graft should be avoided. It is advantageous to align the graft such that its cancellous portion is in contact with the cancellous bone of the recipient bed. Graft survival is enhanced if the recipient bed has been previously prepared, is devoid of necrotic material, and is actively producing new blood vessels and bone (i.e., granulating). The thickness of a free cancellous bone graft should be limited to a maximum of 5 mm.

Rigid fixation of the bone graft is important for successful graft "take" and is preferably accomplished with wires, pins, or plates and screws, although wedging of the graft or packing followed by immobilization of the grafted part or extremity may suffice in certain situations.

CARTILAGE

When compared with bone grafts, cartilage grafts are especially adapted to augmentation of the facial skeleton owing to their resistance to remodeling and resorption. Cartilage is composed of three main elements: chondrocytes, matrix, and bound water. Chondrocytes produce type II collagen and a proteoglycan matrix and are essential for maintaining the viability of cartilage. Chondrocytes are derived from mesenchymal cells containing chondrogenic DNA, which stimulates their differentiation. Mesenchymal cells, myoblasts, and fibroblasts containing the chondrogenic DNA may also be stimulated to differentiate into chondrocytes and form cartilage in the presence of bone morphogenic protein. Chondrocytes reside in lacunae within the cartilage matrix and are not normally replaced during the life of the cartilage.

The bound water in cartilage matrix serves to facilitate the diffusion of nutrients because cartilage has no blood vessels and derives its entire nutritive support from the surrounding perichondrium or synovium. The compressive and tensile forces acting upon cartilage in its normal environment cause migration and shifting of the water layers, which promote the diffusion of nutrients throughout the matrix. This is thought to be a primary mechanism in cartilage nutrition. Immobilization of cartilage (as occurs in cartilage grafting) results in thinning or resorption, and this may be a direct consequence of impaired nutrition.

Chondrocytes produce type II collagen, which is tightly complexed to a proteoglycan matrix. The amount of collagen in cartilage varies according to cartilage type but generally represents 40% to 50% of the dry weight of cartilage. The collagen moiety imparts mechanical strength to cartilage and provides tensile forces that counteract and balance the internal expansive forces caused by proteoglycan hydration. Various amounts of elastin are present in cartilage and impart elasticity to the matrix.

Three types of cartilage are found in the human body and are based on the predominant supporting fiber type: (1) *hyaline cartilage* is the lining cartilage of joints, the thoracic costal cartilage, the supporting cartilage of the tracheobronchial tree, and the nasal septum. This cartilage is uniquely suited to compressive and expansive forces. (2) *Elastic cartilage* has an abundance of elastin in its matrix and is found in the nasal tip, the external ear, and the larynx. Its easy flexibility and shape memory as a scaffold allow for repeated deformation with return to its original shape. (3) *Fibrocartilage* is composed of a predominantly fibrous matrix and is found in the intervertebral disks and in tendon attachments to bone. Fibrocartilage is tough and resilient and is capable of withstanding prolonged compressive and tensile stresses.

Healing and Repair of Autologous Cartilage Grafts

Most cartilage grafts employed for reconstruction are autogenous and are clearly superior to allografts and xenografts. The success of transplantation of an autogenous cartilage graft can be defined in terms of the ultimate survival of the graft and the degree to which its structure and volume are retained at the transplantation site. The maintenance of structure and volume in an autogenous cartilage graft depends on the viability of its chondrocytes, which are necessary for maintaining the collagen/proteoglycan matrix. Unlike bone, collagen does not heal by "creeping substitution" and does not normally become "vascularized." Chondrocytes in a cartilage graft are not replaced by new cells from the recipient bed, and therefore survival of the chondrocytes within the graft depends on the diffusion of nutrients from the surrounding soft tissues, and this is related to the condition of the recipient bed (i.e., well vascularized vs. scarred or irradiated), the adequacy of local mechanical forces in promoting the diffusion and distribution of nutrients, and the size of the graft.

The clinical experience with autogenous cartilage grafts has been characterized by variable rates of resorption depending on the type of cartilage used as a graft, how the graft is prepared prior to implantation, and where it is implanted. For example, hyaline cartilage resists vascular invasion if it is kept in an environment that allows motion (bending, compression, etc.). If rib cartilage is transferred to a relatively immobile site (e.g., nose), vascular invasion and partial resorption will occur. Cartilage grafts placed beneath the periosteum undergo more resorption and ossification than those placed above the periosteum. This may relate to pressure forces and immobilization of the graft in a subperiosteal pocket, both of which are thought to impair graft nutrition. Ear cartilage, which is elastic and is subjected to similar external forces as nasal cartilage, demonstrates less resorption when transferred as a graft to the nose.

Block grafts of autogenous cartilage undergo less resorption than do diced or crushed grafts. Crushing the graft destroys the chondrocytes and thus the ability of the graft to actively maintain its matrix. Autogenous cartilage grafts transplanted with intact perichondrium have a better survival rate and undergo less resorption than do grafts without attached perichondrium. Autografts with attached perichondrium also demonstrate more resorption on the sides having no perichondrium than on the sides with perichondrium. This underscores the importance of the perichondrium as a key source and conduit for nutrient diffusion. Hard freezing of a cartilage autograft destroys the chondrocytes and results in significant resorption of the graft.

Immunology of Cartilage Allografts and Xenografts

Cartilage allografts and xenografts generate mild to severe immunologic reactions; the more severe types of reactions are generally seen in xenografts. The antigens that stimulate immunologic sensitivity to cartilage allografts and xenografts reside primarily in the chondrocytes and are part of the major histocompatibility system. The chondrocytes, which reside within the collagen/proteoglycan matrix, cannot be readily accessed by cell or humorally mediated reactions and are therefore thought to occupy relatively "immunologically privileged" sites within cartilage. This condition changes when the graft is prepared (carved, crushed, etc.) prior to transplantation. The chondrocytes exposed by this preparation process then become inciters of, and targets for, a host immunologic response.

The proteoglycan molecule of the matrix demonstrates at least two antigenic sites on its protein core, which is for the most part protected by the glycosaminoglycans unless exposed by the preparation process.

The host immunologic response to a cartilage allograft or xenograft results in resorption of the graft, and this process is proportional to the intensity of the immunologic reaction. Three major host factors are involved in the destruction of a cartilage allograft or xenograft: lymphocytes, antibodies, and lymphokines.

While allografts and xenografts are characterized by a variable degree of resorption, a common denominator in this process appears to be the method in which cartilage grafts are preserved and stored prior to transplantation. The preservation process is capable of altering the immunogenicity and stability of cartilage grafts as well as their ultimate healing. Cartilage may be preserved fresh in saline or in an antibiotic solution; frozen, which may allow preservation of the chondrocytes; irradiated, which kills the chondrocytes and preserves the matrix; lyophilized (freeze-dried), which kills the chondrocytes, preserves the matrix, and stifles immunogenicity; preserved in thimerosol (Merthiolate) or Cialit, which kills the cells and alters the matrix; or by chemical cross-linking (to create dimensional stability).

Cartilage Allografts

Numerous studies support the efficacy of cartilage allografts in reconstruction. Unfortunately, the majority of these studies are retrospective clinical studies based upon clinical impressions, and most lack scientific objectivity. The experimental studies on cartilage allograft survival can be generally summarized as follows: *Fresh allografts* demonstrate survival of the chondrocytes and a mild immunologic reaction that subsides by 7 to 9 weeks. Resorption of fresh allografts is moderate (20% to 50%) and is greater if the graft is crushed as opposed to being transplanted as a block of tissue. Presumably, crushing of the cartilage allograft exposes more antigenic foci to the host immune mechanism, thereby hastening its destruction and removal. *Irradiated cartilage allografts* demonstrate progressive disappearance of the chondrocytes over time but relatively little inflammatory or immunologic reaction. It appears that irradiated cartilage persists as a nonviable implant that undergoes significant (40% to 100%) resorption and/or calcification. The greatest degree of resorption of irradiated allografts is seen when these grafts are transplanted subperiosteally. Allografts preserved in *Merthiolate* show a variable degree of resorption and interestingly demonstrate the repopulation of the graft to a viable degree with chondrocytes presumably from the host. Despite this observation, a significant amount of resorption is seen in Merthiolate-preserved grafts. *Lyophilized cartilage allografts* have shown a remarkable resistance to resorption (5% to 20%), most likely because of the altered immunogenicity induced by the freeze-drying process (similar to lyophilized bone). These grafts persist as nonviable implants and, similar to other cartilage allografts, undergo calcification if placed subperiosteally.

Despite the above experimental observations, the clinical experience with cartilage allografts has been quite good, with satisfactory clinical results being reported for chemically preserved, lyophilyzed, and irradiated cartilage allografts. The discrepancy between the laboratory and clinical findings may be related to the differences in healing responses between experimental animals and humans, the methods of preparation, and sites of placement of the grafts.

Cartilage Xenografts

The experimental and clinical experience with xenografts has been uniformly poor, with resorption rates as high as 50% to 100%. Recent clinical studies employing irradiated bovine cartilage grafts chemically cross-linked to render them antigenically inert and dimensionally stable have been quite promising. Cartilage grafts treated by the foregoing technique showed minimal absorption at 1 to 4 years, and biopsy specimens revealed fibrous encapsulation, no vascular invasion, and minimal inflammatory reaction.

Influences on Cartilage Graft Warping

Aside from resorption, a common, yet undesirable sequela of cartilage graft transplantation is warping (Fig 4–5). This is particularly applicable to rib or septal hyaline cartilage grafts but may also occur with elastic cartilage grafts. Warping is due to an alteration of the forces within the graft caused by carving or otherwise rendering the graft into a desired shape prior to transplantation. In order to understand this mechanism, it is helpful to examine some biomechanical properties of rib hyaline cartilage. In vivo, cartilage maintains its physical shape and mechanical

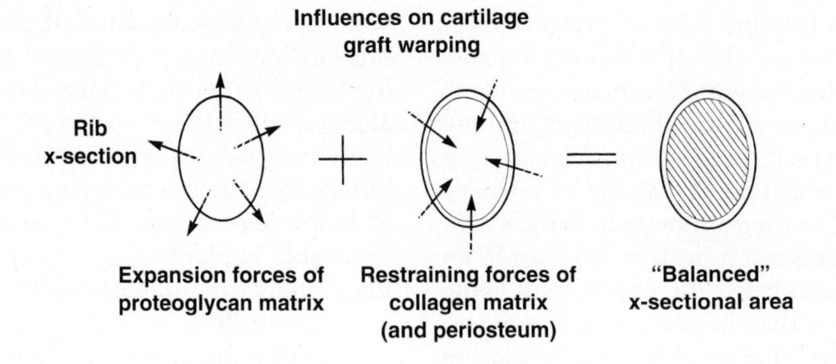

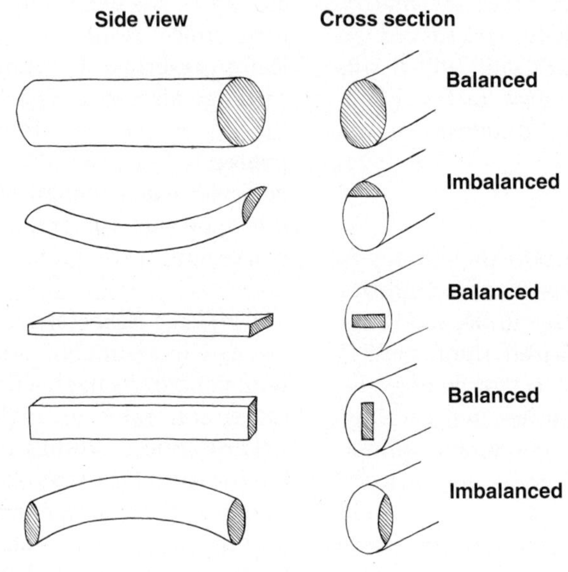

FIG 4–5.
Cartilage graft warping.

properties by virtue of a collagen framework that supports the proteoglycan matrix. The hydrophilic qualities of the proteoglycan matrix allow expansion forces to develop within the cartilage, and this creates turgor and resiliency. Ballooning of the cartilage because of expansion of its proteoglycan moiety as it takes on water is checked by the collagen component of the matrix, which is interspersed throughout the matrix and forms an investing layer at the periphery. When combined with a tightly enveloping perichondrium (although perichondrium is not requisite for this to occur), the cartilage has a *balanced cross-sectional area* with respect to its intrinsic forces, and this allows maintenance of shape and defines the biomechanical properties. Any alteration of the collagen or matrix component will therefore alter the dynamics of the balanced cross-sectional area and alter the shape of the cartilage. For example, if one removes one side of a length of whole rib cartilage, the rib will curve away from its cut side; the cross-sectional area becomes imbalanced with respect to the intrinsic forces. The tethering forces on the cut side are released and allow the expansion forces of the exposed matrix to distort the graft. Similarly, if one removes equal sections from opposing sides of the rib, no distortion will occur; the cross-sectional area remains balanced with respect to the intrinsic forces. By this model it is easy to predict how carved cartilage grafts might warp based upon the distortion of forces in the cross-sectional area. While perichondrium is not necessary for warping to occur, it may accentuate the degree of warping encountered in the graft.

The degree to which a cartilage graft will warp depends to a great extent on its thickness and three-dimensional position within the cross-sectional area. Thinner grafts near the periphery such as shavings tend to undergo more distortion than do thicker grafts; segments of rib composing 50% or greater of the cross-sectional area or grafts from the central portion of the cross-sectional area have little tendency to warp. A dilemma in this observation is encountered clinically: grafts carved from the most central portion of the cross-sectional area are rather flimsy and do not provide good structural support. Similarly, thicker grafts that are more structurally stable may be too bulky to use, for example, in reconstructions of the nasal tip and columella. Some ingenuous technical modifications utilizing rib tip cartilage grafts have been employed to overcome these mechanical and physical shortcomings.

The tendency for a cartilage graft to warp will be manifested within 30 minutes of carving; slight distortion in the graft may progress to significant distortion with further handling or later during the healing process. Methods to stifle the tendency for warping in cartilage grafts include transverse scoring of the graft on its concave side (if perichondrium is attached, both it and the peripheral cartilage layer are scored), crushing of the cartilage graft (which is quite effective but destroys many of the chondrocytes and results in greater graft resorption), and rigid fixation of the graft, which may also lead to its resorption.

Clinical Applications

Cartilage grafts can be employed for a wide variety of clinical reconstructive problems. They are most commonly used in the head and neck region and, in particular, in reconstructive rhinoplasty procedures. As onlay grafts they are superior for augmentation of the nasal dorsum and tip and for correcting minor contour deformities in secondary rhinoplasty procedures. For these purposes, nasal septal cartilage and conchal cartilage grafts from the ear are most commonly employed. For entire dorsal nasal reconstructions, rib cartilage grafts may be employed; their stability is enhanced by including perichondrium on one side of the graft. Because of the thin skin of the nose, sharp edges of a cartilage graft may be visible. To soften the contour, abrading the edges of the graft or crushing the graft has been proposed, although this may theoretically increase the risk for graft resorption.

Autogenous costal cartilage grafts have emerged as the preferred scaffold material for total-ear reconstruction for microtia or for reconstruction of other congenital or acquired ear deformities. In total-ear reconstructions, costal cartilage with attached perichondrium is harvested and carved into helical and scaphoconchal components, which are then assembled with nonabsorbable sutures and inserted into a dissected subcutaneous skin pocket or covered with temporal fascia and grafted with split-thickness skin. These reconstructions have been shown to grow in size as the patient reaches maturity.

As onlay grafts of the facial skeleton, cartilage grafts undergo less resorption when placed above the periosteum. In this position, however, they remain mobile and may therefore be less desirable than bone grafts.

Cartilage grafts have been used to reconstruct joint surfaces destroyed by disease or trauma. The most successful reconstructions have been in children, where nonvascularized, composite toe-joint bone/cartilage grafts with epiphyseal plates have been transferred and have demonstrated prolonged survival and growth. Several successful reconstructions of metacarpophalangeal and interphalangeal joint surfaces have used composite toe-joint cartilage/subchondral cancellous bone grafts. Vascularized whole-joint reconstructions are of recent interest and have been successfully employed for metacarpophalangeal joint reconstruction in the hand and for temporomandibular joint reconstruction.

The use of perichondrium as a graft to promote new cartilage formation has been shown to work experimentally in young animals. This technique has been employed with limited clinical success in the reconstruction of hand joints. Perichondral-cutaneous grafts have demonstrated chondrogenic potential experimentally and have been successfully employed for eyelid reconstruction. Recently, a polyglycolic acid scaffold impregnated with chondrocytes has been shown experimentally to promote new cartilage formation and holds promise for its future application in reconstructive plastic surgery.

ALLOPLASTIC MATERIALS

Numerous types of alloplastic materials have been implanted in the human body over the years to repair tissues, replace structural parts, augment the tissues, stabilize fractures, bond other materials to tissues, etc. The success of implanted alloplastic materials has parallelled our growth in knowledge of the physical/chemical composition of biomaterials, their fabrication, and their reactivity in a biological environment.

All implanted alloplastic materials behave as foreign bodies inflicting trauma to the surrounding tissues and eliciting inflammatory cellular responses. Biocompatibility is a requisite for successful incorporation and retention of an alloplast. This is related to the mechanical, physicochemical, and electrochemical properties of the material as well as its durability. Of key importance are the surface characteristics of the biomaterial and the events that occur at the tissue-biomaterial interface.

The durability of an alloplastic material is often equated with its degree of inertness, but most alloplasts may eventually undergo degradation. This occurs by mechanical and physical events intrinsic to the material itself (i.e., fatigue) and also by the processes of hydrolysis, phagocytosis, and lysis generated by the local cellular milieu. The relevance of alloplast failure assumes importance with regard to time, i.e., the durability of the alloplast vs. the expected life span of the recipient. This aside, important concerns are waged by the undesirable local, regional, and systemic side effects elicited by the microfragmentation of alloplasts in a biological environment, events that may lead to toxic side effects in the host.

Beyond the degree of inertness, a host of factors intrinsic to an alloplast have been found to affect the immediate cellular environment. These include the size and shape of the material and its surface configuration, porosity, and composition. All of these components have an influence on the preferential affinity and adhesiveness of cells to the surface of a biomaterial and define its biocompatibility.

Clinical experience has shown that retention of an alloplastic material is enhanced by its deep placement in tissues, which serves to diffuse the impact of any mechanical or physical disharmony between the material and the surrounding soft tissues. A thin soft-tissue covering may therefore predispose an alloplast to exposure by the simple mechanism of trauma that occasions daily contact with the environment. An ideal alloplast would promote cellular adhesion and regeneration but also have the physical/mechanical properties that complement the viscoelastic nature of the investing soft tissues. These "ideal" properties require further definition.

Tissue responses to biomaterials have been studied primarily in the context of surface-mediated cellular inflammatory reactions generated by native host tissues surrounding implants, and these may vary according to the body site. This surface-mediated cellular response depends upon cellular adherence, which influences (and is influenced by) the type of protein that is initially adsorbed to the surface of the alloplast. Activation of complement on the alloplast surface is thought to be an important step in the pathway to macrophage adhesion and activation, and this in turn plays a pivotal role in modulation of the cellular inflammatory response. The inflammatory cellular reaction to an alloplast decreases over time, thus indicating that a biocompatible alloplast ceases to provide a stimulus for continued inflammatory response. A chronic, "biocompatible" foreign-body response persists to a variable degree around the implant, and the intensity of this reaction is thought to relate to the efficiency of cellular adherence and the physical and chemical stability of the implant. Thus, an implanted biocompatible alloplast material eventually becomes invested by a layer of fibrous tissue and assumes a "steady state" with its biological environment.

Since tissue adherence to an alloplast is widely accepted to be a major factor in its retention in the human body, methods to improve tissue adherence have evolved as important components of the design and manufacturing process. Alloplasts having pore sizes of 30 to 50 μm or greater allow fibrous tissue ingrowth to provide firm anchorage of the material to the surrounding soft tissues. Certain polymers have been fabricated with pore sizes sufficient to allow tissue ingrowth and fixation, and this has been used to advantage in the application of alloplasts for augmentation of the facial skeleton (malar and chin implants) and for repairing fascial defects of the abdominal wall. Alloplast porosity may also serve to promote osteogenic conduction in implanted ceramics where the invasion of the implant by the "creeping substitution" of osteoprogenitor cells is a defined goal. One disadvantage of implant porosity is the substantially increased surface area of the implant that is exposed to the tissues. This may hasten the degradation of the biomaterial or serve to enhance the foreign-body reaction to it. Another potential disadvantage of porosity is the alteration of the physical characteristics of the alloplast such as strength and flexibility.

Surface texturing has been shown to increase soft-tissue adhesion and elicit "biocompatible," foreign-body–type morphologic changes in the macrophages and foreign-body giant cells in contact with the implant (increased cytoplasmic-to-nuclear ratio). The mechanisms by which surface texture initiates these cellular changes are not completely understood.

Textured materials are composed of surface "spikes," and it has been proposed that the radius of the curvature of the spike tip could change the surface energy of cells next to the implant to sufficiently affect the type, rate of adsorption, and conformation of adsorbed proteins, which may then induce morphologic changes in the cells reacting to the implant. Surface texturing may therefore have an influence on the cellular response by mimicking particles; the tip of a surface texture spike elicits a foreign-body reaction. By altering the height and width of surface micropillars (i.e., changing the size and shape of the surface texture spike), different cellular reactions to a biomaterial can be induced.

Surface texturing may cause chronic traumatization of the surrounding soft tissues by the rough surface. This would obviously depend on the size and shape of the texture spike as well as the relative rigidity and motion of the scaffold to that of the soft tissues, problems that have not been well defined. Surface texturing has been shown to cause malignant changes in cells adjacent to implanted biomaterials in rodents, but thus far this has not been observed in humans.

While texturing and porosity have been shown to improve tissue adherence to an implant, these surface characteristics may also promote bacterial colonization, which can result in extrusion of the implant. The preferential affinity of the implant surface to bacteria or eukaryotic cells is thus an important determinant of outcome.

Silicone

Silicone is a generic term for a family of polymers derived from the element silicon. As an implantable biomaterial it is most commonly used in the form of the dimethylsiloxane polymer, which is a large molecule of repetitive units containing silicon, oxygen, and methane. The extent of polymerization determines the viscosity of dimethylsiloxane and hence its physical state: liquid, gel, or solid. Silicone polymers are easily contaminated with heavy metals, low–chain-length polymers, and other impurities during the manufacturing process, and their refinement requires specialized filtration and sterilization. Only medical-grade silicone is approved for implantation in the human body.

By varying the viscosity of silicone to simulate the differing physical and mechanical properties of soft tissues and bone (i.e., liquid, viscous gel, solid), a variety of implants having complex shapes and volumes can be custom-fabricated. The rubbery consistency and flexibility of high-viscosity silicone make it particularly suited as an onlay material for the augmentation of tissues. This type of silicone is also used for fabricating inflatable saline-filled mammary implants and is also the investing layer around gel-filled custom implants and mammary implants. The availability of liquid and viscous gel silicones for human implantation is limited at this time because of concerns over their potential for migration and toxicity in tissues and a presumed but unproven association with human adjuvant disease.

The surface of most implantable silicones is smooth, and this diminishes tissue adherence and may be a prominent factor in implant extrusion, especially if the implant is placed near the skin surface (especially in the nose and ear). Silicone cannot at present be rendered porous in such a way as to improve its incorporation in tissues without substantially altering its physical characteristics. Recently, the concept of texturing of the implant's surface has been introduced as a method to enhance tissue adherence and to modify the fibrous capsule that forms around the implant.

Although dimethylsiloxane polymers are considered to be biologically inert, they do evoke an inflammatory response in humans. The degree of inflammatory response to silicones (especially injectible) having the same density and purity varies widely among individuals, and this may relate to individual immune responsiveness. Medical-grade dimethylsiloxane polymers are used widely in medicine for lubricating disposable syringes and needles and as coatings for suture materials. It is estimated that an insulin-dependent diabetic injects 2 to 5 cc of medical-grade silicone into his body each year as a result of the needles and syringes used for insulin injection.

Although antibodies to medical-grade silicone have never been demonstrated, the particulation of silicone implants has been associated with conditions such as silicone synovitis and siliconoma. In both conditions, the presence of silicone in the tissues is followed by a granulomatous foreign-body reaction, and this appears to be related to the size of the silicone particle. In silicone synovitis, the fragmentation of silicone joint replacement implants (particularly in the wrist and basilar joint of the thumb) is followed by migration of the particles into adjacent synovial spaces and bone. The foreign-body reaction that results from this process produces synovitis with its attendant destruction of joint spaces and tendons and the inflammatory resorption of bone.

Siliconomas (or silicone granulomas) are characterized by the formation of granulomatous inflammatory reactions around particles of liquid silicone. Most cases have been associated with the injection of non–medical-grade liquid silicone or liquid silicone that has been tainted with other substances to increase its inflammatory response and fibrous encapsulation in tissues in the hope of minimizing its migration. Siliconomas may occur at the sites of liquid silicone injection in the skin or subcutaneous tissues, at sites of particle migration, or internally in the major organs such as the liver, spleen, and kidneys. Silicone granulomas are clinically characterized by the appearance of firm, erythematous, ill-defined masses in the skin and subcutaneous tissues. In advanced stages, the skin may assume a *peau d'orange* quality, and there may be tenderness to palpation. The dispersion of silicone from its site of implantation is thought to be due to particulation and migration as well as its transportation by phagocytes. While both mechanisms of silicone dispersion have been demonstrated experimentally in animals and in isolated clinical cases for all viscosities of silicone, the implications of these findings for humans remain to be determined.

In reconstructive surgery, silicone implants are used primarily for augmentation of the bony skeleton and soft tissues and as spacers in joint replacement surgery. The temporary implantation of inflatable silicone implants for soft-tissue expansion has become a well-established technique for reconstruction of soft-tissue defects. When silicone implants are placed subperiosteally for augmentation of the bony skeleton (e.g., chin, zygoma), bone resorption beneath the implant will occur presumably because of the effects of pressure and foreign-body reaction. Less bony resorption follows placement of the implant superficial to the periosteum. Deformation of the calvarial vault and bony thorax has also been observed beneath tissue expanders and silicone implants placed in these areas.

The stability of a silicone implant in tissue resides primarily in fibrous encapsulation of the implant, which as noted above varies among individuals. For solid silicone implants this does not pose a significant problem. In gel- or saline-filled silicone implants used for soft-tissue or breast augmentation, the quality of the reconstruction depends on the softness of the implant in its tissue environment, and this is directly related to the degree of fibrous encapsulation and contraction.

Methyl Methacrylate

Methyl methacrylate, or acrylic, is the polymerized ester of acrylic acid, $CH_2 = CHCOOH$, or an ester of methacrylic acid, $CH_2 = C(CH_3)COOH$. In its cured, polymerized state, methyl methacrylate is a hard, rigid, porous translucent material with low specific gravity. The material does not conduct electricity and is not carcinogenic. It can be shaped by burring and drilled for wire or screw fixation. A great advantage of methyl methacrylate is that it can be prepared intraoperatively and molded in situ before hardening to achieve a desired contour or shape. Powdered granules of polymerized methyl methacrylate polymer are mixed with a liquid monomer; the material is then placed in situ and shaped until it hardens (usually about 7 minutes). Final curing takes an additional 7 minutes. The polymerized monomer bonds to the polymerized polymer to form an acrylic composite. An exothermic reaction generating temperatures of up to 100°C ensues as the material polymerizes, and this serves to sterilize the alloplast. The heat generated by the curing of methyl methacrylate is sufficient to kill cells, and therefore the surrounding tissues must be cooled by irrigation until the polymerization process is complete. Cold curing of methyl methacrylate by this technique has been shown experimentally to limit heat buildup in the immediately adjacent tissues to 68°C, which peaks at about 5 to 6 minutes.

Allergic systemic reactions, hypotension, and cardiac arrest have been reported with the use of methyl methacrylate, and these are due primarily to the escape and absorption of the monomer during the curing process. Once the material has polymerized and the monomer becomes bonded, no further toxicity is seen, although approximately 4% of the monomer remains unbonded in the final acrylic composite. Toxic reactions to methyl methacrylate are associated with the use of large volumes of polymer coming in contact with soft tissues and bone during orthopedic procedures and have rarely been encountered in head and neck reconstructions.

The reactivity of methyl methacrylate in tissues is slightly more than that observed for silicone polymers but is still considered to be relatively mild. A typical foreign-body reaction develops following implantation, and this appears to be related to the size of the polymethyl methacrylate particles on the implant surface. The inflammatory reaction eventually abates as the implant becomes enveloped by fibrous tissue. Adherance of the soft tissues to the implant surface is mostly at the points of surface irregularity since its pore size is insufficient for cellular ingrowth.

Methyl methacrylate has been used extensively in orthopedic surgery as a cement to stabilize joint replacement prostheses in bone. In these situations, new bone formation occurs adjacent to the fibrous capsule enveloping the cement and serves to enhance its mechanical fixation to the bone. The addition of the catalyst tri-*n*-butylborane to methyl methacrylate during the curing process provides a chemical bond of the polymer to bone without any apparent adverse effect on the adjacent bony tissues.

In head and neck surgery, methyl methacrylate implants have been used primarily for the reconstruction of cranial defects. The advantages of methyl methacrylate for this purpose reside in its low morbidity and its ability to be shaped and contoured intraoperatively. As calvarial patch materials, the acrylics have worked quite well owing to the immobility and relatively low stresses intrinsic to this environment. Occasionally, the methyl methacrylate implant loosens and causes erosion of the covering soft tissues, which leads to its exposure and infection. In these situations, the implant must be removed and the defect repaired with autogenous bone or again with acrylic, provided that the reconstruction is performed after the wound has completely healed and the soft-tissue covering is adequate or can be made so.

Other reported disadvantages of methyl methacrylate include seroma, persistent burning sensations in the area of placement because of residual free monomer, and limitations on the ability to keep the surface of the implant smooth when molding it to match the normal cranial contours.

Calcium Phosphate Ceramics

The use of calcium phosphate ceramics in reconstructive surgery has grown considerably over the past 15 years owing to their high level of biocompatibility and desirable qualities as bone substitutes in reconstructive surgery. These materials are composed of crystals of compounded calcium phosphate that are found in nature or synthetically produced. This family of compounds is biologically inert and nontoxic and, in pure form, does not elicit inflammatory or foreign-body responses. Calcium phosphate ceramics share a common ability to become bonded to viable adjacent bone and, depending on their porosity and structure, can serve as osteogenic conductors (*osteoconductive* or *osteophylic*) of new bone formation. This osteoconductive property is dependent on rigid fixation of the material to bone; mobility results in fibrous encapsulation. The major disadvantage of these ceramics is their brittleness and susceptibility to breakage when exposed to load stresses or transplanted to mobile sites. These physical characteristics also have some drawbacks in shaping of the materials prior to implantation, although they can be sawed, burred, or drilled if care is exercised. Two types of calcium phosphate ceramics are commonly used in reconstructive surgery: HA and tricalcium phosphate (TCP).

Hydroxyapatite

HA is a calcium phosphate ceramic that also exists as the major mineral component of bone. It is found in nature as the mineral skeleton of porous coral, which has a morphologic structural configuration and porosity (500 to 600 μm) analogous to human bone. This material can be processed to remove its organic component and leave a pure HA replica of the coral skeleton. In its unimplanted state, this ceramic is weaker than cancellous bone in humans. Following implantation as an onlay or inlay graft in long bones, its large pore size allows tissue ingrowth and osteogenesis to occur by the conductive process. Its ultimate strength in vivo is related to the orientation of its channels in relation to the applied forces. Experimentally it has been shown that this material develops an average mechanical strength three times greater than cancellous bone 6 months following implantation because of the overlay of new bone (representing approximately 30% of the new tissue ingrowth with the remainder being fibrovascular tissue) that has formed on the interstices of the implant. The success of this material in promoting new bone formation is related to its rigid stabilization and close approximation to viable bone. It forms a very tight bond with adjacent bone by an apparently natural cementing mechanism. Up to one third of the porous HA implant may be absorbed over time, although this does not appear to appreciably weaken the implant provided that the deposition of new lamellar bone occurs. Of some concern is the fact that only 30% of available interstices of the porous HA implant eventually become filled with new bone.

Porous corraline HA has been successively employed as a bone substitute in orthognathic surgery (as a filler material for tooth extractions or in mandibular advancements) and as an onlay material for chin and malar augmentation. If the material becomes exposed, the soft tissues do not heal over it, and thus the implant will require partial or complete removal. Porous HA has been used in experimental clinical trials for the grafting of short segmental defects in long bones with encouraging results. As a replacement for calvarial bone its incorporation is incomplete, although new methods of impregnating this substance with osteogenesis-inducing factors (e.g., bone morphogenic protein) are currently being investigated. When compared with onlay bone grafts, porous HA demonstrates less absorption and better maintenance of volume and contour. As noted above, however, the major concern with this material is its variable and incomplete filling with new bone.

HA can be manufactured by various processes to create synthetic ceramics of varying density and porosity. Dense, nonporous HA in block form does not allow cellular infiltration but rather becomes encapsulated similar to other nonporous biomaterials. In this form, the implant has enjoyed limited use as an onlay graft for augmentation of the facial skeleton. Dense HA is hard and brittle and is prone to fracture when subjected to load-bearing stresses. To obviate these shortcomings, the material has been converted to a particulate form that when implanted adjacent to bone becomes invaded by reparative bone and fibrous tissues, thereby improving its viscoelastic properties. The tissue response to HA particles appears to be influenced by the shape of the particles, with smooth particles demonstrating less inflammation than sharp particles. Granular HA has been successfully employed for alveolar ridge augmentation and as a filler substance for dental extractions. This material has also been bonded to tooth implants and has demonstrated good success in rigid fixation of the tooth substitute to alveolar bone.

Tricalcium Phosphate

β-Tricalcium phosphate ($Ca_3[PO_4]_2$) is a specially processed ceramic compound of calcium phosphate that has randomly situated pores of 100 to 300 μm in diameter. In comparison to HA, TCP is gradually absorbed over time, and this constitutes its singular advantage as a ceramic implant. If placed adjacent to viable bone and appropriately stabilized, TCP will promote cellular ingrowth and become eventually replaced by new bone and fibrous tissue. The rate and extent of new bone formation in this material are related to the site of implantation (metaphyseal vs. diaphyseal and cortical vs. cancellous), the availability of local osteoprogenitor cells (i.e., above or below the periosteum), and the quality of fixation to viable bone.

Clinical applications of TCP are at present limited. It has been employed in block form for the repair of long-bone defects with results comparable to HA. The material remains radiodense for many months but gradually blends with the surrounding bone as it is absorbed and new bone forms in its interstices. When implanted into soft tissues, it is gradually absorbed and does not undergo fibrous encapsulation. Further experimental studies are examining the potential applications of TCP and related ceramics for clinical use.

Proplast

Proplast is a composite of Teflon fluorocarbon polymer (polytetrafluoroethylene [PTFE]) and black vitreous carbon fibers (Proplast I) or white aluminum oxide fibers (Proplast II). The addition of vitreous carbon or aluminum oxide to Teflon makes it wettable in tissues and therefore promotes protein adsorption and tissue adherence and ingrowth. Proplast is highly porous (70% by volume), with pore sizes ranging from 70 to 500 μm, which is sufficiently large to allow fibrovascular tissue ingrowth for firm anchorage of the implant in tissues.

Although their biological activities are similar, the two types of Proplast differ in their physical properties. Proplast I is black in color and has a soft spongy consistency, whereas Proplast II is white in color and is harder (although it deforms and compresses more when subjected to equal pressures). Both materials can be cut with scissors or a knife or burred (although Proplast I lends itself to easier shaping because of its softness). Because of its black color, Proplast I can be seen through areas covered by thin skin such as the nasal dorsum and may be less desirable for placement in these areas.

Proplast elicits an initial exuberant and prolonged granulomatous reaction characterized by the presence of histiocytes and foreign-body giant cells. Granulation tissue invades the pores of the implant, and over time the inflammatory reaction subsides and is replaced by fibrous tissue. This fibrous encapsulation and infiltration of the implant firmly anchors it to the surrounding soft tissues, thus making it palpably indistinguishable from bone or cartilage in vivo but also creating substantial technical difficulties if its removal is required.

Proplast has been used extensively for augmentation of the chin, malar region, nasal dorsum, and bony calvarium. Its primary advantages lie in its stability and compatibility in tissues and the firm anchorage achieved by fibrous tissue ingrowth. Proplast implants in the chin have a higher rate of infection and displacement (7.4%) than do implants in other areas of the face. The amount of long-term soft-tissue augmentation achieved with this material is approximately 50% of the original result obtained at surgery, and this appears to remain stable beyond the first year. Although infection infrequently complicates its use, many surgeons advocate the instillation of antibiotic solutions directly into the Proplast implant by means of a needle and syringe, irrigation of the implant pocket with antibiotic solution, and prophylactic systemic antibiotics. As with other alloplasts placed subperiosteally, Proplast has been shown to cause bone resorption, presumably because of a pressure effect.

Other Commonly Used Alloplasts

Expanded PTFE is a pure, microporous form of Teflon that is thin, flexible, and inert and has a high degree of biocompatibility. It has a relatively smooth surface, and the pore size (10 to 20 μm) is insufficient for cellular ingrowth. Expanded PTFE is used as vascular graft and fascial patch material in surgery.

Polyethylene is an inert, lightweight biomaterial with high tensile strength, limited flexibility, and a high degree of biocompatibility. It can be fabricated as a woven or knitted mesh material (Marlex) for the repair of fascial defects or as a porous, three-dimensional material with a large pore size (50 to 100 μm) that allows fibrovascular ingrowth. This material can be carved into complex dimensions and has been used for many years for repair and augmentation of tissue defects.

Polypropylene is a product of polymer chemistry that is not hydrolyzed and resists degradation by tissues. It is the least reactive biomaterial used in surgery with perhaps the exception of stainless steel. This material is strong and lightweight and can be stretched. Polypropylene is most commonly used as a monofilament suture but is also employed in the fabrication of woven fascial patch materials.

BREAST IMPLANTS

For a detailed discussion of the biology, the types, and the clinical applications of silicone breast implants, see Chapter 30.

INJECTABLE MATERIALS

In aesthetic surgery and to a lesser extent in reconstructive surgery, the quest for a substance that can be efficiently and safely injected into the dermal and subcutaneous facial tissues for the purposes of permanently correcting wrinkles or contour deformities has eluded investigators. Materials initially introduced as promising have proved in the long run to be toxic or allergenic, to cause undesirable skin changes, to migrate from their site of implantation, or to undergo absorption. Two materials dominate the current vogue, and each has its defined advantages and disadvantages.

Collagen

Processed bovine collagen (Zyderm) and its glutaraldehyde cross-linked derivitive (Zyplast) have been used for the augmentation of dermal defects of the face since Food and Drug Administration (FDA) approval in 1981. The two materials differ primarily in their rates of absorption from the tissues, a characteristic related to their biochemical stability and antigenicity.

Tissue reaction to injected bovine collagen is characterized by an inflammatory reaction that degrades the implant and replaces it with human collagen. By 4 months Zyderm is not detectable in human dermis. Because of its increased stability produced by cross-linking, Zyplast may persist for up to 6 months. The dermal augmentation that is initially achieved with either product is substantially lost in most cases within 6 to 9 months.

The most important technical factor associated with the use of injectable bovine collagen is the depth of dermal implantation. Zyderm is most effective if placed in the superficial dermis. Zyplast is best suited to implantation in the deeper dermis in thicker-skinned individuals. By this technique, the obliteration or softening of nasolabial, glabellar, periorbital, and lip wrinkles and depressed acne scars may be successfully, albeit temporarily achieved. Bovine collagen is not approved for injection into the deep tissues of the lip for lip augmentation or for use near the orbital rim.

Because of its tendency to be more rapidly absorbed, Zyderm is less likely to undergo encapsulation in the tissues, a process that may produce visible or palpable lumps that may be more unsightly than the original skin problem. For this reason Zyderm may be preferred for the dermal augmentation of thin skin. Because of its longer persistence in the tissues, Zyplast may become encapsulated, and the prolonged inflammatory response may lead to hyperpigmentation of the skin in the area of treatment. Both of the above problems may also be related to the volume of material injected in any one area.

Localized hypersensitivity reactions to bovine collagen develop in approximately 4% of patients. For this reason it is recommended that patients undergoing dermal augmentation by this technique be skin-tested twice at intervals of 8 weeks between tests followed by 8 weeks before the commencement of treatment. Anticollagen antibodies have been identified in patients experiencing localized hypersensitivity reactions to bovine collagen, although there is no known cross-reactivity between bovine and human collagen. Despite this, the injection of bovine collagen has been associated in some reports with the development of autoimmune disease in humans (dermatomyositis, scleroderma, rheumatoid arthritis), but increased rates of the development of autoimmune disease have not been proved to date. Use of injectible bovine collagen is contraindicated in patients having known autoimmune disease and in patients who demonstrate hypersensitivity reactions to skin testing.

Autologous Fat

The injection of autologous fat has recently become a popular but poorly understood method for soft-tissue augmentation of the face. In contradistinction to bovine collagen injections, fat is not injected into the dermis but rather into the subdermis and subcutaneous layers of the integument. Autologous fat injection is therefore used for the correction of contour deformities of the face and has very little effect on fine wrinkling.

The published success rates following autologous fat injections vary considerably, but in the most optimistic circumstances no more than 20% to 40% of the original volume can be expected to remain 1 year following injection. Experimental studies on fat transplantation have shown that a variable number of adipocytes survive the injection process, and this may be related to the method in which the fat is harvested and subsequently implanted into the tissues. Fat for injection is aspirated or suctioned from the subcutaneous tissues of a remote body site such as the abdominal wall or trochanteric region of the hip. Following removal of the supernatant of the aspirate, the "solids" are injected into the facial site. A considerable amount of physical trauma to the fat is generated by harvesting (high negative pressures [1 atm]) and injecting (high positive pressures). The acceleration and deceleration of the injectate as it transgresses the relatively small diameter of the needle to the relatively large diameter of the syringe barrel and vice versa during the aspiration and injection process also cause considerable physical trauma to the fat cells. The cumulative effect of the mechanical trauma imposed by fat aspiration and injection results in a high attrition rate of potentially viable adipocytes. Histologic studies of experimentally aspirated or suctioned fresh fat reveal that approximately 10% of the adipocytes are unchanged, with the remainder of the aspirate consisting of a mixture of ruptured adipocytes, fragmented blood vessels, loose connective tissue, and lipid droplets.

The cellular response to injected fat is typically inflammatory, with phagocytosis and eventual fibrous tissue replacement of the injectate. Areas of fat necrosis may persist and form cystic cavities of lipid encased in fibrous tissue. Experimentally, aspirates of fat demonstrate a higher survival of adipocytes when injected into muscle as opposed to the subcutaneous or subdermal tissues. Current evidence suggests that some lipocytes do survive the transplantation process, but the main components responsible for long-term tissue bulk and volume maintenance are the cystic cavities and fibrous tissue that form following fat injection.

Given the foregoing analysis, the efficacy of autologous fat injections for the treatment of facial contour defects remains uncertain. Despite this, numerous proponents of this technique attest to the benefits of its clinical application. The best results are obtained if small volumes of fat are dispersed into the tissues at repeated intervals. Potential complications are infection, fat necrosis, persistent erythema of the overlying skin, and contour irregularities. The long-term analysis of this technique for soft-tissue augmentation awaits further study.

SUGGESTED READING

Billings E Jr, May JW Jr: Historical review and present status of free fat graft autotransplantation in plastic and reconstructive surgery. *Plast Reconstr Surg* 1989; 83:368.

Burchardt H: Biology of bone transplantation. *Orthop Clin North Am* 1987; 18:187.

Byrd SH: Implantation: Bone, cartilage, and alloplasts, in *Selected Readings in Plastic Surgery,* vol 5, No 4. Baylor University Medical Center, 1988.

Bucholz RW, Carlton A, Holmes RE: Hydroxyapatite and tricalcium phosphate bone graft substitutes. *Orthop Clin North Am* 1987; 18:323.

Donald PJ: Cartilage grafting in facial reconstruction with special consideration of irradiated grafts: *Laryngoscope* 1986; 96:786.

Fisher JC: The silicone controversy—When will science prevail? *N Engl J Med* 1992; 326:1696.

Gibson T, Davis WB: The distortion of autogenous cartilage grafts: Its cause and prevention. *Br J Plast Surg* 1957; 10:257.

Glasgold AI, Silver FH (eds): *Applications of Biomaterials in Facial Plastic Surgery.* Boca Raton, Fla, CRC Press, 1991.

Hanker JS, Giammara BL: Biomaterials and biomedical devices. *Science* 1988; 242:885.

Holmes RE: Bone regeneration within a coralline hydroxyapatite implant. *Plast Reconstr Surg* 1979; 63:626.

Jarcho M: Biomaterial aspects of calcium phosphates. *Dent Clin North Am* 1986; 30:25.

McGrath MH, Burkhardt BR: The safety and efficacy of breast implants for augmentation mammaplasty. *Plast Reconstr Surg* 1984; 74:550.

Rubin LR (ed): *Biomaterials in Reconstructive Surgery.* St Louis, Mosby–Year Book, 1983.

Taylor SR, Gibbons DF: Effect of surface texture on the soft tissue response to polymer implants. *J Biomed Mater Res* 1983; 17:205.

Wolford LM, Wardrop RW, Hartog JM: Coralline porous hydroxyapatite as a bone graft substitute in orthognathic surgery. *J Oral Maxillofac Surg* 1987; 45:1034.

Chapter 5

Special Techniques

Arnold S. Breitbart, M.D.
John W. Siebert, M.D.

CONTENTS

CHAPTER OBJECTIVE

At the end of this chapter the resident understands the principles of a variety of special techniques in plastic surgery, including liposuction, tissue expansion, laser treatment, chemical peel, and dermabrasion, and utilizes the techniques effectively in appropriate clinical settings.

LEARNER OBJECTIVES

On completion of this chapter the resident

1. **Understands the basic principles, the common techniques, and the instrumentation of suction lipectomy.**
2. **Knows the indications for and contraindications to suction lipectomy and is familiar with the principles of preoperative assessment; recognizes the limitations of liposuction and is familiar with alternative techniques.**
3. **Is able to perform preoperative, intraoperative, and postoperative management of the patient undergoing suction lipectomy; is familiar with the complications of liposuction and their management.**
4. **Knows the physiologic principles of tissue expansion.**
5. **Understands the various techniques for tissue expansion and is familiar with the differing expansion devices.**
6. **Knows the principles of management of patients undergoing tissue expansion; recognizes the complications of tissue expansion and is competent in their treatment.**
7. **Understands the physiologic and pathologic principles of dermabrasion and chemical peel; recognizes**

the differences between the two techniques and the indications for choice between the techniques.

8. **Is familiar with the instrumentation and techniques for dermabrasion.**
9. **Understands the principles of preoperative and postoperative management of patients undergoing dermabrasion and chemical peeling; recognizes the complications of the two techniques and their management.**
10. Is familiar with the pharmacologic aspects and the techniques of chemical peeling.
11. Understands the biophysical properties of commonly used lasers and the applications of different lasers for different types of problems.
12. Knows appropriate safety precautions for the use of lasers.
13. Is familiar with the indications for and contraindications to laser treatment, the techniques of laser use, and the various complications of laser therapy and their treatment.

■ CLINICAL PRACTICE ACTIVITIES

During the course of the training program, the resident

1. **Evaluates and treats patients with localized lipodystrophy by using suction lipectomy techniques.**
2. **Evaluates and treats patients with a wide variety of congenital and acquired problems by using tissue expansion techniques.**
3. **Evaluates and treats patients by dermabrasion and/or chemical peeling.**
4. **Evaluates and treats patients with problems amenable to laser therapy.**
5. *Achieves certification in laser use.*

LIPOSUCTION

Suction lipectomy was first popularized in the late 1970s by Kesselring, Ilouz, and Teimourian and today has become one of the most commonly performed plastic surgical procedures. Its usual indication has been for the treatment of fat deposits in patients with good skin elasticity who are unresponsive to exercise and diet, and it has evolved to be a useful adjunct to multiple body-contouring procedures.

Anatomy and Physiology

The primary function of the adipocyte, or fat cell, is lipid synthesis and storage. From birth through adolescence, adipocytes increase in number as well as in size. After adolescence the accumulation of fat is primarily due to an increase in the size of existing adipocytes, except in cases of extreme obesity where adipocyte hyperplasia develops.

Subcutaneous tissue of the torso and thighs is composed of a superficial and deep layer. The superficial layer consists of compact fat bound by a highly organized septal network. The deep adipose layer is made of loose fat within a poorly organized septal arrangement. It is this deep adipose layer for which liposuction is most appropriate.

Apparatus

The equipment used in liposuction consists of a vacuum pump, tubing, and various cannulas (Fig 5–1). The perfect vacuum is 1 atm, or 760 mm Hg; however, in practicality the maximum vacuum that can be generated is slightly less than 760 mm Hg and equal to atmospheric pressure. The tubing used should be thick enough to resist collapse with vacuum.

There are a variety of cannulas currently available. The original cannulas were sharp single-hole curets. The most widely used cannulas today have blunt tips and multiple holes and produce effective liposuction while minimizing trauma to the tissues. The cannula diameter size generally ranges from 1.5 to 6.0 mm. The most popular cannula used today is the three-hole "Mercedes"-type cannula (Fig 5–2). Small-diameter cannulas are used in such areas as the face and neck, whereas larger-diameter cannulas are used on larger suction volumes such as the torso and thigh.

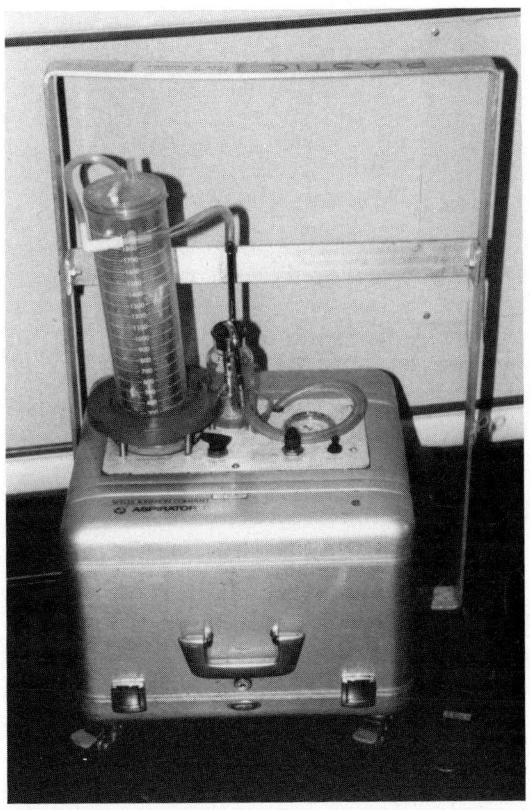

FIG 5–1.
Vacuum pump apparatus with calibrated canister.

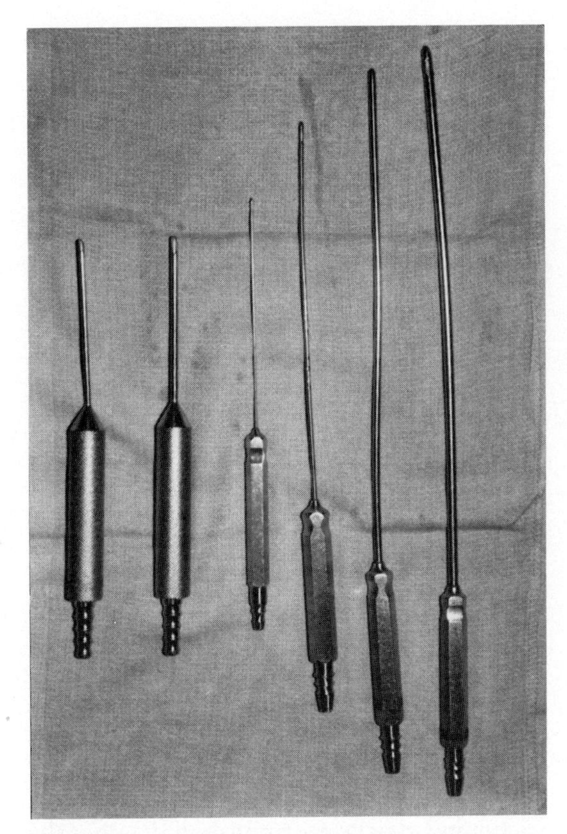

FIG 5–2.
An assortment of liposuction cannulas, including single- and three-holed cannulas, in a variety of sizes.

Technique

General anesthesia is generally used unless the area to be suctioned is small. Some surgeons believe that lidocaine (0.25%) with epinephrine (1:400,000) injected into the sites of suction reduces blood loss. Small stab wound incisions placed in inconspicuous locations such as the groin, umbilicus, and gluteal crease, i.e., along lines of relaxed skin tension, afford access for the suction cannula. Pretunneling, or the insertion and passage of the cannula without suction, may establish and loosen the proper plane in which the liposuction will then be performed. Intersecting tunnels made through adjacent incisions may produce a smoother surface contour (Fig 5–3). Care must be taken to avoid suctioning too superficially in the subdermal plane, which may cause surface irregularity. The wounds are closed with sutures and the patient advised to wear a compression garment for at least 10 days postoperatively.

Face and Neck

Liposuction is very effective in face and neck contouring and is an important adjunct in facial cosmetic surgery. The submental region is particularly amenable to liposuction. Through a submental stab incision a small three-hole "Mercedes" cannula can be introduced to perform liposuction. Alternatively, a longer submental incision can be made and the proper plane of suction established by sharply raising a skin flap. Fat above the platysma can then be suctioned under direct vision. Suctioning should usually be limited to below the jawline in order to achieve optimal contouring. Liposuction of the neck may be accomplished through the submental incision or from a lateral direction beneath the facial-plasty skin flaps. In selected cases the cheeks and jowls may be carefully suctioned.

Abdomen

Abdominal liposuction can be effective alone or in conjunction with an abdominoplasty. Stab wound incisions are made in the umbilicus and pubic area. Large three-hole cannulas are used initially. Smaller cannulas are then used to achieve finer contouring. When there is minimal skin laxity, liposuction alone is effective in the treatment of localized excess fat. When an abdominoplasty is indicated for more severe abdominal deformities, liposuction can be used to thin the abdominal flap as well as contour the flanks.

Extremities

Liposuction is particularly effective in lower-extremity contouring, especially the buttocks, hips, lateral aspect of the thighs ("saddlebags"), medial aspect of the thighs, and medial portion of the knees (Fig 5–4). Suctioning may be accomplished in either the supine or prone position and can be used in conjunction with other contouring procedures, including thigh-plasty and buttock-lifting. The calf and ankle may also be suctioned, but the results are often limited.

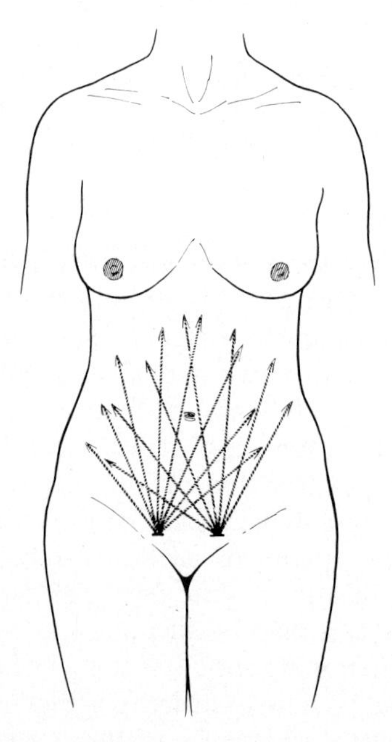

FIG 5–3.
Intersecting tunnels made through separate incisions can help to produce a smoother contour.

Other Indications

The use of liposuction has expanded to include the treatment of gynecomastia resulting from excess fat, breast contouring during breast reduction, flap contour lipoma removal, temporary palliation of lymphedema of the extremities, and the treatment of steroid-induced local fat deposits such as the buffalo hump.

Fat Injection

Autologous fat transplantation has been used in a variety of clinical situations in order to fill creases and smooth surface irregularities. Fat is removed from areas of excess such as the abdomen with a needle or liposuction cannula and injected into an area that requires fullness. Nasolabial creases, glabellar wrinkles, and depressed scars are areas that have been treated with fat injection. Autologous fat has also been used for lip augmentation and for the correction of contour deformities caused by overly aggressive liposuction. It is generally agreed that fat injection, like collagen injection, has only a temporary effect, with resorption of most of the fat in 6 months.

Complications

The overall complication rate of liposuction is approximately 10%. Postoperative surface contour irregularities are usually the result of overly aggressive or too superficial liposuction. Decreased sensation is relatively common, but sensation usually returns within 3 to 6 months. Edema, ecchymosis, and discoloration may also be seen.

Several major complications of liposuction have been reported. These include excessive blood loss, hematoma, seroma, infection, venous thrombosis, pulmonary emboli, skin necrosis, and fat emboli. Aspirated fat contains a significant amount of blood, and a hematocrit drop of 1% can be expected for each 150 cc of fat removed. Blood transfusions are gener-

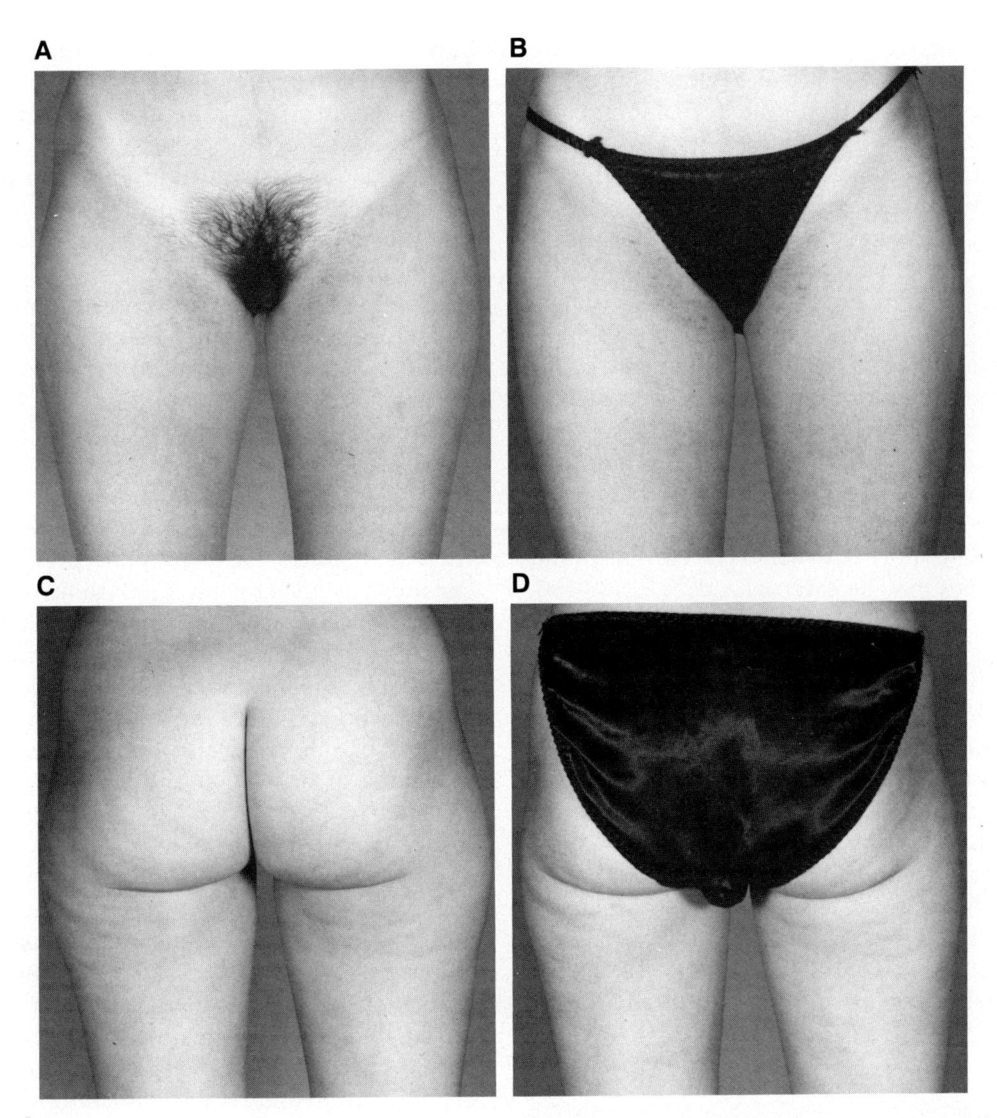

FIG 5–4.
A patient with localized fat of the lateral and medial thighs. **A,** Preoperative front view. **B,** One-year postoperative front view after liposuction of the lateral and medial aspects of the thighs. **C,** Preoperative posterior view. **D,** Postoperative posterior view.

ally not needed unless the volume of aspirated fat significantly exceeds 1,500 cc. In general, fluid resuscitation should approximate 3 cc for every 1 cc of aspirate. Compression garments are useful in preventing the development of seromas. Prophylactic intravenous alcohol has been advocated in order to prevent the development of fat emboli, but this recommendation has not been widely accepted.

In a 5-year experience with over 100,000 liposuction procedures, 11 deaths have been reported. Four of these deaths followed liposuction alone. Two of these were caused by sepsis secondary to necrotizing fasciitis, and 2 were caused by hypovolemic shock and fat embolism.

TISSUE EXPANSION

Since first introduced by Neumann in 1957 and then refined by Radovan and Austad in the 1970s, tissue expansion has developed into a popular and versatile tool of the reconstructive surgeon. Tissue expansion is indicated for a variety of situations in which there is a deficiency in the availability of soft tissue.

Expanders are available in a variety of standard shapes and volumes and can also be custom-fabricated for individual case requirements. Expanders are made of silicone elastomer and inflated with the injection of isotonic saline. Most expanders have a smooth surface, although textured expanders are also available (usually for breast reconstruction) and are believed to minimize the formation of a fibrous capsule around the expander. Expanders generally have a remote filling port that is connected with silicone tubing (Fig 5–5). This port is usually placed subcutaneously but may be externalized.

Histology

The histology of expanded skin has been extensively studied. During expansion the epidermis experiences an increased mitotic rate but no significant change in thickness. Hair follicles and other accessory skin structures are compressed but do not degenerate. The dermis becomes significantly thinner, and there is an increase in the number of fibroblasts and myofibroblasts. There is also a dramatic increase in the vascularity of expanded skin with a resultant increase in the survival of expanded skin flaps as compared with control skin and delayed skin flaps.

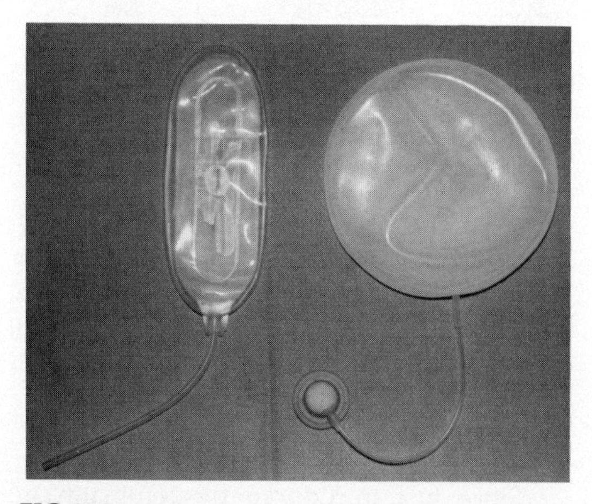

FIG 5–5.
A smooth oblong tissue expander and a textured round tissue expander with attached tubing and filling port.

Muscle and fat atrophy has been noted adjacent to tissue expanders. Depressions are often seen in areas of bone in contact with an expander (e.g., the skull).

The process of tissue expansion results in an increase in tissue surface area. This is due both to a recruitment of adjacent skin and to an increased rate of mitotic activity in the epidermis over the expander.

Technique

The incision for placement of a tissue expander is usually oriented radial to the expander. The location of the incision is dictated by the ultimate incisions required for removal of the expander and flap closure of the defect. Expanders can be placed subcutaneously or submuscularly, depending on the thickness of the skin and the soft-tissue coverage requirements. Multiple expanders can be placed simultaneously.

A small amount of saline is injected intraoperatively to confirm proper placement and function of the expander. Inflation usually begins after a period of 2 to 3 weeks and thereafter at 1- to 2-week intervals. More accelerated inflation schedules have also been used with success. Saline is injected into the expander until there is skin blanching over the expander or the patient experiences discomfort. In order to minimize leaking from the injection port, a 23-gauge or smaller butterfly needle should be used.

Indications

The use of a tissue expander should be considered in the closure of any skin defect that cannot be closed primarily and in which a sensate skin flap with a good color and texture match is desired. Common indications for tissue expansion include staged excision and reconstruction of burn scars, scalp alopecia, and congenital giant nevi.

Tissue expansion has also proved to be a reliable and relatively simple procedure in breast reconstruction. Immediately following mastectomy a tissue expander is placed, usually below the pectoralis major muscle. Inferiorly, the expander should extend just below the inframammary fold, and the base of the expander should be slightly wider than that of the opposite breast. Postoperatively, the expander is inflated incrementally to a volume approximately 30% greater than the size of the anticipated permanent implant. After expansion is complete, the expander is left in place for 2 to 4 months and then replaced with an implant.

Other uses of tissue expansion include the elongation of vessels, peripheral nerves, and tendons for specific reconstruction requirements.

Complications

Complications of tissue expansion can be significant and include deflation, infection, and extrusion of the expander. Deflation is usually caused by inadvertent puncture of the expander or by a leaking injection port. The use of small-gauge needles for injection helps to prevent such leaks. A deflated expander should be removed and replaced.

Infection of an expander can often be treated with systemic antibiotics and externalization of the injection port. When the infection is persistent, however, removal of the expander is warranted.

Extrusion of an expander is caused by placement of the expander too close to the incision, inadequate dissection of the expander pocket, or overly rapid expansion. If exposure occurs early during the expansion process, the implant should be removed and the wound allowed to completely heal. If exposure happens late, topical antibiotics can be used and further expansion performed until the implant is removed.

Particularly high incidences of complications have been observed with tissue ex pansion of the lower extremity. Neuropraxia secondary to nerve compression by the expander has been observed with placement near the sural nerve. Active infection and poor vascularity are considered contraindications to the use of tissue expanders.

CHEMICAL PEELS AND DERMABRASION

Chemical Peels

Chemical peeling is indicated for the treatment of fine facial wrinkles, very superficial acne scarring, and conditions of irregular facial skin hyperpigmentation such as those caused by pregnancy, chloasma, and chronic sun exposure. Patients with fair complexions and thin skin are more favorable candidates for chemical peeling than those with dark skin or thick oily skin. The most popular agents used in chemical peeling are phenol and trichloroacetic acid (TCA).

Phenol

Phenol is the most commonly used agent. One formula often used consists of phenol (USP) 3 cc, tap water 2 cc, liquid soap 8 drops, and croton oil 3 drops. Phenol causes protein precipitation and denaturation and coagulation of keratin. Soap lowers surface tension, and croton oil potentiates the effect of the phenol by increasing local inflammation. Taping of the treated area can help to increase penetration by preventing evaporation.

Phenol is detoxified in the liver and excreted in the urine. The major immediate complication of phenol peeling is cardiac arrhythmias, usually atrial. Thus, cardiac monitoring should be used. These problems have been reported in up to 39% of patients undergoing full face peels, and their incidence can be reduced by peeling the face in small areas at 15- to 20-minute intervals.

Trichloroacetic Acid

TCA is less toxic than phenol and effects a milder chemical peel. Unlike phenol, TCA is not absorbed systemically to any significant degree and can therefore be used in patients with renal, hepatic, or cardiac disease. The depth of penetration and therefore the strength of the peel are proportional to the strength of the TCA solution, which is usually 20% to 35%. This is in contrast to phenol, where increased concentrations tend to coagulate the keratin layer and cause decreased penetration.

Histology

Chemical peels cause homogenization of dermal collagen and an increase in the amount of elastic tissue. Following a chemical peel there is a new band of organized connective tissue 0.2 to 0.3 mm in width that is laid down in the subepidermal region. There is also a decrease in the amount of melanin granules in the epidermis.

Technique

When performing a chemical peel, the skin should first be cleaned with soap and water and an agent such as diethyl ether applied to reduce surface oils. The chemical is best applied with a cotton-tipped applicator and, in order to minimize the line of demarcation of the peel, should extend just into the hairline and vermilion border of the lip. Careful occlusive taping is recommended primarily for full facial peels used for a deeply lined face. A generous layer of petroleum jelly can be applied for regional peels (such as perioral peels) and for those performed for mild wrinkling or hyperpigmentation.

Following a facial peel patients experience a burning sensation for up to 24 hours. In addition there may be significant facial edema. After removal of the occlusive tape at 48 hours, the skin resembles a second-degree burn. A thin crust then forms that should be treated with gentle water cleansing and the application of an ointment such as A&D. As the crust loosens, the underlying skin appears erythematous. This erythema gradually diminishes over a period of 10 to 12 weeks. Direct sun exposure should be avoided for 6 months, and sunscreen use is essential.

Complications

Major complications of chemical peeling include full-thickness skin loss, hypertrophic scarring, and infection. Minor complications include skin bleaching, hyperpigmentation, hypopigmentation, telangiectasias, milia, and persistent erythema. Direct sunlight should be avoided for 6 months after chemical peeling, and topical sun-blocking agents should be used to minimize the possibility of skin hyperpigmentation. Hypertrophic scarring has been noted to occur most commonly after peeling of the neck, trunk, and extremities, and these areas are therefore unfavorable sites for chemical peeling. Chemical peels are contraindicated on acutely raised skin flaps, and it is advisable to wait at least 3 months after a facial-plasty before performing a chemical peel.

Dermabrasion

Dermabrasion is indicated for the treatment of facial wrinkles, acne scarring, traumatic scars, superficial lentigos, superficial dermal tatoos, and the scars of smallpox and varicella.

Histology

The histologic changes associated with dermabrasion are more subtle than those seen with chemical peels. There is no homogenization of dermal collagen, but instead there is partial removal of the dermis, which then

A

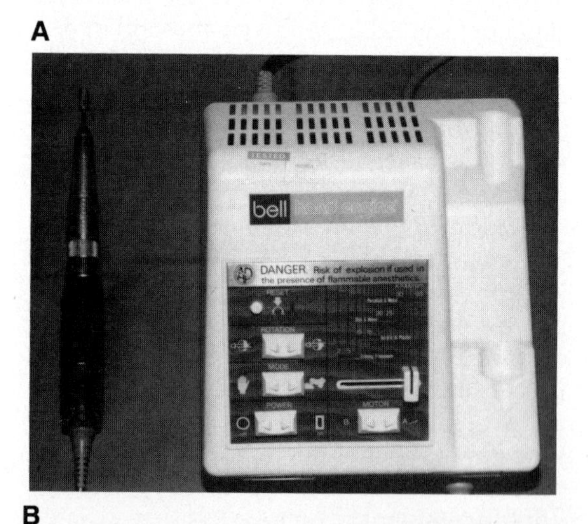

B

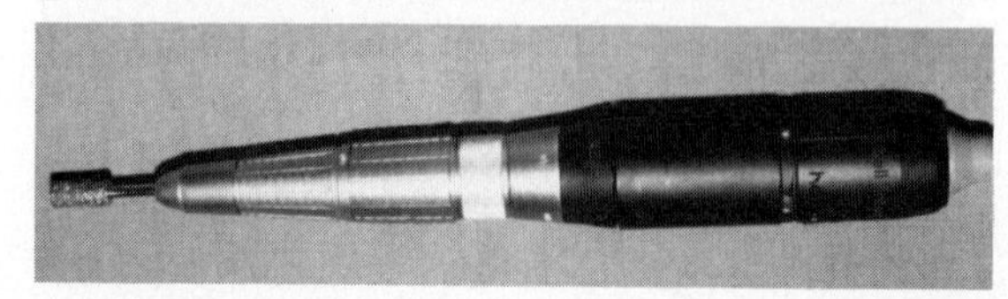

FIG 5–6.
A, Handpiece with motor unit. **B,** Dermabrasion burr attached to handpiece.

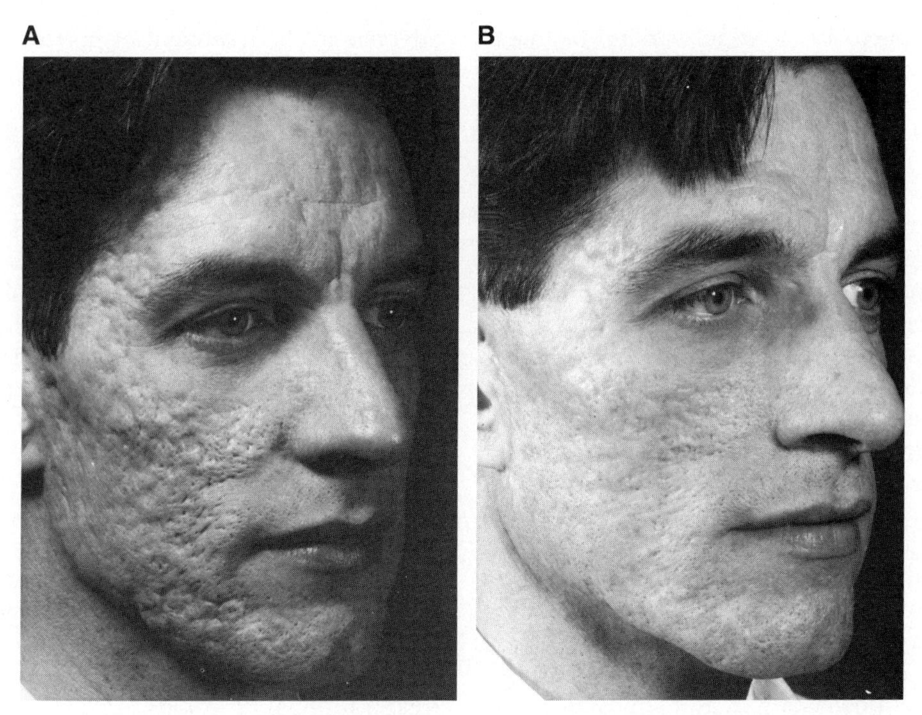

FIG 5–7.
An acne-scarred face treated with punch grafting followed by dermabrasion 6 months later. **A,** Preoperative view. **B,** Postoperative view 6 months after the dermabrasion.

undergoes incomplete regeneration. Optimally, dermabrasion should extend below the epidermis but not below the papillary dermis. Skin regeneration originates from the epithelium of adnexal structures, and therefore skin with the highest concentration of adnexal structures (such as the face, with the exclusion of the eyelids) tends to undergo the most efficient healing. Epidermis generally regenerates within 7 days, whereas dermal regeneration starts at 5 days and continues up to a year.

Technique

The method of dermabrasion utilizes a motor-driven handpiece (12,000 to 15,000 rpm) and various-sized diamond-tipped burrs (Fig 5–6). In order to facilitate the proper depth of dermabrasion, the depth of the area to be dermabraded can be marked with ink, and then dermabrasion proceeds until complete removal of the ink. The appearance of fine punctate bleeding is also a good sign of appropriate dermabrasion. The edges of the dermabrasion can be feathered in order to soften the line of demarcation (Fig 5–7).

Postoperatively, a topical antibiotic ointment can be applied for a week until reepithelialization is complete. Thereafter, as with chemical peels, direct sunlight should be avoided for several months, and sunscreens must be used.

Complications

Complications of dermabrasion are similar to those encountered with chemical peeling. These include hyperpigmentation, hypertrophic scarring, and milia. Skin erythema may also be seen and can last up to 8 weeks. In general, it is prudent to dermabrade or chemically peel small test patches behind the ear before treating extensive areas on the face.

LASER TREATMENT

The history of the laser can be traced to 1917, when Einstein theorized the quantum principle of stimulated emission of radiation. The first laser, a ruby laser, was developed by Maimann in 1960. Since then, the laser has been applied in a wide variety of uses, including recent applications in medicine and surgery.

Physics

Laser is an acronym standing for *l*ight *a*mplification by the *s*timulated *e*mission of *r*adiation. The basis of this stimulated emission of radiation occurs when an atom in a high-energy, or excited, state is struck by a photon and photons of equal energy and wavelength are released.

Laser light has the particular properties of being monochromatic, coherent, and collimated. The single wavelength of the monochromatic beam is determined by the specific laser source. The waves are in phase with each other (coherence) and do not diverge significantly over distance (collimation).

The laser can be adjusted both in the amount of power output and spot size of the beam in order to control the power density of the laser. Laser light can be delivered continuously or in short pulses. Pulsing the beam theoretically results in less surrounding tissue damage.

The effect of a laser on tissue is related to the heat generated. Between 60°C and 100°C proteins are denatured, and photocoagulation of the tissue occurs. Above 100°C there is tissue photoevaporation.

Individual lasers are characterized by their particular wavelength, absorption coefficient, and degree of penetration. The most commonly used lasers in plastic surgery are the argon and CO_2 lasers.

Argon Laser

The argon laser produces blue-green light with a wavelength of 488 to 514 nm. Hemoglobin and pigment particles selectively absorb light at approximately 500 nm, which makes the argon laser suitable for the treatment of vascular and pigment-containing lesions. The argon laser can penetrate to a depth of 2 mm and has been used with much success in the treatment of superficial vascular, pigmented, and inflammatory lesions.

The argon laser has been particularly effective in the treatment of port-wine stains and achieves a 50% to 80% lightening of color in over two thirds of patients, as well as reduced thickness of the lesions. Other vascular lesions successfully treated include telangiectasias, capillary-cavernous hemangiomas, strawberry hemangiomas, and venous lakes. Superficial melanocytic lesions such as the nevus of Ota, as well as superficial tattoos, can be treated with the argon laser. Inflammatory lesions, including granuloma faciale and acne rosacea, are also appropriate for argon laser treatment.

CO_2 Laser

The CO_2 laser produces intense light in the infrared spectrum with a wavelength of 10,600 nm and is selectively absorbed by water. Because biological tissues contain 75% to 90% water, the CO_2 laser can be used to treat a number of lesions.

A major use of the CO_2 laser is as a precise cutting scalpel in the excision of a variety of vascular, pigmented, and malignant lesions, including cavernous hemangiomas, nevi, lentigo, leukoplakia, and superficial basal and squamous cell carcinomas. By focusing the laser to a spot size as small as 0.22 mm, an exact incision can be made with hemostatic control. Blood vessels with lumens up to 0.5 mm in diameter are coagulated and sealed with the laser.

Defocusing the laser beam effects cauterization and can be used to ablate lesions, including tattoos. Laser dermabrasion causing selective ablation of the most superficial epidermal and dermal layers can also be achieved in this defocused mode.

Another advantage of the CO_2 laser is the ability to sterilize infected or contaminated lesions. Viral warts, fungal lesions, and infected pressure sores have been treated with this laser.

Technique and Complications

Laser use may be effected under general or local anesthesia. Epinephrine should not be utilized because vasoconstriction limits tissue absorption of laser light. Prior to definitive laser therapy a test patch is first treated and allowed to heal in order to gauge the expected result and anticipate any wound-healing problems.

The laser stylus is held 2 to 4 cm perpendicular to the skin surface. Following treatment, ice packs are placed to minimize edema. The resultant wound is treated with topical antibiotics and cleansing until separation of the formed eschar is accomplished. Epithelialization is usually completed by 2 weeks. Erythema often persists and can take up to 6 to 12 months to resolve.

When using the laser, safety glasses must be worn to prevent visual injury. Precautions must also be taken to avoid burning the endotracheal tube and drapes.

The most common complications seen with laser therapy are persistent erythema, hypopigmentation, skin texture change, and hypertrophic scarring.

Recent Advances

A new application of laser technology has been in tissue welding. A dye with a specific absorption coefficient is placed on the surface to be welded, and the laser beam is then directed at this site to effect a weld. Skin, nerves, blood vessels, and tendons have been successfully repaired with this technique in experimental trials.

Candela Laser

The Candela pulsed tunable dye laser is becoming the laser of choice in many centers for the treatment of port-wine stains and other vascular ectasias. This laser emits light at a wavelength of 577 nm, which is pulsed at 450 μs.

The advantage of this laser is that it causes very selective vascular destruction while minimizing extravascular damage. This results in effective treatment of many vascular lesions with minimal associated scarring and epidermal textural changes. Port-wine stains have been treated with a greater than 75% response rate and significant lightening of these lesions.

SUGGESTED READING

Apfelberg DB, Maser MR: Laser therapy, in McCarthy JG (ed): *Plastic Surgery,* vol 5. Philadelphia, WB Saunders, 1990.

Argenta LC, Marks MW, Pasyk KA: Advances in tissue expansion. *Clin Plast Surg* 1985; 12:159.

Baker TJ, Stuzin JM: Chemical peeling and dermabrasion, in McCarthy JG (ed): *Plastic Surgery,* vol 1. Philadelphia, WB Saunders, 1990.

Commission on Surgical Suction Lipectomy, Ad Hoc Committee on New Procedures, American Society of Plastic and Reconstructive Surgeons: *Five Year Updated Evaluation on Suction Lipectomy.* Chicago, American Society of Plastic and Reconstructive Surgeons, 1987.

Illouz YG: Body contouring by lipolysis: A 5-year experience with over 3000 cases. *Plast Reconstr Surg* 1983; 72:591.

Litton C, Szachowitz EH II, Trinidad GP: Present day status of the chemical face peel. *Aesthetic Plast Surg* 1986; 10:1.

Pitman GH, Teimourian B: Suction lipectomy: Complications and results by survey. *Plast Reconstr Surg* 1985; 76:65.

Radovan C: Tissue expansion in soft tissue reconstruction. *Plast Reconstr Surg* 1984; 74:482.

Teimourian B: Complications associated with suction lipectomy. *Clin Plast Surg* 1989; 16:385.

PART II

Plastic Surgical Aspects of Specific Related Disciplines

Chapter 6

Medicolegal and Psychiatric Aspects of Plastic Surgery

Mark Gorney, M.D.

CONTENTS

CHAPTER OBJECTIVE

At the end of this chapter the resident has a clear understanding of the medicolegal and psychiatric aspects of plastic surgery practice, regularly obtains informed consent from his patients, and carries out an effective basic psychological evaluation on them when appropriate.

LEARNER OBJECTIVES

On completion of this chapter the resident

1. **Understands the medical and legal perspectives of the contractual agreement between a physician and his patient.**
2. **Understands the concepts of informed consent and implied guarantee.**
3. **Understands the role of the medical record as a legal document.**
4. **Understands the impact that physical deformity can have on patients and their families.**
5. **Knows techniques to explore the motivations of patients seeking cosmetic surgery and how to distinguish acceptable, unacceptable, and pathologic motivations.**
6. Knows legal and ethical ways to sever the physician/patient relationship.
7. Understands the various types of malpractice insurance.
8. Recognizes the basic principles of risk management.
9. Understands psychiatric and psychological treatment options for patients with physical deformities and their families.

CLINICAL PRACTICE ACTIVITIES

During the course of the training program, the resident

1. **Obtains informed consent from all patients; effectively documents the consent agreement.**
2. **Evaluates patients for aesthetic surgery from a physical and psychological perspective.**

3. **Contributes effectively and accurately to the medical record of inpatients and outpatients.**
4. **Treats patients with physical deformity and explores the psychological aspects of their care.**
5. Manages problem patients, including angry patients, dissatisfied patients, "doctor shoppers," "drug seekers," etc.

A plastic and reconstructive surgeon practicing in the United States in the last three decades of the 20th century will find it virtually impossible to end his career unblemished by a claim of malpractice.

However, well over half of the malpractice claims are preventable. Most are based on failures of communication and patient selection criteria, not on technical faults. Patient selection is the ultimate inexact science. It is a melange of surgical judgment, gut feelings, personality interactions, the surgeon's ego strength, and regrettably, economic considerations. Communication, on the other hand, is the sine qua non of building a doctor-patient relationship. Unfortunately, the ability to communicate well is a personality characteristic that cannot be readily learned in adulthood. Regardless of technical ability, someone who appears cold, arrogant, or insensitive is far more likely to be sued than one who relates "humanly."

LEGAL PRINCIPLES APPLIED TO PLASTIC SURGERY

Standard of Care

Malpractice is defined as "treatment which is contrary to accepted medical standards and which produces injurious results in the patient." Since most medical malpractice actions are based on laws governing negligence, the law recognizes that medicine is an inexact art and that there cannot be absolute liability. Thus the cause of action is usually the "failure of defendant/physician to exercise that reasonable degree of skill, learning, care and treatment ordinarily possessed by others of the same profession in the community." In the past, the term "community" was accepted geographically, but now, based on the supposition that all doctors keep up with the latest developments in their field, community is generally interpreted as "specialty community." The standards are now those of the specialty, without regard to geographic location. This is usually referred to as "standard of care."

Warranty

The law holds that by merely engaging to render treatment, a doctor warrants that he has the learning and skill of the average member of his specialty and that he will apply that learning and skill with ordinary and reasonable care. This warranty of due care is legally implied; it need not be mentioned by the physician or the patient. However, the warranty is for service, not for cure. Thus the doctor does not imply that the operation will be a success, that results will be favorable, or that he will not commit medical errors not caused by a lack of skill or care.

Informed Consent

While attempting to define the yardstick of disclosure, the courts divide medical and surgical procedures into two categories:

1. Common procedures that incur minor or very remote serious risk (including death or serious bodily harm), e.g., the administration of antibiotics.
2. Procedures involving serious risks for which the doctor has an "affirmative duty to disclose the potential of death or serious harm and explain, in detail, the complications that might possibly occur."

Affirmative duty means that the physician is obliged to disclose risks on his own, without waiting for the patient to ask. It is the patient, not the physician, who has the prerogative of determining his best interests. Thus the physician is obliged to discuss with the patient therapeutic alternatives and their particular hazards.

How much explanation and in what detail are dictated by a balance between the surgeon's feelings about his patient and legal requirements. It is simply not possible to tell patients everything without scaring them out of their surgery. Rather, the law states that patients must be told the most probable of the known dangers and the percentage of that probability. The rest may be disclosed in general terms while reminding the patient that he also has a statistical possibility of falling down and hurting himself that very same day.

Obviously, the most common complications should be volunteered frankly and openly, and their probability, based on the surgeon's personal experience, should also be mentioned. Finally, any or all of this information is wasted unless it is documented in the patient's record.

PSYCHOLOGICAL AND PSYCHIATRIC ASPECTS OF PLASTIC SURGERY

The growing popularity of cosmetic surgery makes it imperative to establish clear criteria of patient selection; without these, there will be an inevitable parallel increase in patient dissatisfaction and litigation.

Who, then, is the "ideal" candidate for aesthetic surgery? There is no such thing, but the surgeon should note any personality factors that will enhance or detract from the physical improvements sought.

There are basically two categories for rejection for cosmetic surgery. The first is anatomic unsuitability. The second is emotional inadequacy. Since the latter is by far the more important, the surgeon must differentiate between healthy and unhealthy reasons for seeking cosmetic improvement.

Strength of motivation is critical. It has a startlingly close relation with patient satisfaction. Furthermore, a strongly motivated patient will have less pain, a better postoperative course, and a significantly higher index of satisfaction regardless of result.

It is possible to establish some nearly objective criteria of patient selection and liability potential. These can be visualized as illustrated in Figure 6–1.

Figure 6–1 depicts the patient's objective deformity (as judged by the surgeon) vs. the patient's degree of concern with that deformity. Two opposite extremes emerge:

1. The patient with major deformity but minimal concern (lower right-hand corner)
2. The patient with minor deformity but extreme concern (upper left-hand corner)

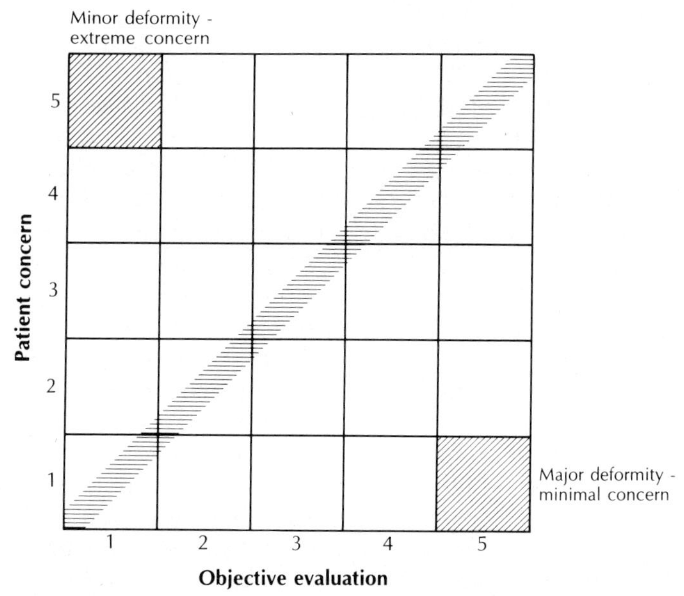

FIG 6–1.
Objective deformity vs. patient concern.

The latter extreme is the poorest candidate, while one seldom sees patients with major deformity and minimal concern. Most who seek aesthetic surgery fit somewhere on a diagonal between the contralateral corners. The closer the patient comes to the upper left-hand corner, the more an unfavorably perceived outcome and a visit to an attorney are likely.

Effective Communication as a Claims Prevention Technique

All litigation in plastic surgery has as a common denominator poor communication. Underlying all dissatisfaction is a breakdown in the rapport between patient and surgeon. This vital relationship is often shattered by the surgeon's arrogance, hostility, coldness (real or imagined), and mostly the fact that "he or she didn't care." There are only two ways to avoid such a debacle: (1) make sure that the patient has no reason to feel that way, and (2) avoid a patient who is going to feel that way no matter what is done.

Although the doctor's skill, reputation, and other intangible factors contribute to a patient's sense of confidence, rapport between patient and doctor is based on forthright and accurate communication. It is faulty communication that most often leads to the inevitable vicious cycle that follows: disappointment, anger, or frustration on the part of the patient; reactive hostility, defensiveness, and arrogance from the doctor; deepening patient anger; and finally, a visit to the attorney.

The art of listening, as well as that of verbal and nonverbal expression, merits serious attention in the effort to reduce malpractice lawsuits.

Expression—Verbal and Nonverbal

Since communication also requires expression, misunderstandings are just as likely to arise from speaking as from listening. The following are ways to improve communication while speaking:

- It is important to speak slowly and clearly to ensure that patients understand what is being said.
- If the message is complex, it is useful to pause frequently, even if no confusion is perceived. A break in speech allows the patient to either digest the message or ask for clarification. There should be repeated invitations for questions.

One of the most common complaints involves physicians' use of complex terminology or medical jargon. Words should be chosen that do not produce anxiety. While "excise" might be misunderstood, "cutting it out" sounds painful. "Removing it" is better.

Various studies show that the average patient retains 35% of what he was told. Thus, it does no harm to repeat, in summary form, the essential points at the end of the consultation or examination. It strongly reinforces what has been said. The anxiety of an office visit often causes patients to forget important questions or information. They should be encouraged to write down any questions and bring them on their next visit.

Starting with the first handshake, nonverbal communication establishes and maintains patient confidence. It becomes absolutely critical if things go wrong.

Physicians should not permit their own emotions or frustrations to be reflected to the patient. The patient's anxiety often magnifies the physician's body language.

Anger: A Root Cause of Malpractice Claims

Patients feel a sense of bewilderment and anxiety when elective surgery does not go smoothly. The borderline between anxiety and anger is tenuous, and the conversion factor is uncertainty—fear of the unknown. A patient frightened by a postoperative complication or uncertain about the future may surmise: "If it is the doctor's fault, the responsibility is the doctor's to correct."

The patient's perceptions may clash with the physician's anxieties, insecurities, and wounded pride. The patient blames the physician, who in turn becomes defensive. At this critically delicate juncture the physician's reaction can set in motion or prevent a natural chain reaction. The physician must put aside feelings of disappointment, anxiety, defensiveness, and hostility and understand that he is probably dealing with a frightened patient who is using anger to gain "control" of the situation. Subsequent developments can be changed by whatever understanding, support, and encouragement seem appropriate to the situation.

The patient's perception that the physician understands the uncertainty and will join with him to help conquer it may decide whether that patient will seek legal counsel. When faced with someone who is upset or angry, it is best to remain silent and let that person talk about the problem. The physician should only respond with noncommittal comments until the emotionally charged patient has calmed down. The technique of attentive silence often defuses angry people. Once the angry speaker has finished expressing his dissatisfaction, it is best to calmly ask the speaker to reiterate part of the message, even though it was fully understood already. The request for additional information or explanation reinforces in the speaker's mind the importance attached to the message.

One of the worst errors in dealing with angry or dissatisfied patients is to try to avoid them. It is necessary to actively participate in the process rather than avoid the issue.

THE MEDICAL RECORD

Accurate Medical Records: The Primary Line of Defense

Regardless of its merits, any medical malpractice suit can be won or lost because of the quality and content of the medical records. Most suits are tried (or settled) years after the critical events.

The following guidelines summarize the simple requirements of a defensible record:

I. *General guidelines*

A. The consequences of illegible handwriting can be costly. Be certain that your entries in all medical records are clear and readable. If possible, dictate long entries that require more than brief or routine annotations.

B. Never "squeeze" words into a line or leave blank spaces of any sort. Draw diagonal lines through all blank spaces after an entry.

C. Never erase, overwrite, or try to ink out an entry. In case of error, draw a single line and write "error" with the date, time, and your initials in the margin.

D. Never add anything at any time unless it is in a separately dated and signed note. Remember that the entry date of ink or type can be accurately determined retrospectively. Also be aware that the plaintiff's attorney may have a copy of the patient's original records, and any alteration after the fact will seriously compromise the defense of your case.

E. The date and time of each entry may be critical. Be sure that each page is dated and bears the patient's name and that each progress note is accompanied by the date and time.

F. Avoid personal abbreviations, ditto marks, or initials. Use only standard and accepted medical abbreviations.

G. Retain your records for a minimum of 7 years from the date of the last entry.

II. *Documentation*

A. General

1. Document when you are absent, with the name of the physician you have signed out to, along with the date and time.
2. Record pertinent observations and follow-up in any abnormal situation.
3. Ensure documentation of laboratory and radiologic examination results with a system that requires that all such reports will be seen, evaluated, and initialed by you or a colleague prior to filing in the patient's chart. This is particularly important when dealing with laboratory or pathology reports, radiographs relating to fractures, or computed tomography (CT) scans.
4. Justify your failure to comply with or reject a consultant's advice.
5. Document in detail your viewpoints and reasons for disagreement on patient care between you and a hospital utilization review

committee or preferred provider organization (PPO).

6. Explain any delayed responses to nurse or house staff calls; enter the dates and times.
7. Respond to nurses' pertinent observations of patient and record follow-up in your progress notes.
8. Document the patient's verbatim statements.
   Wrong: The patient apparently fell.
   Correct: The patient states: "Tried to get up, tripped and hit head on the corner of the bed."
9. Record negative reactions to any treatment or medication.

B. *Office/Hospital Records.* The following entries should appear in the office and/or hospital records of each patient:
1. History and physical examination, especially noting absence of abnormality.
2. Past history, with particular emphasis on current medications, allergies, drug sensitivities, or previous surgery.
3. Specific notation on the patient's experience, if any, with smoking, drug or alcohol abuse, or previous surgeries. If you choose to operate on heavy smokers, you had better record the rationale for doing so.
4. Progress notes, entered after each office visit and on any change in status. If negative, your follow-up should be indicated.
5. Signed and witnessed consent forms for special procedures or surgery.
6. Medications, treatments, specimens (where sent).
7. Patient's response to medications or procedures.
8. Document patient's failure to follow advice or refusal to cooperate or keep appointments. Missed appointments should be logged. Record your follow-up telephone calls and letters.
9. All significant laboratory, pathology, and radiographic reports and the dates when ordered and read.
10. Copies of records of instructions of any kind (including diet) and directions to the family.
11. Consultations with other physicians and their written (or oral) responses with the date and time recorded.
12. Thorough documentation of any patient's grievance, including the date and time. Conversely, file any complimentary notes, letters, and Christmas cards.
13. The critical importance of preoperative and postoperative photographs cannot be over-emphasized. They should be of the same pose, lighting conditions, and quality. In plastic surgical claims, these photographs can spell the difference between the attorney's refusal to take the case or a substantial award to the plaintiff.

C. *Surgical Case Records.* Monitor the following reporting procedures to ensure that they are performed routinely:
1. Anesthesiologist
   a. Accurate entries by the anesthesiologist, including type of monitoring device. A complete record should go in the chart.
   b. Condition of patient on transfer to the recovery ward, including the status of the airway and the position of the patient.
   c. Postanesthesia instructions signed by a responsible person on behalf of the patient.
2. Surgeon
   a. Accurate operative notes of the surgeon dictated *the day of the procedure* and including postoperative orders signed by the operating surgeon.
   b. Postoperative instructions signed by a responsible person on behalf of the patient.
   c. In outpatient cases, a notation by the surgeon of the patient's condition on discharge and a record of a follow-up phone call the evening of surgery.

3. Nursing
   a. Signed and witnessed consent form that conforms to the actual procedure to be performed.
   b. Verification of nothing-by-mouth (NPO) status, allergies, previous anesthetics and surgeries, and physical limitations; results of laboratory, x-ray, and other examinations; status of patient on arrival in the operating room.
   c. Record all preoperative and intraoperative intravenous solutions, blood products, and medications.
   d. Location of electrosurgical grounding pads.
   e. Type of preparation and condition of skin.
   f. Disposition of surgical specimens, tissue, or implant. (Surgical pathology forms must contain appropriate information to ensure adequate examination.)
   g. Identification of all drains, packing, catheters, and especially surgical implants, including type, serial number, amount to fill, and supplementary antibiotics, if any.
   h. Sponge, needle, and instrument count (if irregular, documentation of corrective measures). If product stickers are available, put them in the record. If corticoids are used, record dose and type.
4. Parenteral medications, fluids, intake/output
   a. Record the type and amount of rate of administration, and medications (if any added).
   b. Record the time and site of any injections (intramuscular or subcutaneous) and any untoward reaction.
   c. Record any abnormalities at the site of an intravenous infusion and the time when noticed.
   d. Record the function of draining, including the amount and nature of secretions.
5. Patient instructions
   a. Always record your instructions in writing. Keep a copy in the patient's record.
   b. Review your instructions with the patient and family.
   c. Ensure comprehension. Ask and record whether there are any questions after instructions.
   d. Instructions should include (when applicable) the following:
      (1) Specific wound care.
      (2) Limitations of activity, position, or exercise.
      (3) Dietary restrictions.
      (4) Specific instructions on medications, including possible side effects.
      (5) Follow-up appointments.
   e. Document the following:
      (1) Language limitations, attempts made to overcome them by translators, and your notation if comprehension appears to be questionable.
      (2) Any literature provided to the patient and family and/or video orientations.
      (3) Copy of instructions given.
      (4) Failure to comply with instructions and that the patient was informed of the risks of noncompliance.

Naturally, specific legal requirements may vary from state to state. Adherence to these general principles can nonetheless result in significantly decreased liability.

MANAGING PATIENTS FROM A LEGAL PERSPECTIVE

Claims Prevention in Office Procedures

Not infrequently, the cause of malpractice allegation begins with procedural errors in the office.

Misfiled Reports

Filing of reports not seen by the doctor often leads to malpractice claims. This can result in a delay in diagnosis or treatment of a serious disease.

Patient Noncompliance—Severance of the Physician/Patient Relationship

The staff should chart missed appointments and call them to the physician's attention. If the patient's noncompliance carries the potential for injury, a certified return receipt letter expressing appropriate concern for the patient's welfare and (when indicated) warnings regarding the consequences should be sent.

Suspense files should be set up for all tests, procedures, and consultations. If the tests are not carried out, the staff should call this to the physician's attention, and the patient should be reminded. Patient noncompliance and all callbacks to the patient should be charted. Copies of all letters to the patient should be included.

In the case of continued noncompliance and if circumstances warrant, a certified return receipt letter also should indicate the withdrawal of your care. Notations of all actions and copies of all letters sent to the patient should become a permanent part of the patient's record.

Other Claims Prevention Principles

Another major factor contributing to litigation is the continual billing of an already dissatisfied patient. If a dispute occurs, all billing action should be stopped until resolution. Furthermore, if the patient has indicated dissatisfaction with a treatment or surgical procedure, one should consider forgiving the outstanding balance. This by itself does *not* imply legal guilt!

The physician must identify any drug allergies and display them prominently on a color-coded label placed in a specific location on the outside of the patient's chart. Special labels should also be used for identifying smokers and if the case is a medicolegal or compensation case.

The staff should not discuss the patient's medical problems or records without a release signed by the patient (or legal guardian) and the approval of the appropriate person in your office.

Staff should be encouraged to initiate personal contact with patients by expressing warmth and individual attention. The staff may represent the first, last, and most durable impression patients have of the physician's office.

The physician should be sure that the staff is aware of what has been told to the patient so that there is no confusion.

Avoid Mistakes

Important guidelines for office staff and physicians include the following:

- Double-check the vial or bottle label prior to drawing up any substance. Never permit unlabeled containers in your operating room.
- Make sure that the staff understands dosage—"15" or "50" may sound similar, but the difference may be catastrophic.
- Prior to the administration of any medication by any route, the patient should be asked about allergies to the drug or drugs that are to be injected.
- Everyone should know the location and use of oxygen, the crash cart, and other resuscitative equipment and drugs.
- All personnel dealing directly with patients should be trained in cardiopulmonary resuscitation and should be appropriately recertified.
- Develop guidelines for prescription calls and refills, and always record them with the date and time in the patient's chart.

Equipment Malfunction

Most equipment-related suits involve electrical burns. All electrical equipment should be checked regularly to confirm that it is properly grounded.

There should be a regular schedule of preventive maintenance. A bioengineer should certify safety of electrical equipment on a regular basis. A log of such certification with a reminder of the next scheduled service must be maintained. A desirable place to keep the log is on a label affixed to the instruments themselves.

For a discussion of types of malpractice insurance and for additional perspectives of risk management, see Chapter 35.

SUGGESTED READING

Cole NM: Informed Consent: Considerations in aesthetic and reconstructive surgery of the breast. *Clin Plast Surg* 1988; 15:541–548.

Goldwyn RM: *The Patient and the Plastic Surgeon,* ed 2. Boston, Little, Brown, 1991.

Housman SB: Psychosocial aspects of plastic surgery, in McCarthy JG (ed): *Plastic Surgery.* Philadelphia, WB Saunders, 1990, pp 113–138.

Zupko KA (ed): *Office and Practice Management Notebook.* Chicago, American Society of Plastic and Reconstructive Surgeons, 1992.

Chapter 7

Anesthesia and Critical Care

Warren Garner, M.D.
Pema Dorje

CONTENTS

NOTE: The material in this chapter is frequently covered during the prerequisite training period of many plastic surgery residents. This chapter should serve as a valuable review of important material in such cases. For residents who have not mastered this material previously, this chapter is essential.

CHAPTER OBJECTIVE

At the end of this chapter the resident understands the indications, principles, techniques, and complications of local, regional, and general anesthesia in a wide variety of clinical settings; is thoroughly familiar with the principles and techniques of critical care; and effectively manages critically ill burn, trauma, and postoperative patients.

LEARNER OBJECTIVES

On completion of this chapter the resident

1. **Demonstrates knowledge of common agents for local anesthesia (esters and amides), regional anesthesia, and general anesthesia (intravenous agents, inhalation agents, muscle relaxants, antiemetics, etc.)**
2. **Knows the principles and the techniques for administration of local anesthesia.**
3. **Is familiar with the emergency care of burn and trauma patients, including diagnostic techniques and management principles.**
4. **Is skilled in the postoperative management of all plastic surgical patients.**
5. Knows the principles and techniques for regional anesthesia, particularly

A. Digital block
B. Wrist block
C. Brachial block
D. Bier block
E. Ankle block

The resident is also generally familiar with the principles of spinal and epidural anesthesia.

6. Has basic knowledge of the principles and techniques for general anesthesia using different anesthetic techniques.
7. Knows the indications for various modes of anesthesia that relate to:
   A. procedure
   B. patient conditions
8. Is generally familiar with the type and the incidence of complications from various kinds of anesthesia and the cause for morbidity and mortality and their occurrence in local anesthesia, regional anesthesia, general anesthesia, and hypotensive anesthesia.
9. Is competent in the management of critically ill patients in the surgical intensive care unit.

CLINICAL PRACTICE ACTIVITIES

During the course of the training program, the resident

1. **Participates in the decision as to which technique of anesthesia should be used on his patients.**
2. **Utilizes the techniques of local anesthesia.**
3. **Carries out emergency management of burn and trauma patients.**
4. **Manages all plastic surgical patients postoperatively.**
5. Utilizes the techniques of regional anesthesia.
6. Becomes familiar with all monitoring equipment in facilities used for general anesthesia, regional anesthesia, and local anesthesia.
7. Participates in the treatment of complications from anesthesia.
8. Manages complications of local anesthesia when these occur.
9. Manages burn and trauma patients in the intensive care unit.

EMERGENCY CARE OF TRAUMATIZED PATIENTS

The initial management of critically ill, traumatized patients is based on the "ABC" management sequence: airway, breathing, and circulation. Airway obstruction caused by tissue swelling, loss of mandibular support, or disruption of normal anatomy is treated by tracheal intubation or, if this is technically not possible, cricothyroidotomy. A lack of patient-initiated breathing is cause to begin positive-pressure ventilation, initially with an Ambu bag. Only when patients are stable should they be placed on a ventilator. Tissue perfusion is the goal of circulation and should be accomplished by optimizing preload first, then improving cardiac contractility, and finally improving afterload. In most patients, this means resuscitation with Ringer's lactate and blood. If this resuscitation does not restore circulation, invasive monitoring should be used to accurately direct further treatment.

The clinical diagnosis of critical illness in an adult is based on clinical findings such as abnormal vital signs or altered mental status. Treatment requires diagnosis of both the emergent problem and its underlying cause.

Many patients undergoing limited reconstructive or grafting procedures are healthy individuals and therefore require only basic monitoring procedures. On the other hand, patients with established systemic illness or massive injury such as major burns have a significantly greater risk of perioperative mortality and should receive intensive preoperative evaluation and monitoring.

MONITORING

Noninvasive measurement of oxygen saturation by use of pulse oximetry is a major advance in the ability to monitor patients. The technique utilizes the differential absorption of oxyhemoglobin and reduced hemoglobin to determine the hemoglobin saturation. This technology allows continuous real-time measurement of both arterial and mixed venous hemoglobin saturation. Arterial pulse oximeters provide accurate information about patients' respiratory status. They should also be used during procedures when the patient is sedated.

The specific information needed to treat life-threatening cardiopulmonary dysfunction is obtained by invasive monitoring. Arterial catheters, used to provide real-time measurements of arterial blood pressure and allow blood sampling, are usually inserted in the radial artery since the ulnar artery and the palmar arches provide collateral circulation to the hand. (An Allen test should be performed before every radial artery catheter placement.) Alternate placement sites include the femoral, dorsalis pedis, and axillary arteries. The most common complication is infection. Thrombosis is less common but more serious. It is more common with catheters larger than 20 gauge, in surgically inserted catheters, and in smaller arteries. Most thrombosis (96%) is asymptomatic, and recanalization usually occurs.

Development of the flow-directed pulmonary artery (PA) catheter by Swan and Ganz resulted in a major advance in monitoring potential. PA catheters should be used in all patients with significant cardiopulmonary dysfunction. PA "wedge" pressure is useful as the best available approximation of left ventricular end-diastolic volume. Cardiac output measurements can be used to titrate vasoactive and inotropic drugs. Probably the most useful determinant is the mixed venous oxygen content since this value reflects overall cardiac and pulmonary performance.

RESPIRATORY FAILURE

There are multiple causes of respiratory failure in plastic surgery patients. These are a neurogenic inability to breathe, airway compromise, hypoxic respiratory failure, and inadequate ventilation. Traumatic brain injury may occur in patients with facial fractures. Airway compromise is common in patients with significant head and neck trauma and in patients with inhalation injury. Acute respiratory failure (ARF) is usually the result of sepsis and is most common in the postoperative period. ARF after thermal injury is often due to inhaled toxic products of combustion and is frequently a contributor to mortality in these patients.

AIRWAY MANAGEMENT

Airway management is of central importance in critically ill patients. Indications for tracheal intubation include inability to maintain or protect the airway, the need to provide airway pressure support to improve hypoxia, and inability to effectively ventilate. In some patients undergoing major operative procedures in the head and neck, tracheostomy is appropriate to maintain a secure airway. In patients with massive facial trauma or significant airway burns, early intubation may be necessary to prevent incipient airway obstruction. When emergent airway control is needed and intubation is not possible, a cricothyroidotomy should be performed. There is little role for emergency tracheostomy.

For most patients, airway management means tracheal intubation during the early phases of illness and tracheostomy for patients with prolonged respiratory failure. The timing of transition to tracheostomy is controversial. Previous recommendations have been based on retrospective analysis and personal experience. A recent prospective study found that tracheostomy before 7 days decreased mechanically ventilated days and hospital days. Our practice is to place a tracheostomy in a patient likely to require more than a week of mechanical ventilation.

RESPIRATORY SUPPORT

Effective management of ARF first requires a diagnosis of the need for ventilation and/or oxygenation support. These two needs can be differentiated by an arterial blood gas (ABG) determination. A Pao_2 less than 60 combined with low $Paco_2$ suggests problems with oxygenation. An elevated $Paco_2$ and a Pao_2 less than 60 indicate ventilatory dysfunction. Most surgical patients with ARF have difficulties in oxygenation, not ventilation, although alterations of lung compliance may necessitate ventilatory support as well. Therefore, it is critical to determine the need for ventilatory and oxygenation support independently and provide the particular type of support each patient needs.

Ventilatory failure reflects an inadequate patient ability to maintain the needed amount of air movement. It results from decreased respiratory effort, decreased lung compliance, or increased ventilatory requirements in the face of limited ability to increase respiratory efforts. Any patient who demonstrates clinical evidence of inadequate ventilation should have immediate treatment with positive pressure. A tidal volume of 10 to 15 cc/kg and a respiratory rate of 8 to 12 provides adequate minute ventilation in most patients. The adequacy of delivered minute ventilation is determined by an ABG study demonstrating a normal $Paco_2$ and pH at a respiratory rate of less than 30. Additional improvement in a patient's ability to ventilate can sometimes be achieved by the use of positive end-expiratory pressure (PEEP) or continuous positive airway pressure (CPAP) to improve lung compliance. Treatment of the underlying causes of ARF may decrease the need for ventilatory support.

There is controversy about the best method to provide positive-pressure ventilation. Intermittent mandatory ventilation (IMV), synchronized intermittent mandatory ventilation (SIMV), and assist-control (A/C) ventilation all have proponents. In most cases the mode chosen to deliver positive-pressure ventilation is based on physician training and familiarity. Our practice is to encourage spontaneous breathing by using limited IMV or SIMV. The increased use of spontaneous breathing, sometimes augmented by a pressure support assist device, decreases mean and peak airway pressures and improves ventilation-perfusion matching. In addition, low-pressure ventilation limits pressure-induced pulmonary damage and subsequent pulmonary fibrosis. This decreases the risks of barotrauma and cardiac compromise. The increased work of breathing needed for this protocol is seldom clinically relevant.

Inability to effectively oxygenate is a problem distinct from ventilatory failure. Hypoxia in the face of adequate ventilation is usually due to cardiac failure or adult respiratory distress syndrome (ARDS). The diagnosis is based on measurements of intravascular pressures as previously described. There are many conditions associated with ARDS, and the pathophysiology is complex. Treatment is designed to maintain oxygenation with therapy that is not toxic to the lung. The methods for achieving this are controversial. Increased inspired oxygen content will increase arterial po_2 in patients with normal lungs; however, mismatched ventilation and perfusion limit the effectiveness of this technique in patients with ARDS. In addition, while oxygen toxicity is defined for patients with chronic pulmonary insufficiency, the "safe" level of inspired oxygen is not established for septic or recently traumatized patients. PEEP is an effective alternative to improve oxygenation and can be used to limit the administration of toxic oxygen levels. Because PEEP increases intrathoracic pressure, compromised cardiovascular performance can result from its use. At levels above 18 to 20 cm H_2O, some degree of cardiac compromise is predictable; therefore, hemodynamic monitoring is essential. In patients with severe ARDS, complex decisions between toxic oxygen levels, cardiac compromise, and acceptable levels of tissue oxygen delivery are necessary and generally require the input of an experienced intensivist.

CARDIOVASCULAR DYSFUNCTION

Critically ill patients most often manifest cardiac dysfunction as inadequate tissue perfusion. Improving performance requires correction of specific pathologic factors such as ischemia and pericardial tamponade. General cardiac function is improved by normalizing intravascular volume, increasing contractility with inotropes, and normalizing vascular tone. In most patients accurately treating these processes requires invasive monitoring with a PA catheter. The end point of therapy is adequate tissue perfusion clinically evidenced by urine output of at least 30 cc/hr. In complicated situations we utilize mixed venous oxygen saturation as an indicator of total-body perfusion. Treatment of cardiac arrhythmias is indicated if the dysrhythmia results in impaired hemodynamic performance or is likely to do so. Asymptomatic tachycardias or bradycardias indicate a need for diagnosis and treatment of an underlying cause.

FLUID RESUSCITATION

The fluid requirements of a critically ill patient are extremely variable and must be individualized. They can be divided into fluid needed to resuscitate a patient and daily fluid replacement. When fluids are required to replenish inadequate intravascular or extracellular fluid spaces, Ringer's lactate is usually used. This fluid is chosen because its electrolyte composition reflects that of the missing fluid, it is effective, and it is cheap. While experimental evidence has documented the efficacy of colloid-containing fluids or hypertonic saline for specific clinical indications, their increased cost and potential for complications limit their general use.

CARDIOVASCULAR SUPPORT

Treatment of poor cardiac performance assumes adequate fluid resuscitation. Additional improvements in cardiac function require the use of inotropes or assist devices. Dobutamine and dopamine are the most commonly used inotropes. Dobutamine is a selective β_1-agonist and increases cardiac output without increasing myocardial oxygen requirements. It must be used cautiously in patients with sepsis since it can cause vasodilation. Because dopamine is a vasoconstrictor at higher doses (>10 μg/kg/min), it is an alternative in this patient population. The role of digoxin as an inotrope in the intensive care unit (ICU) is limited. Inotropes should be used with arterial and PA monitoring. The end point of therapy is a cardiac index sufficient to maintain tissue perfusion, not a specific blood pressure. This is determined by normalization of mixed venous oxygen tension. In patients with pathologic vasodilatation caused by sepsis or liver disease, tissue perfusion can be improved with the judicious use of vasoconstrictors such as norepinephrine. The goal of this therapy is to increase the afterload toward the normal range. It is critical that patients treated in this fashion first undergo complete fluid resuscitation and optimization of myocardial performance.

The intra-aortic balloon pump (IABP) is a percutaneously inserted balloon catheter used in cases of reversible cardiac dysfunction. The IABP increases diastolic aortic pressure, usually decreasing afterload, increasing coronary blood flow, and increasing the cardiac index. Its effectiveness is limited to patients with short-term, reversible cardiac failure.

VENOUS DISEASE

Deep venous thromboembolic disease (DVT) is important as a predecessor of pulmonary embolism (PE). Risk factors include patient immobility, pelvic or hip surgery, malignant disease, obesity, and a past history of DVT or PE. The clinical signs and symptoms of PE are nonspecific, and the diagnosis should be considered in any patient with unexplained dyspnea or hypoxia. ABG analysis will demonstrate hypoxia. The diagnosis is made by using ventilation-perfusion scans or, if these are not diagnostic, pulmonary angiography. Treatment with heparin prevents clot extension and improves symptoms in most patients. Continued anticoagulation with warfarin for 3 months is recommended. Thrombolytic therapy is not used because of the high rate of hemorrhagic complications. The best treatment is prevention. The risk of PE can be significantly reduced with low-dose heparin or warfarin or the use of intermittent pneumatic calf compression.

INFECTION AND SEPSIS

Localized subcutaneous infections after traumatic injury are usually the result of bacterial contamination at the time of injury. Debridement of necrotic tissue, irrigation to reduce bacterial load, and short-term antibiotic administration reduce the rate of infection. Prophylactic antibiotic use for longer than 48 hours does not improve results. When localized infections develop, they should be drained. Systemic sepsis results from untreated local infection and requires more intensive antibiotic therapy in addition to treatment of the local problem.

Nosocomial infections such as pneumonia, catheter infection, or urinary tract infection are common in critically ill patients and should be considered when patients become febrile. Evaluation should be symptom directed and empirical antibiotic therapy based on the sensitivities of organisms likely to cause an infection. The fever itself is seldom a problem and should rarely be treated. Moreover, most immunologic processes are more effective at elevated temperature. Temperatures below 104°F cause sequelae only in patients with severely compromised cardiopulmonary function or brain injury, patients in whom the increase in metabolic rate is not tolerated.

NUTRITION

Nutrition support is an essential component of a complete treatment plan because without support patients will catabolize structural proteins as a caloric source and decrease both muscle mass and their ability to respond to infection. The survival and complication rates of burned and traumatized patients improve with early feeding. The need for nutrition support in other patients is less well defined. Patients with significant weight loss and decreased delayed cutaneous hypersensitivity, lymphocyte counts, and serum protein levels, such as patients with head and neck cancer and a long-standing inability to eat, benefit from preoperative nutrition support. Patients who are able to resume a diet within 7 days of a surgical procedure probably do not require nutrition support. If a longer period of starvation is expected, support should be started. Alimentary tract feedings are the preferred route of administration since they are more effective in reestablishing nutritional balance, are cheaper, help to maintain bowel mucosal integrity and decrease bacterial translocation, and are associated with fewer complications. Total parenteral nutrition should be reserved for patients whose gastrointestinal tract is unavailable or is unable to tolerate an enteral diet.

Our practice is to place a feeding tube in all traumatized or burned patients on admission and begin feedings within 24 hours. In patients undergoing extensive procedures in the head and neck region, a feeding tube should be placed at the time of surgery and tube feedings begun in the early postoperative period. Nutrition support should be provided to maintain the patient in a positive nitrogen balance. Estimation of a patient's caloric requirements is complex. The best formula to estimate caloric needs utilizes the Harris-Benedict equation, but this is not accurate in stressed patients. Our method of choice is the specific measurement of a patient's caloric needs by using indirect calorimetry. There is no simple method to estimate protein requirements. Studies of protein requirements have shown that administration rates of 2 g/kg/day are sufficient in most patients. The efficacy of the nutrition provided should be documented in all patients since the individual patient's nutritional needs, ability to absorb the tube feeding, and metabolic state will vary. Weekly measurement to confirm increasing concentrations of acute-phase proteins like prealbumin and retinol-binding protein are useful for this purpose.

HEMATOLOGIC DISORDERS

Disordered coagulation can result from preexisting abnormalities of coagulation factors or platelets. These abnormalities are usually ascertained by a thorough history and physical examination. Acquired defects can be more subtle and include aspirin-induced platelet dysfunction, decreased factor synthesis from occult liver disease, or antibiotic-induced vitamin K deficiency. Preoperative delay and judicious replacement will allow correction of most problems. Coagulation deficiencies caused by massive transfusion occur after one–blood volume exchanges and should be treated with replacement of 2 units of fresh frozen plasma and 8 units of platelets for each 10 units of red blood cell (RBC) replacement.

At this time transfusions are linked to overwhelming patient concern about contaminated blood. Transfusions to replace massive blood loss are accepted. Patients with chronic blood loss or marginal hematocrit values are a more difficult problem. Thorough discussion of the benefits and risks is essential. Currently, the risk of human immunodeficiency virus (HIV) transmission is 1 in 100,000 in most major institutions, and the risk of hepatitis developing is about 0.1%, although this may decrease with improved testing for hepatitis C.

ANESTHESIA FOR PLASTIC SURGERY

Modern anesthesia care begins with preoperative assessment and extends well into the postoperative period. The result is that the overall risk of death from anesthesia is now estimated to be 1 to 2 in 10,000.

Drugs Used in General Anesthesia

Induction Agents

Induction agents (e.g., thiopental, methohexital, propofol, etomidate, ketamine) are used to produce the initial unconscious state. They are usually administered intravenously, reach the brain in high concentrations, and produce anesthesia. The drugs are then redistributed to less vascular areas of the body, and their brain effect decreases. Anesthesia is then maintained by using a combination of opioid and inhalational agents. The exact mechanism of action of these drugs is not known, but they are believed to work through γ-aminobutyric acid (GABA) receptors. These agents depress cardiovascular function to a variable degree. Benzodiazepines may also be used as induction agents in special circumstances. Propofol can be given by infusion for prolonged sedation or to maintain total intravenous anesthesia.

Inhalational Agents

Inhalational agents are halogenated vapors (halothane, isoflurane, and enflurane) or nitrous oxide. The minimum alveolar concentration (MAC) of a vapor is a measure of its anesthetic potency. MAC is defined as the alveolar concentration at which 50% of the subjects move in response to a noxious stimulus. All inhalational agents produce dose-related cardiovascular and respiratory depression, although the depressive effect of nitrous oxide is small. The pharmacology of these drugs is determined by the inspired concentration of the agent, the agent's solubility in blood, the patient's cardiac output and minute ventilation, and the pressure gradient for diffusion from the alveolus to blood. The less-soluble agents change alveolar concentration more quickly because less is added to or from the blood. Hence, less-soluble agents have a rapid induction and recovery time—a desirable feature. Currently, nitrous oxide is the only agent that is gaseous at ambient temperature and is therefore administered by using a flowmeter instead of a special vaporizer. It must be administered in high concentrations because of its low potency. It is the only inhalational agent that has analgesic properties.

Narcotics

Narcotics are adjuncts to intravenous and inhalational anesthetics and include morphine, meperidine, fentanyl, sufentanyl, and alfentanyl. They act on opioid receptors in the brain and spinal cord. Narcotics are respiratory depressants, have little action on the heart, but can cause hypotension in hypovolemic patients. Opioids are highly bound to plasma proteins, mainly to α_1-acid glycoprotein, an acute stress protein. During illness the concentration of this protein is elevated, and a higher proportion of the narcotic is in the bound inactive form. Liver disease and renal insufficiency can prolong opioids' clinical effects. Fentanyl and very dilute solutions of bupivacaine can be infused in the thoracic epidural space to control postoperative pain. This combination has the advantage of not producing muscle paralysis, hypotension, and sedation.

Muscle Relaxants and Reversal Agents

Muscle relaxants block the transmission of the nerve impulse to the muscle by occupying the acetylcholine receptors in the postsynaptic muscle cell membrane. The muscle relaxants are water soluble, quaternary ammonium compounds and have a structural similarity to acetylcholine. There are two types of neuromuscular blocking drugs, depolarizing and nondepolarizing agents. Succinylcholine is a depolarizing muscle relaxant with a rapid onset (1 minute) and a short duration of action

(5 minutes). It is metabolized by plasma cholinesterase, and prolonged effects are seen in patients with abnormal cholinesterase levels. Complications include myalgia, bradycardia, and asystole. Patients with burns, wounds or traumatized tissue, or neurologic conditions may respond to succinylcholine with lethal hyperkalemia, so these conditions contraindicate the use of succinylcholine. The nondepolarizing muscle relaxants (curare, vecuronium, atracurium, pancuronium, etc.) have a slower onset (3 minutes) and a longer duration of action (30 to 45 minutes). Vecuronium and atracurium have no cardiovascular effect, whereas pancuronium increases the heart rate because of its vagolytic effect. Neostigmine and edrophonium are inhibitors of the enzymes that metabolize acetylcholine at the neuromuscular junction. The resultant increased levels of acetylcholine compete with muscle relaxants for the acetylcholine receptors. Moderate levels of neuromuscular blockade by nondepolarizing muscle relaxants can be reversed with one of the above anticholinesterases. The desirable effects of the reversal agents at the nicotinic receptor always come with the undesirable effects at the muscarinic receptors, such as bradycardia, bronchospasm, and increased secretions.

Antiemetics

Low-dose droperidol (0.25 mg) given soon after induction of anesthesia has proved to be effective in reducing the incidence of nausea and vomiting. Prochlorperazine (5 to 10 mg by slow intravenous route) is widely used in the recovery room. The drug is a mild α-receptor blocker and may therefore produce hypotension. Because it can cause dystonia, a total dose of 40 mg should not be exceeded in any 24-hour period.

Preoperative Evaluation of the Patient

Preoperative evaluation of the patient will ensure that he is optimally prepared for anesthesia. The evaluation should include a review of the history, physical examination, and laboratory results. The patient may then be allotted to one of the classes of the physical status classification of the American Society of Anesthesiologists (ASA). The ASA classification is used mainly for descriptive purposes, but it also has some outcome-predictive value (Table 7–1).

During the preoperative history it is important to note concurrent medications that may have an influence on anesthetic management, such as antihypertensives, monoamine oxidase inhibitors, and family history of abnormal sensitivity to drugs that is suggestive of cholinesterase deficiency. Physical examination focuses on the airway and major organ dysfunction. A previous history of difficult intubation, limited mouth opening and neck extension (e.g., from burn contractures), a prominent upper jaw and teeth, and a small receding mandible are some of the features that suggest difficult airway management. When regional anesthesia is planned, the ease of identifying landmarks and any evidence of infection at the site of injection are noted.

TABLE 7–1.

Physical Status Classification of the American Society of Anesthesiologists

Class	Physical Status
1	Patient has no organic, physiologic, biochemical, or psychiatric disturbances.
2	Patient has mild to moderate systemic disturbances that may or may not be related to the disorder requiring surgery (e.g., essential hypertension, diabetes mellitus).
3	Patient has severe systemic disturbance that may or may not be related to the disorder requiring surgery (e.g., heart disease that limits activity, poorly controlled essential hypertension).
4	Patient has severe systemic disturbance that is life-threatening with or without surgery (e.g., congestive heart failure, persistent angina pectoris).
5	Patient is moribund and has little chance for survival, but surgery is to be performed as a last resort (resuscitation effort) (e.g., uncontrolled hemorrhage, as from a ruptured aneurysm).
6	Patient requires an emergency operation.

Laboratory investigation is ordered for specific indications. A clinically healthy person less than 40 years of age should not need any laboratory investigation, although women need a hemoglobin level determination.

Nulla Per Os Policy

All elective patients should have no *solid* food after midnight before the day of surgery and should not be fed on the day of surgery. Juice with pulp (e.g., orange, grapefruit) and milk should be considered solid food. Clear noncarbonated *liquids* may be permitted up to 3 hours prior to anesthesia in unrestricted amounts. Examples of clear liquid include water, apple juice, black tea, and black coffee. An easier policy to implement is that nothing is permitted by mouth after midnight prior to surgery.

Monitoring During Anesthesia

As a minimum, an electrocardiograph (ECG) and pulse oximeter should be continuously observed during anesthesia and the blood pressure checked at least every 5 minutes during general or regional anesthesia and for monitoring and pharmacologic support (MAPS). The delivered oxygen content, end-tidal carbon dioxide, neuromuscular blockade, and urine output should be monitored in most patients. There must be a reliable ventilatory disconnection alarm. Body temperature must be monitored except in very short procedures. Critically ill patients, those with preexisting cardiopulmonary disease, or patients undergoing extensive procedures may be candidates for invasive cardiovascular monitoring.

The Conduct of Anesthesia

Anesthesia is usually induced with an intravenous agent and then maintained with a combination of opioid and inhalational agent. In most cases the airway is managed by intubating the trachea after induction of anesthesia and paralyzing the patient. Manual ventilation of the lung by using a mask before the intubation is not necessary and may be hazardous. However, the patient must breathe 100% oxygen through a well-fitting mask for about 3 minutes before the induction. For short cases in which no muscle relaxation is required to facilitate surgery, anesthesia may be maintained by allowing the patient to breathe spontaneously with a mask. If there is a high risk aspiration of gastric contents, a rapid-sequence method of anesthesia is performed by using an intravenous agent and a muscle relaxant that has a rapid onset of action (succinycholine) to allow the trachea to be intubated without any delay. To prevent gastric contents from reaching the pharynx before the airway is secured with an endotracheal tube, an assistant must occlude the esophagus between the cricoid cartilage and the vertebral column by manual pressure on the cricoid cartilage. A high-performance suctioning device must be within easy reach during this period. If the patient's airway is expected to be difficult to maintain, awake intubation using fiber-optic endoscopy should be considered. It is essential that the anesthesiologist be able to ventilate or intubate the patient after intravenous induction. Adequate intravenous access to deliver drugs and replace blood and fluids rapidly is essential, particularly when anesthetizing patients for debridement of burns. Previously checked blood, prewarmed fluids, and good communication between the anesthesia and surgical teams will limit hypovolemia, hypothermia, and other complications.

Methods to Reduce Blood Transfusion

Autotransfusion. Autotransfusion can be done in one or more ways: preoperative removal and storage, removal of blood and hemodilution just before the start of surgery, and intraoperative blood salvage and retransfusion. The main risk of retransfusing the salvaged blood is the transmission of infection and cancer cells back to the patient.

Deliberate hypotension. In deliberate hypotension the blood pressure is electively reduced and maintained at the lowest safe level. The technique is employed in plastic surgery to minimize blood loss and to facilitate delicate surgery by reducing blood in the surgical field. Patients with carotid artery disease, cardiac disease, or uncontrolled hypertension and acutely ill burn patients are not suitable candidates for induced hypotension.

Monitored Anesthesia Care

Plastic surgery is often performed on awake patients under nerve blocks and local infiltrations by the surgeon. This trend is to be encouraged because it is safe, simple, and cheap and the patient is not exposed to the side effects of anesthesia such as nausea and vomiting, which can affect the outcome of the plastic surgery. The amount of local anesthesia required can be substantial, and the infiltration of anesthesia can be painful and unpleasant. Hence the patient must be monitored and given pharmacologic support as needed. Preparation and monitoring for nerve blocks and infiltration are performed in the same way as for general anesthesia. O_2 must be administered via a nasal cannula. The exact technique of sedation varies. Midazolam may be given for anxiolysis; narcotics are generally avoided because they can cause nausea and/or vomiting. The unpleasant part of the experience usually comes at the time of local infiltration. A deeper level of intravenous sedation at this point is obtained by using propofol. If the airway becomes obstructed with this sedation, it is only temporary and can be overcome by jaw support and neck extension by the surgeon or anesthesiologist. A level of sedation can be maintained by using small doses of midazolam and an infusion of propofol.

Complications of General Anesthesia

Postoperative Nausea and Vomiting

Postoperative nausea and vomiting are more common among younger, particularly female patients. The type and technique of anesthesia can influence the incidence of nausea and/or vomiting. Narcotics and inhalational agents can cause postoperative nausea in a high proportion of patients. Hypoxia and hypoperfusion of the brain can induce nausea and vomiting, and therefore patients must be checked before rushing to prescribe antiemetics. Regional anesthesia is associated with a very low incidence. Straining, retching, and coughing increase the risk of hematoma formation under skin flaps in the head and neck area, and therefore their occurrence should be minimized.

Hepatotoxicity

The development of massive hepatic necrosis after halothane anesthesia has been described but is very rare. It is diagnosed by a process of elimination of other causes of hepatitis in the postoperative period.

Malignant Hyperthermia

Malignant hyperthermia is a rare, genetically inherited, life-threatening hypermetabolic disorder precipitated by triggering factors such as stress and certain anesthetic drugs. There seems to be a loss of the ability of the sarcoplasmic membranes to resequester calcium from sarcoplasm. The high calcium level leads to increased and persistent muscle contracture, which may account for the hypermetabolic state. Certain muscle diseases such as Duchenne's muscular dystrophy and periodic paralysis may have a higher association with malignant hyperpyrexia. Treatment of malignant hyperthermia consists of withdrawal of the triggering agents, limitation of the ongoing surgical procedure to minimize further stress, and administration of dantrolene. The patient will require active cooling and intensive respiratory, circulatory, and renal support.

Local Anesthesia

Local anesthetics are drugs that produce a reversible block of impulse conduction in nerve fibers. The conduction block occurs as the local anesthetic acts on the sodium channels, which are membrane proteins spanning the double layer of phospholipid molecules forming the axolemma. The binding of local anesthetics to the sodium channels prevents the conformational change that is necessary for impulse conduction.

The basic structure of the commonly used local anesthetics is similar. One of the hydrocarbon groups of a tertiary amine (hydrophilic) is joined by an amide or ester linkage

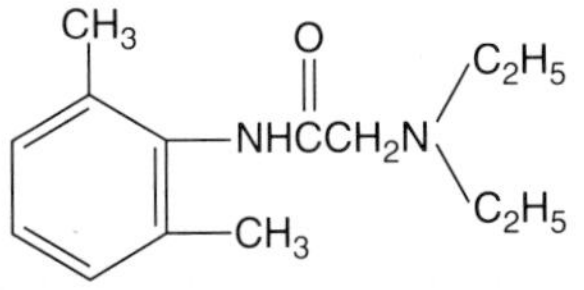

FIG 7–1.
Lidocaine, an amino amide.

to an aromatic group (lipophilic) (Fig 7–1).

The type of linkage allows classification into two groups: amino esters (procaine, chloroprocaine, and tetracaine) and amino amides (lidocaine, bupivacaine, and mepivacaine). The two groups differ in their site of biotransformation and in their potential for adverse reactions. Amino esters are hydrolyzed in the plasma and in the liver by cholinesterase. The rate of hydrolysis of chloroprocaine is rapid, but that of tetracaine is much slower. Amino amides are cleared by hepatic biotransformation. Lidocaine biotransformation parallels hepatic blood flow.

Adverse reactions to local anesthetics involve primarily the central nervous system (CNS) and the cardiovascular system. The toxicity of a local anesthetic may be due to accidental intravascular or intrathecal injection, to relative overdosage, or to epinephrine effects. Symptoms of CNS toxicity occur at lower concentrations and include lightheadedness, dizziness, and visual and auditory disturbances. Objective signs include shivering and twitching progressing to convulsions and ending in generalized CNS depression including the respiratory and cardiovascular centers. The clinical picture of toxicity is initially excitatory in nature, even though the drugs cause CNS depression. The inhibitory neuronal pathways are more susceptible to the depressive effect of local anesthetics and result in unopposed activity of the facilitatory neurons. If the dosage is very high or if the patient is already under the influence of sedative medication, the picture may be that of CNS depression. Respiratory acidosis increases cerebral blood flow, reduces the plasma protein binding of the drug, and reduces intracellular pH. These effects increase drug delivery to the brain, increase the free fraction of the drug, and facilitate its intracellular diffusion by ion trapping. Management must address three areas of concern: (1) hypoxia, hypercarbia, and acidosis can develop rapidly during convulsions; (2) pulmonary aspiration of gastric contents may occur; and (3) skeletal injury can result from the convulsion. Treatment usually consists of a small dose of thiopental (100 to 150 mg) and hyperventilation with 100% O_2 from a mask. Intubation of the trachea must be done by an experienced hand if it becomes necessary. The patient's ECG and blood pressure must be monitored for evidence of cardiotoxicity.

Local anesthetics reduce the maximum rate of depolarization in Purkinje and ventricular muscle fibers by acting on the fast Na^+ channels. The more potent local anesthetics such as bupivacaine produce this effect to a greater extent, and the recovery from it is much slower. This electrophysiologic effect of bupivacaine results in the reentrant type of conduction abnormality, which can cause severe cardiac arrhythmia, including ventricular fibrillation. Cardiac toxicity may be associated with peripheral vasodilatation and pulmonary vasoconstriction. The enhanced cardiac toxicity of these more potent agents is due to greater myocardial uptake. Cardiac resuscitation must be vigorous and prolonged when bupivacaine administration is the cause.

Liver disease, reduced liver blood flow from congestive heart failure (CHF) or anesthesia, hypovolemia, metabolic and respiratory acidosis, hypoxia, and pregnancy are some of the conditions that increase the likelihood of a toxic reaction. The site of anesthetic injection is also a very important factor. Intercostal nerve block, topical anesthesia of the tracheobronchial tree, and epidural analgesia may rapidly result in high serum levels. The use of epinephrine, 1:200,000, can reduce the rate of absorption. The maximum recommended dose of an anesthetic is usually given in terms of body weight, but doses should be individualized with the above-mentioned factors taken into consideration (Table 7–2).

Local anesthetics are basic drugs dissolved in an acidic solution, and this acidity is the reason for the burning sensation when injected subcutaneously. True allergies to local anesthetics are very rare; allergic reactions are usually due to preservatives in multidose vials.

Techniques of Regional Anesthesia

Before the administration of any local anesthetic, it is very important to ensure that the bed can be tilted and that there is good intravenous access for fluid and drug therapy. A functioning suction apparatus, oxygen, equipment for manual ventilation, drugs such as thiopental, succinycholine, diazepam, and vasopressors drugs, and intravenous fluid must be available.

Infiltration Anesthesia

Many plastic surgery procedures in the head and neck region can be done under selected nerve blocks and infiltration anesthesia by the surgeon. Using epinephrine (1:200,000) in the local anesthetic solution reduces the rate of systemic absorption and prolongs the duration of action, thus increasing the maximum recommended dose that can be used (Table 7–2). The doses in Table 7–2 are for a 70-kg adult. Epinephrine also reduces bleeding in the surgical field.

Spinal Anesthesia

Spinal anesthesia is relatively simple to perform and has a rapid onset of action. The dose of local anesthetic is small, and hence the patient is not exposed to its toxic effect. The most commonly used agents are lidocaine, bupivacaine, and tetracaine, and their durations of action are about 1, 2½ and 4 hours respectively. Adding small amounts of vasoconstrictors can increase anesthetic duration of action. The spinal cord usually ends at the level of the second lumbar vertebra, and the needle must not be inserted higher than the L2–3 interspace so as not to transfix the cord. Contraindications of spinal anesthesia are local infection, coagulopathy, raised intracranial pressure, and hypovolemia. Patients who have severe obstructive lung disease may not tolerate high spinal anesthesia. Complications of spinal anesthesia are hypotension, urine retention, spinal headache, and meningitis. Injection of the wrong drugs into the cerebrospinal fluid (CSF) can have disastrous results. Hypotension is managed by administration of oxygen, fluid, and ephedrine. Elevating the patients' legs temporarily is also a useful maneuver. Spinal headache is characteristically bitemporal and nuchal and is made worse by sitting, straining, or coughing. It is believed to be due to low CSF pressure and traction on intracranial contents. Fluid intake is encouraged, and an epidural blood patch should be considered. It is important to rule out intracranial infection as the cause of the headache. If the patient has a fever or leukocytosis, then an epidural blood patch may not be wise.

Epidural Anesthesia

Epidural anesthesia is achieved by injecting local anesthetic into the extradural space, usually into the lumbar region. The anesthesia level and duration can be controlled through a catheter inserted in the epidural space. Epidural anesthesia by continuous infusion can be used for postoperative analgesia. The catheter for this purpose may need to be placed at the lumbar or low thoracic level, depending on the site of pain. The anesthetic agent may consist of a mixture of low concentrations of a local anesthetic (bupivacaine, 0.125% or 0.0625%) and an opioid (fentanyl, 0.5%). This combination tends to cause less hypotension, and muscle function is mini-

TABLE 7–2.
Maximum Dose and Duration of the Two Most Commonly Used Local Anesthetics (for a 70-kg Adult)

		Plain Solution		Epinephrine-Containing Solution	
Anesthetic	Concentration (%)	Max Dose (mg)	Duration (min)	Max Dose (mg)	Duration (min)
Lidocaine	0.5–1.0	300	30–60	500	120–360
Bupivacaine	0.25–0.5	175	120–240	225	180–420

mally affected. In caudal anesthesia the epidural space is entered from the sacral hiatus rather than from the lumbar intervertebral space. Accidental dural puncture and total spinal and intravenous injection of local anesthesia are the main complications of epidural anesthesia.

Brachial Plexus Block

Peripheral nerve blocks are most commonly used in the upper extremity. There are three main approaches to block the brachial plexus: the axillary, supraclavicular, and interscalene approaches. The median, radial, and ulnar nerves can be blocked at the elbow or the wrist. An interscalene block produces ideal anesthesia in the shoulder and arm but has a tendency to miss the ulnar nerve. The major risks of an interscalene block are the injection of a large quantity of local anesthetic in the subarachnoid space, in the epidural space, and in the vertebral artery. The phrenic nerve usually gets blocked in the interscalene approach to the brachial plexus and hence is best avoided in patients with severe lung disease. A supraclavicular block may produce a phrenic nerve block and pneumothorax. An axillary block frequently misses the musculocutaneous nerve. In any of these approaches to the brachial plexus, the intercostobrachial and medial cutaneous nerve of the arm are blocked by an arc of subcutaneous infiltration in the axillary surface of the arm to eliminate pain from the tourniquet.

Intravenous Regional Anesthesia (Bier Block)

The Bier block is an elegant and simple technique of producing anesthesia of the upper limb by intravenously injecting local anesthetic to an exsanguinated limb below an artery-occluding tourniquet. The limb is exsanguinated by elevating it and applying pressure with elastic bandage in a distal-to-proximal direction. If it is not practical to use the bandage because of pain or other reasons, then limb elevation and digital compression of the brachial artery are helpful. However, if the limb is not properly exsanguinated, high intravenous pressure can build after local anesthetic injection, and the drug can get past the inflated cuff into the systemic circulation. The tourniquet is inflated to 2½ times the systolic pressure and is tested for adequate occlusion. Through a previously placed intravenous cannula on the dorsum of the hand, 40 to 50 mL of 0.5% lidocaine is injected into the vein. The cannula is then removed. There will be discoloration of the arm and tingling and numbness of the limb at the onset of anesthesia. Adequate anesthesia is usually obtained within 10 minutes. A Bier block is not suitable for surgery that takes much longer than 45 minutes because of the pain and discomfort from the tourniquet pressure. Double-cuff tourniquets are available to reduce this problem. The proximal cuff must be inflated first. At the time of switching over to the distal cuff to reduce tourniquet pain, the distal cuff must be inflated before deflating the proximal cuff. After injecting local anesthesia the cuff must stay inflated for at least 20 minutes before it can safely be deflated. The patient must be closely observed at the time of cuff deflation. Bupivacaine is not recommended for use in the Bier block.

Nerve Blocks Around the Elbow

The ulnar nerve can be palpated and blocked in the groove between the medial condyle of the humerus and the olecranon. Local anesthetic solution (4 mL) is injected next to but not into the nerve. The median nerve is blocked by injecting 5 to 7 mL of solution at the level of the elbow crease just on medial side of the brachial artery. The nerve lies deep to the deep fascia, and frequently a "pop" can be felt as the needle pierces the fascia. The radial nerve can be blocked at the elbow, but it is easier to block above the elbow at the lateral border of the humerus where the nerve can frequently be palpated on the bone in the groove between the brachialis and the brachioradialis muscles. The needle is inserted as far as the bone and then moved up and down to elicit paresthesia.

Nerve Blocks at the Wrist

Nerve blocks in this region are simple to perform once the anatomic locations of the nerves are known. The ulnar nerve lies between the flexor carpi ulnaris tendon and the ulnar artery. The median nerve can be blocked by injecting 5 to 7 mL of solution between the palmaris longus and the flexor carpi radialis at the level of the proximal palmar crease. To block the radial nerve at the wrist, 4 mL of local anesthetic is injected between the flexor carpi radialis and the radial artery, and then from the same site a subcutaneous wheal of local anesthetic extending just beyond the midline is raised on the dorsum of the hand. The digital nerves are blocked by infiltrating 3 mL of local anesthetic between the skin and bone on each side of the base of the finger. Excessive volume and epinephrine should be avoided.

Chapter 8

Immunology and Transplantation

Bruce M. Achauer, M.D.
Ramon Llull, M.D., Ph.D.

CONTENTS

NOTE: The material in this chapter is frequently covered during the prerequisite training period of many plastic surgery residents. This chapter should serve as a valuable review of important material in such cases. For residents who have not mastered this material previously, this chapter is essential.

CHAPTER OBJECTIVE

At the end of this chapter the resident understands the basic principles of immunology and utilizes tissue transplantation techniques for treatment of common plastic surgical problems.

LEARNER OBJECTIVES

On completion of this chapter the resident

1. **Understands the physiology of skin graft take and the immunology of allograft rejection.**
2. Understands the basic immune response including antibody recognition of foreign antigens, first-set rejection, and second-set rejection.
3. Understands the cellular response to foreign tissue or material, including the role of lymphocytes, macrophages, and T cells.
4. Understands the actions of and proper usage of pharmacologic agents to alter the immune response, including cyclosporine, azathioprine (Imuran), steroids, and monoclonal antibodies.
5. Understands the role of immunology in host responses to tumor, including lymphocytic infiltration of melanoma, basal cell carcinoma, and squamous cell carcinoma.
6. Knows the role of immunology in response to foreign materials and regional or systemic reactions, e.g., "silicone synovitis," capsular contractures.
7. Is familiar with the difference between skin transplantation and the

transplantation of heart and solid organs.
8. Knows current information regarding human immunodeficiency virus and associated diseases.

CLINICAL PRACTICE ACTIVITIES

During the course of the training program, the resident

1. Manages plastic surgical problems in patients with autoimmune and collagen vascular diseases such as lupus erythematosus.
2. Identifies patients who are at risk for malignancy because of their immunosuppressed condition and provides screening and education to these patients.
3. Identifies and treats patients whose condition warrants allografting (e.g., large body surface burn).
4. Performs pre- and postoperative management of immunosuppressed patients undergoing plastic surgical procedures.

BASIC PRINCIPLES OF IMMUNOLOGY

The human immune system consists of a number of organs and several different cell lines that have evolved to accurately and specifically recognize nonself antigens *irrespective* of the nature of these antigens (microbial, foreign bodies, oncologic, self-antigens). The immune system has two functional divisions: the innate and the adaptive immune system. The former acts as a first line of defense against pathogens. If these innate defensive mechanisms are breached, the adaptive immune system is activated, produces a specific reaction to each pathogenic agent, and remembers how to react toward such a specific agent in subsequent encounters. Thus, the two key features of the adaptive immune system are specificity and memory (Table 8–1).

Phases of specific humoral and cellular immune responses may be divided into *cognitive, activation,* and *effector* (Figs 8–1 and 8–2). The first two phases make up the afferent arm of the immune response, whereas the third, the effector phase, corresponds to the efferent arm. Both humoral and cellular-mediated immunity are dependent upon populations of lymphocytes and macrophages.

IMMUNOMODULATION AND IMMUNOSUPPRESSION

Pharmacologic

The immune response can be downregulated by immunomodulatory drugs. They readjust the immune response back to normal levels following unwanted immune activation. Historically, their action was nonspecific, such as with corticosteroids and cytotoxic agents. More recently, however, some agents have obtained a certain degree of specificity

TABLE 8–1.
The Major Elements of the Immune Response*

	Innate (Natural) Component	Adaptive (Acquired) Component
Physical barriers	Skin, mucous membranes	Cutaneous and mucosal immune system Antibodies in mucosal secretions
Soluble factors	Lysozyme Complement Acute-phase proteins Cytokines (α- and β-IFN†, TNF†)	Antibodies Lymphokines (interleukins)
	Phagocytes (macrophages, monocytes, hystiocytes and PMNs†) Natural killer cells	T lymphocytes B lymphocytes

* There is considerable interaction between the two systems (see Fig. 8–1).
† IFN = interferon; TNF = tumor necrosis factor; PMNs = polymorphonuclear neutrophils.

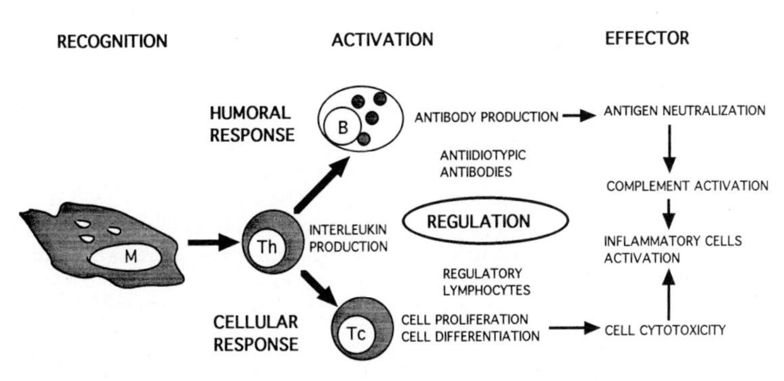

FIG 8–1.
During the cognitive phase, T-helper cells recognize antigen in the context of major histocompatibility complex (MHC) determinants. The antigen presentation requires two signals that are mediated by macrophages: MHC restriction and synthesis and release of interleukin-1. The activation phase mainly consists of T-helper *(Th)* interleukin production (i.e., interleukin-2) and differentiation and clonal expansion of T and B lymphocytes. The effector phase is mediated through antibody production and activation of T-cytotoxic *(Tc)* cells. (*M* = macrophages; *B* = B cell.)

(cyclosporine, antilymphocyte serum, monoclonal antibodies, FK 506, rapamycin). They have dramatically opened up a new era in clinical organ transplantation. Additionally, many of these drugs have demonstrated excellent efficacy in experimental allotransplantation of skin and musculoskeletal tissue in rodent and primate experimental models. Side effects and clinical complications of drugs

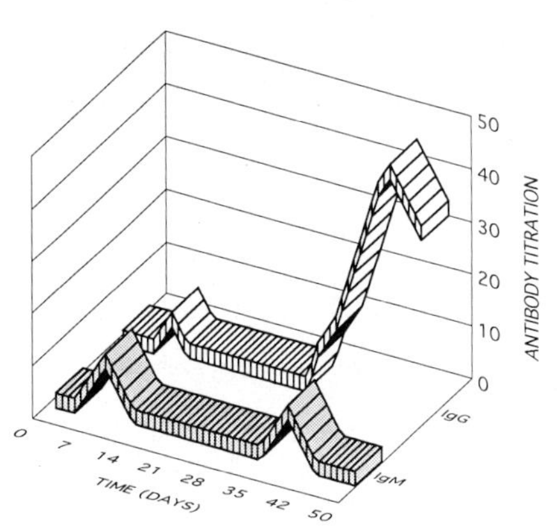

FIG 8–2.
A primary humoral immune response (days 3 to 7) occurs following the first exposure to antigen (day 0) and is composed mainly of the synthesis of IgM antibodies. If a sufficient length of time elapses after the primary antigenic stimulation, serum antibody levels will decrease. However, following subsequent antigen exposure (day 30), a secondary response will ensue because of the presence of long-lasting memory cells that were generated during the first exposure. Additionally, antibody production shifts to IgG with higher antigen affinity.

currently in clinical use are summarized in Table 8–2.

Corticosteroid therapy is the mainstay in the treatment of many immune diseases. *Cytotoxic* drugs like cyclophosphamide, azathioprine, chlorambucil, and methotrexate are effective antineoplastic agents. Periods of no therapy permit recovery of the normal turnover of nonneoplastic cells. Considerable toxicity forces these drugs to be reserved for protocols that do not respond to corticosteroid therapy. *Monoclonal antibodies* such as murine anti-CD3 are currently used to reverse acute allograft rejection. The anti-CD3 antibody targets surface determinants that are associated with the antigen recognition site of T cells and are essential in signal transduction. Circulating CD3+ T lymphocytes are removed from the circulation within minutes following intravenous administration. Cyclosporine A (CsA) has proved very successful in suppressing allograft rejection. Its mechanism of action is thought to be due to inhibition of lymphokines, interferon-γ, B-cell differentiation factors, and inhibition of the response of lymphocytes to interleukin-2.

Immunodeficiency and Immunosuppression

Defects in one or more components of the immune system can lead to serious and often fatal disorders (Table 8–3). The primary immunodeficiencies are genetic defects that re-

TABLE 8–2.
Clinical Complications of Immunosuppressive Drugs

Drug	Complication
Corticosteroids	Cushing's syndrome, osteoporosis
Cyclophosphamide	Myelosuppression, hemorrhagic cystitis
Methotrexate	Myelosuppression, gastrointestinal disturbances
Azathioprine	Myelosuppression, lymphoproliferative diseases
Cyclosporine	Nephrotoxicity, hepatotoxicity, neurotoxicity, lymphoproliferative diseases
Monoclonal antibodies	Pyrexia, dyspnea, chest pain, diarrhea, headache, tachycardia
FK 506 and rapamycin	Still under investigation

sult in increased susceptibility to infections, frequently manifested early in infancy. It is estimated that in the United States approximately 1 in 500 individuals is born with a defect in some component of the immune system, although only a small sample is clinically relevant. Secondary immunodeficiencies develop as a consequence of malnutrition, metabolic disorders, disseminated cancer, immunosuppressive treatment, or infections of immunocompetent cells (acquired immunodeficiency syndrome [AIDS]). Features of an immunosuppressed patient include increased susceptibility to infections, malignancies, and autoimmune diseases.

Acquired Immunodeficiency Syndrome

AIDS is a severe T-cell immunodeficiency caused by infection with the human immunodeficiency virus (HIV). This virus selectively infects CD4+ T lymphocytes and causes depletion of these cells by direct lysis as well as several indirect mechanisms that lead to death, defective maturation, and abnormal function of uninfected cells (Fig 8–3). Depletion of T cells results in greatly increased susceptibility to infection by a number of opportunistic microorganisms, including *Pneumocytis carinii,* mycobacteria, and various fungi and viruses. Patients have a propensity to tumors, particularly Kaposi's sarcoma and Epstein-Barr virus–associated lymphomas, and encephalopathy frequently develops (the mechanisms of which are not yet fully understood).

IMMUNOLOGY OF TUMORS

Principles of Tumor Immunology

Cellular oncogenic processes are accompanied by changes in the antigenic profile

TABLE 8–3.
General Classification of Immunodeficiencies and Associated Signs

Primary*
- *Cellular.*—Positive familial history, chronic viral infections, failure to thrive, chronic diarrhea and anorexia, atrophic lymphoid organs, alopecia, lymphopenia
- *Humoral.*—Recurrent bacterial infections, recurrent arthritis refractory to NSAIDs†, chronic diarrhea and malabsorption, severe hepatitis, failure to thrive, atrophic lymphoid organs
- *Complement.*—Recurrent meningococcal meningitis, chronic gonococcal infections, auto-immune diseases, recurrent skin infections, hypergammaglobulinemia
- *Phagocytic function.*—Mucosal and skin infections, abscesses, pneumonias, granulomas, hypergammaglobulinemia.

Secondary
- Coexisting diseases
- Trauma
- Alcoholism, drug addiction
- Malnutrition
- Drug therapies

* Primary immunodeficiencies frequently give rise to secondary immunodeficiencies thus making the diagnosis more difficult and worsening the prognosis.
† NSAIDs = nonsteroidal anti-inflammatory drugs.

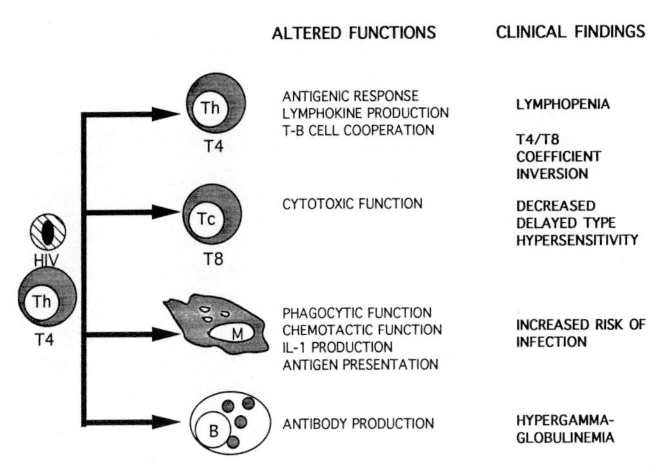

FIG 8–3.
Functional alterations and clinical findings following HIV infection. *IL-1* = interleukin-1; *Tc* = T-cytotoxic cell; *Th* = T-helper cell; *M* = macrophage; *B* = B cell.

of the cells. These neoantigens may be found in the nucleus, cytoplasm, or cell membrane and can elicit immune responses to that particular tumor. Both specific (cell and humoral mediated) and nonspecific immune responses are involved in antitumor surveillance (Table 8–4). Unfortunately, tumors have developed mechanisms to escape such a surveillance (Table 8–5). Cytotoxic T cells appear in response to tumor-specific antigens (TSAs) or viral antigens. Antibody formation, although present, is not very effective in causing tumor rejection, particularly in solid tumors. Antibody-dependent cellular cytotoxicity (ADCC) is mediated by killer cells that recognize IgG antibodies on the target cell. This process is complement independent. Complement-mediated cytolysis is also mediated by antibodies, particularly IgM. Natural killer (NK) cells are present in tumor immune responses. NK cells may bear Fc and T-cell receptors. Therefore, they are capable of simultaneous ADCC and direct cytolytic interaction. Phenotypically they are non–T, non–B cells and are morphologically associated with large granular lymphocytes. Macrophages can be activated by TSAs and lead to tumor cell killing. Macrophages release antitumor products such as hydrolytic enzymes, interferons, tumor necrosis factors, oxidative products, and complement components.

TABLE 8–4.
Mechanisms of Antitumor Immune Response

Cellular
Macrophages
Natural killer cells
Lymphokine-activated killer cells
Polymorphonuclear cells
Humoral
Antibodies
Complement

Basal Cell Carcinoma

Basal cell carcinomas are common, slow-growing tumors that rarely metastasize. They are directly related to chronic sun exposure, especially in lightly pigmented people. The incidence of basal cell carcinoma rises sharply

TABLE 8–5.
Mechanisms of Tumor Escape

Selection of less antigenic tumor cell lines
Antigen release to the extracellular compartment
Modulation of the antigen expression
Production of suppressor factors
Generation of suppressor cells

with immunosuppression and in patients with inherited defects in DNA replication or repair (i.e., xeroderma pigmentosum). A marked inflammatory infiltrate of T lymphocytes usually accompanies these tumors. The belief that local immunity is important in limiting the growth of these easily curable tumors is fostered by hyperplasia of Langerhans' cells, apposition of T cells to necrotic tumor cells, and markers of functional activation of these T cells.

Squamous Cell Carcinoma

Squamous cell carcinoma is the most common tumor arising on sun-exposed sites of older people. Implicated as predisposing factors, in addition to sunlight, are industrial carcinogens, chronic ulcers, draining osteomyelitis, old burn scars, ingestion of arsenicals, ionizing radiation, and in the oral cavity tobacco and betel leaf chewing. Patients with xeroderma pigmentosum and immunosuppressed individuals also have a high incidence of this neoplasm. Sunlight, in addition to its effect on DNA, also seems to have a direct and at least a transient immunosuppressive effect on skin by affecting the normal surveillance function of antigen-presenting Langerhans' cells in the epidermis.

Melanoma

Malignant melanomas are aggressive, frequently metastatic and fatal tumors from melanocyte or melanocyte-related nevi. They make up 3% of all skin cancers. Melanomas are among the most thoroughly characterized human tumors. Melanoma TSAs include chrondroitin sulfate proteoglycan and gangliosides. Melanoma tumor-associated antigens (TAAs) have been identified during developing stages of melanoma. They include major histocompatibility complex (MHC) antigens, growth factor receptors, matrix-binding molecules, cation-binding proteins, gangliosides, and nevomelanotic differentiating factors. Antibodies to a few melanoma TAAs are detected in the serum of patients with melanoma, yet there is no evidence that immune responses to these antigens play any role in antimelanoma immune surveillance. Nevertheless, monoclonal antibodies specific for melanoma TAAs are used for immunodiagnostic purposes and have been tried with limited success for immunotherapy.

AUTOIMMUNE DISEASES

Systemic Lupus Erythematosus

Systemic lupus erythematosus (SLE), a chronic remitting and relapsing inflammatory disease, appears to result from an immune dysregulation brought about by the interaction of genetic, hormonal, and environmental factors. These interactions most likely act on the immunoregulatory T-cell circuits that ultimately control the production of antibodies, including autoantibodies. The prominent clinical manifestions (glomerulonephritis, vasculitis, arthritis, thrombocytopenia, and hemolytic anemia) are attributed to the many different autoantibodies found in patients with SLE (against DNA, ribonucleoproteins, histones, and nucleolar antigens). Once the systemic disease has been brought under appropriate therapy, operative management of associated lesions has been uneventful. Reconstructive skin grafts and flaps in patients with SLE have been successful with steroid coverage. The benefits of steroid therapy for suppressing the vasculitis far exceed the risks of delayed wound healing when dealing with these patients.

Rheumatoid Arthritis

Rheumatoid arthritis (RA) is a chronic systemic destructive inflammatory disease of unknown etiology that is characterized by progressive involvement of joints, hand deformity, and eventually, variable degrees of incapacitation. Despite many years of research, the etiology of RA remains unclear. Endocrine, metabolic, nutritional, geographic, occupational, and psychosocial factors have been studied. While they may be implicated in the course of the disease, they cannot specify its cause. RA is characterized by destruction of the joint cartilage and inflammation of the synovium, with a morphologic picture suggestive of local immune response. T4 cells, activated B lymphocytes, and plasma cells are found in the inflamed synovium, and in severe cases, well-formed lymphoid follicles with germinal centers may be present. Numerous cytokines, including interleukin-1, tumor necrosis factor, and interferon-γ have been detected in the synovial fluid.

Systemic Rheumatoid Diseases Associated With Plastic Surgery Procedures

Reports have recently appeared in the literature that relate the development of rheumatic diseases to the placement of biomaterials in plastic surgical procedures (e.g., breast augmentation). The reported complications include human adjuvant disease, scleroderma, lupus erythematosus, rheumatic arthritis, gout, Hashimoto thyroiditis, and anticardiolipin syndrome. The association between surgical procedures involving biomaterials and the development of such diseases was suggested by the fact that the disease developed following prosthesis implantation. However, the proof of cause and effect remains elusive even after retrospective analysis. In the case of breast augmentation, prosthesis removal was reportedly followed by improvement in only 60% of patients.

SKIN TRANSPLANTATION

Free autotransplantation of skin is widely used in plastic surgery and produces excellent results under normal conditions. However, when a patient has a loss of full-thickness skin coverage exceeding 30% of the body surface as a result of burns or mechanical trauma, autografts may not be available in sufficient quantity or could be obtained only at considerable disadvantage. Temporary coverage can be obtained by means of skin allografts from living donors or recently deceased individuals. This is often a lifesaving procedure. However, in order to avoid rejection, skin allografts applied as biological dressings must be changed every 2 to 3 days. Skin allografts also serve as dressings for infected burns or wounds, which rapidly become sterile and develop well-vascularized granulation on which autografts will engraft readily. Skin allotransplantation in patients with massive burns who receive systemic cyclosporine coverage has been proved successful.

Skin Graft Transplantation

Transplantation of living tissues involves the surgical removal of viable cells from a donor area and subsequent transfer to a recipient site. Whether or not the transplanted cells survive and propagate a lineage of living cells in the recipient site depends on the nutritive supply, metabolic waste removal, and immunogenetic relationships between donor and recipient. The survival of any skin graft (allograft or autograft) is dependent on rapidly acquiring a blood supply adequate for nutrition and disposal of metabolic waste products. In the time interval between transplantation and actual engraftment, survival of anoxic graft cells appears to be maintained by the absorption of fluid from the host. This phase may be described as a period in which the graft vessels fill with a fibrinogen-free fluid and cells from the host bed. Endothelial ingrowth from the host progresses until a definitive vasculature is established. The stagnant fluid absorbed by the graft during the early phase of serum imbibition is apparently drained off by the newly established blood and lymphatic circulation.

Skin Allograft Rejection

The orderly sequence of events that lead to the rejection reaction of skin allografts begins with mononuclear cell infiltration, accompanied by polymorphonuclear cells at the host-graft junction. The graft undergoes progressive edema and dilation of the graft vascular system with a gradually diminishing blood flow and terminates with an inflammatory reaction along with thrombosis and rupture of graft vasculature. The graft undergoes hemorrhagic necrosis and eventually sloughs as a hard, dry scab. The lymphatic vessels draining the site of skin allografts are the principal access of antigenic stimuli to the host regional lymph nodes, where immunologically competent cells are activated by graft antigens. Following confrontation with the antigenic material, these cells settle in the regional lymph nodes and are transformed into immunoblasts, which in turn rapidly proliferate into a clone of effector lymphocytes, eventually enter the blood vasculature via efferent lymphatic vessels, and initiate allograft rejection.

IMMUNOLOGY OF MUSCULOSKELETAL TISSUES

Cartilage and Bone

Cartilage is among the few types of mammalian cell tissues that can be allografted without rejection, apparently because the sparse population of chondrocytes is walled off from immune surveillance by the relatively avascular cartilaginous matrix. Bone grafting is widely used for bridging and fracture stabilization in orthopedic procedures, but (except for autografts) no viable donor cells survive in the recipient. However, the remaining dead matrix has bone-inducing capacity that stimulates neighboring osteoblasts to recolonize the matrix. Allografts are preserved by freezing and glycerolation (preserves chondrocytes) and transplanted with no pharmacologic immunosuppression. Patients develop anti-HLA antibodies, yet no cartilage degradation occurs.

Composite Tissue Allografts

The development of microsurgical techniques has supplied plastic surgery with the opportunity to transfer tissue to nearly any recipient site in the body. Classic grafting methods still have their value but also possess limits in many circumstances. Free tissue transfer has demonstrated its advantages, especially in covering defects in the lower extremity. Microsurgical techniques have also gained ground in reconstructive surgery of the head and neck, female breast, abdominal wall, and hands. Furthermore, microsurgical technology increases the feasibility of free transfer of allogeneic grafts. The prospect of successfully transplanting composite tissue allografts (CTAs) remains one of the last frontiers in clinical transplantation. A CTA consists of a composite of various tissues, predominantly of ectodermal and mesodermal derivation, in contrast to visceral organs. CTAs can include transplantation of complex modules diverse in composition such as a complete limb, abdominal wall, or craniofacial structures.

It has been proposed that CTAs or substructures thereof would be useful for functional and structural reconstruction or restoration following massive burns, birth defects, traumatic injuries, or oncologic diseases. In the future, composite tissue allotransplantation may become incorporated into plastic surgeons' armamentarium for the treatment of severe cosmetic and functional defects. In fact, with the present technology and surgical expertise, human CTAs probably could be performed. However, much remains to be done at both the basic science and clinical trial levels, including investigating tissue immunogenicity of CTAs, novel immunosuppressive regimens, tolerance induction unique to CTA modules, specific molecular targets that trigger the CTA rejection process, possibilities for functional restoration, and potential adverse effects. This effort will open new strategies for immunosuppression and the ultimate design of CTA modules possessing the highest reconstructive potential and chances for success.

IMMUNOLOGY OF BIOMATERIALS

Silicone Implants

Silicone implants have proved to be long lasting, physiologically inert, and generally well tolerated in the majority of recipients. Postsurgical histologic changes have typically included a subclinical inflammatory response with fibrotic encapsulation. More recently, however, investigators have noted that implantation of biomaterials (such as silicone or paraffin) is associated with the development of implant capsule contracture (breast implants), inflammatory arthritis (silicone synovitis), and rheumatic diseases (see the section on autoimmune diseases). The presence of an immune response to biomaterials is of great interest in understanding the biological properties of that agent, but it must be viewed in conjunction with clinical performance.

It is commonly suggested that the inflammatory cell infiltrate evoked by silicone devices represents a nonspecific foreign-body reaction that is part of normal wound healing. However, there is evidence that the inflammatory infiltrate also responds to an immunologic reaction mediated by immunocompetent cells being sensitized by protein-silicone complexes. The identity of these complexes remains controversial. The immune response to silicone products involves exposure of an antigenic determinant on a denatured protein absorbed to the otherwise immunologically nonreactive silicone moiety, thus making the silicone-protein complex antigenic.

Silicone Synovitis

Silicone synovitis, a relatively rare complication of implant surgery, generally develops 3 to 5 years postoperatively and ranges in severity from a mild synovitis to an erosive arthropathy. Recently, however, a high incidence of reactive synovitis with lytic bony lesions has been reported in association with silicone joint implants.

It is suggested that excessive usage causes microtears of the implant and consequent migration of free silicone particles to the synovium. The typical findings of silicone synovitis are those of an inflammatory monoarthritis, including erythema, heat, swelling, and painful limitation of motion. The erythrocyte sedimentation rate may be normal or elevated, while rheumatoid factor and fluorescent antinuclear antibodies are negative. Synovial fluid appears cloudy or bloody. Polymorphonuclear neutrophils (PMNs) may predominate, even in the absence of overlapping infection. Cultures for bacteria and fungi are sterile, except when there is a superimposed infectious process. Radiographically, soft-tissue swelling, bony sclerosis, and periarticular osteopenia are seen. Histologically, proliferative granulomatous synovitis with giant cells, papillary hyperplasia, and birefringent intracellular fragments is found. Removal of the prosthesis, synovectomy, curettage, and bone grafting of the lytic lesions may be required. In all patients with Silastic implants, close clinical follow-up and x-ray studies are indicated.

Collagen-Derived Biomaterials

The biocompatibility of collagen for medical applications has long been recognized. The medical applications include augmentation of soft tissue (injectable collagen), treatment of acute and chronic wounds (artificial skin), and regeneration of bone (bone graft substitutes). The most widely characterized collagen application is injectable collagen for correcting soft-tissue contour irregularities caused by trauma, aging, or congenital deformities. Hypersensitivity to the initial skin exposure to injectable collagen develops in 3% of the population and occurs during the first 72 hours, thus indicating presensitization to bovine collagen. In addition, localized hypersensitivity responses to subsequent treatment with injectable collagen develops in 1% of subjects. Wound dressings prepared with atelocollagen (obtained by selectively removing the telopeptide atelocollagen, which is the major antigenic epitope residing in the nonhelical portion of the collagen molecule) did not induce either an Arthus reaction or a delayed-type hypersensitivity response. Collagen membranes have been used as a short-term skin substitute in burn patients to cover split-thickness donor graft sites. Donor sites so treated exhibit improved healing and a modest decrease in pain when compared with synthetic dressings. A slight inflammatory response has been reported in association with collagen dressings used in wound sites. Used as a hemostatic agent, collagen has low immunogenic potential with minimal adverse effects. However, moderate granulomatous inflammatory responses have been observed following application of hemostatic agents.

Bone allografts and xenografts are composed in large part of collagen and mineral. Type I collagen is the major structural protein in bone and composes approximately 90% of its organic matrix.

Collagen has been used as bone substitute for bridging bony defects or as coating for ceramic and metallic implants to increase attachment. Collagen serves as a conductive matrix for the ingrowth of bone-forming cells to produce new bone formation. Collagen materials have been used with little evidence of immunologic adverse effects.

In summary, whereas an immune response to xenogeneic and allogeneic collagen-derived materials has been demonstrated in both animal and human models, the data clearly suggest that the immunity per se is not associated with significant adverse effects in vivo. Indeed, in most cases, the presence of antibodies to collagen is an epiphenomenon and not a source of implant rejection.

Acknowledgment

This work was supported by a Fulbright Commission–Ministry of Education, Spain, Scholarship and a 1992 Plastic Surgery Educational Foundation Fellowship.

SUGGESTED READING

Achauer BM, et al: Immunosurgery. *Clin Plast Surg* 1985; 12:293.

DeLustro F, Dasch J, Keefe J, et al: Immune responses to allogeneic and xenogeneic implants of collagen and collagen derivatives. *Clin Orthop* 1990; 260:263.

Fisher JC: *Report From the Research Committee for Silicone Implants.* Arlington Heights, IL, Plastic Surgery Educational Foundation, 1992.

Gallo RC, Montagnier L: AIDS in 1988. *Sci Am* 1988; 259:41.

Herlyn M, Koproski H: Melanoma antigens: Immunological and biological characterization and clinical significance. *Annu Rev Immunol* 1988; 6:283.

Llull R, et al: Composite tissue allotransplantation: Perspectives concerning eventual clinical exploitation. *Transplant Rev* 1992; 6:42.

Roit I, Brostoff J, Male D: *Immunology,* ed 2. Philadelphia, JB Lippincott, 1990.

Rosen FS, et al: The primary immunodeficiencies. *N Engl J Med* 1984; 311:235.

Schumacher HR (ed): *Primer on Rheumatic Diseases.* Atlanta, Arthritis Foundation, 1988.

Wingard LB, et al: *Human Pharmacology. Molecular to Clinical.* St Louis, Mosby–Year Book, 1991.

Worsing R, Engber MD, Lange TA: Reactive synovitis from particulate Silastic. *J Bone Joint Surg Am* 1982; 64:581.

Chapter 9

Pharmacology/Therapeutics

W. Thomas Lawrence, M.P.H., M.D., F.A.C.S.
David B. Brothers, M.D.
John W. Decorato, M.D.

CONTENTS

Pharmacology
- Antibiotics
- Analgesics
- Anti-inflammatory agents
- Steroids
- Chemotherapeutic agents
- Extravasation

Bacteriology of wounds
- Bacteriology
- Skin infections
- Head and neck infections
- Breast infections
- Surgical wound infections
- Hand infections
- Bite wounds

NOTE: The material in this chapter is frequently covered during the prerequisite training period of many plastic surgery residents. This chapter should serve as a valuable review of important material in such cases. For residents who have not mastered this material previously, this chapter is essential.

CHAPTER OBJECTIVE

At the end of this chapter the resident understands the pharmacology of drugs commonly used in plastic surgical practice, including antibiotics, anti-inflammatory agents, analgesics, and steroids and effectively utilizes such drugs in a wide variety of settings.

LEARNER OBJECTIVES

On completion of this chapter the resident

1. **Knows the common pathogens producing infections of the skin, head and neck structures, breast, and hand.**
2. **Knows the special pathogens related to infections caused by human and animal bites and infections resulting from farm injuries.**
3. **Understands the indications and proper antibiotics for treatment of the problems noted in items 1 and 2 above.**
4. **Knows the principles of use (including dosage and complications) of common analgesics.**
5. **Understands the pharmacology and clinical use of steroids in plastic surgery patients (including scar treatment, hand problems, steroid-dependent patients).**
6. Is familiar with the pharmacology of the major types of antibiotics and the indications for their use.
7. Knows the pharmacology of common analgesics (oral and parenteral).
8. Is familiar with the commonly used anti-inflammatory agents, including dosage and mechanism of action.
9. Is familiar with the pharmacology, complications, and clinical use of common chemotherapeutic agents for treatment of skin and head and neck malignancies.
10. Understands the principles of management of extravasation injuries involving chemotherapeutic agents and other drugs.

CLINICAL PRACTICE ACTIVITIES

During the course of the training program, the resident

1. **Diagnoses and treats patients with surgical wound infections.**
2. **Evaluates and treats patients with infections of the head and neck, breast, skin, and hand.**
3. **Prescribes analgesics for postoperative care and for pain management.**
4. **Prescribes anti-inflammatory agents for appropriate cases.**
5. **Utilizes steroids to treat a variety of plastic surgical problems and in the postoperative care of steroid-dependent patients.**
6. Participates in the management of patients undergoing chemotherapy for head and neck and/or skin malignancies.
7. Manages patients with localized extravasation injuries.

PHARMACOLOGY

Antibiotics

Antibiotics are chemical substances that, in dilute solutions, inhibit the growth of or kill microorganisms. Early antibiotics were all products of microorganisms, although most newer antibiotics are synthetic. When choosing an antimicrobial agent to treat an infection, the physician should consider the infecting organism, the site of infection, and host factors affecting drug metabolism and toxicity such as hepatic and renal function, pregnancy, and age. Drug-related factors such as cost, toxicity, efficacy, and possible allergy must also be considered. Selection of antibiotic therapy in clinical infection is ideally based on culture and sensitivity results, although empirical therapy must frequently be initiated before culture results are available. If the agent causing an infection is not known, antimicrobials should be directed at the most likely pathogen.

Antibiotics may be given prophylactically as well as to treat infection. Antibiotic prophylaxis can be justified if the risk of infection outweighs the potential hazards of the drug. Prophylactic antibiotics are usually given 1 hour preoperatively so that peak serum concentrations are present at the time of the surgical incision. The antibiotics utilized should be directed at the bacteria most likely to produce infection in the given clinical setting.

In order to eradicate an infection, adequate concentrations of an antimicrobial must be delivered to the site of infection. Orally administered antibiotics can achieve adequate levels to treat mild infections, although severe infections often require parenteral antibiotics, which produce higher tissue levels. Infections of poorly vascularized soft tissues and bone are particularly refractory to antimicrobial treatment and may therefore require treatment for prolonged periods.

Some antimicrobial agents, e.g., vancomycin and the aminoglycosides, have narrow therapeutic ranges. These agents require monitoring of peak and trough serum levels to ensure effective concentrations and prevent accumulation and toxicity. Most other antimicrobials do not require measurement of serum concentrations unless renal function is compromised.

Although the majority of infections can be treated with a single antimicrobial agent, combination therapy is sometimes indicated. Combination therapy is often indicated to treat polymicrobial infections, to prevent the emergence of resistant organisms, and to provide broad-spectrum coverage for patients with compromised host defenses. Disadvantages of polypharmacy include an increased likelihood of superinfection with unusual organisms (particularly fungi) and an increased likelihood of drug reactions and other metabolic side effects.

Antibiotics interfere with bacterial proliferation by different mechanisms. Vancomycin and β-lactam antibiotics (such as penicillins, cephalosporins, imipenem, and aztreonam) interfere with bacterial cell wall biosynthesis. Aminoglycoside antibiotics (gentamicin, tobramycin, amikacin, and kanamycin), chloramphenicol, erythromycin, clindamycin, and the tetracyclines (tetracycline, oxytetracycline, methacycline, doxycycline, and minocycline) all interfere in different ways with protein synthesis. Metronidazole and the quinolones (nalidixic acid, oxolinic acid, cinoxacin, ofloxacin, norfloxacin and ciprofloxacin) interfere with DNA by different mechanisms. Sulfonamides interfere with folic acid metabolism. Some antibiotics are bacteriostatic, while others are bactericidal, although this is generally not an important consideration if the agent is effective against the bacteria being treated. The drugs of choice for infections caused by most bacteria are listed in Table 9–1.

Analgesics

There are two broad categories of analgesics, opioid and nonopioid. Nonopioid anal-

TABLE 9–1.
Drugs of Choice in Serious Infection*

Organism	Drug of Choice	Alternate Drugs
Gram-positive cocci		
Staphylococcus aureus or *Staphyloccus epidermidis*		
Penicillin sensitive	Penicillin G	Cephalosporin, vancomycin, or clindamycin
Pencillinase producing	Oxacillin or nafcillin	Cephalosporin, vancomycin, or clindamycin
Methicillin resistant	Vancomycin	TMP/SMZ†
Nonenterococcal streptococci	Penicillin G	Cephalosporin, vancomycin, or clindamycin
Enterococci	Penicillin or ampicillin + aminoglycoside	Vancomycin + aminglycoside
Pneumococcus	Penicillin G	Cephalosporin, vancomycin, chloramphenicol, erythromycin
Gram-positive bacilli		
Listeria monocytogenes	Ampicillin	Chloramphenicol, tetracycline
Bacillus anthracis	Penicillin	Tetracycline, erythromycin
Clostridium difficile	Vancomycin	Metronidazole
Clostridium tetani	Penicillin	Tetracycline
Clostridium perfringens	Penicillin	Cloramphenicol, clinamycin, metronidazole, tetracycline
Corynebacterium diptheriae	Erythromycin	Penicillin
Corynebacterium	Vancomycin	
Proprionobacterium species	Penicillin	Clindamycin, erythromycin
Actinomyces israelii	Penicillin G	Tetracycline
Nocardia asteroides	Sulfonamide	TMP/SMZ, minocycline, ampicillin + erythromycin
Gram-negative cocci		
Branhamella catarrhalis	Amoxicillin-clavulanic acid	TMP/SMZ, ceftriaxone, erythromcyin, tetracycline
Neisseria gonorrhoeae	Penicillin G	Spectinomycin
Neisseria meningiditis	Penicillin G	Chloramphenicol, cefuroxime, TMP/SMZ
Enteric gram-negative bacilli		
Bacteroides		
Oral flora	Penicillin	Clindamycin, cefoxitin, metronidazole
Bowel strains	Clindamycin or metronidazole	Cefoxitin, mezlocillin, piperacillin, imipenem, chloramphenicol
Citrobacter	Gentamicin or cephalosporin	Gentamicin, amikacin, chloramphenicol, piperacillin, aztreonam, imipenem
Enterobacteriaceae	Gentamicin or cephalosporin	Gentamicin, amikacin, chloramphenicol, piperacillin, aztreonam, imipenem

* Adapted from Crawford CE: An approach to use of antimicrobial agents, in Civetta JM (ed): *Critical Care.* Philadelphia, JB Lippincott, 1988, pp 769–783.
† TMP/SMZ = trimethoprim/sulfamethoxazole.

(Continued.)

TABLE 9–1 (cont.).
Drugs of Choice in Serious Infection*

Organism	Drug of Choice	Alternate Drugs
Escherichia coli	Gentamicin or cephalosporin	Gentamicin, ampicillin, amikacin, imipenem, aztreonam, piperacillin
Klebsiella	Gentamicin or cephalosporin	Gentamicin, amikacin, chloramphenicol, piperacillin, aztreonam, imipenem
Proteus		
P. mirabilis	Ampicillin	Gentamicin, cephalosporin, tobramycin, amikacin, chloramphenicol, piperacillin
Other *Proteus* species	Cephalosporin or gentamicin	Tobramycin, amikacin, chloramphenicol, piperacillin, aztreonam, imipenem
Providentia	Second- or third-generation cephalosporin	Gentamicin, amikacin, piperacillin, aztreonam, imipenem, TMP/SMZ
Salmonella typhosa	Chloramphenicol	Ampicillin, TMP/SMZ
Other *Salmonella*	Ampicillin	Chloramphenicol, TMP/SMZ
Serratia	Gentamicin	Cephalosporin, imipenem, aztreonam, piperacillin, TMP/SMZ
Shigella	TMP/SMZ	Ampicillin, chloramphenicol
Yersinia enterocolitica	TMP/SMZ	Gentamicin, tetracycline, third-generation cephalosporin
Other gram-negative bacilli		
Acinetobacter	Gentamicin	Imipenem, amikacin, piperacillin, TMP/SMZ, tetracycline
Eikenella corrodens	Ampicillin	Erythromycin, tetracycline
Francisella tularensis	Streptomycin	Tetracycline, chloramphenicol
Fusobacterium	Penicillin	Clindamycin, metronidazole, chloramphenicol
Haemophilus influenzae	Chloramphenicol	Ampicillin, cephalosprin, TMP/SMZ
Legionella	Erythromycin	Rifampin, tetracycline
Pasturella multocida	Penicillin	Tetracycline, cephalosporin
Pseudomonas aeruginosa	Antipseudomonal penicillin + gentamicin	Aztreonam or cephalosporin + amikacin
Pseudomonas cepacia	TMP/SMZ	Chloramphenicol
Spirillum minus	Penicillin G	Tetracycline, streptomycin
Streptobacillus moniliformis	Penicillin G	Tetracycline, streptomycin
Vibrio cholerae	Tetracycline	TMP/SMZ
Yersinia pestis	Streptomycin	Tetracycline, chloramphenicol
Chlamydia		
C. trachomatis	Tetracycline	Erythromycin, sulfonamide
C. psittaci	Tetracycline	Chloramphenicol
Mycoplasma	Erythromycin	Tetracycline
Rickettsia	Tetracycline	Chloramphenicol
Spirochetales		
Treponema pallidum	Penicillin	Tetracycline, erythromycin
Borrelia	Penicillin	Tetracycline

gesics include nonsteroidal anti-inflammatory drugs (NSAIDs), which will be discussed separately. Opioid analgesics function by binding to one of several related receptors in the central nervous system and blocking the transmission of pain signals. These agents do not eradicate awareness of painful stimuli, although they effectively dull the severity of the pain. Morphine and codeine are naturally occurring opioids, and they can be directly extracted from opium, the dried juice of the poppy plant. Most of the other opioid analgesics are semisynthetic derivatives of these naturally occurring agents.

Opioid analgesics include the agents listed in Table 9–2. Parenterally administered agents are generally more effective against severe pain than oral agents are, and agents administered intravenously usually take effect more rapidly. Morphine and meperidine are the two agents most commonly utilized for parenteral analgesia, and they are efficacious in 70% to 80% of patients with moderate to severe pain. There are no clear advantages to one or the other of these agents in most circumstances. Individuals may have unpleasant side effects with one agent and not another, although this is not predictable. A particular agent may have advantages in certain clinical situations, however. Meperidine, for example, is less likely to induce biliary spasm than morphine is and may be more useful in patients with biliary colic.

Fentanyl is 80 times as potent as morphine, and it has a much shorter duration of action, which makes it popular for use during anesthesia. It also produces less hemodynamic disruption than morphine does. The most commonly used oral agents are codeine and oxycodone, which are effective and have a limited number of side effects. Methadone is sometimes preferred as an oral analgesic because its long half-life allows less frequent administration and more constant analgesia once an adequate serum level has been achieved. The onset of action of methadone is slow, however.

Agents such as pentazocine, nalbuphine, and butorphanol are classified as mixed agonist-antagonists. The agonist-antagonists have less abuse potential than the other opioid narcotics. In addition to providing an analgesic effect, they block the effects of other morphine-like drugs, although each of the agonist-antagonists is unique in the way that it interacts with other agents. Pentazocine, for example, is effective in individuals tolerant to other agents, although it can generate a withdrawal reaction in addicts.

Opioid analgesics produce a significant number of side effects. They increase intestinal smooth muscle tone, delay gastric emptying, and decrease peristalsis. The most common clinical presentation of this action is constipation. Opiates can also cause urinary retention and slow uterine contraction during

TABLE 9–2.
Opioid Analgesics

Generic Name	Trade Name	Route*	Dose (mg)
Morphine		iv	4–10
		im, sc	5–20
		o	10–30
Hydromorphone	Dilaudid	im, sc	1–4
		o	1–4
Levorphanol	Levo-Dromoran	im, sc	1–3
		o	1–3
Methadone	Dolophine	im	2.5–10
		o	2.5–15
Meperidine	Demerol	iv	25–100
		im, sc	50–100
		o	50–150
Fentanyl	Sublimaze	iv	0.05–0.1
		im	0.05–0.1
Codeine		im	30–60
		o	30–60
Hydrocodone	Vicodin	o	5–10
	Lorcet Plus	o	5–10
Oxycodone	Percocet (with Tylenol)	o	5–10
Propoxyphene	Darvon	o	65
Pentazocine	Talwin	iv	20–60
		im, sc	20–60
		o	50–100
Nalbuphine	Nubain	iv	10
		im	10
Butorphanol	Stadol	iv	1
		im	2

* iv = intravenous; im = intramuscular; sc = subcutaneous; o = oral.

labor. Probably the most dangerous consequence of opioid use is a decrease in the sensitivity of the respiratory center to CO_2. Large doses of opioids induce contraction of bronchial smooth muscle in addition, which exacerbates respiratory problems. In acute opioid poisoning, respirations are extremely slow, and mechanical support may be required. Pinpoint pupils, another opioid effect, may aid in diagnosing the problem. If the diagnosis is suspected, intravenous naloxone, an opioid antagonist, should be administered immediately at a dose of 0.4 to 2.0 mg. It will promptly improve respiratory and circulatory functions with virtually no adverse effects.

Tolerance may develop to the analgesic effects of opioids, although this rarely occurs unless the agents are used in the absence of pain. Addicts have been known to tolerate up to 20 times the lethal dose. The possibility of addiction is another problem with these agents. The use of these agents in the postoperative period should not be limited because of concerns regarding addiction, however. The drug-seeking behavior seen in addicts rarely develops in patients who use narcotics when pain is present.

The most effective delivery system for these agents in the postoperative setting is patient-controlled analgesia (PCA). The patient can titrate the dose of narcotic received to pain and more effectively prevent pain from becoming severe. With more traditional narcotic delivery systems, 75% of patients fail to receive adequate analgesia. This is partially due to wider swings in serum drug levels with the more common intramuscular route of drug administration and partially the inability of the nurse to give the drug at precisely the right time. For pain in the lower extremity, lower part of the abdomen, or perineal area, epidural opioid narcotics may be effective while limiting opioid-induced respiratory depression. Other blocks are useful in the upper extremity and other areas.

Anti-inflammatory Agents

The prototype of the anti-inflammatory agents is aspirin, and collectively the agents are referred to as NSAIDs. Some of the more common NSAIDs are listed in Table 9–3. NSAIDs produce their anti-inflammatory effects by inhibiting the enzyme cyclooxygenase. Cyclooxygenase catalyzes one of the early steps in the arachidonic acid cascade that generates prostaglandins. Prostaglandins are primary mediators of the inflammatory response.

TABLE 9–3.
Nonsteroidal Anti-inflammatory Drugs

Generic Name	Trade Name	Dosage Range (mg)
Aspirin	Bayer Bufferin	650–1,300 q4–6h
Diflunisal	Dolobid	250–750 bid
Flubiprofen	Ansaid	50–100 tid
Ibuprofen	Motrin	400–800 qid
Indomethacin	Indocin	25–50 tid
Naproxen	Naprosyn	250–500 bid
Piroxicam	Feldene	20 qd
Sulindac	Clinoril	150–200 bid

NSAIDs have analgesic activity in situations where pain is the result of inflammation and injury. Inflammation causes sensitization of pain receptors to normally painless mechanical and chemical stimuli. Inhibition of prostaglandin synthesis by NSAIDs controls the pain response to these stimuli. These agents also have the ability to control the febrile response in that prostaglandins mediate the pyrexic response in the hypothalamus.

NSAIDs are used mainly in the treatment of musculoskeletal disorders such as rheumatoid arthritis, osteoarthritis, tendonitis, and bursitis. They have also been effective in dysmenorrhea. Although these agents provide symptomatic relief from pain and inflammation, they generally do not treat the responsible disease process.

NSAIDs can also produce untoward side effects, which can limit their usefulness. Gastric and intestinal ulceration may result because the inhibition of prostaglandin synthesis results in a decrease in submucosal blood flow and a decrease in the production of cytoprotective mucus and bicarbonate in the bowel. Ibuprofen produces the least gastrointestinal side effects. NSAIDs limit the formation of another arachidonic acid metabolite, thromboxane A_2 (TXA_2), a potent platelet-aggregating agent. They can therefore produce hemorrhagic complications.

They also interfere with renal function through inhibition of the production of vasodilatory prostaglandins. This can produce renal ischemia and a decreased glomerular filtration rate, which in extreme cases can proceed to renal failure. Fluid retention can also result from this decrease in renal function. Patients with congestive heart failure, hepatic cirrhosis with ascites, and hypovolemia are more susceptible to the renal complications of NSAID use. Sulindac affects renal prostaglandin synthesis the least and may be the safest to use in these settings and in hypertensive patients, although it is one of the more likely drugs to produce gastrointestinal side effects. Hepatotoxicity is another possible complication of these agents.

The choice of NSAIDs for the treatment of inflammatory disorders is largely empirical. More experience exists with the older agents such as aspirin and indomethacin, and the effect of these agents may be more predictable. Large variations are possible in response to the different NSAIDs, and therefore multiple trials may be necessary before the optimal therapeutic response is achieved for a given patient.

Steroids

The term "steroids" refers to a group of biologically active compounds synthesized in the adrenal cortex and their synthetic analogs. Corticosteroids affect nutrient metabolism, fluid and electrolyte homeostasis, the immune response, and the physiology of numerous organ systems. Commonly used steroids are shown in Table 9–4.

TABLE 9–4.
Steroid Preparations

Generic Name	Relative Equivalent Potency	Daily Dosage*	
		mg	mg/day
Hydrocortisone	1.0	20.0	80–160
Cortisone	0.8	25.0	100–200
Predinsone	4.0	5.0	20–100
Methylprednisolone	5.0	4.0	16–80
Triamcinolone	5.0	4.0	16–80
Dexamethasone	25.0	0.75	3–15

* The daily dose range is based on the severity of illness.

Steroids are primarily utilized clinically for their anti-inflammatory properties. The precise mechanism of action of the anti-inflammatory effects is not known, however. The different agents vary in their anti-inflammatory potency and duration of action, as well as in the amount of coexistent sodium-retaining mineralocorticoid effect they produce. The anti-inflammatory effect remains consistent regardless of the agent responsible for the inflammation. These effects are generally palliative, and the underlying condition that elicited the inflammation often remains untreated.

Steroids are used for the treatment of a large number of clinical conditions. Oral, parenteral, ophthalmic, and topical agents are available. Oral steroids such as prednisone are effective at ameliorating the pain associated with rheumatoid arthritis. Intra-articular injections have been used since 1950 for osteoarthritis. Steroids have also been injected locally in involved tissue to treat entrapment neuropathies such as carpal tunnel syndrome, tenosynovitis (including de Quervain's tenosynovitis), tendinitis, and neuromas. These injections are not uniformly efficacious and, in some locations, carry risks of damage to adjacent structures such as tendons and nerves if the injections are not precisely localized to the offending structures.

At present, triamcinolone, a longer-acting agent, appears to provide the best long-term results for local injections. Up to 40 mg is injected, with repeat injections dispensed according to patient response. Topical 0.05% to 2.5% hydrocortisone ointment is effective in the treatment of contact dermatitis and a large number of other dermatologic disorders. Steroids have also been placed both inside and outside breast prostheses to try to decrease capsule formation after breast augmentation. They have been administered, both intralesionally and systemically, with some success to children with rapidly growing hemangiomas, such as those threatening to interfere with a visual field. They have been utilized for patients with large hepatic hemangiomas causing congestive heart failure as well.

Steroids are used in a variety of circumstances to decrease edema formation. They are used for that purpose after head trauma and are also sometimes used to decrease edema after elective surgery. Steroids of various types have been utilized to treat or prevent keloids in that they interfere with virtually all aspects of the wound healing process and, in addition, indirectly increase collagenase activity. Intralesional triamcinolone in doses up to 120 mg have produced responses in approximately 80% of patients.

Steroid treatment is not without risk. Complications of steroid use can affect virtually every organ system. More common complications of systemic steroids include peptic ulceration, hyperglycemia and new-onset diabetes, a cushingoid habitus, growth retardation, amenorrhea, osteoporosis, hypertension, infections secondary to immune impairments, and wound healing complications. Local injections can produce thinning of tissues with vitiligo.

Patients with adrenal insufficiency and patients receiving exogenous steroid therapy for other problems require steroid supplementation in the perioperative period to prevent acute adrenal insufficiency. Normally the adrenal gland produces three to four times the normal amount of cortisol in response to the stress of major surgery, with the maximal secretion occurring during anesthetic reversal and extubation. A number of regimens have been used to cover patients receiving steroids during the perioperative period. One regimen that is effective is to administer 25 mg of hydrocortisone hemisuccinate intravenously preoperatively, 100 mg intravenously intraoperatively, and 50 mg intravenously every 8 hours for the first postoperative 24-hour period. For the second postoperative 24-hour period 25 mg is given every 8 hours. The dosage should be tapered 50% each day until the maintenance dose is reached if the postoperative course is uncomplicated. Lower doses are required for minor surgery.

Chemotherapeutic Agents

Chemotherapy can be given (1) as palliative therapy for patients with advanced disease, (2) as adjunctive therapy to local treatment for tumors where the likelihood of failure with local treatment alone is high, and (3) as primary therapy for individuals with responsive tumors. For a chemotherapeutic agent to be effective, the cancer cells must be sensitive to the agent, the agent must reach the cells at the appropriate time during the cell cycle, and the malignant cells must be destroyed before drug resistance emerges. Antineoplastic drugs exert their cytotoxic effects by interfering with normal metabolic activities of tumor cells such as DNA synthesis, RNA synthesis, and protein synthesis. They only affect cells that are actively dividing, so quiescent cells are not affected. A higher percentage of cells in small tumors is dividing, and therefore chemotherapeutic agents are most effective when the tumor burden is low. Most acute toxicities of chemotherapeutic agents are also expressed in rapidly dividing tissues or organs such as bone marrow, intestinal mucosa, and hair follicles.

Chemotherapeutic agents differ from many other drugs in that they follow log kill kinetics and kill a constant percentage of the cells, not a constant number as antibiotics do. For example, a particular dose of an agent will reduce 10^{10} cells to 10^7 or 10^5 cells to 10^2. If the number of cells is too high, it is impossible to administer an adequate amount of drug to eradicate the tumor. The effectiveness of chemotherapeutic agents is also hindered because spontaneous mutations in cancer cells frequently render the agents ineffective. Combinations of agents are frequently utilized to maximize cell kill within the toxicity tolerated for each drug, to provide broader coverage for resistant cell lines, and to slow the development of resistant lines. Combinations are most effective when all agents are effective against the neoplasm being treated in the doses administered, when cellular metabolism is affected in different ways by the different agents, when cross-toxicity is limited, and when the mechanism of tumor cell resistance is different.

With the exception of lymphoma, chemotherapy alone for head and neck cancers is rarely curative, and it is usually combined with surgery and/or radiation. The cytotoxic agents are generally given intravenously, and most antitumor protocols involve multidrug therapy. The most effective drugs for treating malignancies of the head and neck are methotrexate, bleomycin, 5-fluorouracil (5-FU), cisplatin, carboplatin, and vincristine. Although a significant number of tumors respond to regimens utilizing one or more of these agents, survival in either the adjunctive setting or in the palliative setting has not been significantly improved.

Chemotherapy for cutaneous cancers has also been disappointing. Chemotherapy has no proven role in the primary treatment of basal or squamous cell carcinomas. Topical treatment with 5-FU has been abandoned because of poor cure rates and high morbidity. Chemotherapeutic regimens have been used as palliation for patients with metastatic disease, although with limited benefit. Similarly, no agents have been demonstrated to be efficacious in the adjuvant setting for malignant melanoma, although a number have been tried. Results with L-phenylalanine mustard (L-PAM or melphalan) as a surgical adjuvant have been encouraging in patients with disease isolated to a limb when the agent is administered in an isolated hyperthermic limb perfusion, however. Imidazole carboxamide (dacarbazine or DTIC) is currently being used to treat metastatic melanoma with some promising results. Nitrosoureas are also melanoma active and are often used in combination with DTIC.

Extravasation

A frequent, yet often overlooked complication of chemotherapy is extravasation injury. Although extravasation injuries can also occur with drugs other than chemotherapeutic agents, some of the most devastating extravasation injuries are caused by agents used for chemotherapy. Doxorubicin produces perhaps the worst extravasation injuries. It is a vesicant and has a cytotoxic effect when it extravasates. The cytotoxicity is perpetuated by the doxorubicin-DNA complex that is released from cells when they die; this complex continues to affect viable cells and causes a deep, slow-healing ulcer.

The majority of extravasation injuries occur in the upper extremities at and distal to the antecubital fossa. The sequelae of extravasations depend upon the anatomic location and the toxicity of the agent used as well as the concentration and volume of the extravasate. Tissue reactions range from localized erythema to full-thickness necrosis requiring operative debridement and, rarely, amputation. Epidermal blistering often precedes full-thickness skin loss. Clinical symptoms of an extravasation injury include pain, redness, and swelling around the intravenous site. These injuries can be complicated acutely by compartment syndromes and less acutely by infection.

Prevention of severe injuries requires trained personnel knowledgeable in intravenous insertion and early recognition of the problem when it begins to develop. Central access catheters and ports have reduced the incidence of injuries. Proper initial treatment of an extravasation includes careful documentation and initial assessment of the injury. The involved extremity should be elevated, the intravenous catheter removed, and serial examinations performed to rule out neurovascular compromise. Compressive dressings frequently help reduce edema. Cold compresses for 15 to 60 minutes three to four times per day may further diminish the swelling and tissue damage. Certain drugs may be useful as antidotes for some extravasations. Phentolamine (Regitine), an α-blocking agent, can counteract the effects of vasopressors, and sodium thiosulfate may limit skin damage resulting from nitrogen mustard. Hyaluronidase (Wydase) has been used to facilitate rapid diffusion of many extravasated agents. A large number of additional treatment modalities have been used for extravasation injury, including locally injected steroids of different types, topical dimethyl sulfoxide (DMSO), topical DMSO with vitamin E, and local injections of sodium bicarbonate, phentolamine, and local anesthetics, although none has been proved effective in careful trials.

Common intravenous solutions generally resorb with nonsurgical treatment without complication. Hypertonic solutions such as hyperalimentation solution, solutions containing vasopressors such as dopamine, and solutions with cytotoxic agents are much more likely to produce tissue damage and need to be monitored more carefully. There is no way to accurately predict the clinical course of any extravasation injury when it is first seen, and consideration of surgery should generally be postponed until the extent of the injury is clearly defined. Most infiltrations, even with vesicants, resolve with nonsurgical management and few sequelae. Early surgery is only required for neurovascular compromise. When surgery is required as a consequence of tissue necrosis and persistent pain, surgical excisions for doxorubicin extravasations must be radical and include a margin of normal skin and subcutaneous tissue; otherwise, adjacent unexcised doxorubicin-damaged tissue can lead to a persistent ulcer.

BACTERIOLOGY OF WOUNDS

Bacteriology

Humans do not live in a sterile environment, and no body structure exposed to the outside environment is free of bacteria. The number and type of bacteria vary between anatomic locations. Dry skin contains 10^1 to 10^3 bacteria per gram of tissue, while skin in moist areas contains up to 10^5 bacteria per gram of tissue. The variation in bacterial flora between anatomic areas is a result of differences in temperature, pH, moisture content, oxygen, oxidation-reduction potential, and other factors related to the local cellular and biochemical environment.

Under normal conditions, the number of bacteria in each location remains relatively constant, and bacteria do not invade surrounding tissues. Bacterial proliferation and invasion require that the bacteria be able to adhere to an epithelial or endothelial surface and survive. Adherence and survival of bacteria are limited by defense mechanisms specific to each anatomic location. In skin, the superficial keratin layer limits bacterial attachment and invasion. The keratin is sloughed every 14 days, which limits the time in which an adherent bacterium may invade if it becomes attached. Bacterial growth in the skin is inhibited by dryness in most areas as well, although when skin becomes extremely dry, it can crack and allow bacteria to penetrate. Skin cells produce a number of products that limit bacterial proliferation. Bacteria-inhibiting substances produced by skin cells include fatty acids, polar lipids, glycosphingolipids, lysozymes, lactic acid, and uric acid. These cellular products help maintain an acidic pH, which is at least one of the mechanisms by which bacterial proliferation is limited. Sebaceous gland secretions include bactericidal and fungicidal fatty acids, which limit bacterial proliferation in skin as well. IgA and IgG are secreted by the eccrine sweat glands and help prevent infection by both direct bactericidal effects in conjunction with complement and by limiting bacterial adherence. The skin also assists with T-cell activation and differentiation. The skin is therefore protected against bacterial invasion in many ways.

In addition to local factors, circulating immune cells contribute to the control of bacterial proliferation. Neutrophils and macrophages phagocytize bacteria, T lymphocytes are cytotoxic to bacteria and other foreign cells, and B lymphocytes produce antibodies that kill bacteria in the presence of complement. The resident bacteria in specific locations inhibit proliferation of exogenous bacteria through the production of bacteriocins, blockage of attachment sites, depletion of nutrients, production of toxic products, and other mechanisms.

Infection represents a condition where the normal homeostasis between resident bacteria and the body's defense mechanisms is disrupted. A change in the number or type of bacteria or a defect in some aspect of the defense system allows the bacteria to proliferate and invade the local tissue. Under normal conditions, infection exists when there are greater than 10^5 bacteria per gram of tissue. The only exception to this rule is β-hemolytic *Streptococcus,* which is able to proliferate and invade local tissues even if present in lesser numbers. When the body is immunocompromised (as with acquired immunodeficiency syndrome [AIDS], diabetes, or steroids), the number of bacteria required to generate infection is less than 10^5 per gram of tissue.

A Gram stain of tissue or drainage is an inexpensive, rapid method of identifying many bacteria and fungi. Quantitative cultures of wound biopsy samples provide definitive information regarding whether or not greater than 10^5 bacteria per gram of tissue are present in a wound, although 24 to 48 hours is required to generate a diagnostic result. The rapid slide technique can diagnose the presence of greater than 10^5 bacteria per gram of tissue in less than an hour, although the rapid slide technique does not identify the species of bacteria present. *Staphylococcus aureus* is reliably cultured from the abscesses it produces, although swab cultures of wounds or wound exudates can sometimes be misleading and identify resident or transient flora as infecting agents. Swab cultures of wound exudate or pus suggest a polymicrobial origin for the majority of infections, although tissue cultures more commonly grow a single organism.

Skin Infections

Skin infections are generally initiated by a break in epidermal integrity produced by surgery or trauma or by maceration resulting from excess moisture. Infections are often caused by endogenous resident bacteria, although the normal resident bacteria, which include *Staphylococcus epidermidis* and other staphylococcal species, *Corynebacterium* species (aerobic diptheroids), anaerobic gram-positive bacilli such as *Propionibacterium acnes* (anaerobic diptheroids), and *Pityrosporum* species (a lipid-requiring yeast), rarely produce infections. The most common bacteria producing skin infections are *S. aureus* and β-hemolytic streptococci. *S. aureus* colonizes 10% to 35% of normal people and is frequently found in the nares of carriers. The infection can be confined to the skin, although other structures can be seeded through bacteremia. Staphylococcal skin infections are generally characterized by abscesses. Staphylococcal organisms can produce multiple small pustules (impetigo), which it does most commonly in children, infection around hair follicles (folliculitis), infection in nail folds (paronychia), deep abscesses (furuncles), or very deep abscesses (carbuncles). Definitive treatment requires drainage of the abscess, removal of any foreign body or necrotic tissue that may be potentiating the infection, and appropriate antimicrobial therapy, which usually involves a penicillinase-resistant penicillin. *S. aureus* can also produce toxins that can lead to staphylococcal scalded skin syndrome and toxic shock syndrome as well. The primary infection can sometimes be relatively inocuous in the toxin-related skin diseases.

Group A β-hemolytic streptococci are another common cause of skin infections. Involved tissue becomes erythematous, edematous, and tender, although the involved area is often not clearly demarcated. In erysipelas-type infections, the involved tissue becomes indurated, and the area of involvement is well demarcated with a raised reddish or purplish border. Erysipelas is a result of partial or complete lymphatic obstruction secondary to the infection. Streptococcal impetigo is relatively common in children and is characterized by multiple small vesicles or pustules filled with clear fluid and surrounded by a limited amount of erythema. Streptococcal infections are frequently accompanied by regional adenopathy and systemic signs such as fevers and chills. Streptococci can frequently be isolated from vesicles if they exist, although the diagnosis must often be made on clinical grounds. The infections are effectively treated with penicillin or first-generation cephalosporins. Toxins of group A *Streptococcus* occasionally produce scarlet fever and toxic shock syndrome.

The likelihood of a particular species of bacteria being isolated depends on the location of the wound or abscess. *S. aureus* is especially common on the leg, neck, and hand, although it is relatively common in most locations. Group D streptococci, *Escherichia coli,* and *Neisseria gonorrhoeae* are aerobic organisms commonly isolated from the external genitalia and perirectal area. *Haemophilus influenzae* is most commonly seen on the head and neck. More anaerobes are isolated from the head and neck and perirectal area as a result of proximity to the oral cavity and gastrointestinal tract. Anaerobic bacteria predominate when pyogenic drainage from cutaneous abscesses is cultured, with the most common species of anaerobes being *Bacteroides, Peptostreptococcus, Clostridium,* and *Fusobacterium.* The predominant aerobic bacteria are *S. aureus,* group A streptococci, and *E. coli.*

Fungi can produce skin infections as well. Various species of *Trichophyton* produce tinea pedis in the feet, tinea manuum of the hands, tinea cruris in the groin, tinea capitis in the scalp, tinea unguium in the nails, and tinea at other sites. Tinea, in most locations, is characterized by scaling, pruritis, and often redness. In the toenail there may be a hyperkeratotic reaction. *Trichophyton* can generally be isolated on culture. When tissue scrapings are mounted in KOH, hyphae are often visible. Most are well treated by topical antifungal agents such as undecylenic acid, tolnaftate, haloprogin, clotrimazole, and miconazole, although sometimes with tinea unguium, systemic therapy with griseofulvin is required. *Candida* is a normal inhabitant of the gastrointestinal tract and vagina, and it can occasionally produce infections with white plaques in the mouth, red confluent patches on the buttock, or swelling without purulence in the nail fold. *Candida* infections are most commonly seen in macerated areas, and they are also more common in patients who are immunosuppressed. *Sporothrix schenkii* can produce subcutaneous infections that ulcerate. These ulcers are associated with lymphadenopathy and occasionally subcutaneous nodules along the lymphatics. Individuals at risk are those who work around the plants and soil where the organisms reside such as forestry workers and farmers. The infection is diagnosed by culturing the organism and treatment involves the use of potassium iodide. Fungi rarely produce deep infections.

Nontuberculous mycobacteria may cause systemic or pulmonary infections, although cutaneous infections may be the first or only sign of such infections. The nontuberculous myobacteria responsible for most cutaneous disease in North America are *Mycobacterium marinum, Mycobacterium fortuitum, Mycobacterium chelonei, Mycobacterium kansasii,* and *Mycobacterium avium-intracellulare.* (*M. avium* and *M. intracellulare* are two very closely related mycobacteria that are usually considered together.) *M. marinum* has been isolated from water in fish tanks, swimming pools, and other moist environments, and infections generally occur after lacerations or abrasions at the seashore or a lake. These infections are characterized by papules or nodules and ulcers that may invade deeply. The lesions may be quite indolent and exist as an encrusted lesion for 1 year or more. The mycobacteria will not survive at body temperature, so infections tend to be localized to extremities. *M. marinum* must be cultured at 30 to 33° C, which distinguishes it from other mycobacteria and bacteria. *M. fortuitum* and *chelonei* tend to contaminate open wounds, often in immunocompromised hosts, and cause granulomatous nodules, ulcers, abscesses, cellulitis, or disseminated disease. Skin manifestations of *M. avium-intracellulare* and *M. kansasii* generally develop in patients with pulmonary disease, and infections with *M. avium-intracellulare* are uncommon in humans. The diagnosis of mycobacterial infections requires clinical suspicion to ensure that histologic staining for acid-fast organisms and appropriate cultures are carried out. Treatment involves antituberculous drugs such as isoniazid, ethambutol, and rifampin.

Viruses can also produce cutaneous infections in humans. The more common infective agents are herpes simplex types 1 and 2 and varicella-zoster virus, which is also known as herpes type 3. Herpes simplex usually occurs as a result of direct inoculation of skin or a mucosal surface. The virus may produce systemic symptoms such as fever, headaches, malaise, myalgias, or lymphadenopathy. The primary cutaneous lesion is a vesicle, which usually ruptures after 3 days and leaves an ulcer that lasts 4 to 15 days. The ulcers then crust and limit viral shedding. After an infection, the virus travels up the sensory nerve and establishes latent infection in the dorsal root ganglion. The lips and buccal mucosa are most commonly infected with herpes simplex 1, while herpes simplex 2 more regularly infects the genitalia, although either virus can infect either location. Acyclovir has become the mainstay of treatment for herpes infections. Individuals exposed to orotracheal secretions may get "herpetic whitlow" of the hand, which is characteristically manifested as painful vesicles filled with clear fluid. The vesicles eventually ulcerate and crust as with herpes elsewhere. Herpes type 1 or 2 is causative and can be cultured from the vesicles. The Tzanck smear is often diagnostic, and the infections are generally not treated.

Varicella-zoster virus produces a vesicular eruption in children that lasts 7 to 14 days. The diagnosis is usually made on clinical grounds, although a Tzanck smear or culture can be performed to corroborate the diagnosis. Zoster is seen in older individuals who were previously exposed to the varicella-zoster virus as children but in whom incomplete immunity developed. It is manifested as paresthesias, itching, burning, and pain in a radicular pattern along with fever, malaise, and nausea. Virus can be cultured from the open vesicles, and a Tzanck smear can also be diagnostic. Varicella is generally not treated, although acyclovir can be used for zoster.

The most severe skin infection that can develop is a necrotizing infection. Bacterial necrotizing infections involving fascia and skin can be produced by (1) *Clostridium perfringens* alone, (2) a combination of microaerophilic streptococci and *S. aureus,* or (3) a polymicrobial mixture of aerobic and anaerobic organisms. *Streptococcus* and *S. aureus* are commonly components of the polymicrobial infections, although enteric bacteria such as *Enterococcus* and *Bacteroides* are also frequently seen. Occasionally, severe infections with group A *Streptococcus,* staphylococci, or coliforms can be necrotizing, although in these cases the necrosis is usually limited to the skin. Reported mortality rates from necrotizing infections range up to 64%. The diagnosis must be made early to facilitate immediate aggressive debridement of all infected tissue, careful hemodynamic monitoring, and appropriate antimicrobial therapy.

Head and Neck Infections

The head and neck include some of the most highly contaminated parts of the human body. The excellent blood supply to the head and neck region limits the ability of bacteria to produce infection in that location, however. Bacterial invasion is also limited by the inhibitory effects of the endogenous flora; the mucosal barrier that includes IgA; the mechanical clearing of structures by swallowing, breathing, and blinking; and enzymes present in saliva and tears that kill bacteria or limit their growth. The species of bacteria present within the oral cavity vary slightly between the tongue, the cheek, and the gingival area, but all areas are heavily laden with a wide variety of both aerobic and anaerobic bacteria, with anaerobes predominating. Saliva contains in excess of 10^8 bacteria per milliliter. The skin of the head and neck usually becomes infected as a result of a break in the skin or mucosa. There are special concerns for infections in this anatomic area. There are a number of interconnections between superficial veins in the head and neck area and intracranial veins through valveless emissary veins. Infections in these areas can lead to intracranial venous thrombosis. The points of connection include (1) the anterior facial vein which connects to the cavernous sinus through the superior ophthalmic vein; (2) the deep facial vein, which connects to the cavernous sinus via the pterygoid plexus through the vesalian vein; (3) a large sagittal emissary vein from the scalp to the superior sagittal sinus; and (4) mastoid emissary veins to the sigmoid sinus. Thrombosis of the cavernous vein can limit flow in the adjacent internal carotid and ophthalmic artery and can also compromise cranial nerves III, IV, V, and VI. The areas of concern for potential spread to the cavernous sinus are the upper lip, the tip of the nose, and the medial parts of the cheeks. Infections in the scalp can extend to the sagittal sinus and cause thrombosis and increased intracranial pressure. Infections in the mastoid region can also lead to intracranial infection. Orbital cellulitis can be dangerous because of the possibility of damage to the eye if the infection is not quickly controlled with antibiotics and, on occasion, surgical drainage.

Deep infections in the neck are generally a result of oral flora that obtain access to the deep spaces through a break in the intraoral mucosal barrier. They are commonly initiated by an odontogenic infection. Infections in the submandibular, lateral pharyngeal, and retropharyngeal-prevertebral spaces can compromise the airway and be potentially life-threatening. These infections are characteristically necrotizing and rapidly spreading, thus necessitating early diagnosis and treatment. The infections are most commonly polymicrobial and generally involve anaerobes as would be expected from the normal oral flora. Infection in the submandibular space, known as Ludwig's angina, is a woody cellulitis without suppuration that can produce mouth pain, dysphagia, drooling, and a stiff neck as well as airway compromise. Infections in the prevertebral space differ from the other deep infections in this region because bacteria generally reach the area through the adjacent cervical spine, usually as a complication of trauma. Oral flora are therefore less commonly involved.

Infections in the submandibular, lateral pharyngeal, and retropharyngeal-prevertebral spaces can be diagnosed by computed tomography (CT), ultrasound, and sometimes lateral neck films. Direct aspiration of the involved area can also sometimes be diagnostic. Surgical drainage and antibiotics are required for infections in all of these locations.

Breast Infections

The breast is differentiated from skin in other locations in that milk ducts provide direct passageways from the surface to deep within the breast tissue. This unique characteristic does not modify the endogenous bacterial flora, however. Infections in nonlactating breasts are most likely initiated by blockage of the lactiferous ducts by keratinaceous debris, although infections may arise de novo, at least at times, from subepidermal glands of the areola. These infections are manifested as pain, erythema, and often suppuration in the subareolar area. If no suppuration is present, antibiotics alone may suffice, although suppuration necessitates drainage. Simple incision and drainage result in a 38% recurrence rate, which has encouraged some to recommend excisional treatment of all suppurative lesions. Patients with recurrent, chronic periareolar abscesses generally have fistulous connections between the abscess cavity and the periareolar area as well as with the nipple. Successful treatment of chronic fistulas generally requires complete excision of the fistulous tract. Acute infections are most commonly a result of *S. aureus,* while chronic infections most commonly involve *S. epidermidis,* with *S. aureus* being the next most common organism isolated.

Surgical Wound Infections

Approximately 5% of all surgical wounds become infected. Clean cases become infected 1% to 2% of the time, while clean-contaminated cases (e.g., bowel cases without spillage of enteric contents), become infected in 7% to 8% of cases. A case where there is spillage of the enteric contents is considered a contaminated case, and these become infected 15% to 16% of the time. A dirty case with gross pus will lead to a wound infection in 40% of patients. Shaving preoperatively increases the infection rate as compared with patients whose hair is clipped. Other factors associated with a higher rate of wound infections are a long preoperative stay, older patients, long operations, and the lack of a preoperative shower. Interestingly, adhesive drapes, the length of time the surgeon scrubs, punctures in surgical gloves, laminar flow, and the use of electrocautery have not been associated with a difference in the rate of wound infection.

In the majority of cases, the organism causing the infection is endogenous. As mentioned, different parts of the body harbor different resident bacteria, and therefore the likelihood of a particular bacteria being causative for an infection varies with the part of the body undergoing surgery. Overall, the most common organism responsible for postoperative wound infections is *S. aureus,* which causes 30% to 40% of all such infections. *E. coli* and *Pseudomonas aeruginosa* are the next most common.

Hand Infections

The hand is particularly susceptible to injury because it is used for so many activities. The normal bacterial flora of the hand is similar to that in other locations, and the hand is not unusually prone to infections. Randomized prospective trials of prophylactic antibiotics for routine hand injuries demonstrated no advantage to the antibiotics. The development of infection in the hand generally requires a break in the intact skin such as a laceration, injection, or a crack in a callus. Injections are more likely to generate infections than are lacerations because the bacteria are localized in a closed space. Injuries that involve damage to a great deal of tissue such as high-compression injection injuries, burn injuries, and crush injuries are more prone to infection. Farm injuries and particularly human bites are contaminated with large quantities of virulent bacteria and have a greater likelihood of becoming infected. The anatomy of the hand makes infections in certain locations more likely to involve adjacent areas. Infections that involve the flexor tendon sheath spread all along the sheath. In the thumb and small finger the sheath extends into the wrist, while in the index, long, and ring fingers, the sheath ends at the base of the finger. The thenar and midpalmar spaces also tend to be involved in their entirety if infected. The most common organism involved in hand infections is *S. aureus,* although the prevalence of *S. aureus* infections is decreasing. β-Hemolytic streptococci have remained the second most common organism found in hand infections. Mixed infections with gram-positive and gram-negative organisms have been increasing in frequency, and the *S. aureus* infections that have occurred are less frequently sensitive to penicillin. Treatment for hand infections involves elevation, immobilization, drainage if suppuration is present, and antibiotics. Heat and dressing changes are also frequently used, depending on the clinical situation.

Certain groups and types of injuries have unusual characteristics. Infections in diabetics more commonly involve both gram-positive and gram-negative organisms. Diabetics are less often successfully treated with the usual treatment modalities, more commonly have deeper infections and osteomyelitis, and more commonly require amputations. The elderly are also more prone to having mixed infections. Mutilating injuries and farm injuries are also prone to bacterial infection. Farm injuries are more frequently contaminated with gram-negative organisms than gram-positive organisms in contrast to the usual home and industry injuries. Prophylactic antibiotics are not necessarily required in farm injuries, although aggressive wound management is essential.

Bite Wounds

Human bite wounds are contaminated with saliva, which harbors 10^8 bacteria per milliliter. Human bite wounds need to be considered infected from their inception, and they should generally not be closed. Most human bites occur on the hand or arm, usually as a result of a fist to the mouth. Anaerobes predominate in infections resulting from human bites, although the infections are characteristically polymicrobial. The most common anaerobes isolated are peptostreptococci, *Fusobacterium* species, and *Bacteroides melaninogenicus.* The most common aerobic bacteria isolated are *S. aureus, S. epidermidis,* streptococcal species, *Corynebacterium* species, and *Eikenella corrodens.*

Animal bite wounds are characteristically less severely contaminated than human bite wounds. Dog bites make up 80% to 90% of animal bites, and the upper extremity is the body part most commonly injured. Aerobic bacteria predominate in dog and cat bites. *Pasturella multocida* has been isolated from 26% of dog bite wounds and 50% or more of cat bite wounds. Other commonly isolated aerobic bacteria include *S. aureus, S. epidermidis,* streptococci, and corynebacteria. The most common anaerobes isolated are peptostreptococci, fusobacteria, and *Bacteroides* species.

Animal and human bite wounds require cleansing, irrigation, and debridement. Human bites should generally not be closed, although closure may be considered for wounds of the face if antibiotics are given and the wound is adequately irrigated and debrided prior to closure. Wounds created by human bites, especially in the hand, need to be carefully evaluated for deep injuries to bone, joints, and tendons, and surgical debridement in the operating room may be required.

Animal bites may be considered for closure after adequate irrigation and debridement. Prophylactic antibiotics have been shown to be unnecessary for dog bites, although this is not universally accepted. Dicloxacillin or cephalexin are appropriate antibiotics if they are to be given. Although it was previously felt that hospitalization was mandatory for parenteral antibiotics, even for uninfected human bites, the efficacy of this treatment has been questioned. If the patient is not treated with parenteral antibiotics, penicillin VK or amoxacillin is a reasonable antibiotic choice.

When infections develop secondary to animal bites, penicillin, to which *P. multocida* ,is sensitive, is usually adequate. Human bite infections generally require treatment with penicillin and a penicillinase-resistant penicillin such as dicloxacillin, penicillin plus an aminoglycoside, or a second- or third-generation cephalosporin.

Tetanus prophylaxis must be considered for all bite wounds. Rabies must also be considered, especially for bat and skunk bites. Dogs and cats should be watched for signs of the disorder for 10 days if they bite an individual. The brain of potentially infected animals can be examined for Negri bodies in the motor neurons, which are diagnostic if they are found. For suspected rabies, the patient should undergo a series of injections with both diploid cell rabies vaccine and rabies immunoglobulin.

SUGGESTED READING

Bier J: Chemotherapy for squamous cell carcinomas of the head and neck. *Int J Oral Maxillofac Surg* 1990; 19:232–234.

Brook I: Human and animal bite infections. *J Fam Pract* 1989; 28:713–718.

Brook I, Frazier EH: Aerobic and anaerobic bacteriology of wounds and cutaneous abscesses. *Arch Surg* 1990; 125:1445–1451.

Crawford CE: An approach to use of antimicrobial agents, in Civetta JM (ed): *Critical Care.* Philadelphia, JB Lippincott, 1988, pp 769–783.

Cruse PJE, Foord R: The epidemiology of wound infection: A 10-year study of 62,939 wounds. *Surg Clin North Am* 1980; 60:27–40.

Fitzgerald RH, Cooney WP, Washington JA, et al: Bacterial colonization of mutilating hand injuries and its treatment. *J Hand Surg* 1977; 2:85–89.

Gilman AG, Rall TW, Niles AS et al: *Goodman and Gilman's The Pharmacological Basis of Therapeutics,* ed 8. New York, Pergamon Press, 1990.

Heggers JP: Natural host defense mechanisms. *Clin Plast Surg* 1979; 6:505–513.

Larson DL: What is the appropriate management of tissue extravasation by antitumor agents? *Plast Reconstr Surg* 1985; 75:397–405.

Lewis RC: Infections of the hand. *Emerg Med Clin North Am* 1985; 3:263–274.

McGrath MH: Local steroid therapy in the hand. *J Hand Surg [Am]* 1984; 9:915–921.

Napolitano LM, Chernow B: Guidelines for corticosteroid use in anesthetic and surgical stress. *Int Anesthesiol Clin* 1988; 26:226–232.

Pariser DM: Cutaneous viral infections: Herpes simplex and varicella-zoster. *Primary Care* 1989; 16:577–589.

Patino JF, Castro D: Necrotizing lesions of the soft tissues: A review. *World J Surg* 1991; 15:235–239.

Robson MC, Krizek TJ, Heggers JP: Biology of surgical infection. *Curr Probl Surg* 1973; 10:1–62.

Street ML, Umbert-Millet IJ, Roberts GD, et al: Nontuberculous mycobacterial infections of the skin. *J Am Acad Dermatol* 1991; 24:208–215.

Stromberg B: Changing bacterial flora of hand infections. *J Trauma* 1985; 25:530–533.

Thadepalli H, Mandal AK: Anatomic basis of head and neck infections. *Infect Dis Clin North Am* 1988; 2:21–34.

Watt-Boolsen S, Rasmussen NR, Bilchert-Toft M: Primary periareolar abscess in the nonlactating breast: Risk of recurrence. *Am J Surg* 1987; 153:571–573.

PART III

Plastic Surgery of the Integument

Chapter 10

Anatomy/Physiology/Embryology

Noel S. Tenenbaum, M.D.
David J. Smith, Jr., M.D.

CONTENTS

CHAPTER OBJECTIVE

At the end of this chapter the resident is thoroughly familiar with the histology, function, and development of the skin.

LEARNER OBJECTIVE

On completion of this chapter the resident

1. Demonstrates knowledge of the structure and function of the epidermis.
2. Demonstrates knowledge of the structure and function of the dermis.
3. Demonstrates knowledge of the structure and function of the skin appendages.
4. Demonstrates knowledge of the structure and function of subcutaneous tissues and fascial layers.
5. Knows the embryologic origin of the skin and at which gestational age the various components of the skin appear.
6. Understands the differentiation of the stratum germinativum into surface cells and appendages and the differentiation of the dermis.
7. Demonstrates knowledge of the structure and function of the nails.

CLINICAL PRACTICE ACTIVITIES

During the course of the training program, the resident

1. Reviews histologic slides of normal skin and pathologic processes.
2. Regularly reviews pathology slides of skin lesions from specific patients.
3. *Participates in the preparation and review of frozen sections in selected cases.*

ANATOMY AND EMBRYOLOGY OF THE SKIN

The integument serves as a barrier between the host cells and various environmental agents. Additional functions include the regulation of fluid loss and temperature, immunologic surveillance, and protection from radiation and ultraviolet (UV) light.

The various components of the integument are embryologically derived from the ectoderm or mesoderm. Embryologic development of the integument occurs early in gestation. Sensory fibers have been noted as early as 5 weeks of gestation. Skin appendages such as hair follicles, sebaceous glands, and sweat glands develop following epidermal invasion of the dermis at 3 months of gestation and have completed development at 5 months.

The skin is composed of epidermis and dermis and may vary in thickness from 0.5 to 6 mm, depending upon the anatomic location and age of the patient. The epidermis is composed of four layers, the stratum germinativum, stratum spinosum, stratum granulosum, and superficial stratum corneum. The basal layer, or stratum germinativum, is the only proliferating layer of the epidermis. Melanocytes are also located within this layer. Immediately superficial to the stratum germinativum is the prickle layer known as the stratum spinosum. Cells are larger here and are joined by tonofibrils. In this layer the majority of viable cells, known as keratinocytes, produce keratin, precursor proteins, and granules. The stratum granulosum features mature keratinocytes containing cytoplasmic granules and is the site of protein synthesis. A clear band known as the stratum lucidum separates the stratum corneum from the underlying stratum granulosum.

As the outermost layer, the stratum corneum varies in thickness from 10 to 20 μm and is thickest in the palms and soles. This layer consists of nonviable, keratinized cells that are highly interdigitated and 10 to 15 cells thick and serve primarily as a protective barrier. The stratum corneum also regulates water balance by transporting water passively to the skin surface where it evaporates. Normal water loss is 0.1 to 0.5 mL/cm^2 hr but may increase dramatically to 10 to 12 mL/cm^2/hr after injury to the stratum corneum.

Another function of the stratum corneum is the inhibition of bacterial invasion. Resident bacteria (such as *Streptococcus* and *Staphylococcus,* which are normally present in concentrations of 10^3 organisms per gram of tissue) or transient flora may penetrate the integument. Such action is generally inhibited by sebum, which is secreted by the sebaceous glands. Sebum, which contains fatty acids such as oleic acid, is bactericidal to *Streptococcus* and *Staphylococcus.* Inflammation of the epidermis involving increased serum accumulation and edema inactivates sebum, thus allowing for streptococcal proliferation.

Aside from keratinocytes, the epidermis also contains several other cell types. Melanocytes are nonreplicating, neural crest derivatives. The melanin they produce absorbs UV light and traps photochemically activated free radicals. The mesenchyme-derived Langerhans' cells provide an immunologic role by identifying and processing antigens for other immunocompetent cells of the immune system. They are thought to originate in the bone marrow. Merkel cells function as mechanoreceptors. These nonreplicating cells are thought to be of neural crest origin.

The epidermal-dermal junction is an undulating boundary that increases the contact area and diminishes the shearing potential at the junction. The basement membrane serves as a barrier to molecules greater than 40 kilodaltons and is a site for immune complex deposition. Inflammatory and neoplastic cells as well as bacteria are capable of penetrating this layer.

The dermal layer represents approximately 95% of the total skin thickness. It contains two layers, the more superficial papillary and the deeper reticular dermis. Many structures are contained within the dermis, including nervous, vascular, and lymphatic tissue as well as the skin appendages (Fig 10–1). Perhaps most significant are the fibrous proteins responsible for the bulk, density, and tensile properties of the dermis. Collagen fibers synthesized by fibroblasts are found in the dermis and are of the type I and III variety in a 5:1 ratio. Each collagen fiber is composed of hundreds of finer fibrils. A fibril consists of many triple-helical spiraled collagen molecules. At rest, the collagen fibers are convoluted and relaxed. Upon stretching these fibers straighten, eventually becoming parallel if enough force is applied.

Elastin fibers, also produced by fibroblasts, are finer than collagen and contain two components: microfibril bundles and a dense elastin matrix. These fibers also differ from collagen in that they contain end-to-side junctions and restore the skin and its deformed collagen to its relaxed position. These fibers are responsible for the naturally occurring resting skin tension.

The nonfibrous molecules of the dermis, known as the amorphous ground substance, provide an easy milieu for cell migration and integration while also influencing protein and collagen polymerization as well as the osmotic properties of the dermis. Synthesized by fibroblasts, the mucopolysaccharide ground substance contains hyaluronic acid, dermatan

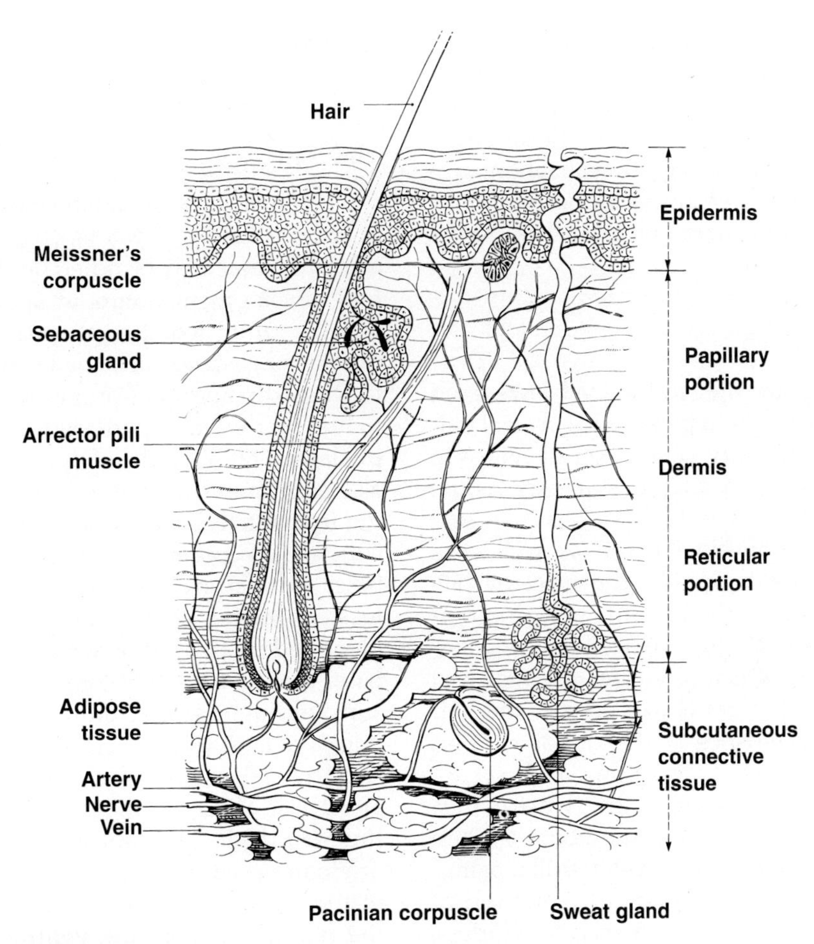

FIG 10–1.
Cross section of human skin including subdermal plexus.

sulfate, as well as chondroitin sulfate. These nonfibrous molecules may also undergo phagocytosis by macrophages.

A rich vascular supply separates the thicker reticular dermis from the overlying papillary dermis. This plexus regulates body temperature and can affect integument viability if significant vasoconstriction occurs. The dermis also contains nervous tissue as well as a high concentration of lymphatic channels that produce lymphedema upon obstruction. The epidermal appendages terminate in the reticular dermis.

The fibrous components of the dermis are the principal determinants of a variety of viscoelastic properties such as stress relaxation and skin creep. Skin creep is particularly important and is exhibited when a constant stretching force is applied to produce skin extension. As dermal fibers undergo alignment, tissue fluid and dermal ground substances are progressively displaced and produce skin extension. Naturally, the greater the prestretch dermal fluid composition, the greater the degree of skin creep. If greater forces are applied, skin blanching occurs secondary to compression of the dermal plexus. If still greater tension is applied, dermal rupture occurs with subsequent striae formation, which may occur during pregnancy, body building, or rapid growth.

The resting state of tension of the elastin fibers is diminished with advancing age. Skin tension varies with anatomic location and is particularly high in all directions at the shoulder and sternum. As a result, hypertrophic scarring or wound stretching is more prevalent at such sites. The skin appendages located within the dermis are the end product of epidermal invasion of the dermis during the third month of fetal life. In addition to their other functions, these structures are vital to the reepithelialization process that occurs after partial-thickness injury such as abrasion, burn, or partial-thickness skin graft harvest.

Skin Appendages

The hair of the scalp, eyebrows, and eyelashes represents a persistence of fetal hair or lanugo. At puberty, coarse hair develops in the axillary and pubic regions, as well as the male facies. The hair follicle sheath is surrounded by connective tissue as well as a bundle of smooth muscle, the arrector pili. Upon contraction, the arrector pili promotes hair orientation changes as well as the secretion of sebum, which lubricates the hair and skin surface. Skin grafts will possess the hair growth characteristics of the donor site, including hair follicle orientation.

Eccrine glands such as the sweat glands may be found throughout the body. Certain anatomic sites such as the eyelid, axilla, palms, and feet have an increased concentration of these tubular glands, which secrete odorless, hypotonic fluid. These glands are thought to represent a phylogenetically older group of glands and respond to emotional stimuli. The phylogenetically younger sweat glands found throughout the remainder of the body are predominantly thermoregulatory in nature. At puberty, apocrine sweat glands begin to function and secrete an odorous fluid that results from bacterial decomposition.

Sebaceous glands are holocrine glands that are appendages of hair follicles and drain into the pilosebaceous canal. These glands are found in increased size and concentration at the forehead, nose, and cheek and reach concentrations of 400 to 900 glands per square centimeter of skin surface. The normal concentration of sebaceous glands is approximately 100/cm^2. The gland lobules fill with fat granules that eventually disintegrate and produce sebum. Secreted sebum lubricates hair and skin alike; it reduces friction and allows the skin to be impervious to moisture. Sebum secretion is not mediated by the central nervous system.

The Nail

The first stage of nail development occurs at approximately 10 weeks of gestation when a dorsal plume may be noted on the fetus. Nail fold development occurs at approximately 3 months and actual nail production at 4 months of gestation. The nail serves to protect the fingertip inasmuch as it is closely adherent to the underlying periosteum of the distal phalanx. This specialized epidermal structure also contributes to tactile sensation, thus aiding in manual dexterity. The eponychium, or cuticle, is an epidermal shelf located at the nail base. The paronychium is the region of skin located lateral to the nail. The lunula is identified as the white semicircle at the nail base. Together, the nail complex, nail bed, and surrounding paronychium are termed the perionychium (Fig 10–2).

The nail originates in the germinal matrix at the base of the nail fold and grows out along the nail bed. The dorsal nail component originates predominantly from the dorsal roof of the nail fold. The intermediate portion of the nail arises from the ventral floor of the fold. Finally, the ventral nail layer arises from the nail bed itself. The nail is composed of onychin, which is similar in nature to keratin and is highly resistant to infection. The arterial supply emanates from branches of the volar digital artery, which forms sinuses beneath the nail bed and regulates flow to the region. Venous drainage is located dorsally and proximal to the nail fold. The nerve supply arises from dorsal branches of the digital nerve. Nail growth occurs at approximately 0.1 mm/day, and complete nail turnover ranges from 70 to 160 days.

THERMAL INJURY

The integument tolerates heat up to 40°C for relatively long periods of time. Above 40°C, tissue destruction occurs in logarithmic fashion, depending upon actual temperature and duration (Fig 10–3). Heat injury occurs via two

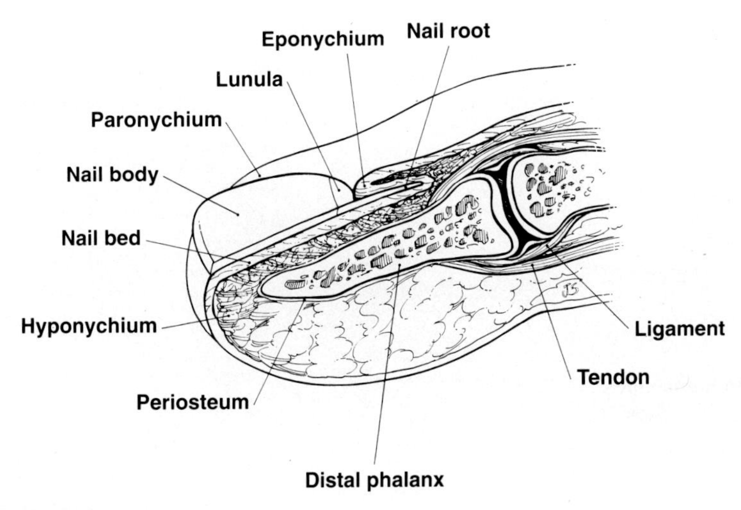

FIG 10–2.
Saggital view of distal fingertip including nail and nail bed.

pathways: direct cellular injury occurs when cell temperature rises above 45°C and protein denaturation exceeds cell repair capacity; a delayed pattern of cellular injury results from dermal ischemia.

Thermal injury of the integument features three concentric zones of injury (Fig 10–4). The central area, or zone of coagulation, includes nonviable coagulated tissue and is surrounded by the zone of stasis, which features injured but potentially viable cells. Survival in the zone of stasis is adversely affected by the progression of dermal ischemia or local infection. The peripherally located zone of hyperemia features hyperemic tissue with minimal injury. This zone will recover within 7 to 10 days unless an additional insult occurs.

The cellular response to thermal injury features the redistribution of intracellular fluid to the nucleus followed by membrane rupture and pyknosis. The cytoplasm becomes progressively granular and progresses to coagulation. Finally, protein denaturation pro-

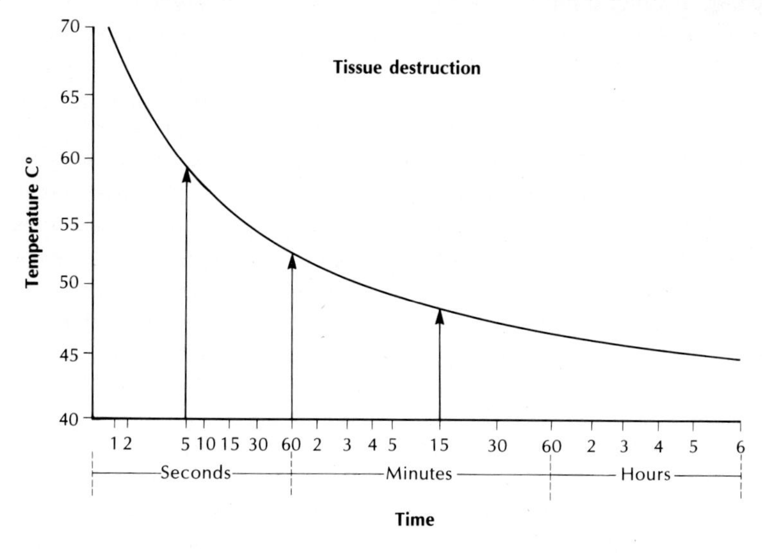

FIG 10–3.
Tissue destruction as a function of time and temperature. (From Robson MC, Krizek TJ, Wray RC: Care of the thermally injured patient. In Zuidema GD, Rutherford RB, Ballinger A (eds): *Management of Trauma.* Philadelphia, WB Saunders, 1979. Used by permission.)

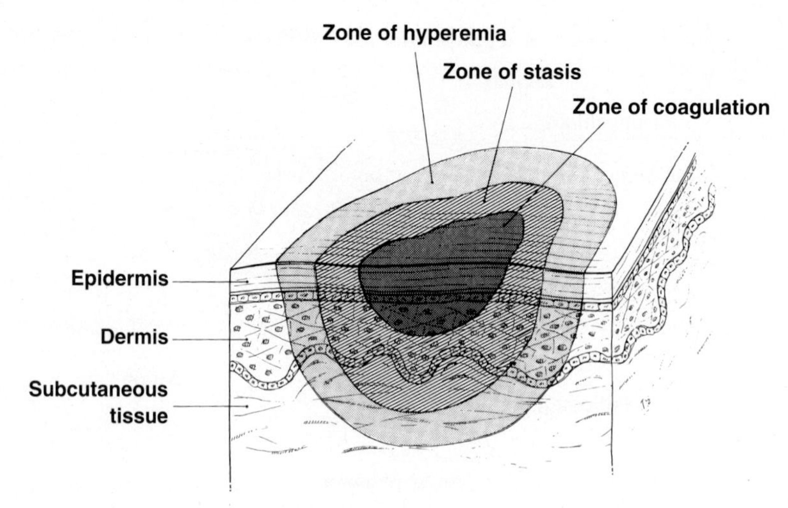

FIG 10–4.
Diagrammatic representation of concentric zones of injury in a burn wound, showing areas of decreasing damage more peripherally.

gressively reduces enzyme activity until a 50% reduction has occurred, which results in cell death.

Progressive dermal ischemia may convert an area of stasis to a zone of devitalized tissue following thermal injury. Physical factors implicated in the creation of secondary injury in the zone of stasis include pressure, desiccation, and infection. Such circumstances may be avoided by adequate hydration, wound coverage with skin or skin substitutes, and appropriate topical antimicrobials.

Inflammatory mediators have also been implicated in the progression of dermal ischemia and the expansion of the zone of coagulation following thermal injury. Prostaglandins have been isolated from lymph tissue draining a burn wound, and thromboxane has been isolated from burn bullae. Thromboxane is a potent platelet aggregator and vasoconstrictor. Indeed, progressive dermal ischemia has been prevented by thromboxane synthetase inhibition by such agents as imidazole, dipyridamole, and methimazole in experimental animals. Other inflammatory mediators that potentiate progressive dermal ischemia include leukotriene B_4, which stimulates leukocyte adherence and thromboxane release, as well oxygen free radicals.

The physical characteristics of the integument in response to thermal injury include painful, erythematous tissue for first-degree burns and erythema and bullae in partial-thickness injuries or second-degree burns. Insensate skin resembling parchment is noted in full-thickness or third-degree burns. A so-called fourth-degree burn features thermally injured tissue extending into the subcutaneous tissue, fascia, or bone.

COLD INJURY

Frostbite may encompass four phases of tissue pathology. A freeze phase features tissue cooling without crystal formation. Transendothelial plasma leakage and vasospasm occur. Ice crystals appear in the freeze-thaw phase. The vascular stasis phase produces vasodilation, plasma leakage, and spasticity and eventually progresses to stasis, coagulation, and shunting. A late ischemic phase features thrombosis, gangrene, and autonomic dysfunction.

At the cellular level, dehydration and cell shrinkage occur along with intracellular ice formation. Intracellular electrolyte concentrations also run awry, followed by lipid-protein complex denaturation. Although a skin injury may be reversible, progression often results secondary to microvascular changes.

Factors affecting the extent of cold injury

to the skin include duration of exposure, level of humidity, wind chill, history of previous cold injury, smoking, peripheral vascular disease, and immobility. Late sequelae of frostbite include pain, paresthesias, cold sensation, depigmentation, as well as joint stiffness and nail growth abnormalities. These patients often exhibit hyperhidrosis secondary to an abnormal sympathetic nervous system.

MEDIATORS OF SKIN INJURY

Actinic damage caused by UV light, be it local and direct or indirect and systemic, is universally recognized as a risk factor for skin cancer. Protection from skin cancer would appear to be facilitated by a high melanocyte content of the skin. The incidence of skin cancer is high among those of Celtic ancestry as well as other fair-skinned populations.

The UV light band rests in the middle of the electromagnetic spectrum and contains three varieties. The ozone layer absorbs all UVC light (1 to 290 nm) and the majority of UVB light (290 to 315 nm). Although 95% of the solar light passing through the ozone layer is UVA light (315 to 400 nm), it is the UVB light that produces acute and chronic sun damage. UVA light, however, can exacerbate an already damaged integument. The integument may be protected by a variety of sunscreens such as zinc oxide, a reflector of all UV light, and para-aminobenzoic acid (PABA), which absorbs the UV light.

Since its discovery in 1895 by Roentgen, x-rays have been used in diagnostic and therapeutic modalities. The effects of radiation therapy are secondary to ionizing radiation in the form of α-, β-, or γ-rays and are expressed as rads of energy.

Acute radiation injury to the skin produces dry, painful, erythematous skin, often resembling a thermal injury. Swelling and pruritus are frequent. With progression of injury, ulceration, sloughing, and frank necrosis may occur secondary to obliterative endarteritis. Subacute injury is manifested by woody, indurated skin. Histologic changes include the loss of rete pegs, fragmentation of elastic fibers, hyperpigmentation, and dermal fibrosis. Chronic radiation histologic changes resemble those of acute and subacute injury.

SKIN INFECTION

The development of skin and subcutaneous infections represents an alteration in the homeostatic balance that exists between pathogens and host-defense mechanisms. Pathogen delivery to the skin may occur via direct inoculation, extension of a local infectious process, or hematogenous dissemination. The severity of the infectious process will be dependent upon the quantity and virulence of the pathogen, as well as the successful delivery and effectiveness of various local and systemic mediators of the host's defense response.

Cellulitis is a nonsuppurative inflammatory process of the skin and subcutaneous tissue that extends along connective tissue planes. Cellulitis is classically caused by hemolytic *Streptococcus* infection and results in erythema, swelling, and tenderness of the integument. Treatment consists of bed rest, elevation, and intravenous antibiotics.

Lymphangitis is characterized by an inflammatory process involving the lymphatic channels and features erythematous streaks along the integument. This process, typically caused by hemolytic streptococci, is also treated with bed rest, limb elevation, and intravenous antibiotics. Erysipelas caused by *Streptococcus pyogenes* produces a butterfly pattern rash on the malar region of the face. Characteristic findings also include fever, chills, and prostration. Treatment consists of bed rest, intravenous antibiotics, and close monitoring.

A furuncle, or "boil," is an abscess of the sweat gland or hair follicle that may or may not produce surrounding cellulitis. Treatment consists of incision and drainage, as well as supplementation with antibiotics sensitive to *Staphylococcus*.

Furunculitis may extend into the subcutaneous tissue and produce a multiloculated suppurative process known as carbunculosis.

Often located on the neck or back, such collections should be treated by incision and drainage as well as antibiotic coverage.

CHEMICAL INJURY

Chemical injuries to the integument tend to occur at exposed body sites in addition to body parts that handle such substances such as the hand. The degree of injury observed depends on chemical toxicity, concentration, volume, and duration of integument exposure. Local toxicity will continue until the substance is washed away, neutralized, or exhausted by tissue reaction. Systemic toxicity such as hypercalcemia may occur with chemicals like oxalic and hydrofluoric acid and phosphorus. Initial treatment generally consists of copious water irrigation.

Acid burns are painful and produce erythematous changes as well as an eschar characteristic of deeper injury. Initial therapy consists of copious water irrigation. Following initial treatment, wound management consists of debridement and skin grafting for full-thickness injuries. Hydrofluoric acid contains elemental fluorine and is used in the production of plastics, pottery, and rust removers. Direct cell injury occurs secondary to an increased hydrogen ion concentration, which alters barrier mechanisms. Soluble fluoride ions may produce subcutaneous liquefaction and bone decalcification. Treatment consists of water irrigation and the application of calcium gluconate via topical, local injection or intra-arterial methods.

Alkalis are the most common home chemicals and are frequently used in drain and oven cleaners. In the early stages, these solutions produce less damage than acids do. Their late effects, however, are more serious because of fat liquefaction and cell death, followed by cellular alkali release with progressive tissue penetration and destruction. Irrigation is therefore required for a prolonged period of time followed by occlusive dressings and topical mafenide (Sulfamylon). Cement burns are particularly caustic, with pH values ranging up to 12, and produce symptoms up to several hours following exposure. Treatment again consists of early excision and grafting for full-thickness injuries.

Phosphorus injuries occur most frequently in military personnel, fire fighters, and those handling insecticides. These particles undergo an oxidative, exothermic reaction with 1% copper sulfate solution that produces a precipitate and facilitates phosphorus removal. Copper toxicity may be avoided by copious irrigation.

Injection injuries frequently follow infiltration of an intravenous medication and typically occur in the hands and limbs. The subsequent inflammatory reaction depends on the solution toxicity, concentration, and volume. Osmotically active agents such as Ca^{+2} and K^{+} disrupt cell transport and produce cellular imbibition and death. Other solutions such as TPN or Renograffin 60 produce intracellular dehydration and death. Catecholamines and pressors such as epinephrine, norepinephrine, and dopamine produce ischemic necrosis. Treatment consists of excision and grafting where necessary.

Direct cellular toxicity occurs upon infiltration of antineoplastic drugs, the most common of which is doxorubicin (Adriamycin). Adriamycin combines with DNA and inhibits nucleic acid synthesis. Following cell death, the chemotherapeutic agent is picked up by viable cells, and the cycle is repeated. A "recall phenomenon" has been reported whereby the extent of the tissue destruction at a site of infiltration injury is enhanced by the resumption of Adriamycin administration. The morbidity of vesicant infiltration is determined by location, concentration, volume, and toxicity of a given agent. The development of epidermal blisters in such cases is indicative of full-thickness loss, unlike a thermal injury.

The treatment of chemotherapeutic infiltration injury includes removal of the intravenous line, elevation, and cold pack application to produce vasoconstriction, thereby localizing the toxic material. In contrast, the vinca alkaloids increase their toxic effects upon cold pack application. In such cases, warm pack application will produce beneficial vasodilation and increase agent absorption, especially if hyaluronidase (Wydase) has been utilized. Specific antidotes utilized include hyaluronidase, which can increase the diffusion rate of an irritant solution such as 10% dextrose in water ($D_{10}W$), Ca^{+2}, K^{+}, aminophylline, as well as radiocontrast material. Phentolamine (Regitine), an α-blocker, may aid in the treatment of vasoconstrictor infiltration. The use of dimethyl sulfoxide (DMSO) and corticosteroids in the management of infiltration injuries is controversial.

SUGGESTED READING

Jackson DM: The diagnosis of the depth of burning. *Br J Surg* 1953; 40:388.

Larsen DL: Treatment of tissue extravasation by antitumor agents. *Cancer* 1982; 49:1796.

McCarthy JG: *Plastic Surgery.* Philadelphia, WB Saunder, 1990, pp 207–224, 851–857, 5435–5443.

Odland GF: Structure of skin, in Goldsmith LA (ed): *Biochemistry and Physiology of Skin.* New York, Oxford University Press, 1983.

Robson MC, Krizek TJ, Wray RC: Care of the thermally injured patient. In Zuidema GD, Rutherford RB, Ballinger A, (eds): *Management of Trauma.* Philadelphia, WB Saunders, 1979.

Zook EG, et al: Anatomy and physiology of the perionychium. *J Hand Surg* 1980; 5:528.

Chapter 11

Benign and Malignant Skin Lesions

Frank R. Rogers, M.D.
Robert Hardesty, M.D.

CONTENTS

CHAPTER OBJECTIVE

At the end of this chapter the resident has a thorough understanding of benign and malignant skin lesions, recognizes the morphologic and histologic features of the more common lesions, and effectively manages small and large skin tumors by using a variety of treatment modalities.

LEARNER OBJECTIVES

On completion of this chapter the resident

1. **Is familiar with the clinical presentation of benign and malignant cutaneous lesions and generalized skin disorders.**
2. **Understands the natural history of both treated and untreated benign and malignant cutaneous lesions and generalized skin disorders.**
3. **Fully comprehends histologic grading and clinical staging systems currently in use for malignant and premalignant skin tumors.**
4. **Is able to provisionally evaluate both simple and complex cutaneous lesions and proceed with diagnostic steps necessary to secure a definitive diagnosis.**
5. **Formulates a definitive treatment plan for the particular lesion in question by choosing a surgical or nonsurgical treatment modality that best suits the lesion (based on size, anatomic location, and physical condition of the patient).**
6. **Is familiar with other treatment modalities including (but not limited to)**

x-ray therapy, Mohs' micrographic surgery, cryotherapy, laser therapy, and topical chemotherapy.

7. **Is able to explain in a comprehensible but simplified manner to the patient the nature of the lesion, its extent, treatment options, and long-term results.**
8. **Can formulate a definitive treatment plan for regional or distant spread of malignant cutaneous tumors.**
9. Is familiar with the histologic characteristics of benign and malignant cutaneous lesions.

CLINICAL PRACTICE ACTIVITIES

During the course of the training program, the resident

1. **Evaluates a variety of cutaneous lesions and recommends an approach to therapy based on the lesion's size, clinical characteristics, and location.**
2. **Performs all invasive diagnostic studies including (but not limited to) direct incisional and excisional biopsy, needle biopsy, and punch biopsy; recognizes under which circumstances each should be used.**
3. **Executes extirpative surgery of a variety of benign and malignant cutaneous lesions and associated locoregional disease by choosing the optimal surgical incision or excision for the particular region to be treated.**
4. **Executes complex procedures for the reconstruction of surgically created wounds (including skin grafts, local or distant flaps, or free tissue transfer) resulting from skin tumor extirpation.**
5. Prescribes pharmacologic agents for the care of cutaneous lesions not deemed appropriate for surgical extirpation.

TUMORS ARISING PRIMARILY IN THE EPIDERMIS

Benign, Premalignant, and In-Situ Malignancies of the Epidermis

- Seborrheic keratosis
- Verruca vulgaris
- Actinic keratosis
- Cutaneous horn
- Leukoplakia/erythroplakia
- Keratoacanthoma
- Bowen's disease
- Extramammary Paget's disease

Seborrheic keratosis (also known as verruca senilis and pigmented papilloma) arises from the basal cell layer of the epidermis and consists of layers of well-differentiated basal cells interspersed with many cystic inclusions or "horn cysts" of keratinous material. The lesions typically exhibit hyperkeratosis, acanthosis, and papillomatosis. They contain melanocytes and may show mononuclear inflammatory infiltration.

Seborrheic keratoses are commonly seen on the head, neck, and trunk of persons in later life. Frequently multiple, they are sharply demarcated and classically have a "stuck-on" appearance. The surface is soft, verrucoid, and occasionally pedunculated and is said to have a "greasy" feel. The lesions range from a few millimeters up to about 5 cm.

Seborrheic keratoses require no specific treatment, but patients may request removal for aesthetic reasons. This can be accomplished by the "shave" technique or cryotherapy. Pigmented or inflamed lesions, especially solitary lesions, may be mistaken for pigmented basal cell carcinoma or melanoma and therefore require excisional biopsy for diagnosis.

Verruca vulgaris (the common "papillary wart") is probably a reactive lesion associated with the human papillomavirus rather than a true neoplasm. Clinically, these occur as single small lesions or clusters of lesions on the upper extremity and occasionally on the face, most commonly in children or adolescents. They exhibit a rough surface surmounted by friable keratotic material. Although the lesions may persist for several months, they are generally self-limiting and spontaneously regress. Histologically verruca vulgaris is characterized by hyperkeratosis and parakeratosis and arises from the stratum granulosum of the epidermis. The involved cells typically have basophilic inclusion bodies thought to be of viral origin, and an inflammatory cell infiltrate is typical.

Topical treatment (cryotherapy or chemical application) is often effective; excision is rarely necessary and is usually reserved for troublesome or recurrent lesions. The patient should be forewarned that verrucae may promptly recur along the lines of the excision. Other verrucoid skin lesions closely associated with human papillomavirus include plantar warts and condyloma acuminata, or "anogenital warts."

Actinic keratosis (also known as solar keratosis and senile keratosis) occurs almost exclusively on sun-exposed skin. Typical lesions are multiple and usually small (1 cm). They are manifested as minimally elevated, erythematous, and hyperkeratotic or "scaly" patches.

Histologically this very common precursor of squamous carcinoma is characterized by dyskeratosis and has varying degrees of atypia in the basal layer of the epidermis and the adjacent stratum corneum. The squamous cells may show hyperchromasia, nuclear pleomorphism, and increased mitosis. Hyperkeratosis and subepidermal inflammation are typical. However, the lesions are not invasive, and the dermal-epidermal junction remains distinct. Actinic keratosis may progress to squamous carcinoma. It is estimated that invasive squamous carcinoma of the skin will develop in 20% of patients with these lesions at some point.

The presence of multiple actinic keratoses suggests a field change in the areas of sun-damaged skin and indicates the need for increased surveillance and prompt biopsy of any suggestive lesions to ensure early diagnosis of invasive malignancy. Actinic keratosis is well managed by surface treatment, including electrodesiccation and curettage, cryotherapy, and topical 5-fluorouracil. Surgical excision with pathologic examination is appropriate in cases where the diagnosis is unclear.

The *cutaneous "horn"* is an unusual hyperkeratotic lesion, generally well circumscribed and conical in shape. It consists of built-up cornified material and, by definition, exceeds in height its own radius. The histologic picture at the base of the lesion is usually that of an actinic keratosis, but invasive squamous carcinoma may also occur. Management is by local excision with careful histologic evaluation of the base.

Leukoplakia is a mucosal lesion consisting of a white plaque on stratified squamous epithelium that cannot be removed. Clinically the lesions most typically arise on oral mucosa and are associated with chronic irritation, sometimes mechanical, but most often caused by tobacco and alcohol. Lesions in similar form can occur on the mucosal surfaces of the genitalia. Microscopically the lesions appear as a benign thickening of the stratum corneum characterized by hyperkeratosis, parakeratosis, and chronic inflammation. About 20% of the lesions will show varying degrees of atypia. Leukoplakia is usually reversible with removal of the offending irritants, which is the treatment of choice. However, the ultimate development of invasive squamous carcinoma in 7% to 17% of cases suggests that excision or (in the case of larger areas) incisional biopsy is indicated for diagnosing a persisting area of leukoplakia. A less common but more often malignant lesion is *erythroplakia.* The mucosal surface is red because of the loss of normal surface orthokeratin. The etiology, histology, and treatment are comparable to that for leukoplakia.

Keratoacanthoma occurs typically as a solitary lesion on the head and neck or other sun-exposed areas of hair-bearing skin in older individuals. The lesion begins as a firm dome-shaped nodule and grows to a size of 1 to 3 cm within a period of 6 to 8 weeks. Mature lesions are characterized by a raised nodule with a prominent "horn-filled" central depression. The natural history is then one of spontaneous resolution over a period of up to 6 months, with a small residual cutaneous scar left. Histologically the mature lesion demonstrates a large central crater filled with keratin and surrounded by thickened epidermis that extends over the lip and sides of the crater. At a deeper level the lesion demonstrates a hyperplastic epidermis, frequently with some cellular atypia and increased mitosis. The base of the lesion exhibits a dense inflammatory infiltrate and becomes well demarcated, extending no further than the sweat gland appendages of the dermis. The lesion may be difficult to differentiate from invasive squamous cell carcinoma. Although the lesions are self-limiting, in some areas a rapid proliferation may be locally destructive and indicate removal, particularly on the face. Failure of the tumor to follow a typical course or to resolve completely and promptly or any recurrence of the lesion demands clinical management appropriate for squamous carcinoma.

Bowen's disease is a form of in situ or intraepidermal squamous cell carcinoma. Microscopically, the epidermis is thickened, and the squamous cells exhibit malignant characteristics, but the dermal-epidermal border remains distinctly intact. Clinically Bowen's disease manifests itself as a slowly enlarging, irregular, but well-demarcated erythematous patch with scaling and crusting. The lesion occurs anywhere on the body surface but is most common on the trunk and extremities. Erythroplasia of Queyrat is a histologically identical lesion occurring on the glans penis of uncircumcised men. In many patients, the lesions remain as slowly progressive in situ lesions for years. The development of invasive squamous cell carcinoma in Bowen's disease has been estimated to occur in 3% to 11% of cases. Much has been made of an association of Bowen's disease with other visceral neoplasms, but recent studies have not confirmed this association. Bowen's disease is most appropriately managed surgically by excision and direct closure or resurfacing, generally skin grafting.

Extramammary Paget's disease is a form of intraepidermal adenocarcinoma. The characteristic Paget's cell is probably of epidermal glandular origin and is the same as that encountered in mammary Paget's disease. Because these cells have some characteristics in common with malignant melanocytes, differentiation from superficial spreading melanoma must be made. Clinically this disease appears as a pruritic, crusting, slowly enlarging reddish patch with a sharp but irregular border. It may occur secondarily as an extension of an adjacent adenocarcinoma of genital or anal origin or independently in previously normal skin, most commonly in areas of apocrine gland concentration such as the axilla and genital areas. Management is similar to that for Bowen's disease. Twenty percent of cases demonstrate invasive malignancy at excision.

Epidermal Cysts

- Epidermal inclusion cysts
- Trichilemmal cysts
- Congenital dermoid cysts
- Synovial cysts
- Milia

One of the most common benign lesions is the *epidermal inclusion cyst* (commonly but incorrectly termed "sebaceous" cyst). An epidermal inclusion cyst is lined with true stratified squamous epithelium that is filled with keratin debris. Fibrosis, foreign-body reaction, and giant cells are present in cysts that are inflamed or ruptured. Epidermal inclusion cysts may arise spontaneously from the infundibulum of hair follicles or from traumatic implantation of viable epithelium. The clinical history is that of a well-circumscribed, elevated, round firm lesion 1 to 5 cm in size that is slow growing and either intraepidermal or subcutaneous in location. Treatment is excision or local enucleation. When infected, the lesion may first require incision and drainage, followed by delayed excision to remove remnants of the cyst wall and avoid recurrence.

Trichilemmal cysts (also known as pilar cysts or pilosebaceous cysts) exhibit similar histology to epidermal inclusion cysts except that the lining cells show characteristics of hair follicle epithelial differentiation. A related proliferative lesion with solid elements predominating is referred to as a *trichilemmoma.* Trichilemmal cysts have a clinical presentation similar to the epidermal inclusion cyst and differ only in frequency and distribution. Ninety percent occur in the scalp, and the lesions are multiple in 70% of cases. Treatment is also similar.

The *dermoid cyst* is distinguished histologically from an inclusion cyst by its lining, which contains all types of epidermal skin appendages, at least in vestigial form. Closely resembling the epidermal inclusion cyst or pilar cyst clinically, the dermoid cyst is congenital in nature and is noticed at birth or in early childhood. The lesions are most often in the supraorbital ridge or lateral brow area. Treatment is by simple enucleation or excision. Care must be taken with lesions that occur on or near the midline since these may actually be more complex congenital rostral neural tube defects that have sinuses or other connections to the central nervous system or dura.

Synovial cysts (also known as mucoid cysts) are degenerative cysts bearing similarities to the so-called "ganglion" of joints and tendon sheaths. They demonstrate a lining of compressed fibrocytes rather than a true epithelium and are filled with clear mucinous fluid, presumably of joint origin. Clinically the most typical synovial cysts occur over the dorsum of the distal interphalangeal joints proximal to the nail fold and are usually associated with underlying degenerative joint abnormality. Although they actually arise from deeper tissues, these lesions may thin the overlying dermis and present at the skin surface. They may also rupture and become infected or distort nail growth. Surgical treatment involves local excision with preservation of the eponychium and the dermal matrix of the nail. Debridement of the underlying joint is necessary to prevent recurrence. Rarely, skin grafting or coverage procedures are necessary.

Milia are tiny retention cysts resulting from epithelial proliferation in response to injury and, in most cases, arise from adjacent eccrine ducts. They appear clinically as small (1 mm or less), numerous, firm, white-yellow round lesions in areas of dermal healing, frequently following burns, skin grafting, and particularly, dermabrasion or chemical peeling. A primary form occurring without injury also exists. Treatment is nonsurgical and generally consists of unroofing the lesions with mildly abrasive wound management.

Malignant Epidermal Neoplasms

Basal Cell Carcinoma

Pathology. The malignant basal cell is an ovoid cell with a large oval nucleus and a small amount of spineless cytoplasm. The cells are uniform and occur in closely packed nests lacking intercellular bridges. Mitoses are common. The nests of basal cells are typically rimmed by a single vertically oriented cell layer. This feature is called "palisading" and is a dominant characteristic. The majority of basal cell carcinomas contain identifiable melanocytes and melanin. Many also exhibit keratin production. Typically, basal cell carcinoma arises in the basal layer of the epidermis or in the deeper portions of subadjacent hair follicles. An important variant of basal cell carcinoma termed "sclerosing" or "morpheaform" basal cell carcinoma is characterized by increased connective tissue components in a dense hyalinized stroma showing marked desmoplasia or fibrosis. Some investigators believe this tumor variant to be more biologically aggressive.

The classic basal cell carcinoma is an elevated nodule with "pearly" translucent edges and a central depression with telangiectasis. Later appear central ulceration and a rolled edge characteristic of subepidermal spread—the typical "rodent ulcer." In addition to this noduloulcerative type, other morphologic variants including a superficial type and the morpheaform or sclerosing type are recognized grossly. The former occurs in flat, scaly, erythematous patches with superficial crusting rather than ulceration and has a "thread-like" border. Lesions with these characteristics are noted predominantly on the trunk. The morpheaform type appears as a white or yellowish indurated plaque with only slight elevation; it rarely ulcerates. These lesions are said to be "scar-like."

Biological Behavior. Basal cell carcinoma typically exhibits slow but relentless locally erosive growth. True metastasis of basal cell carcinoma is exceedingly rare.

Basal cell carcinoma occurs almost exclusively on hair-bearing skin and probably does not arise in mucous membrane. In the United States, up to 85% of the lesions occur in the head and neck areas, but overall, up to a third of basal cell carcinomas occur on non–sun-exposed body surfaces, most commonly in older Caucasian persons. Basal cell carcinoma is rare in blacks and Asians. Exposure to ultraviolet light has been epidemiologically shown to be one predisposing factor in the development of basal cell carcinoma. Other environmental factors include ionizing radiation and exposure to arsenic and chronic chemical exposure, particularly to aromatic hydrocarbons. Basal cell carcinoma has also been associated with chronic wounds and with immunosuppression. It is also strongly associated with several specific genetic syndromes and inherited cutaneous dysplasias. Although basal cell carcinoma most frequently arises de novo in previously normal skin, specific premalignant lesions include the nevus sebaceus of Jadassohn (discussed later) and localized types of porokeratosis.

Patient Evaluation and Treatment. Excisional techniques for basal cell carcinoma include cold knife excision, usually with rapid frozen section control of the margins, and Mohs' micrographic technique. In primary lesions, the 5-year control rates for basal cell carcinoma treated with both techniques exceed 90%. Because of the virtual absence of metastasis of basal cell carcinoma, local control becomes synonymous with cure. The subclinical spread of basal cell carcinoma beyond the visible borders of smaller primary lesions rarely exceeds one tumor radius. For these lesions, a 3- to 5-mm margin generally results in greater than 90% local control. In larger or more aggressive lesions and in recurrent tumors, the margin must be increased in size, and careful histopathologic study of the margin becomes more important. Mohs' technique (see the section on treatment techniques at the end of the chapter) probably offers the most rigorous form of intraoperative margin assessment.

In very large and invasive tumors, samples for frozen section must be taken from the deepest areas of invasion, particularly at points of expected spread along tissue planes, *e.g.*, along major peripheral nerve trunks.

Studies have documented a 67% clinical recurrence of basal cell carcinoma when the postexcisional surgical margin is found to be grossly involved with the tumor. Other reviews have indicated a 33% local recurrence rate when the margins were described as "close" or "microscopically involved." Sixty percent of the postexcisional recurrences were evident at 2 years. In most cases, prompt reexcision of such lesions with more adequate margins is indicated rather than observation.

Squamous Cell Carcinoma

Pathology. *Squamous cell carcinoma* arises from the keratinocytes of the epidermis. Microscopically, irregular nests of malignant epidermal cells infiltrate downward into the dermis and beyond. These cells vary from near-normal keratin-producing cells to highly anaplastic spindle shapes. Most tumors show variable amounts of inflammation in the dermis, and well-differentiated "nests" of tumor cells with central keratin production ("keratin pearls") are seen. Squamous cell carcinoma can be histologically graded in a four-step system that has a rough correlation to its overall biological behavior and prognosis. The essential features in grading are the degree of keratinization in individual cells, the number of pleomorphic or spindle cells in the tumor, and the number of mitotic figures.

Squamous cell carcinoma most often begins in sun-damaged skin or in a preexisting actinic keratosis. The lesions characteristically crust and then ulcerate. A few squamous carcinomas arising in skin are exophytic. Squamous cell cancers arising in long-standing chronic wounds are usually heralded by an increase in activity or thickness of the wound margin and are accompanied by increased pain or drainage.

Biological Behavior. Squamous cell carcinoma arising in skin occurs almost exclusively in areas exposed to ultraviolet light. Other causative factors closely related to squamous carcinoma include radiation injury and chemical carcinogens such as aromatic hydrocarbons, coal tar, and arsenic. Squamous cell carcinoma has been observed to occur with increased incidence in patients who are medically immunosuppressed and also those receiving antineoplastic drugs for other tumors. Potential patients may be genetically predisposed to squamous cell carcinoma by inheriting racial characteristics such as light skin or inheriting specific disease states such as xeroderma pigmentosum, the latter condition involving an enzymatic defect that causes faulty DNA repair after ultraviolet injury to the skin (see Chapter 13).

Squamous cell carcinoma has long been associated with chronic wounds. Classic Marjolin's ulcer involves tumor development in a nonhealing ungrafted burn wound after a very long lag time (up to three decades). Squamous carcinoma has been reported in other chronic wounds including pressure sores, chronic fistulas, osteomyelitis, and hidradenitis suppurativa. It has been reported that squamous cell carcinoma developing in such chronic wounds is biologically more aggressive and exhibits more anaplasia, metastasis, and a higher mortality rate.

Basal cell carcinoma is about four times more common than squamous cell carcinoma. However, squamous carcinoma is biologically diverse and exhibits a more variable clinical course. Aggressive tumors may cause death by local invasion, hemorrhage, invasion of the central nervous system, or distant metastatic spread. The incidence of metastatic disease in squamous carcinoma of the skin overall is about 2%, while the incidence of local recurrence following treatment is about 20%. Certain tumor characteristics correlate with both increased local recurrence and metastatic disease. These include increasing tumor size, higher tumor grade, greater depth of invasion, and the microscopic characteristic of perineural invasion. Squamous cell carcinoma typically spreads first to regional lymph nodes. Nodal spread diminishes the outlook for survival despite treatment. Systemic metastasis primarily involves lung, bone, and more rarely, other viscera. Involvement of the central nervous system may occur by direct extension or by metastasis.

Patient Evaluation and Treatment. Squamous cell carcinoma of the skin is defined by direct physical examination and confirmed by excisional or incisional biopsy. Knowledge and evaluation of the specific regional lymph nodes draining the site of any particular primary lesion are important. Symptoms related to neural involvement by tumor include paresthesia, numbness, paresis, and/or disproportionate local pain. Imaging workup is primarily guided by clinical examination and the patient's symptomatology.

Clinical tumor staging assumes equal importance with histologic grading of the squamous cell carcinoma in evaluation, treatment planning, and prognosis. Current international guidelines to TNM tumor staging of squamous cell carcinoma are listed in Table 11–1.

For invasive squamous cell carcinoma, surgery is the mainstay of treatment; radiation therapy is an adjunct only. For small primary lesions, both excision and Mohs' micrographic surgery are approximately 95% effective for local control. Although the excision margin is not the only factor in determining local recurrence of original spread of squamous carcinoma, it is the most important. Added margin is necessary for local control as the tumor increases in size.

In general, the clinical use of rapid frozen sectioning and margin control is similar to that in basal cell carcinoma. Mohs' micrographic technique, where applicable, offers the same advantages with respect to the evaluation of surgical margins. For management of local recurrent disease, surgical reexcision, however

TABLE 11–1.

Simplified Tumor Staging for Squamous Carcinoma of Skin by the American Joint Committee on Cancer Staging

TNM classification	
T1	≤2 cm
T2	2–5 cm
T3	>5 cm
T4	Invading underlying muscle or bone
M0	No metastatic disease
M1	Distant metastatic disease
N0	No nodal involvement
N1	Regional lymph nodes involved
G1	Low grade
G2	Moderately differentiated
G3	High grade or highly anaplastic
Clinical staging summary	
I	T1, N0, M0
II	T2-3, N0, M0
III	T4, N0, M0 *and* any T, N1, M0
IV	Any T, any N1, M1(+)

extensive and difficult, is preferred. With lymph node involvement, standard radical lymph node dissection techniques are indicated.

TUMORS ARISING FROM EPIDERMAL SKIN APPENDAGES

- Hair follicles
  - Trichofolliculoma
  - Trichoepithelioma
  - Pilomatricoma
  - Trichilemmoma
- Sebaceous glands
  - Sebaceous hyperplasia
  - Nevus sebaceus of Jadassohn
  - Adenoma sebaceum
  - Sebaceoma
  - Sebaceous carcinoma
- Sweat glands
  - Apocrine
  - Hydradenoma/hidrocystoma
- Syringal cystadenoma papilliferum
- Cylindroma
- Eccrine poroma
- Spiradenoma
- Sweat gland adenocarcinoma

A variety of cutaneous neoplasms may arise from the epidermal skin appendages. Skin appendages are of three types: hair follicles, sebaceous glands, and sweat glands (apocrine and eccrine). A number of different classifications and varying theories of histogenesis for skin appendage tumors have been advanced. The nomenclature associated with skin appendage tumors is confusing. In the following section, the histologic appearance and clinical presentation of only a few selected lesions that are more likely to come to the attention of a plastic and reconstructive surgeon will be discussed.

Among tumors of hair follicle origin, the *trichoepithelioma* is a "skin-colored" nodule 2 to 8 mm in size, generally multiple and occurring on the face, particularly on the nasolabial folds, nose, upper lip, and forehead. Rarely, these lesions may be solitary or ulcerated. Histologically the tumor is composed of basaloid cells, masses of which are surrounded by fibroblasts, suggestive of hair follicle differentiation. The other major components of the lesion are "horn" cysts filled with keratinized debris.

The significance of trichoepithelioma is that it is easily confused with basal cell carcinoma, both clinically and microscopically. Management is by simple excision.

Pilomatricoma, also known as "calcifying epithelioma of Malherbe," is a sharply demarcated lesion occurring in the lower dermis and subcutaneous fat. It consists of basaloid cells that sometimes occur in a syncytial mass. Tumor islands of these cells show a gradual transition to "shadow cells," which demonstrate a gradual loss of nuclei and transition to eosinophilic hylanized cytoplasm. Calcification is common, and metaplastic ossification also occurs. These characteristics account for the mobile, but unusually firm character of these lesions, which usually occur on the face and upper extremities. Rarely, the lesions will erode overlying skin and be manifested as a dark red nodule or even extrude in the form of a hematoma. This is a common lesion of children, with 40% of the lesions occurring in children under the age of 10 years. The diagnosis can usually be suspected on clinical grounds but is established by excisional biopsy, which is the only required treatment.

Nevus sebaceus of Jadassohn is a congenital hamartoma of sebaceous gland origin. In childhood, the lesion is seen as a solitary raised, hairless, linear or elongated plaque-like lesion, usually occurring on the scalp or head and neck area. It is brown to yellow in color and "waxy" in surface texture. After puberty, the lesion changes markedly in appearance and becomes verrucous and nodular. During adolescence, the lesion is characterized microscopically by a large number of sebaceous glands with adjacent papillomatous hyperplasia of the epidermis. The lesions contain hypoplastic hair structures as well as ectopic apocrine glands.

Postpuberty, Nevus sebaceus of Jadassohn exhibits a degenerative change to basal cell carcinoma in 5% to 15% of cases. Other skin appendage tumors also occur in significant numbers. Because of this, it is recom-

TABLE 11–2.
Classification of Skin Appendages (Type of Differentiation)*

			Sweat Gland	
Tumor Type	Hair Follicle	Sebaceous	Apocrine	Eccrine
Hyperplasia/ hamartoma		Sebaceous hyperplasia *Nevus sebaceus of Jadassohn*		
Adenoma	Trichofolliculoma	Adenoma sebaceum	Hydradenoma/ hidrocystoma *Syringocystadenoma papilliferum*	
Benign epithelioma	Trichoepithelioma Trichilemmoma Pilomatricoma	Sebaceoma		Poroma Spiradenoma Cylindroma
Carcinoma	Some classify basal cell carcinoma in this group	Sebaceous carcinoma	Sweat gland adenocarcinoma Apocrine, eccrine, and adenoic cystic variants	

* Adapted from Lever WF, Schaumburg-Lever G: *Histopathology of the Skin*, ed 7. Philadelphia, JB Lippincott, 1990. Used by permission.

mended that the lesions be excised during childhood.

Classification of benign tumors of sweat gland origin by apocrine or eccrine differentiation is difficult. Often, benign tumors showing glandular or adenomatous characteristics are lumped together, as are tumors showing ductal (or "syringal") morphologic characteristics. In the former category are eccrine and apocrine *cystadenoma.* These lesions are also referred to as "hydrocystomas" or "hidradenomas." These lesions are seen clinically as solitary, 1- to 3-cm, translucent cystic nodules on the face, sometimes with a blue hue; microscopically they exhibit large cystic spaces in the dermis lined with papillary projections of typical secretory epithelium. Simple excision is adequate.

Benign sweat gland neoplasms of "syringal" (ductal) origin occasionally encountered include *syringal cystadenoma papilliferum.* The clinical presentation and management of this lesion is very similar to that for sweat gland adenomas. The *eccrine poroma,* also known as "papillary syringoma," is seen as a single, raised or pedunculated tumor commonly found on the skin and soles of the feet and palms of the hand and composed of intraepidermal proliferations of cells of eccrine sweat duct origin. Another closely related neoplasm is the eccrine *spiradenoma,* also referred to as "lobular syringoma," which is composed of compact lobulated groups of "lymphocytoid" epithelial cells and appears as a solitary, firm, cutaneous nodule that is distinguished by exquisite tenderness or associated pain.

The *cylindroma,* known as "turban tumor," is a variant of the eccrine spiradenoma and is frequently multiple and involves the scalp. It may be extensive enough to cover the entire scalp.

Sweat gland adenocarcinoma of either the apocrine or eccrine type has varying degrees of differentiation. In general, the tumors are low grade but may metastasize (Table 11–2).

LESIONS ARISING PRIMARILY AT THE DERMAL-EPIDERMAL JUNCTION

Melanocytic Nevi

- Acquired melanocytic nevi and variants
- Congenital melanocytic nevi
- Dermal melanocytic hamartoma
    - Blue nevus
    - "Nevus of Ota"
    - "Nevus of Itoh"

Acquired melanocytic nevi are common, generally pigmented skin lesions present in virtually all Caucasian individuals and, more occasionally, on the less pigmented body surfaces of the darker-skinned races. Nevus cells arise from the epidermal melanocytes of neural crest origin and exhibit variation from round "epithelioid" or "lymphocytoid" cells to spindle-shaped cells resembling fibroblasts. The cells occur in "nests" or clusters in the basal portion of the epidermis. Three types of acquired nevi are recognized on the basis of their internal architecture and, specifically, the relationship of the clusters of nevus cells to the dermal-epidermal junction. In the *junctional nevus,* cellular proliferation occurs at the dermal-epidermal junction. Junctional nevi are flat or slightly elevated, variably pigmented common moles typically appearing in adolescence or early adulthood. The *intradermal nevus* exhibits little activity at the dermal-epidermal junction and is composed of quiescent-appearing nevus cells with less melanin production deep within the dermis. The intradermal nevus is characteristically an elevated, dome-shaped, lightly pigmented or nonpigmented, usually hair-bearing lesion and is the dominant type of mole occurring in older adults. The *compound nevus* has both junctional and intradermal components and is probably a transitional form between the other two types, thus suggesting that these nevi undergo a natural evolution from the junctional to the intradermal form as the patient ages. The active junctional nevus is the most difficult to differentiate from melanoma, which also begins at the dermal-epidermal junction.

Several variants of melanocytic nevi distinguishable both by histologic and clinical characteristics have been described. The *halo nevus* is seen clinically as a melanocytic nevus surrounded by a distinct depigmented zone of skin or "halo" around the nevus. Microscopically, the depigmented zone is characterized by an intense inflammatory infiltrate of lymphocytes, macrophages, and degenerating melanocytes. The depigmentation is believed to be the result of immunologic activity against the nevus cells. Occasionally, complete disappearance or resolution of the pigmented portion of these nevi has been seen.

The *Spitz nevus* is a benign pigmented nevus arising in children and originally but incorrectly referred to as "juvenile melanoma." Microscopically it exhibits increased cellularity and pleomorphism among the nevus cells. It has been considered difficult to differentiate histologically from malignant melanoma, although there are specific microscopic characteristics that define the two. The typical Spitz nevus is a pink to dark brown, raised, asymptomatic small (<1 cm in size) nodule occurring in the face or distal part of the lower extremities. Seventy-five percent occur in persons under 14 years of age.

Dermatopathologists refer to some acquired melanocytic nevi with particular architectural characteristics as *dysplastic nevi* or, more recently, *"nevi with architectural disorder."* Dysplastic characteristics include irregularity of the nevus cell "nests" at the dermal-epidermal junction, an abnormal pattern of melanocyte growth, melanocytic nuclear atypia, and particularly, radial extension of nevus cells in the epidermis. All stages of transformation occur in a continuum from a typical acquired melanocytic nevi to in situ melanoma.

Clinical features that suggest that a given pigmented lesion may be a nevus with architectural disorder include an irregular outline, an indistinct border, fading into the surrounding skin, and frequent central darker pigmentation. Color is often variegated, and a pink or erythematous background color is common. They may be multiple, are frequently larger than 6 mm in diameter (that is, larger than the usual acquired melanocytic nevus), and may occur in any body part.

Over the years, a group of Caucasian individuals with multiple nevi having dysplastic characteristics have been identified who are believed to have an increased risk of development of malignant melanoma and other skin cancers. In addition, this syndrome exhibits a dominant inheritance pattern in some family groups. Therefore, patients with multiple nevi having architectural disorder require special follow-up, including complete skin examination for other possibly dysplastic lesions and perhaps evaluation of first-order relatives (Table 11–3).

Congenital melanocytic nevi of at least 1.5 cm in diameter are found in at least 1% of Caucasian newborns. They are arbitrarily di-

TABLE 11–3.
Management of Individuals With Dysplastic Nevi*

Careful family history concerning melanoma and moles
Examination of the entire skin and careful evaluation of atypical moles
Removal of the two most atypical nevi, if any are present
Examination of first-degree relatives recommended if melanocytic dysplasia histologically confirmed
Overview and close-up photography (preferably life-size or 1:1)
Follow-up examination and photography, depending on lesional stability, number of lesions, and genetic basis (*e.g.* every 3–6 mo for familial dysplastic nevus syndrome, less often for "sporadic" cases)
Patient self-examination of skin every 1–2 mo
Avoidance of unnecessary sun exposure and the development of redness
Avoidance of exogenous hormonal preparations (especially estrogens)
Patient education with respect to self-examination of skin, potential changes in pigmentary lesions requiring medical attention, and the need for continued periodic surveillance

* Adapted from Barnhill RL, Hurwitz S, Duray PH, et al: *Plast Reconstr Surg* 1988; 81:280. Used by permission.

vided into "giant" and "nongiant" types on the basis of size, with the latter being smaller than 3 cm in greatest diameter and a majority of the "giant" lesions greater than 10 cm. The "giant" lesions tend to have intradermal components and more complex morphology. In clinical presentation, the "nongiant" nevi are raised and moderately pigmented, while the "giant" lesions typically occur in "garment" distribution such as the "bathing trunk" nevus, which covers the lower portion of the torso and buttock area widely. Satellite lesions may occur, and the lesions may exhibit hair growth.

Congenital melanocytic nevi are significant because of cosmetic disfigurement related to the larger lesions and because malignant degeneration occurs in both types. For "nongiant" lesions, there is approximately a 1% incidence of malignancy over a lifetime, while in the "giant" lesions, estimates range from 6% to 12%. The tumors that develop in these nevi may be typical malignant melanoma or more anaplastic tumors with characteristics of neurosarcoma. Since invasive melanoma occurring in these lesions is virtually always fatal, prophylactic treatment of larger lesions, usually with staged excision and/or extensive resurfacing, may be required.

Dermal Melanocytic Hamartoma

The *blue nevus* is a small (generally smaller than 1 cm), smooth, very dark blue or blue-black lesion, most often occurring on the dorsum of the hands and feet or the buttock area. The nevus cells have an extremely elongated slender wavy appearance and are filled with melanin granules. They occur in densely cellular-like irregular bunches oriented with the long axis parallel to the dermal-epidermal junction and are actually melanocytes of neural crest origin.

Other congenital lesions with similar cellular characteristics to the blue nevus but without the dense cellularity include the *"nevus of Ota,"* which is generally a unilateral congenital pigmented facial lesion covering the periorbital, temporal, and nasal-malar areas. It may also involve ipsilateral eye abnormalities and tends to occur in Asian individuals. Another variant called the *"nevus of Itoh"* appears to be virtually identical but occurs in a supraclavicular, scapular, or deltoid distribution.

Malignant Melanoma

- Superficial spreading melanoma
- Nodular malignant melanoma
- Acral lentiginous melanoma
- Lentigo maligna melanoma

Malignant melanoma may arise de novo or in preexisting nevi. Initially, compact masses of melanocytes showing malignant morphology spread radially from the dermal-epidermal junction and eventually invade the dermis. The amount of melanin and pigment varies in malignant melanoma and is not of prognostic significance. Four morphologic types of malignant melanoma are recognized grossly. *Superficial spreading melanoma,* accounting for 70% of body surface tumors in Caucasians, is characterized by a long superficial radial growth phase prior to deep invasion. Fifteen percent of malignant melanomas in Caucasians are *nodular malignant melanomas,* which are deeply invasive and usually ulcerated lesions. *Acral lentiginous melanoma* develops primarily in the glabrous skin of the palms or soles, in the distal parts of the extremities, and in subungual locations; they account for 8% of melanomas in Caucasian patients but encompass the majority (60%) of lesions in the darker-skinned races. Finally, *lentigo maligna melanoma* is an invasive melanoma arising in a precursor lesion called *"lentigo maligna,"* or the "melanotic freckle of Hutchinson." These lesions cover portions of the head and neck and develop in lighter-skinned individuals during the sixth and seventh decades. They account for 5% of cases of melanoma in Caucasian patients. Unusual primary sites for melanoma include the choroidal portion of the retina of the eye and melanoma arising in congenital melanocytic nevi. Transplacental spread of melanoma to a fetus has also been reported.

Current diagnosis of melanoma, treatment planning, as well as prognosis depend almost entirely on the characteristics and microstaging of the primary lesion. Clark's microstaging system is based on the level of dermal invasion by the melanoma; Breslow's concept of microstaging is based on tumor thickness (Tables 11–4 and 11–5).

Biological Behavior

Malignant melanoma is a lethal disease of young and middle-aged adults with an average age at diagnosis of 45 years. It is one of very few tumor types showing a rapid sustained increase in both men and women over the past four decades; it is increasing in incidence at the rate of 4% per year. The patient at highest risk for malignant melanoma is an individual with light skin, blue eyes, and a history of sun exposure. Malignant melanoma is rare in blacks and Asians; in Hispanic individuals, it occurs only a sixth as commonly as in Caucasians (Table 11–6).

There are differences between the sexes as regards the usual distribution of melanoma on the body surface. Different primary sites for malignant melanoma have been linked with differences in prognosis. Extremity sites other than the hands and feet have the most favorable outlook, while lesions on the trunk are the worst, with head and neck sites being intermediate. Lesions arising in the mucosa of genital and anal areas have a uniformly dismal

TABLE 11–4.
Microstaging Systems

Clark's Levels*	5-Year Mortality Rate†	Breslow Tumor Thickness‡	5-Year Survival
I	*In situ* lesion		
II	8%	<0.85 mm	99%
III	35%	0.85–1.69 mm	94%
IV	46%	1.70–3.60 mm	78%
V	52%	>3.65 mm	42%

* Adapted from McGovern VJ, Mihm MC Jr, Bailly C: *Cancer* 1973; 32:1446–1457.
† Mortality trends confirmed 10 years posttreatment.
‡ Adapted from Day et al: *Ann Surg* 1982; 195:44

TABLE 11–5.
Simplified Tumor Staging System for Cutaneous Melanoma by the American Joint Committee on Tumor Staging

TNM classification

Tis	Melanoma *in situ,* not an invasive lesion *Clark's level I*
T1	Tumor 0.75 mm or less in thickness *Clark's level II*
T2	Tumor >0.75 mm but not >1.5 mm in thickness *Clark's level III*
T3	Tumor >1.5 mm but not >3 mm in thickness *Clark's level IV*
T4	Tumor >3 mm in thickness or adjacent cutaneous satellites *Clark's level V*
N0	No nodal involvement
N1	Involved lymph node 3 cm or less in greatest dimension
N2	Involved lymph node > 3 cm and/or contralateral or bilateral
M0	No distant metastasis
M1	Distant metastasis present

Clinical staging summary

I-A	T1–2, N0, M0
I-B	T3–4, N0, M0
II	Any T, N1, M0
III	Any T, N2–3, M0
IV	Any T, any N, M1

TABLE 11–6.
Summary of Risk Factors for the Development of Cutaneous Melanoma*

Risk Factor	Relative Risk†
Persistently changed or changing mole	Very high
One or more large or irregularly pigmented lesions	
Dysplastic mole(s) and familial melanoma	148
Dysplastic mole(s) but no familial melanoma	27
Lentigo maligna	10
Congenital mole	21
Caucasian race (*vs.* black)	12
Previous cutaneous melanoma	9
Cutaneous melanoma in parents, children, or siblings	8
Immunosuppression	4
Sun sensitivity	3
Excessive sun exposure	3

* Adapted from Rhodes, et al: *JAMA* 1987; 258:3146. Used by permission.
† Expected baseline risk for a Caucasian individual = 1X.

prognosis. Increasing age generally worsens the prognosis in melanoma except for the lentigo maligna variety. Female patients generally have greater long-term survival than do men overall, but they also have more extremity lesions.

Patient Evaluation in Melanoma

In 80% of cases malignant melanoma is diagnosed in a localized clinical stage. In primary lesions smaller than 2 cm in diameter, the diagnosis should be established by excisional biopsy. Incisional biopsy, including active nodular ulcerated areas and areas bordering normal skin, may be indicated in very large lesions. Destructive biopsy techniques or "shave" biopsies should not be used. Indications for biopsy of pigmented lesions (other than cosmetic considerations) are based on (1) the characteristics of the lesion itself, including its gross appearance (see the discussion of dysplastic nevi); (2) symptoms of virtually any kind related to the pigmented lesion itself; and (3) the location of the pigmented lesion. Lesions located in areas that are subject to chronic irritation may be removed. Lesions occurring on the glabrous skin of the palms and soles, the subungual areas, and those occurring on mucosal surfaces of the genital or gastrointestinal tract are at high risk for development of melanoma and should be removed. It is also advisable to consider removal of new pigmented lesions arising in adult patients over the age of 30 years and in those with an identified genetic predisposition, a history of dysplastic nevus syndrome, or personal history of melanoma.

During physical examination of patients with biopsy-confirmed melanoma, careful attention to the regional lymph node area draining the primary lesion site is important, as is evaluation of the entire body surface for other atypical pigmented skin lesions. Chest x-ray and liver function studies are the only recommended tests in an asymptomatic patient. Specific guidelines for metastatic work-up in symptomatic patients based on specific symptoms or physical findings are outlined in Table 11–7.

Patient Treatment in Melanoma

Surgery is the mainstay of therapy in all skin surface melanomas. In local excision of primary melanoma, it appears logical to base the size of the surgical margin on the thickness of the lesion that correlates directly with the risk for local recurrent disease. Large retrospective reviews have established that a 1-cm margin is adequate for melanomas less than 0.75 mm in thickness, while others have shown no improvement in either rates of local recurrence or metastatic disease in any thickness of melanoma when surgical margins are extended beyond 3 cm. The local recurrence rate in melanoma is about 3%, with most recurrences evident within 3 to 5 years following primary treatment. Local recurrence portends a poor prognosis and is frequently associated with systemic metastatic spread.

Studies such as the technetium 99 radioisotope lymphangiogram are commonly used to reveal the primary lymph node drainage of a primary site that is on a "watershed" area between nodal drainage systems. Radical lymph node dissection techniques for the neck, axilla, and the superficial groin nodes are accepted as standard treatment for patients having clinically involved lymph nodes (therapeutic lymph node dissection). Lymph node dissection in patients without clinically involved regional nodes is referred to as

TABLE 11–7.
Evaluation of Specific Signs or Symptoms*

Abnormal chest x-ray or physical examination findings
- Tomograms (detect lesions down to 6 mm in diameter)
- CT scan (lesions as small as 3 mm in diameter)
- Bronchoscopy with biopsy (when diagnosis of a lesion is questionable)
- Mediastinoscopy (if lymph nodes are accessible for biopsy)
- Thoracentesis or pleural biopsies (for evaluating effusions)
- Thin-needle biopsy (under CT control to establish a histologic diagnosis in selected cases only)

Abnormal liver function test or physical examination results
- Abdominal CT, ultrasound, or NMR

Bone pain
- Radionuclide bone scan

GI symptoms such as epigastric distress, nausea, anorexia or weight loss, melena, or bowel obstruction
- Stool guaiac (anemic patients or those with a change in bowel habits)
- Endoscopy
- Contrast studies

Headaches, memory loss, personality change, or focal neurologic defect
- CT scan with contrast enhancement
- Carotid arteriogram (to rule out vascular anomalies)
- NMR (may replace CT scan)
- Skull films (only to identify bony metastases)
- Spinal tap (may be dangerous in the face of increased intracranial pressure)
- Stereotactic-guided biopsy (if a histologic diagnosis is required for further treatment management)

* From Anderson RG, O'Brien JC: Skin tumors II: Melanoma, in *Selected Readings in Plastic Surgery*, vol. 7. 1988, p. 18. Used by permission.

"*elective*" or "prophylactic" lymph node dissection. Current treatment may involve use of elective lymph node dissection in specifically selected cases based on tumor microstaging. This approach is based on several studies showing improved survival in groups having intermediate-thickness primary lesions and treated with elective node dissection vs. groups having no node dissection but matched for tumor thickness, sex, and other characteristics. The differences in these groups are particularly noticeable 5 years and more posttreatment.

Late therapeutic lymph node dissection after regional nodes become clinically involved has been associated with a 5-year survival rate less than 20%. Current recommendations would be that lymph node dissection be considered in patients with melanomas 1.5 to 4.0 mm in thickness and, possibly, in lesions 0.76 to 1.5 mm in thickness occurring in men and in nonextremity sites.

Aggressive, widespread metastatic disease is relatively common in melanoma. Treatment failure and death most commonly result from metastatic disease, usually from respiratory failure. Ninety-five percent of patients dying of melanoma have multiple organ metastasis.

Therapy for metastatic disease in melanomas is extremely limited. In localized lesions, some palliation may be obtained with radiotherapy given with high-dose per-fraction techniques; melanoma is only intermediately radiosensitive. Immunotherapy has been tried in a number of different forms. Currently, therapeutic antitumor vaccines are in experimental development. The chemotherapy response for melanoma remains poor, with response rates of 20% or less. Limb perfusion techniques using chemotherapy with and without hyperthermia have shown promise for salvage in extremity melanomas.

TUMORS ARISING PRIMARILY IN THE DERMIS AND SUBCUTANEOUS TISSUES

Hemangioma and Vascular Malformations

- Hemangioma
- Vascular malformations
    - Capillary vascular malformations
    - Venous vascular malformations

- Lymphatic vascular malformations
- Arterial vascular malformations
- Arteriovenous malformations

Currently, vascular lesions are divided into two major categories (Table 11–8): (1) true hemangiomas, which are benign, proliferative neoplasms of vascular origin, and (2) vascular malformations, which represent congenital morphogenetic anomalies. Hemangiomas and vascular malformations may be similar, but the former tend to involute and rarely require treatment, while the latter may be progressive and symptomatic and do not involute.

Hemangiomas, also called hemangioendotheliomas, arise from vascular endothelial cells and are typically composed of compact masses of independently proliferating, well-differentiated cells arising from the dermis and extending into the subcutaneous tissue. Increased numbers of mast cells and erythrocyte-filled vascular spaces are noted.

The clinical appearance of a true hemangioma depends on its depth in relation to the dermis and the growth phase in which it is observed. Early proliferating lesions are elevated with a bright red irregular surface, often referred to as "strawberry" hemangiomas. Deeper lesions may be blue or show no color. Involution typically begins with the fading of color to purple and the development of colorless or gray areas with softening of the mass and then shrinkage. The end result is often a scar consisting of redundant, wrinkly skin of "crepe paper" texture.

The typical hemangioma may go unnoticed at birth or may be evident as a faint "herald" patch. Rapid proliferative growth may occur during the first year of life, involution usually beginning prior to 18 months.

Clinical studies suggest that hemangiomas of varying size can be detected in 1% to 2½% of all neonates and that the lesions are multiple in 15% to 20% of patients. There is a

TABLE 11–8.
Differences Between Hemangioma and Vascular Malformations*

Hemangioma	Vascular Malformations
Clinical	Clinical
30% herald patch at birth	Present at birth although may be missed on examination, especially if deep
Rapid postnatal proliferation in the first year and slow involution thereafter in 75%–90%	Grows with child (may change in response to sepsis and hormonal stimulation)
F:M = 3:1	F:M = 1:1 (many syndromal/genetic associations)
Histologic	Histologic
Hypercellular	
Endothelial proliferation	Flat nonproliferative endothelium
Hyperplastic, well-differentiated, multilaminate basement membrane	Normal basement membrane
Increased cell turnover	Slow turnover
Increased number of mast cells	Normal number of mast cells
Endothelial cells grow and show capillary tubule formation in tissue culture	Poor in vitro cellular growth
Platelet trapping	
Thrombocytopenia (Kasabach-Merritt)	Localized consumptive coagulopathy
Radiographic	Radiographic
Angiogram	Angiogram
Well circumscribed on angiography	
Lobular parenchymal staining	No parenchymal pattern on angiography
	Low-flow lesions—ectatic channels with phleboliths
	High-flow lesions—enlarged tumor arteries with arteriovenous shunting
Skeletal Effects	Skeletal Effects
Hypertrophy rare	
"Mass effect" on adjacent bone uncommon	Distortion hypertrophy or destructive/erosive damage

* Adapted from Mulliken JB, Young AE: Hemangiomas and malformations, in *Vascular Birthmarks.* Philadelphia, WB Saunders, 1988. Used by permission.

decreased incidence in darker-skinned races, and the lesion is three times more common in females than in males. Hemangiomas may occur anywhere in the body, but the majority are on the body surface, and 60% are on the head and neck area.

Most clinical problems, complications, and indications for intervention or treatment in hemangioma occur during the early proliferative growth phase. These include coagulopathy and bleeding, congestive heart failure, hemorrhage, ulceration, infection, obstruction of visual fields, and airway obstruction. Coagulopathy associated with hemangioma has been called the "Kasabach-Merritt syndrome," its primary cause being thrombocytopenia associated with platelet trapping in large hemangiomas. Congestive heart failure is caused by shunting through the hemangioma and occurs with only very large visceral lesions or in neonates overwhelmingly involved with multiple hemangiomas. Hemorrhage in hemangiomas may be associated with ulceration of a surface lesion or a systemic coagulopathy. Fewer than 5% of hemangiomas show significant ulceration. Hemangiomas occurring in the periorbital area may obstruct the visual fields and cause deprivation amblyopia. Total obstruction of one visual field for greater than 1 week during the first year of life may result in permanent visual impairment. Problems with hemangiomas in the orbit may require an ophthalmologic evaluation.

The majority of true hemangiomas require no specific treatment. Management of the complications is primarily nonsurgical. Preventive local measures involving hygiene and the avoidance of irritation are extremely important. Systemic use of corticosteroids may induce resolution of true hemangiomas in 50% to 90% of patients. Short-term, high-dose steroid regimens in the very young have not been associated with acute or long-term problems such as growth disturbance. More recently, intralesional use of steroids has been shown to be effective in small critical lesions, for example, tumors involving the periorbital areas.

Surgical excision of hemangiomas during the proliferative phase is rarely necessary. Some lesions are surgically unresectable. The primary use of surgical treatment of hemangiomas occurs postinvolution in the management of abnormally textured or redundant skin and scar left behind.

Vascular malformations are considered to arise from embryologic errors in the formation of vascular elements at about 8 weeks of embryonic life. Vascular malformations have histologic characteristics suggesting a steady state without increased cellular proliferation or turnover. Vascular malformations represent a spectrum of types and are frequently classified by the dominant type of vascular channel composing the lesion: venous, arterial, lymphatic, or capillary. Vascular anomalies are frequently associated with related congenital syndromes (see Table 11–9).

The intradermal version of the *capillary vascular malformation* ("port-wine" stain) appears at birth as a flat, smooth, intense purple stain, most frequently on the head and neck areas and often within the area served by the first and second branches of cranial nerve V. With age, the surface of these lesions becomes nodular and hyperkeratotic. The reported incidence of capillary vascular malformation of this type is about 0.3% in the Caucasian population. Treatment considerations in the "port-wine stain" are typically cosmetic. The primary therapy has use of the tunable dye laser at a wave length of approximately 577 Å, which offers the best compromise between scar formation and appropriate penetration for selective vessel ablation. The laser has yielded improved results, with proponents advising early treatment before nodularity and skin changes occur.

Venous vascular malformations cover a spectrum from limited lower extremity hypoplasias and obstruction to complex large venous malformations of visceral and retroperitoneal vessels. Venous malformations on the body surface are seen as compressible "spongy" or "rubbery" surface lesions, blue in color, that tend toward swelling or enlargement when dependent. Phleboliths are a distinguishing radiographic feature. The incidence of venous malformations of all types may be as high as 4% in the general population. Venous malformations are associated with an increased incidence of thromboembolic phenomena as well as cosmetic deformity. Larger localized

Syndromes Associated With Vascular Malformations

Anomalad, Sequence, or Syndrome	Vascular Malformation Type	Other Components of the Syndrome	Type of Inheritance	Significant Factors in Management
Sturge-Weber	Capillary malformation or "port-wine" stain in (trigeminal) cranial nerve V_1 distribution	CNS disorders, seizures, sometimes hemiparesis, mental retardation, ipsilateral leptomeningeal calcification and cortical atrophy, glaucoma, and visual field defects	Unknown Appears to be sporadic	"Port-wine" stain or capillary malformation in trigeminal nerve $V_1 + V_2$ distribution requires CT head scan and neuro-ophthalmologic evaluation
Klippel-Trenaunay-Weber	"Port-wine" and/or venous-lymphatic malformation of the extremities with skeletal hypertrophy frequently in a single extremity	Frequent deep venous anomalies "Persistent lateral vein" often in the lower extremity Venous malformation results in swelling, edema, and intermittent venous thrombosis	Unknown Sporadic	Symptoms vary with the extent of venous involvement Pneumatic sequential compression, compression garments, and symptomatic care are often helpful
Parkes-Weber	Similar to Klippel-Trenaunay but associated with arteriovenous malformation—more morbidity and worse prognosis		Unknown Sporadic	
Bannayan	Multiple vascular malformations rare (first described in 1971)	Vascular malformation associated with microcephaly and multiple lipomatosis	Autosomal dominant inheritance	
Riley-Smith	Similar to Bannayan	Similar to Bannayan but no lipomatosis; pseudopapilledema is a consistent feature		
Osler-Weber-Rendu (hereditary hemorrhagic telangiectasia)	Multiple vascular malformations of the skin and viscera including bowel and mucous membranes with large ectatic vessels; vascular malformations appear after puberty and increase with age; epistaxis, hematuria, and upper and/or lower gastrointestinal bleeding are common features		Autosomal dominant with variable expression	Hemorrhage the main clinical problem CNS symptoms predominate with bleeding intracranially or into cord
Von-Hippel-Lindau	Chief characteristic is vascular malformation involving retinas and cerebellum; other viscera sometimes involved; the disorder is rare; retinal and CNS manifestations most often after the age of 25 yr	Cerebellar cysts sometimes cystic change in pancreas, liver, adrenals, and lower part of kidneys; may develop cerebellar hemangioblastoma and renal cancer	Autosomal dominant with varying expression	25% renal cancer often bilateral
Maffuci	Small papillary or pedunculated vascular malformations in skin and subcutaneous tissue; sometimes visceral involvement with vascular malformations as well, usually capillary or venous malformations with high incidence of phlebitis	Multiple skeletal enchondroma (60% bilateral) in digits and proximal extremities; also associated with malignant intracranial tumors; 15%–20% incidence of chondrosarcoma	Sporadic	Thrombosis of dilated venous channels often a problem; pathologic factors related to enchondromas or malignant chondrosarcoma
Blue "rubber-bleb" nevus syndrome	Venous malformations involving skin and frequently bowel; lesions tend to be bluish, compressible, and rubbery to palpation; liver, spleen, and CNS are sometimes involved; most frequently lesions are manifested at adolescence; rare disorder		Pattern unknown	Skin lesions may be painful; angiography demonstrating typical bowel lesions aids diagnosis; palliative resection of involved bowel segments or local excision of skin

lesions may develop into functionally limiting masses. The mainstay in managing the local pain and edema is compression therapy. Other nonsurgical treatment includes intralesional sclerosing agents such as hypertonic saline, sodium tetradecyl sulfate and, more recently in Europe, Ethibloc. Lesions producing a mass or cosmetic deformity may be treated by local surgical excision. Although not truly invasive, lesions may intimately surround vital neurovascular structures. Delineation of lesions with angiography is helpful prior to surgery.

Lymphatic vascular malformations are frequently referred to as lymphangiomas. Localized "simplex" types have been identified, while larger deeper lesions, frequently occurring in the head and neck area with cavernous cystic spaces, are often called "cystic hygromas." Lymphatic vascular malformations may communicate with the venous system and coexist with elements of venous malformations. Clinically, lymphatic malformations are manifested as fairly deep compressible "spongy" masses. Most are evident at birth, and virtually all are diagnosed by the age of 3 years. Head and neck sites predominate, particularly the floor of the mouth, the tongue, and the cheek, while other commonly involved areas include the neck, axilla, and prepectoral areas. Clinically, rapid changes in the size and consistency are frequently noted and are accounted for by lymphatic obstruction or venous connection as well as recurrent bouts of inflammation and scarring.

Problems related to lymphatic vascular malformations include airway obstruction with bulky lesions in the head and neck area in infants and infection. The structure of the lesions and related edema predispose them to cellulitic infections with *Streptococcus* or *Staphylococcus.*

Treatment options center around the aggressive treatment of infection and airway protection. Surgical treatment might include tracheostomy and, in a few cases, surgical excision or debulking of the lymphatic lesion. Complete surgical excision of a lymphatic vascular malformation is very difficult because the lesions tend to proliferate through the surrounding tissues in a way that makes excision without sacrifice of vital structures difficult. Surgical morbidity is increased by prolonged drainage and wound healing difficulties.

Arterial vascular malformations include tortuous and anomalous vasculature, hypoplasia, and duplication or congenitally stenotic vessels in the arterial circulation. Most of these lesions are asymptomatic, and the diagnosis is most frequently made during evaluation in later life for coexisting vascular occlusive disease.

Arteriovenous malformations are complex lesions with arterial input and high vascular flow. The associated pathophysiology caused by unregulated arteriovenous shunting dominates the clinical picture, including pulsation, increased temperature, vascular thrill, and bruit. The effects of the arteriovenous shunting are manifested by alterations in blood pressure, increased blood volume, and increased cardiac output. In addition, there may be direct local tissue destruction from the expanding lesion or limb hyperplasia. Distal extremity ischemia may be due to the "steal" effect of the arteriovenous shunt or the increased venous pressure produced directly by the lesion. Other significant problems include consumptive coagulopathy as well as skeletal distortion and growth disturbance.

Selective angiography can define the anatomy and hemodynamics of these lesions. Surgical management is difficult and often associated with high morbidity. The lesions are rarely resectable without recurrence. It has been noted that simple ligation of the vessels feeding an arteriovenous anomaly is contraindicated because of rapid opening of new vascular channels and further expansion of the lesion. Treatment by embolization of vessels feeding the lesion is either palliative or used in preparation for extirpative surgery. A few extremity lesions are best managed by amputation (see Table 11–9).

Other Tumors of Vascular Origin

- Pyogenic granuloma
- Glomus tumor
- Hemangiopericytoma
- Angiosarcoma/lymphangiosarcoma
- Kaposi's tumor

Other tumors of vascular origin, both benign and malignant, typically arise either from the capillary endothelial cells or from specialized perivascular cells of neural crest origin. *Pyogenic granuloma* is a reactive lesion caused by chronic inflammation. Histologically it appears most like hemangiomas. Most lesions are small (0.5 to 1.5 cm), raised, pedunculated, soft red nodular lesions showing superficial ulceration which bleed easily when traumatized. The lesions are most common on the hands and face. A "collarette" of epidermis growing around the base of the lesion is typical. The lesions grow fairly rapidly. Treatment consists of surface destructive methods such as simple cautery or silver nitrate and discontinuation of the surface irritation. Other lesions respond to excision and cautery at the base or excision and careful closure.

The *glomus tumor* arises from a subcutaneous arteriovenous shunt known as the Sucquet-Hoyer canal, or "cutaneous glomus." These shunts are seen microscopically on the skin of the extremities, particularly the fingertips and most especially in the corium of the nail bed.

The typical solitary glomus tumor is a small purple nodule (a few millimeters in size). Most typically, the nodule is extremely tender, and disproportionate pain may be triggered by seemingly insignificant stimulation of the lesion, including cold exposure. The subungual variety may be nearly invisible and can cause paroxysmal digital hand pain (see Chapter 22).

A hemangiopericytoma arises from the pericyte, a cell found throughout the body around capillaries and vessels. It is situated peripheral to the periendothelial reticular membrane. It differs from the glomus cell because of its unusual location and because it lacks myofilaments. Microscopically, it is characterized by branching endothelial-lined tubules surrounded by packed, moderately anaplastic but identifiable pericytes with spindle-shaped nuclei. Clinically, the tumor presents as red, indurated plaques or nodules that are often locally invasive. The behavior of a hemangiopericytoma is difficult to predict on a historic basis. Of those that do metastasize, up to 50% are ultimately fatal, which is usually a result of pulmonary involvement.

Angiosarcoma is also referred to as "malignant angioendothelioma." Tumor variants arising from lymphatic endothelium have been referred to as *"lymphangiosarcoma"* or "lymphangioendothelioma." This is a rare, highly malignant tumor arising from the endothelial cells. Two clinical presentations are described. In the first, the lesion is seen as a spreading erythematous plaque with papules and macules on the face and scalp of elderly individuals, later becoming nodular and ulcerative; in the second, the tumor develops in lymphedematous tissue, particularly an extremity. These tumors exhibit rapid local proliferation and early systemic spread. Early radical surgery, in particular amputation, has been advanced as the only appropriate surgical treatment for some cases. For the plastic and reconstructive surgeon who participates in the care of patients with lymphedema, both acquired and congenital, a high index of suspicion for any cutaneous nodule with these characteristics and prompt biopsy are important.

Kaposi's sarcoma is a malignant proliferative tumor arising from the vascular endothelial cells. Opinions differ as to whether it is a true metastasizing sarcoma or a vascular tumor that is multifocal in origin. It has become prominent because of its association with acquired immunodeficiency syndrome (AIDS). Clinically, Kaposi's sarcoma in early stages is manifested as red or brown, indurated, plaque-like annular serpiginous lesions on the lower extremities. Progression to nodularity and finally ulceration generally occurs over time. Widespread visceral lesions and mucosal oral lesions are frequently noted. Diagnosis is by careful history and incisional biopsy. Plastic and reconstructive surgeons may encounter such lesions during the evaluation of unusual nonhealing wounds and lower extremity ulcerations. Optimal treatment is nonsurgical.

Tumors of Neural or Neuroendocrine Origin

- Neurofibroma
- Neurilemmoma/ganglioneuroma

- Neurosarcoma
- Merkel cell tumor

Tumors in this group generally arise from cells of the embryologic neural ectoderm. The typical *neurofibroma* is a benign tumor consisting of Schwann cells and endoneurial fibroblasts. Microscopically they exhibit multidirectional collagen strands interspersed with uniform spindle-shaped cells with ovoid nuclei. They typically appear as well-circumscribed but not encapsulated tumors arising from peripheral nerves. They may infiltrate dermis or surrounding tissue.

Clinically the lesion occurs in solitary form or in multiple form associated with cutaneous "café au lait" spots in hereditary von Recklinghausen's disease. Such surface lesions are clinically similar. They are soft, flesh-colored tumors involving the skin, sometimes globular or pedunculated. Neurofibromas also occur in deeper tissue planes and are attached to major cranial and peripheral nerves. In von Recklinghausen's disease, central nervous system or spinal cord involvement occurs in 5% to 10% of patients, and malignant degeneration to fibrosarcoma or neurosarcoma may occur in 3% to 4% of such patients. Neurofibromas may cause digital gigantism. Severe craniofacial involvement may cause gross distortion of the involved cranium and facial skeleton. Solitary cutaneous lesions may be locally excised. Lesions associated with major peripheral nerves may be difficult to remove without nerve sacrifice because of their infiltrative nature. A suspicion of malignant degeneration is also an indication for surgical excision and/or biopsy.

A *neurilemmoma* is a biphasic, well-encapsulated spindle cell neoplasm. Clinically, neurilemmomas are solitary, generally subcutaneous tumors occurring along the course of a major peripheral nerve. Most common in the head and neck, the lesions are 2 to 4 cm in size and are usually asymptomatic. Simple excision of these encapsulated lesions suffices for diagnosis and treatment, with nerve preservation usually possible.

Neurosarcoma is a highly malignant spindle cell neoplasm difficult to differentiate from fibrosarcoma and other high-grade spindle cell tumors and shares with them a poor prognosis. It usually arises in deeper tissue planes but may develop in preexisting neurofibromas. It has a tendency toward longitudinal spread along involved nerves and early distant metastasis.

The *Merkel cell tumor* arises from a cell recently identified as a neuroendocrine cell arising from the neural crest and differentiating as part of the APUD (amine precursor uptake dependent) system. This cell also has a capability for epithelial differentiation. Merkel cell tumors arise in the dermis and consist of small "lymphocytoid cells" that extend to the epidermis. Clinically the lesion is a solitary or locally multiple, pink to red nonulcerated nodular lesion on the head or scalp and, more rarely, on the extremities. The tumors are aggressive with a tendency toward subclinical radial spread and metastatic dissemination. Death occurs in over 25% of patients. Local excision analogous to treatment for melanoma is usually warranted. Subclinical involvement of regional lymph nodes is as high as 50% at the time of initial treatment, thus suggesting the need for radical lymph node dissection.

Tumors of Mesenchymal Origin

Benign tumors of mesenchymal or connective tissue origin are very common, while malignant sarcomas are relatively rare. Some of the malignant sarcomas appear to arise in preexisting benign precursor lesions, but most appear de novo. Enzinger and Weiss have noted a strong age relationship with the peak incidence of the more common sarcomas (Fig 11–1).

With the exception of rhabdomyosarcoma in infancy and childhood and the primary bone tumors, histologic grading correlates well with biological behavior. Sarcomas arising in deep tissue planes of extremities or in the retroperitoneum and thorax tend to exhibit a higher histologic grade and more aggressive behavior and are larger at the time of diagnosis. In general, sarcomas exhibit great variability in the degree of differentiation in diverse areas within the same tumor. Often, when they are locally recurrent, they show increasing anaplasia and dedifferentiation with each clinical recurrence.

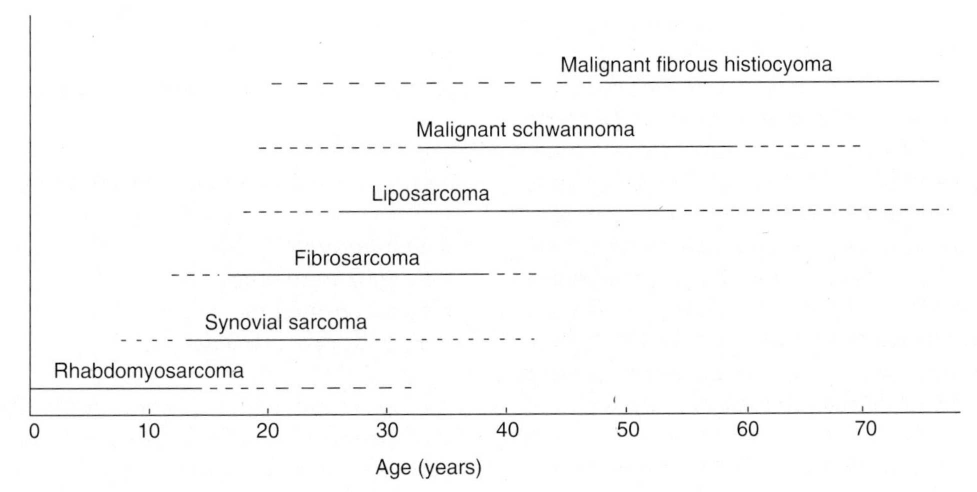

FIG 11–1.
Approximate age at the incidence of various types of sarcomas. *Solid lines* indicate peak incidence of tumor; *Dotted lines* indicate reduced incidence of tumor. (From Enzinger FM, Weiss SW: *Soft Tissue Tumors.* St Louis, Mosby–Year Book, 1983, p. 3. Used by permission.)

A predilection for hematogenous metastasis to viscera, particularly the lung, is common with high-grade soft-tissue sarcomas. Pulmonary metastases are the most usual site of treatment failure and the most frequent cause of death. Pseudo-encapsulation is characteristic of many soft-tissue sarcomas and is a hazard inviting incomplete surgical excision. Wide subclinical extension is the rule, and the grossly apparent border of these tumors is very deceptive. Histologic evaluation of the margins in soft-tissue sarcomas is difficult, and rapid frozen sections are generally not reliable. When operating with curative intent, radical excision, usually including complete resection of the entire soft-tissue muscular compartment containing the tumor or, in the case of some extremities, amputation, is the rule. Clinical staging for such sarcomatous lesions, including those arising in the skin, according to the American Joint Commission on Cancer Staging in the TNM system, is outlined in Table 11–10.

Multidisciplinary treatment is important. When all soft-tissue sarcomas are included, long-term control is achieved in only approximately a third of patients.

Tumors of Fibrous Connective Tissue

- Cutaneous fibroma (dermatofibroma)
- Dermatofibrosarcoma protuberans
- Fibrosarcoma
- Fibroxanthoma/histiocytoma
- Fibroxanthosarcoma
- Epithelioid sarcoma

The typical *cutaneous fibroma,* or *dermatofibroma,* is a small (<2 cm), red to brown cutaneous nodule frequently seen on the

TABLE 11–10.
Simplified Tumor Staging for Soft-Tissue Carcinoma

TNM classification	
T1	<5 cm
T2	5 cm or greater
T3	Tumor that grossly invades bone, major vessel, or major nerve
N0	No histologically verified regional lymph node metastasis
N1	Histologically verified regional lymph node metastasis
M0	No distant metastasis
M1	Distant metastasis
G1	Low
G2	Moderate
G3	High
Clinical staging summary	
I	T1–2, N0, M0, G1
II	T1–2, N0, M0, G2
III	T1–2, N0–1, M0, any G
IV	Any N, any G, T3, M0

extremities. It is a cellular tumor consisting primarily of fibroblast-like cells and is rarely symptomatic. Local excision or excisional biopsy will suffice for diagnosis and treatment.

Dermatofibrosarcoma protuberans is an unusual low-grade sarcoma consisting of malignant fibroblasts. Clinically the lesion is seen as a slowly enlarging, raised, flesh-colored, plaque-like surface lesion that is minimally symptomatic and typically occurs on the extremities or trunk of older people. Dermatofibrosarcoma protuberans may attain a large size, and reconstruction is frequently required after suitably wide local excision. Local control is problematic because the margins of the tumor are indistinct and difficult to verify microscopically. There is typically a very long interval, frequently lasting years, between primary management and local recurrence or manifestations of metastatic disease.

Fibrosarcoma is the definitive and highly malignant anaplastic spindle cell neoplasm of fibroblast origin. It generally appears as a deep, rapidly progressive, infiltrating subcutaneous mass rather than involving the skin directly.

The *fibroxanthoma* or *histiocytoma* is a benign tumor of fibrous tissue and histiocytic cells.

Fibroxanthosarcoma ("malignant fibrous histiocytoma") is a malignant lesion containing both cell types. The lesions are highly cellular with extreme pleomorphism and contain large polygonal irregularly shaped cells, bizarre "giant cells," and lipid-laden macrophages, or "foam" cells, as well as more typical anaplastic spindle-shaped cells. It is probably the most common soft-tissue sarcoma of elderly patients. Fibroxanthosarcoma is most often seen clinically as a subcutaneous lesion but will occasionally invade the skin and ulcerate. Cutaneous lesions are most common in the thigh and buttock area. Even the lower-grade lesions are highly prone to local recurrence, and radical surgical resection is indicated.

Epithelioid sarcoma arises from undifferentiated cells capable of both mesodermal and epithelial differentiation. The invasive nature of the tumor is obvious microscopically, with perivascular and perineural invasion being extremely common. Epithelioid sarcoma is frequently seen as an intradermal or subcutaneous nodule on the distal extremities, most particularly the hands and feet, including the digits and palmar skin (see Chapter 22).

Mesenchymal Tumors of Muscle Origin

- Leiomyoma
- Angioleiomyoma
- Leiomyosarcoma
- Rhabdomyosarcoma

A benign *leiomyoma* arises from smooth muscle cells in the skin, particularly from the arrectores pilorum associated with hair follicles. Others arise from cutaneous smooth muscle of tissues of the genital tract such as the vulva or scrotum or from the mammillary muscles of the areolar area of the breast. Despite their location, the tumors are similar histologically and consist of thick interlacing bundles of near-normal–appearing smooth muscle cells interspersed with collagen.

Clinically, these lesions are multiple, but localized and are manifested as groups of red or brown intradermal nodules of up to 2 cm in size. They are frequently tender and occasionally are spontaneously painful. Local complete excision is adequate for diagnosis and treatment of these benign lesions.

Leiomyosarcoma occurring in skin is usually low grade and composed of atypical but recognizable smooth muscle cells with increased nuclear pleomorphism and mitotic activity. Higher-grade leiomyosarcomas are anaplastic spindle cell neoplasms. The cutaneous version most likely also arises from the arrectores pilorum and is manifested as a painful intradermal nodule that ulcerates. Radical excision is the treatment of choice for leiomyosarcoma. Regional lymph nodes have been successfully managed in low-grade lesions by lymph node dissection, while higher-grade tumors cause death by hematogenous distant metastasis in at least a third of the cases.

Rhabdomyosarcoma is a highly malignant and undifferentiated neoplasm arising from striated muscle cells or their precursors. It almost never involves skin directly and is the most common sarcoma in children and neonates.

Mesenchymal Tumors of Adipose Tissue

- Lipoma
- Angiolipoma
- Liposarcoma

The common *lipoma* arises from the adipocyte and is histologically composed of mature normal-appearing adipose tissue that grows independently and is typically surrounded by a loose connective tissue capsule.

A lipoma is a typical soft, round or lobulated, mobile subcutaneous lesion of widely variable size. Lipomas are generally asymptomatic, but angiolipomas may be painful. The lipoma is probably the most common solid tumor of adulthood.

Excision by enucleation or "shelling out" of the encapsulated lesion usually suffices for diagnosis and treatment. Liposuction has been advocated but has resulted in occasional recurrence, and the material obtained thereby for histologic evaluation is of extremely limited quality.

Liposarcoma is the most common malignant sarcoma of soft tissue. It may arise in a preexisting lipomatous lesion but most typically occurs de novo and, most commonly, in deeper, intramuscular, fascial, or retroperitoneal tissue planes. Histologically, liposarcomas exhibit highly variable degrees of dedifferentiation from only slightly pleomorphic fat cells to poorly differentiated spindle cells and bizarre lipoblasts. Clinically, liposarcoma may occur at any age and is typically seen as a deep, rapidly enlarging mass. Occasionally, it may be manifested as a diffuse nodular infiltration of subcutaneous tissue and skin. Lower-grade lesions tend to recur locally, while higher-grade lesions tend to rapid distant visceral metastasis by hematogenous spread. Surgical treatment generally involves radical resection or amputation.

MYELOGENOUS NEOPLASMS HAVING MAJOR SKIN MANIFESTATIONS

- Lymphomas
    - Hodgkin's and non-Hodgkin's types
    - Malignant histiocytosis
    - Mycosis fungoides
- Leukemias and multiple myelomas
    - Leukemia cutis
    - Plasmacytoma (extramedullary myeloma)

Lymphomas are malignant neoplasms derived from lymphocytes or, occasionally, macrophages/histiocytes. Clinically significant groupings include *Hodgkin's* and *non-Hodgkin's lymphomas, malignant histiocytosis,* and *mycosis fungoides. Leukemias* and *multiple myeloma* are neoplastic diseases involving monoclonal cell lines of lymphocytes, neutrophils, and plasma cells. All of these diseases frequently demonstrate both nonspecific and specific cutaneous lesions. So-called nonspecific cutaneous lesions common to the group include toxic erythroderma, lichenification secondary to generalized pruritus, and abnormal pigmentation, as well as petechiae, ecchymosis, and purpura associated with the hemorrhagic diathesis of bone marrow failure. Specific lesions represent direct cutaneous infiltration by malignant cells of the underlying neoplasm. The clinical significance of this is that the skin manifestations may precede the onset of systemic disease in lymphomas or leukemia. In that setting, incisional biopsy of the skin lesion may result in early diagnosis.

Mycosis fungoides is an unfortunate misnomer for a very slowly progressive form of lymphoma primarily arising in and involving the skin. Biopsy is often diagnostic in the later phases of the disease, and treatment is nonsurgical.

SKIN INVOLVEMENT WITH METASTATIC TUMOR

Direct involvement of the skin by *metastatic tumor* without evidence of the underlying primary neoplastic focus is rare. Tumor types in which it is difficult to determine whether they are metastatic or primary in skin include lymphomas, multicentric Kaposi's sarcoma, myeloma, and melanoma. Metastatic adenocarcinoma to skin may sometimes be confused with the primary cutaneous carcinoma of sweat gland origin or extramammary Paget's disease.

True cutaneous metastasis to skin may arrive by lymphatic or hematogenous spread. The most common carcinomas metastasizing to skin include breast, lung, adenocarcinomas of the gastrointestinal tract, endometrial carcinoma, pancreatic carcinoma, thyroid carcinoma, and prostate cancer.

TREATMENT OPTIONS AND TECHNIQUES IN THE MANAGEMENT OF SKIN CANCER

Biopsy and Tissue Sampling Techniques

- Excisional biopsy
- Incisional biopsy
- Punch biopsy
- "Shave" biopsy

Excisional biopsy is the usual method for sampling skin lesions that are less than 2 cm in diameter. On most body surfaces, such lesions can be excised full thickness with simple direct skin closure. Orientation of the resulting scar should be along the lines of least skin tension, and care should be taken to completely encompass smaller lesions so that those that show benign pathology will not require further treatment.

Incisional biopsy generally denotes a partial sampling technique for larger surface lesions that cannot be completely removed without leaving unacceptable defects or necessitating complex reconstructive techniques. In most instances, the incisional biopsy specimen should be taken from the portion of the lesion showing the greatest pathologic activity or change and, most often, should include an area of any active border so that the interface of the lesion with normal skin can be studied histologically.

Punch biopsy is generally a minute form of incisional biopsy. A 3 to 5 mm punch sample from various parts of any skin lesion can be taken under local anesthesia. Care must be taken to not transfer biopsy instruments from one site to another and to avoid macerating these relatively small tissue samples by using proper technique.

"Shave" biopsy involves tangential removal of the upper layers of skin around or under a lesion and is appropriate only for lesions that are confined to the epidermis and appear characteristic and benign, such as seborrheic keratosis or verruca vulgaris. It would also be appropriate for obtaining small surface samples from larger lesions associated with generalized skin disorders or dermatoses or to obtain a specimen for culture. Atypical pigmented lesions, in particular, should not be subjected to a "shave" biopsy technique because the quality of the tissue obtained is frequently insufficient for definitive diagnosis and, in the case of melanoma, histologic study of the full thickness of the lesion is necessary for appropriate diagnosis and treatment planning. Some low-grade skin cancers such as basal cell carcinoma display a falsely reassuring tendency to epithelialize and appear to heal over following partial biopsy techniques such as "shave" or punch biopsy.

Nonsurgical Treatment Modalities for Skin Cancer (basal cell carcinoma and squamous carcinoma)

- Radiotherapy
- Topical chemotherapy
- Cryosurgery
- Electrodesiccation and curettage

In basal cell carcinoma and squamous carcinoma of smaller size, radiation treatment has produced 5-year control rates nearly equal to excisional therapy. *Radiotherapy* appears to be a noninvasive technique appropriate for a few patients who are not surgical candidates. It has its role as adjunctive treatment with surgery in extensive cases of basal cell and squamous cell carcinoma and in a variety of other skin malignancies of both epidermal and dermal/mesenchymal origin. As with excisional therapy, the cure rate with therapy diminishes with increasing tumor size. Although there is less immediately evident tissue destruction with radiotherapy, there is evidence that the "scar" produced by ionizing radiation may slowly worsen with time. Because there is no direct margin control with radiotherapy, treatment portals must be widened slightly to ensure that all parts of a particular lesion are covered. Acute complications of radiotherapy include radiation dermatitis and, occasionally, osteitis or chondritis.

Since radiation itself is known to be carcinogenic, its use is unappealing in younger patients. It is well known that the indiscriminate use of radiotherapy for benign skin conditions has resulted in a multitude of serious complications in later life, including secondary malignant tumors. A long latent interval between recurrence from initial treatment to local recurrence following radiation therapy for basal cell carcinoma of 7 to 12 years has been noted.

Topical chemotherapy with 5-fluorouracil cream (Efudex) was widely applied for skin cancer and a variety of nonmalignant surface skin lesions. Its efficacy in basal cell carcinoma is poor. Treatment indications are now primarily limited to the management of actinic keratosis. 5-Fluorouracil cream produces an intense inflammatory reaction and if used over large surface areas, may be very uncomfortable or even debilitating, particularly for elderly patients. The inflammatory reac-

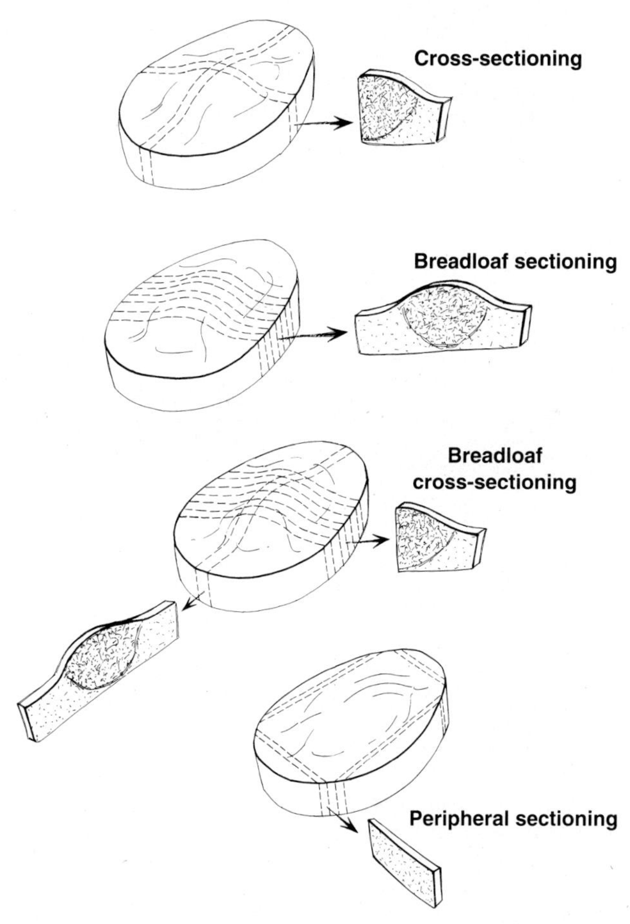

FIG 11–2.
Conventional sectioning techniques. Many surgeons combine cold-knife excision of skin cancers with intraoperative rapid frozen sections to assure complete excision. This is particularly helpful when reconstruction will follow in a single operative stage, in areas where tissue conservation is an issue (e.g., facial lesions), and/or tumor extension is difficult to estimate visually. Regardless of the type of sectioning used, it is imperative to maintain spatial orientation of the specimen and to establish reference points relating to the excisional defect.

tion must be allowed to subside before its therapeutic effect can be assessed. This requires close follow-up of patients over a significant period of time. Treatment cycles with 5-fluorouracil typically last about 6 weeks.

Cryosurgery using liquid nitrogen has resulted in reasonable local control of small basal cell carcinomas and is appropriate for treatment of other common surface lesions such as actinic keratosis. However, the use of cryosurgery for basal cell carcinoma has contraindications. Proponents have suggested that it should not be used on large lesions, on recurrent lesions, on lesions in certain anatomic areas, and on certain histologic types of basal cell carcinoma, particularly the sclerosing type. Cryosurgery is contraindicated in individuals with any type of cold intolerance. Besides the inability to confirm a diagnosis or control margins, other drawbacks include a relatively long healing time and significant

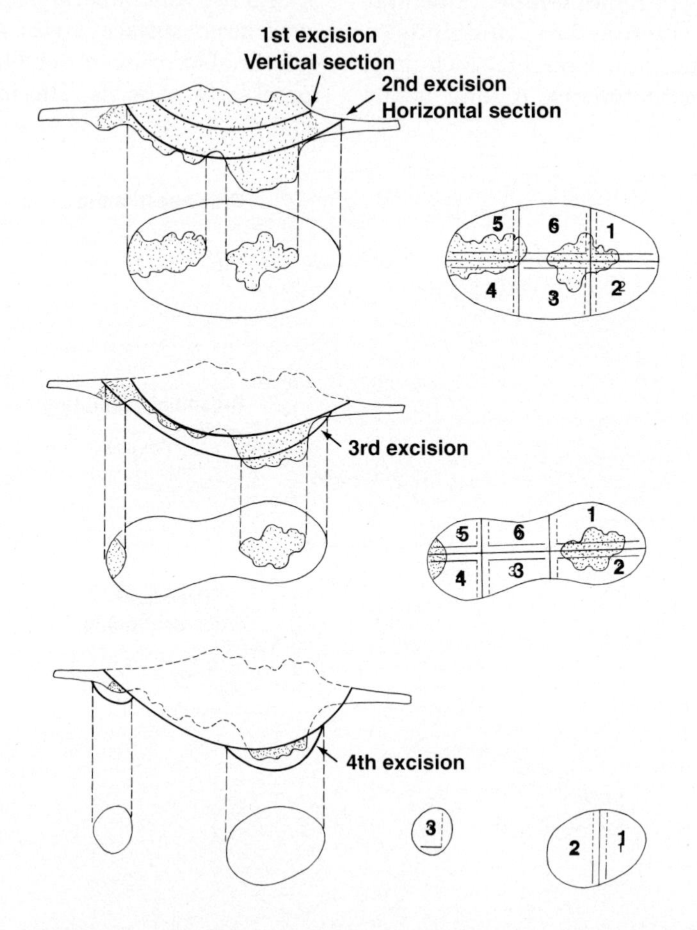

FIG 11–3.
Mohs' micrographic sectioning. The essence of the Mohs' technique is uniform tangential excision of skin surface lesions combined with careful orientation and microscopic evaluation of each layer of tissue removed. Each subsequent excision can be narrowed to conserve uninvolved areas or widened to encompass lateral tumor spread. Successively deeper layers are removed until the deepest extension of tumor is reached. In the diagrams at (left/right opposite), a vertical cross section of a hypothetical skin lesion with lateral and deep extension from the skin surface is presented on the left. A corresponding horizontal projection of excised tissue is on the right. As each excision is made, the undersurface of each tissue layer is mapped as shown. The specimen may then be marked with tissue stains and subdivided into as many parts as necessary for microscopic evaluation. As the limits of tumor extension are reached, the excisions narrow and the last sections removed are free of tumor on both lateral and deep edges. (Adapted from Helm F, Milgrom H, Phelan JT, et al: *Dermatol Wochenschr* 1964; 150:451–458.)

pigment change. This is a particular problem with treatment in facial areas.

Electrodesiccation combined with curettage is probably the most widely applied treatment for small basal cell carcinomas and some benign skin lesions. Problems include the fact that it is a destructive technique that provides no tissue to confirm the diagnosis and does not allow rigorous margin control. Like other surface destructive methods, its efficacy in larger tumors is greatly reduced.

Surgical Excision Techniques for Basal and Squamous Cell Carcinoma

- Cold knife excision
- Mohs' micrographic histosurgery

Two options for surgical excision exist in most primary basal and squamous cell carcinomas: (1) cold knife excision and (2) Mohs' histosurgical or "micrographic" technique. Both techniques offer excellent control in both basal cell and squamous carcinoma. Standard rapid frozen sectioning is the usual method used for intraoperative margin control with *cold knife excision.* Successful use requires cooperation between surgeon and pathologist. For surgery of difficult lesions or those requiring immediate complex reconstruction techniques, frozen sections must be verified in a manner that involved margins can be reresected and checked again. The surgeon should have specific knowledge of the types of frozen section techniques used by his pathologist. (Commonly used techniques are demonstrated in Figure 11–2.) In basal or squamous cell carcinoma that requires reconstruction, excision with rapid frozen section margin control as a single-stage technique often appears to be the best compromise between time and expense, patient tolerance, and improved accuracy in surgical excision.

In the 1930s Frederic Mohs, M.D., developed a special technique of serial tangential excision of skin cancers that allows careful mapping of marginal areas of tumor involvement. The current method of *Mohs' micrographic histosurgery* is accomplished with "fresh tissue technique." Layers of tissue from the tumor are tangentially excised, generally under local anesthesia, and then carefully oriented and mapped (Fig 11–3). Areas of residual tumor involvement are specifically located on each successive layer of tissue until all areas of the tumor are completely removed. Disadvantages to Mohs' micrographic histosurgery are primarily logistic in nature and include the time and expense involved and the practical need for delayed reconstruction. A practical limitation is the difficulty in applying it to the most extensive and difficult cases of basal and squamous cell carcinoma, particularly deeply invasive lesions involving bone. Most problems with Mohs' technique, such as the time lag before reconstruction and patient discomfort, can be minimized by careful preplanning between the surgeon performing the Mohs' technique and the reconstructive surgeon. Mohs' surgery can be effective in treating some cases that are very difficult to manage with cold knife excision such as sclerosing or morpheaform basal cell carcinoma and carcinoma recurrent in a previously scarred or irradiated area.

SUGGESTED READING

Abide JM, Nahai F, Bennett RG: The meaning of surgical margins. *Plast Reconstr Surg* 1984; 73:492.

American Cancer Society: *Cancer Facts and Figures, 1992.* American Cancer Society.

Anderson RG, O'Brien JC: Skin tumors II: Melanoma, in *Readings in Plastic Surgery,* vol 5. Dallas, University of Texas, 1988.

Anderson WAD, Kissane JM: In Allen AC (ed): *Pathology,* ed 7. St Louis, Mosby–Year Book, 1977, pp 1802–1873.

Balch CM, Milton GW: *Clinical Management and Treatment Results Worldwide.* Philadelphia, JB Lippincott, 1985.

Beahrs, et al (eds): *Manual for Staging Cancer,* ed 3. Philadelphia, JB Lippincott, 1988.

Bechtel MA, Callen JP, Owen LE, et al: Etiologic agents in the development of skin cancer. *Clin Plast Surg* 1980; 7:265.

Breslow A: Thickness, cross-sectional areas, and depth of invasion in the prognosis of cutaneous melanoma. *Ann Surg* 1978; 172:902–908.

Burns J, Rohrich J: Vascular anomalies and lymphedema, in *Selected Readings in Plastic Surgery,* vol 5. Dallas, University of Texas, 1988.

Cottel WI: Skin tumors I: Basal cell carcinoma and squamous cell carcinoma, in *Selected Readings in Plastic Surgery,* vol 6. Dallas, University of Texas, 1990.

Enzinger FM, Weiss SW: *Soft Tissue Tumors.* St Louis, Mosby–Year Book, 1983.

Fitzpatrick TB, et al: Primary melanoma of the skin: Recognition and management. *J Am Acad Dermatol* 1980; 2:179.

Lever WF, Schaumburg-Lever G: *Histopathology of the Skin,* ed 7. Philadelphia, JB Lippincott, 1990.

McGovern VJ, Mihm MC Jr, Bailly C: The classification of melanoma and its historical reporting. *Cancer* 1973; 32:1446–1457.

Mohs F: Chemosurgery. *Clin Plast Surg* 1980; 7:349.

Mulliken JB, Young AE: Hemangiomas and malformations, in *Vascular Birthmarks.* Philadelphia, WB Saunders, 1988.

Shanoff LB, Spira M, Hardy SB: Basal cell carcinoma: A statistical approach to rational management. *Plast Reconstr Surg* 1967; 39:619.

Chapter 12

Burns and Trauma

John O. Kucan, M.D.

■ CONTENTS

NOTE: The material in this chapter is frequently covered during the prerequisite training period of many plastic surgery residents. This chapter should serve as a valuable review of important material in such cases. For residents who have not mastered this material previously, this chapter is essential.

■ CHAPTER OBJECTIVE

At the end of this chapter the resident understands the physiology of burns and soft-tissue injury, the principles of burn resuscitation, and the techniques of burn wound repair and reconstruction and performs comprehensive, long-term management of burn and soft-tissue injuries.

■ LEARNER OBJECTIVES

On completion of this chapter, the resident

1. **Understands normal skin anatomy and circulation.**
2. **Understands the physiologic changes that occur with thermal injury, including the relationship between duration of exposure and temperature and the specific changes that occur in the zone of coagulation, stasis, and hyperemia.**
3. **Recognizes the rule of nines, the use of more detailed body surface charts, and the difference in relative body surface area in children vs. adults.**
4. **Knows the parameters that define major, moderate, and minor burns.**
5. **Knows the various factors in addition to body surface area that affect the prognosis of a patient with a thermal injury.**
6. **Understands the pathophysiology and treatment of inhalation injuries and carbon monoxide poisoning.**

7. **Understands the principles and techniques of fluid resuscitation, including isotonic and hypertonic techniques, and the principles of monitoring resuscitation.**
8. **Understands the pathophysiologic changes unique to chemical burns, including acid burns, alkali burns, chemotherapy extravasations, hydrofluoric acid burns, etc.**
9. **Recognizes injuries and sequelae associated with electrical injuries, including cardiac dysrhythmias, central nervous system damage, intra-abdominal injury, vascular injury, cataracts, etc.**
10. **Knows the anatomy and physiology pertinent to the excisional treatment of burns and treatment by split-thickness skin grafting.**
11. **Understands principles pertinent to burn rehabilitation and reconstruction, including aesthetic units of the face, tissue expansion, hair transplantation, hand splinting, etc.**
12. **Understands the pharmacology and utilization of topical antibacterial agents, analgesics, and antibiotics in the treatment of burns.**
13. Understands the basic theories pertaining to current flow, energy disposition, and the location and extent of injury associated with conductive and arc injuries from electrical current.
14. Understands the pathophysiology of acute and chronic radiation damage.
15. Understands the pathophysiology of frostbite and its natural history.

■ CLINICAL PRACTICE ACTIVITIES

During the course of the training program, the resident

1. **Evaluates patients with minor, moderate, and major burns of chemical, electrical, and thermal origin.**
2. **Manages outpatient burns operatively and nonoperatively.**
3. **Performs surgical treatment of acute burns, including escharotomies, fasciotomies, excision, grafting, etc.**
4. **Manages patients with burns of the hand, including operative treatment, postoperative therapy, and late reconstructive surgery.**
5. Manages inpatients with major burns, including resuscitation, treatment of inhalation injury, and rehabilitation.
6. Evaluates and treats patients with acute and chronic radiation injuries.
7. Manages patients with chemical burns, including intravenous infusion injuries.
8. Performs reconstructive surgery on burn patients, including functional and aesthetic procedures.
9. Manages patients with frostbite injuries.

Thermal injury continues to be a significant cause of morbidity and mortality. Burns affect all age groups and may be caused by a variety of agents, including heat, chemicals, electricity, and radiation. Extreme cold resulting in frostbite can also produce injury to the skin and deeper structures and give rise to considerable morbidity. The first priority in caring for a burned patient at the scene of the accident is to stop the burning process. The contact of smoldering clothing or clothing soaked with chemicals may result in ongoing injury unless the clothes are promptly removed. In the case of flame burns, prompt extinguishing of the flame is imperative and can be accomplished by the technique of stop, drop, and roll with the application of a blanket or other smothering agent or the use of water or other extinguishing liquids.

The last two decades have witnessed a significant improvement in the overall care of the burned patient. These advances are the direct result of a continuously expanding body of knowledge relative to the pathophysiology of thermal injury and its systemic consequences. Likewise, the rapid growth of medical technology and improved anesthesia and surgical techniques have had a major impact upon the treatment of these injuries.

These advances are reflected by a decreased mortality rate among those sustaining major thermal injury. In addition, the development and utilization of the burn team concept has produced highly positive results in the management of burn victims.

The objectives of burn care constitute the basic outline for management of thermally injured patients. The first objective is to do no harm. Other objectives include prevention and treatment of shock, control of bacterial growth, conversion of an open wound to a closed wound, preservation of body function and appearance, and attainment of these goals within a minimal amount of time. In seeking to attain these objectives, the preservation of the mental and emotional equilibrium of the patient is an equally important goal.

Over 2 million people sustain burn injuries in the United States every year. Between 100,000 and 150,000 of these patients require hospitalization. The number of people that die from burn injuries ranges from 7,000 to 10,000 annually. The areas of the body most frequently burned are the upper extremity (70%) and the head and neck region (55%), and the potential for disfigurement and functional loss resulting from injuries to these anatomic areas is clearly apparent.

Treatment of the burned patient is predicated upon the goals and objectives of burn care and requires a knowledge of the pathophysiology of thermal injury, an understanding of the impact of major comorbid factors, and the specific physiologic needs of the burn victim.

FUNCTION OF THE SKIN

The skin serves multiple functions. It is our major protection against the environment, prevents the loss of body fluids, and controls body temperature. In addition, it functions as an organ of excretion and sensation as well as providing cosmesis and identity. Thermal injury results in destruction or significant blunting of these major skin functions. The degree of impairment in the functions of the skin primarily depends on the depth of the burn injury and the total body surface area burn.

PATHOPHYSIOLOGY OF BURN WOUNDS

During the past decade, the burn wound has been the subject of intense scrutiny. Research in this area has demonstrated the burn wound itself to be the major culprit and primary causative agent of the numerous systemic problems that plague patients following major thermal injury.

The skin is a highly complex organ. The ability of the skin to regenerate following thermal injury depends on the depth of injury. Besides serving the important functions outlined earlier, the skin is also a component of the immune system. In addition to providing mechanical protection, it is involved in antibody production and is an element in both the cellular and humoral portions of the immune response to injury. Therefore, injury to the skin provokes significant immunologic changes in the patient. The contribution of the skin to the overall defense mechanisms is now becoming more apparent.

Injury to the skin is directly related to time and temperature. Once the temperature of 45°C has been exceeded, irreversible protein coagulation occurs (Fig 12–1). In 1953, Douglas Jackson described the three classic zones of burn injury. These include a central zone of irreversible injury, the zone of coagulation; a peripheral or marginal zone of reversible injury, the zone of hyperemia; and finally, a middle, potentially reversible zone of injury that may heal if the proper environment for healing can be achieved, the zone of stasis (Fig 12–2). The zone of stasis is the pivotal area of burn injury. Within this area, the microcirculation is profoundly affected. It is in this zone that progressive circulatory deterioration occurs from 24 to 48 hours following thermal injury. If effective treatment to the zone of stasis could be developed, the progressive deterioration of the burn wound could be halted. The result would be a significant decrease in the depth and extent of thermal injury.

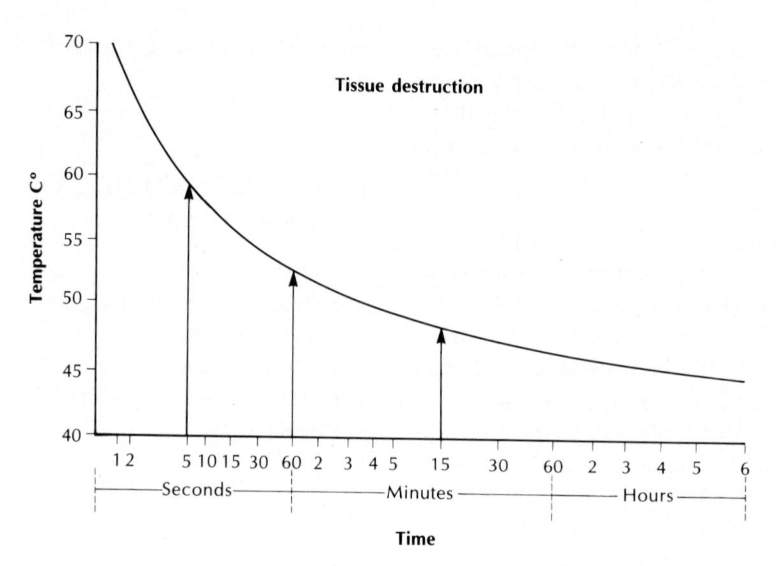

FIG 12–1.
Temperature duration curve. Tissue destruction proceeds logarithmically with increasing temperature as a function of time exposure. (From Robson MC, et al: 1979. Used by permission.)

The changes in the microcirculation following burning are not limited to the burn wound itself. A number of models for assessing the microcirculation at a distance from the burn wound reveal profound microcirculatory changes. These include neutrophil adherence and aggregation to the endothelium, sludging of red blood cells, development of edema in adjacent tissues, and an overall decrease in tissue perfusion. Another consequence of thermal injury is bacterial translocation through the intact gut of experimental animals following major burn, which may result in profound septic complications.

Thermal injury exerts direct effects on the cells of the burn wound. These direct effects of heat include immediate cell destruction and coagulation necrosis. In addition, there is intravascular destruction of red blood cells, so a population of red blood cells is effectively removed from the circulation. Also, additional red blood cells that pass through the damaged endothelium of the burn wound are altered, destroyed, or trapped in the burn wound. This produces a further decrease in the effective

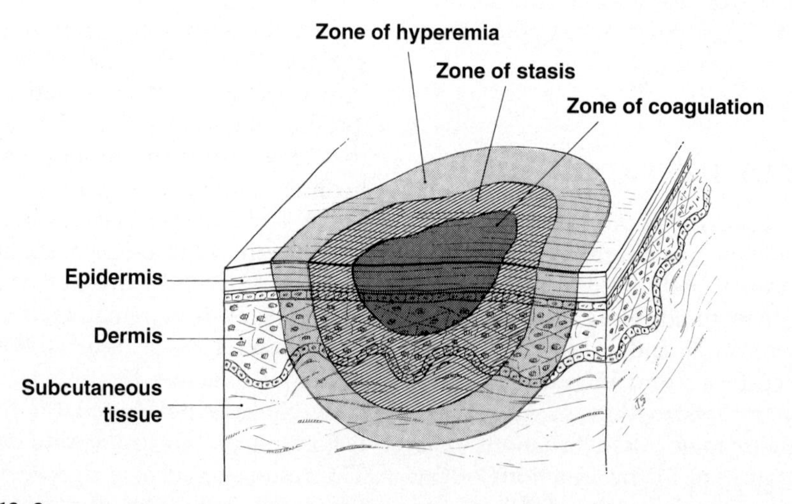

FIG 12–2.
Jackson's representation of the three classic zones of injury within the burn wound.

red blood cell volume and results in decreased oxygen carrying capacity and a diminished survival rate of red blood cells. Coupled with a marked decrease in red cell production, the problem of reduced oxygen carrying capacity becomes apparent in both the immediate and later phases of burn injury. The increased vascular permeability and obligatory edema of the burn wound itself further contribute to cessation of the microcirculation.

Following thermal injury, the local effects of cellular injury also become apparent. Injured cells liberate a variety of vasoactive substances. Thus, the normal transmembrane potential of the injured cells is reduced, which results in an influx of sodium ions and the obligatory movement of water into cells to correct the hyperosmolar state. The net result is tissue edema. The burn wound also induces numerous systemic effects. There is a general alteration of the normal hormonal milieu with elaboration of stress hormones by the neurohumoral axis. Numerous toxic substances are liberated into the circulation, and the immunologic alterations of thermal injury become apparent. Complement is activated by the alternative pathway. Stimulation of neutrophils results in the release of oxygen-derived free radicals, which produce additional microcirculatory damage. A rapid depletion of circulating immunoglobulins and clotting factors along with an altered lymphocyte population and helper/suppressor cell ratio is seen.

A number of biochemical mediators are released from the burn wound, and these induce both local and systemic changes. The initial vasoconstriction is followed by histamine-mediated vasodilation. Kinins and serotonin are produced. The liberation of arachidonic acid metabolites resulting in either leukotriene or thromboxane production results in additional neutrophil aggregation and vasoconstriction. The release of oxygen-derived free radicals further contributes to microvascular injury and subsequent thrombosis. The net results of thermal injury are local and systemic changes that have profound effects on the physiologic response of the burn victim (Table 12–1).

Thermal injury exerts a direct tissue effect and a generalized systemic effect. Further

TABLE 12–1.
Mediators of the Inflammatory Response

Histamine
Kinins
Serotonin
Arachidonic acid metabolites
Prostaglandins
Thromboxane
Leukotrienes
Oxygen-derived free radicals
Lipid peroxidases

progress in burn care will be the result of pharmacologic manipulation of the zone of stasis and interruption of the effects of vasoactive substances at both the local and systemic levels. Presently, cooling of the burn wound is the only available modality for limiting some of the microcirculatory changes in the burn wound. Cooling, when initiated within the first 30 minutes of injury, has been shown to significantly decrease the progression of the burn wound. This method is applicable in the emergency treatment of small burn wounds. However, the risk of hypothermia and metabolic consequences precludes the use of cooling in patients with extensive body surface area burn wounds.

Traditionally, the depth of the burn wound has been classified in degrees of injury (Fig 12–3). *First-degree* burn wounds involve only the outer layer of the epidermis and are characterized by erythema and mild discomfort. There is minimal tissue damage, and the protective functions of the skin are essentially intact. Pain usually resolves in the first 48 to 72 hours, and healing occurs rapidly. There is no residual scarring. First-degree burns are not included in the calculation of total body surface area burn. *Second-degree* burns are classified as those that involve the entire thickness of the epidermis and variable portions of the dermis. A more appropriate method of classifying such injuries is to refer to them as *partial-thickness injuries*. Therefore, a superficial second-degree burn, also classified as a superficial partial-thickness burn wound, involves heat destruction of the upper levels of the dermis. The microvasculature in this area is injured, and tissue permeability is altered. This results in leakage of large amounts of plasma into the interstitium, blis-

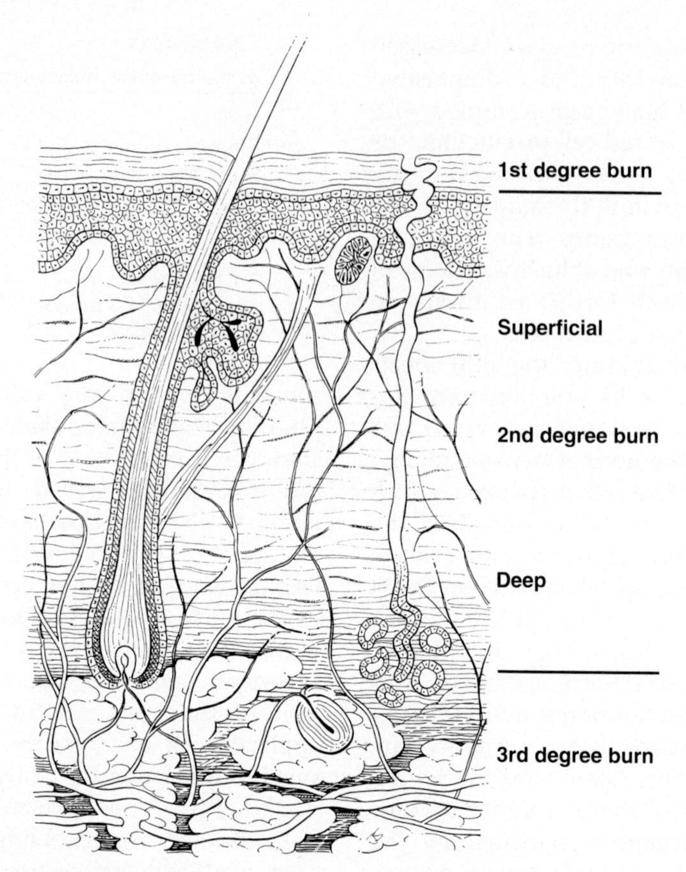

FIG 12–3.
Scheme of normal skin histology and the categorization of burn injury.

ter formation, and the development of obligatory tissue edema. Such burn wounds are extraordinarily painful since a large number of sensory nerve endings are exposed. These wounds, however, generally heal within 7 to 14 days, provided that desiccation of the wound and secondary bacterial infection are prevented. In most cases, scarring following such injuries is minimal.

Intermediate and deep second-degree partial-thickness burn wounds involve a significant thickness of the dermal layer, and injury to the epidermal appendages is considerable. Therefore, reepithelialization in such wounds is generally slow and unpredictable. Blister formation does not occur. A large amount of necrotic tissue is present, and this may result in a wound that is grossly indistinguishable from a *third-degree* or full-thickness injury. The blood supply in such wounds may be marginal, and progression to a deeper injury is frequently noted. Pain is present in variable degrees but is far less than that seen with more superficial injuries, given the destruction of neurosensory organs. The metabolic effects and fluid losses that are characteristic of deep dermal burn wounds are essentially the same as those seen following third-degree injury. Substantial scar formation is frequently observed when such wounds are allowed to heal by secondary intention. The functional and cosmetic results following spontaneous healing of deep, partial-thickness burn wounds is predictably poor, and the tendency toward hypertrophic scar formation is great.

Full-thickness or *third-degree* burns are defined as those in which the entire dermis is destroyed. This results in absence of epidermal appendages within the dermis and thus an inability to heal by reepithelialization. Healing of such wounds is possible only by replacement of the devitalized tissue by skin grafting. Healing by secondary intention may be possible when these wounds involve only small areas of the body and where the functional consequences of such healing are minimal. Most often, however, spontaneous healing of full-thickness burns results in severe deformity or functional disorders, e.g., burn scar contractures. In a full-thickness burn wound, completely coagulated dermal blood vessels result in a totally avascular burn wound. The burned tissue has a waxy, white, or charred appearance. Occasionally, a cherry-red appearance is noted (particularly in young children or elderly patients); this does not represent viable tissue but rather fixed carboxyhemoglobin within the tissues.

SEVERITY OF BURN INJURIES

Several factors exert a profound influence on patient outcome following thermal injury. These include the size and depth of the burn injury, the location of the injury, the patient's age, the presence of associated injuries, the presence of preexisting or coexisting diseases, and inhalation injury. The total body surface area burned in addition to the depth of injury and the age of the patient are major parameters that have an influence on survival. Inhalation injuries superimposed upon thermal injury profoundly affect the prognosis for survival and greatly increase the mortality rate in these patients.

The extent of the burned surface area can be estimated by using the rule of 9s. Each arm constitutes 9% of the total body surface area; each leg, 18%; the anterior portion of the trunk, 18%; the posterior portion of the trunk, 18%; and the head and neck, 9%. In small children, modification of this rule is necessary, for the head size in very young children approaches 18% of the total body surface area. The depth of burn is a significant prognostic factor; patients with deeper burn wounds fare worse than do patients with more superficial burn wounds of the same body surface area. Age is an important comorbid factor because patients in the extremes of age (children under 3 years of age, adults over 60 years of age) tolerate burn injury poorly. A number of factors are operative in these patients. In the very young, the higher mortality rate is the result of several factors, including an incompletely developed immune system, immature organs, and an underdeveloped physiologic response to major trauma. In the elderly, the general deterioration of body systems and the reduced ability to deal with major physiologic stress in combination with numerous preexisting medical diseases result in an increased mortality rate.

The American Burn Association has categorized burn injuries into major, moderate, and minor categories (Table 12–2). This classification is helpful in deciding the level of care needed for patients following thermal

TABLE 12–2.
Categorization of Burn Injuries (American Burn Association)

Feature	Major Burn	Moderate Burn	Minor Burn
Size—partial thickness	>25% adults >20% children	10%–25% adults 10%–20% children	<15% adults <10% children
Size—full thickness	>10%	2%–10%	<2%
Primary areas	Major burn if involved	Not involved	Not involved
Inhalation injury	Major burn if present or suspected	Not suspected	Not suspected
Associated injury	Major burn if present	Not present	Not present
Comorbid factors	Poor-risk patients make the burn major	Patient relatively good risk	Not present
Miscellaneous	Electrical injuries		
Treatment environment	Usually specialized burn care facility	General hospital with designated team	Often managed as an outpatient

injuries. In general, those patients who have sustained a large body surface area burn, those with extensive full-thickness involvement, and any patient with significant comorbid factors or involvement of special areas, including the hand, the face, the feet, and the perineum, should be cared for in a specialized burn care facility.

A more precise way to determine the extent of burn injury is to use a burn diagram known as the Lund-Browder chart (Fig 12–4). Careful mapping of the distribution of the burn wound in conjunction with an estimate of depth and calculation of the total area of involvement will produce a reasonably accurate estimation of the burn size. In addition, the various complications and comorbid factors can be tallied on this sheet. This provides a useful starting point for planning fluid resuscitation, developing a prognostic index, and initiating a needs assessment and plan of action for the burn victim.

INHALATION INJURY

It has been estimated that between 15% and 25% of patients admitted to burn centers in the United States have sustained at least some degree of inhalation injury. Currently, pulmonary complications following thermal injury constitute the primary cause of mortality in burn patients and are responsible for up to 70% of thermal injury–related deaths (Table 12–3). Pulmonary complications in burn patients may be the result of inhalation injury or may arise in conjunction with a purely thermal cutaneous burn. The management of these life-threatening problems is virtually identical. Patients who sustain inhalation injury may demonstrate a spectrum of symptoms ranging from minimal to severe. Even those patients who show minimal initial symptoms may deteriorate and have severe life-threatening complications. Therefore, the identification of inhalation injury and institution of prompt and directed treatment are imperative.

Therapy begins with the diagnosis of inhalation injury based on an accurate history. A history of closed-space injury or extrication of an unconscious patient from a fire in an enclosed space should strongly suggest the possibility of inhalation injury. Physical examination may elicit specific physical signs suggestive of inhalation injury, including circumoral burns, burns or injection of the pharynx, singeing of nasal hairs, respiratory distress, progressive hoarseness, bronchorrhea, production of carbonaceous sputum, and conjunctivitis. Although initial chest x-ray studies may be normal, this does not exclude the diagnosis of inhalation injury. Fiberoptic bronchoscopy can positively identify injuries to the large airways and has both diagnostic and therapeutic value. Xenon 133 lung scanning may also be employed and reveals injury to the smaller airways. In general, however, macroscopic bronchoscopic findings will positively identify upper airway changes consistent with inhalation injury and often precludes the need for xenon lung scanning.

Three classic stages of inhalation injuries have been described: (1) acute respiratory distress occurring immediately after inhalation injury or arising within 12 hours of injury, (2) adult respiratory distress syndrome (ARDS) beginning within 1 to 5 days following injury, and (3) bronchial pneumonia developing as early as 3 days or as late as 10 days following inhalation injury. The presence of an inhalation injury in conjunction with thermal injury generally doubles the mortality rate of thermal injury alone, whereas development of bronchial pneumonia following thermal injury may carry a 60% to 70% mortality rate.

Pulmonary injury is generally the result of inhaling incomplete products of combustion and the consequent development of a chemical pneumonitis. True burns of the airways below the level of the larynx are extremely uncommon since the upper airway readily buffers the heat of smoke and the injury is usually confined to the larynx and upper part of the trachea. The primary exception is the inhalation of live steam, which has a heat carrying capacity 400 times that of dry air.

In the immediate period following exposure to smoke, carbon monoxide poisoning is a major concern and a frequent cause of death. Since carbon monoxide has a binding affinity for the hemoglobin molecule that is 210 to 240

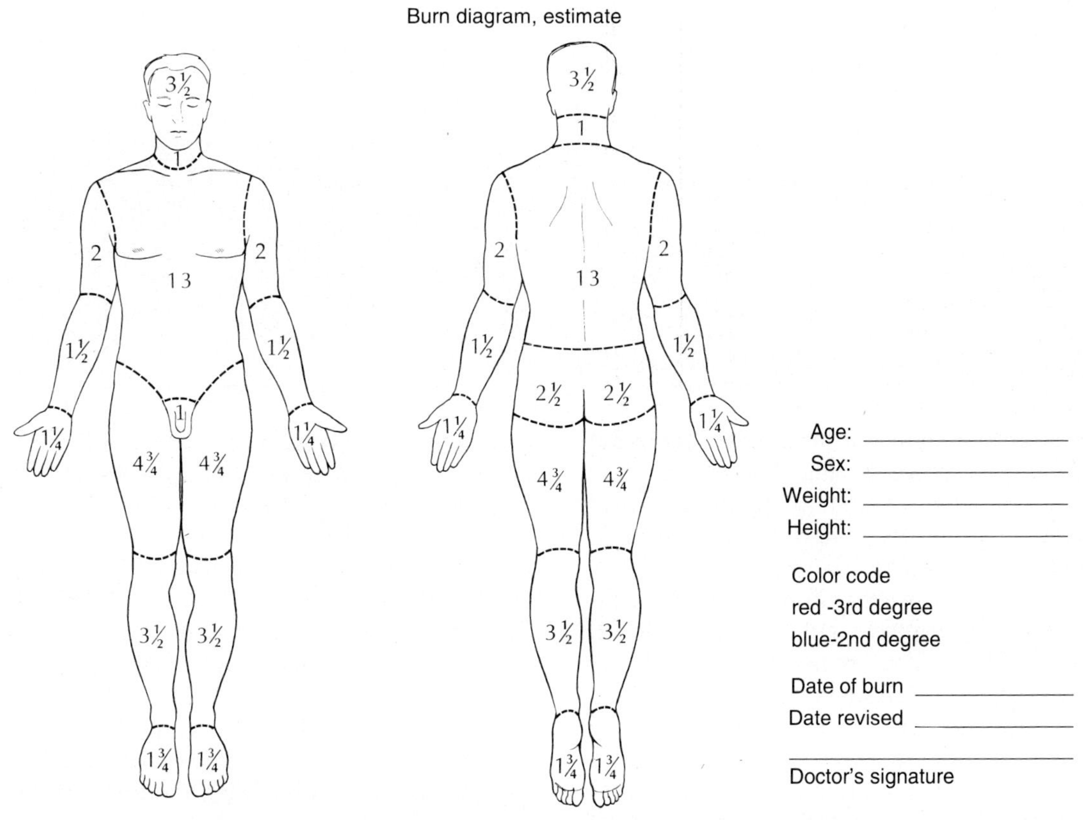

Area	Infant	1–4	5–9	10–14	15	Adult	2°	3°	Total	COMPLICATIONS LIST
Head	19	17	13	11	9	7				1.
Neck	2	2	2	2	2	2				2.
Anterior trunk	13	13	13	13	13	13				3.
Posterior trunk	13	13	13	13	13	13				4.
Right buttock	2½	2½	2½	2½	2½	2½				5.
Left buttock	2½	2½	2½	2½	2½	2½				6.
Genitalia	1	1	1	1	1	1				7.
Right upper arm	4	4	4	4	4	4				8.
Left upper arm	4	4	4	4	4	4				9.
Right lower arm	3	3	3	3	3	3				10.
Left lower arm	3	3	3	3	3	3				11.
Right hand	2½	2½	2½	2½	2½	2½				
Left hand	2½	2½	2½	2½	2½	2½				
Right thigh	5½	6½	8	8½	9	9½				
Left thigh	5½	6½	8	8½	9	9½				
Right leg	5	5	5½	6	6½	7				
Left leg	5	5	5½	6	6½	7				
Right foot	3½	3½	3½	3½	3½	3½				
Left foot	3½	3½	3½	3½	3½	3½				
						Total				

Lund-Browder chart

FIG 12–4.
Lund-Browder chart to estimate the extent of burn injury.

TABLE 12–3.
Incidence and Mortality of Inhalation Injury as Related to Total Body Surface Area Burn*

			Mortality (%)	
TBSA Burn (%)	No. of Patients	With Inhalation Injury (%)	Without Inhalation Injury	With Inhalation Injury
0–20	627	2	1	36
21–40	200	11	2	38
41–60	102	20	18	50
61–80	56	32	24	67
81–100	33	55	47	63

* Both the incidence and mortality rate increase with increasing size of the burn.

times greater than that of oxygen, the resultant displacement of the oxygen molecule from hemoglobin results in significant tissue hypoxia. In addition, high concentrations of carbon monoxide have been shown to directly interfere with the cytochrome system, further augmenting the toxic effects. In addition to carbon monoxide, frequently encountered toxic substances of smoke include hydrogen cyanide, nitrogen dioxide, carbon dioxide, hydrogen chloride, benzene, acrolein, chlorine, and phosgene (Table 12–4). These components of smoke are carried into the airways and may be highly soluble and cause severe local irritation. In addition, the inhalation of suspended particulate material may produce further damage as a result of their mechanical effects. Many of these substances initiate acute bronchospasm, while others such as hydrogen chloride and acrolein produce acute pulmonary edema.

Indications for endotracheal intubation in the burn patient include the presence of supraglottic edema and inflammation on bronchoscopy, progressive hoarseness or air hunger, coma or respiratory depression, acute respiratory distress, full-thickness burns of the face or circumoral region, circumferential neck burns, and a blood gas picture indicative of respiratory distress or failure.

A number of pathologic processes may act in concert to produce respiratory failure following thermal injury. These include the direct toxic effects of smoke, the development of atelectasis and shunting, and numerous iatrogenic factors such as fluid overload, patient position, narcotics, and controlled ventilation. Aspiration, a low-flow state, and the trapping of neutrophils with liberation of free oxygen radicals also contribute to pulmonary dysfunction. All of these elements may act together to produce a profound, vicious cycle that frequently results in death. The effect of smoke on lung surfactant results in greatly diminished pulmonary compliance, reduced oxygen exchange, atelectasis, and respiratory failure. The addition of a circumferential chest burn may restrict chest expansion, thus contributing to ventilatory difficulty (Fig 12–5).

Laboratory studies to aid in the diagnosis include arterial blood gas analysis and determination of carbon monoxide levels. When pure carbon monoxide poisoning is encountered, it should be treated aggressively with

TABLE 12–4.
Common Toxic Products of Combustion

Substance	Toxic Products
Polyvinylchloride	Hydrogen chloride, phosgene, chlorine
Wood, cotton, paper	Acrolein, acetaldehyde, formaldehyde, acetic acid, formic acid
Petroleum products	Acrolein, acetic acid, formic acid
Nitrocellulose film	Oxides of nitrogen, acetic acid, formic acid
Nitrogen-containing compounds (polyurethane)	Isocyanate, hydrogen cyanide
Polyfluorocarbons (Teflon)	Octafluoroisobutylene
Melamine resins	Ammonia, hydrogen cyanide

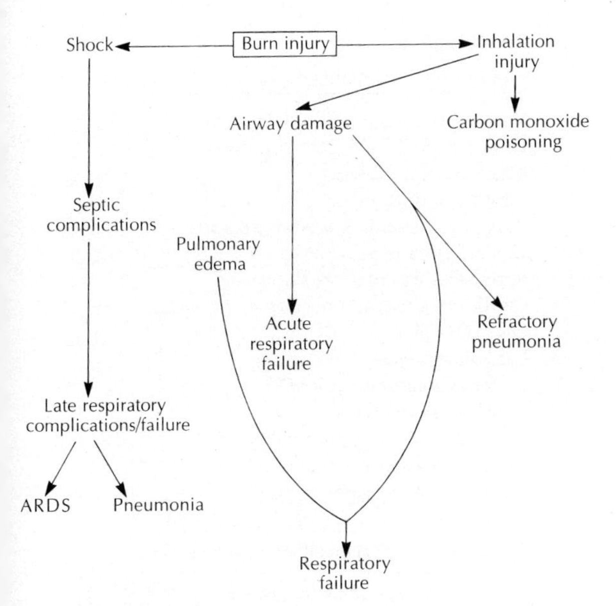

FIG 12–5.
Scheme of pulmonary complications (ARDS = adult respiratory distress syndrome).

100% oxygen until the carboxyhemoglobin levels have fallen below 10%. The use of hyperbaric oxygen for carbon monoxide poisoning has been described, but the overall utility of this modality has not been assessed in a prospective fashion. Carbon monoxide levels frequently serve as reasonable, indirect indicators of the severity of inhalation injuries. Likewise, the presence of hypoxemia, hypercarbia, and acidosis provides additional important information regarding the presence and potential severity of inhalation injury. An assay of complement C5a to detect inhalation injury has been described.

The treatment of inhalation injury and other pulmonary complications of thermal injury is primarily supportive and expectant. There are few hard and fast rules. However, treatment should be implemented before the establishment of a definitive diagnosis. Foremost is the provision of an adequate airway. One hundred percent humidified oxygen should be administered as soon as possible. The administration of intravenous bronchodilators may be helpful in countering the acute irritation of smoke on the tracheobronchial tree. Control of the upper airway must be achieved by prompt endotracheal intubation, where indicated, and ventilatory support established. Early tracheostomy in these patients should be avoided because of the demonstrated twofold to fourfold increase in pulmonary septic complications.

Fluid resuscitation should be carefully monitored but should be adequate to maintain a normal cardiac output. Recent studies have demonstrated that hypovolemia in the presence of inhalation injury may increase margination of neutrophils in the pulmonary vascular beds, thus setting the stage for possible reperfusion injury and increased severity of microcirculatory damage in the pulmonary vasculature. Hypertonic saline resuscitation may be employed in these patients to minimize the potential for hypervolemia. The use of invasive monitoring should be employed on a case-by-case basis. Diuretics may be required. Sputum cultures and sputum surveillance by Gram stains are obtained at the initiation of therapy and then on a regular basis. This permits bacteriologic monitoring of the tracheal bronchial tree and institution of appropriate antibiotic therapy based upon positive culture data. Prophylactic antibiotics should not be used, and steroids should be avoided. Serial bronchoscopy is an important adjunct to critical care of these patients. The use of bronchodilators may be effective in treating airway obstruction. Recently, heparinized saline lavage of the tracheobronchial tree has been shown to be a useful adjunct in caring for patients with inhalation injury.

Despite maximum supportive care, the development of fatal complications is not infrequent. Nevertheless, prompt institution of appropriate therapy based upon a high index of suspicion and adherence to the aforementioned guidelines may help to salvage even those patients who have sustained significant pulmonary injury.

FLUID RESUSCITATION

Fluid resuscitation is an essential component of initial care. Placement of a peripheral intravenous line through nonburned tissue is the preferred route for fluid administration. It is generally accepted that patients with burn wounds exceeding 15% of their total body surface area require fluid resuscitation and resuscitation should be individualized and based upon the patient's response (burn formulas serve only as guides for the initiation of fluid resuscitation). Successful resuscitation requires continual monitoring with frequent corrections and adjustments in the rates of fluid administration.

Resuscitation begins with a calculation of the patient's weight and an accurate determination of the extent of body surface area burn. A large-bore intravenous catheter is placed and fluid replacement initiated. Another component of initial therapy is the placement of a nasogastric tube in patients with burns exceeding 20% of the total body surface area or in patients who have sustained facial burns, especially children. A Foley catheter should also be inserted.

A number of formulas have been described and successfully employed in resuscitating burned patients. The objective of initial fluid resuscitation is to restore and maintain tissue reperfusion, avoid organ ischemia, and preserve viability in the zone of stasis within the burn wound. The failure rate for initial volume resuscitation is less than 5% in major burn centers. The historic problem of hypovolemia, which is now aggressively corrected, has been replaced by the problem of generalized burn edema formation, which is the result of overresuscitation. The consequences of fluid overload include decreased oxygen delivery, further ischemia to already damaged cells, and pulmonary insufficiency as a result of chest wall edema or pulmonary edema. Thus, overhydration may be as serious a problem as underhydration.

The success of fluid resuscitation is based upon frequent and appropriate monitoring of the patient (Table 12–5). Arterial blood pressure, because of the initial catecholamine response, is not a sensitive measure of adequate fluid replacement. The pulse rate is usually more helpful. In older patients, however, the pulse rate may be less reliable because the heart is unable to increase its rate in response to volume deficits. The direct measurement of intracardiac filling pressure or pulmonary capillary wedge pressure may be misleading in patients who have sustained burn injuries exceeding 25% to 30% of their total body surface area. Because burns of this magnitude are accompanied by generalized capillary leakage, it is not possible to accurately replace fluids by attempting to increase filling pressures to an arbitrary number. Measurements of cardiac output may be very helpful in this situation. It should also be remembered that complications of central and Swan-Ganz lines are far greater in a burn patient than in a critically ill patient without cutaneous burn injuries. Urine output has been found to be a very useful guide since maintenance of renal blood flow will reflect adequate perfusion to other organs as well. A urine output of 0.5 to 1 mL/kg of body weight per hour in an adult and 1 mL/kg of body weight per hour in a child is considered adequate.

TABLE 12–5.
Monitoring Parameters

Vital signs, sensorium, anxiety level*
Urine output*
Mean arterial pressure
Cardiac output/index*
Pulmonary capillary wedge pressure
Central venous pressure
Peripheral vascular resistance
Continuous tissue probes (pH, O_2, CO_2)
Laser Doppler
Laboratory tests
Hemoglobin/hematocrit*
Serum electrolytes*
Serum and urine osmolality
BUN, creatinine
Arterial blood gas*
Urinalysis

* Most useful clinical monitoring parameters.

The maintenance of acid-base balance is also a good measure of tissue perfusion since a persistent base deficit is indicative of inadequate tissue perfusion. In cases of inhalation injury, titration of fluid to the amount necessary to maintain organ perfusion is essential. In the presence of hemoglobinuria or myoglobinuria as seen in large body surface area burns of significant depth or following high-voltage electrical injury, an increase in the amount of fluid administered and the addition of mannitol and alkalizing agents (e.g., Na^{2+}

bicarbonate) to the intravenous fluids are necessary. In general, fluids that contain salt but are free of glucose are appropriate for resuscitation following burn injuries. The intravenous route is necessary in burns exceeding 20% of the body surface area since a paralytic ileus usually accompanies burns of this or greater size. Lactated Ringer's solution with a sodium concentration of 130 mEq/L is most popular. In children under the age of 3 years, the use of a dextrose-containing resuscitation fluid such as 5% dextrose in lactated Ringer's solution is appropriate because of the limited glucose stores in very young patients.

Edema formation, which is characteristic of thermal injuries, produces a loss of intravascular volume with leakage of significant quantities of protein from the intravascular space. The result is an osmotic gradient into the injured tissues. In burns exceeding 25% to 30% of the body surface area, this capillary leak becomes generalized as the result of markedly increased vascular permeability. Thus, overall edema in burn patients is evident. Furthermore, an alteration in the normal cell membrane potential produces an intracellular migration of sodium, which in turn draws water into the intracellular space and results in cellular swelling. The net result is edema of the interstitial tissue, which becomes maximal 12 to 18 hours following thermal injury and then gradually stabilizes and begins to recede. The restoration of normal membrane potentials occurs at approximately 24 to 36 hours after injury, depending upon the adequacy of volume resuscitation and restoration of tissue perfusion. The provision of colloid during the period of maximum edema formation, usually 24 to 30 hours following injury, will increase the intravascular oncotic pressure, thus drawing the edema fluid from the interstitium back to the intravascular space. Complete restoration of intravascular volume during the acute phase is not possible despite adequate fluid resuscitation as evidenced by progressively rising hematocrit values during the first 24 hours following burn injury.

Crystalloid resuscitation is based primarily on the calculated deficit in sodium ion that is lost from the intravascular space. This has been estimated to be 0.5 to 0.6 mEq per percent body surface area burn per kilogram of body weight. Therefore, 4 mL of lactated Ringer's solution per kilogram of body weight per percent body surface area burn will be required in the first 24 hours (Table 12–6). The rate of fluid administration is initially calculated by giving half of the 24-hour volume over the first 8 hours and the subsequent half over the succeeding 16 hours. It should be emphasized, however, that the rate of fluid infusion must be dictated by the patient's response and the variables employed for monitoring. The formula, in effect, sets the first hour's infusion rate.

Sodium is the major element in crystalloid resuscitation, with water serving as the solvent. Solutions with increased sodium concentrations have a theoretical advantage over isotonic or hypotonic solutions. The hypertonic salt solutions used clinically have a concentration of 400 to 600 mOsm/L and can generate osmotic pressure of several thousand millimeters of mercury in excess of normal. Therefore, use of hypertonic solutions is thought to decrease the net fluid flux into the burn wound. Hypertonic sodium solutions have been reported to increase myocardial contractility, produce precapillary dilatation, and decrease vascular resistance. Theoretical advantages of hypertonic fluid resuscitation include decreased edema formation as well as a lower incidence of paralytic ileus. Indications for the use of hypertonic resuscitation include patients with inhalation injury, patients with burn wounds in excess of 40% of

TABLE 12–6.
Parkland Formula

Adults	
LR*, 4 mL/kg/% BSA* burn	
½ over first 8 hr	
½ over second 16 hr	
Children	
LR, 3 mL/kg/% BSA burn	
½ over first 8 hr	
½ over second 16 hr + maintenance	
(100 mL/kg for first 10 kg)	per 24 hr
(50 mL/kg for second 10 kg)	per 24 hr
(20 mL/kg for over 20 kg)	per 24 hr

* LR = lactated Ringer's solution; % BSA = percent body surface area.

their body surface area, and hemodynamically unstable patients in whom fluid overloading will be poorly tolerated such as the elderly. The disadvantages of hypertonic resuscitation include relative complexity and the requirement of careful monitoring. Complications include hypernatremia, hyperosmolar coma, renal failure, and alkalosis with a left shift of the oxygen dissociation curve. Serum sodium levels must be monitored closely in patients receiving this form of resuscitation, and sodium levels should not be allowed to exceed 160 mEq/L. If this degree of hypernatremia does occur, a slightly hypotonic solution such as lactated Ringer's should be infused until the hypernatremia has been corrected.

Colloid infusions generally commence 12 to 24 hours after the burn injury and are given at a rate of 0.35 to 1 mL/kg per percent body surface area burn. The amount given depends upon the magnitude of injury, the degree of hemodynamic stability, and the overall concern over excess edema formation. Colloid infusion is usually provided over a 6-hour period. Fresh frozen plasma is preferred because it contains protein fractions that produce both oncotic and nononcotic properties. Fresh frozen plasma also contains the clotting factors necessary to assist early burn wound excision, as well as fibronectin, an important opsonin for circulating microaggregates.

Following administration of crystalloid and colloid during the first 24 to 30 hours after a burn injury, one may anticipate a restoration of the altered cell membrane potential, a gradual decrease in capillary endothelial leakage, and a gradual sodium diuresis. As fluid losses into the burned and unburned tissue diminish, a second major source of fluid loss becomes readily apparent. Because the skin loses its normal barrier function, evaporation from the burn surface occurs. The magnitude of this loss depends on the depth of the burn and the character of the burned tissue. Initially, thick dry eschar has less net water loss than a moist eschar or one that contains viable dermis. These additional insensible losses must be taken into consideration and replaced. A reasonable estimate of such losses can be quantitated by the following formula: evaporative loss (mL/hr) = 25 + percent body surface area burn × surface area (m^2) (e.g., 25 + 40% body surface area burn × 1.73 m^2 = 112 mL/hr, or 2,699 mL/24 hr). Therefore, maintenance fluid in the form of dextrose and water should be provided during this period. Dextrose is necessary because the glucose stores have been depleted during the initial catecholamine release and volume resuscitation. Potassium replacement may also be necessary. The serum sodium concentration should be monitored every 4 to 6 hours and free water either provided or restricted based on the serum sodium concentration. The need for blood replacement may become apparent during this period, and blood transfusions should be given to maintain a hematocrit of 30% to 35%.

Careful assessment of the status of circumferentially burned extremities, the chest wall, and the neck is important during the initial postburn resuscitation. A restricting eschar that overlies the burn wound in deep partial-thickness or full-thickness injuries may interfere with circulation and restrict chest wall movement. Patients who have sustained circumferential burns of the extremities must be monitored carefully for signs of impending compartment syndrome. Clinical observation alone may be insufficient, while the use of Doppler measurements may provide erroneous information. Direct muscle compartment measurements may need to be carried out in circumferential burned extremities.

The patient's ability to adequately ventilate in the presence of circumferential chest and neck burns must be carefully assessed. Chest wall escharotomies may be necessary in patients who have an endotracheal tube but require continual increases in ventilator pressure in order to provide adequate ventilation. Surgical escharotomies should be carried out with attention to detail so that a complete escharotomy with effective hemostasis is achieved. An incomplete escharotomy is of no benefit. Occasionally, especially in the lower extremities, escharotomy may be insufficient, and fasciotomy may be necessary. High-voltage electrical injuries generally mandate fasciotomies with decompression of major neural structures in areas of known compression neuropathies such as the carpal tunnel and the canal of Guyon. The morbidity associated with surgical escharotomies may be significant. This is generally the result of inadequate hemostasis along with significant and occasionally life-threatening hemorrhage from escharotomy sites and the later development of septic complications in surgical escharotomy wounds.

An alternative to surgical escharotomy is a chemical or medical escharotomy employing sutilains ointment (Travase). The application of sutilains ointment to an acute burn wound can achieve effective decompression of circumferential extremity and thorax burns. This method is ineffective in charred full-thickness burn injuries, in wounds that are dry and desiccated, or in situations where the time from injury to treatment is significantly prolonged.

CARE OF BURN WOUNDS

Closure of burn wounds remains the primary goal in the management of burned patients. However, before closure of the burn wound can be achieved, proper care must be delivered to the wound to enhance healing of superficial partial-thickness wounds, to prevent conversion of deeper wounds to full-thickness injury, or to prepare deep burn wounds for ultimate closure. Additional tissue damage must be avoided by the prevention of desiccation and infection.

The majority of infections in burn patients are endogenous. Normal skin contains relatively large numbers and numerous varieties of bacteria, all of which are capable of producing invasive burn wound sepsis. Following thermal injury, the resulting avascular burn wound serves as an excellent culture medium for bacterial proliferation. Because of the avascular nature of the burn wound, systemic antibiotics are ineffective in controlling bacterial growth in this area. Thus topical antibacterial agents are necessary to control bacterial proliferation in the burn wound. There is no single ideal topical antibacterial agent (Table 12–7). All may be useful adjuncts in the care of the burn wound, but all have specific deficiencies. Silver sulfadiazine cream is the most widely employed topical antimicrobial agent in the United States. Although it is generally safe and effective in controlling bacterial growth, it does not penetrate the burn wound to any great extent, and therefore its activity is primarily limited to the surface of the burn wound. Silver sulfadiazine cream is painless and nontoxic and is generally well tolerated by patients. Although it does not produce any metabolic side effects, it has been associated with neutropenia in burn patients and has been shown to delay healing of burn wounds. Mafenide acetate (Sulfamylon cream) with an active concentration of 11.2% was the first topical agent shown to be effective against *Pseudomonas* burn wound sepsis. This agent, however, has been relegated to second-line status in the management of burn injuries because of metabolic side effects and pain associated with its application to partial-thickness wounds. Sulfamylon cream produces a metabolic acidosis with a compensatory respiratory alkalosis because it is a potent carbonic anhydrase inhibitor. Also, it results in hyperventilation and may produce irreversible pulmonary edema in patients with inhalation injuries. It is a strong desiccating agent on wounds because of its high osmolality (2,000 mOsm/L). Nonetheless, Sulfamylon cream remains the "gold standard" for topical antimicrobial therapy because of its ability to penetrate intact eschar, its broad spectrum of activity, and its potency against gram-positive as well as gram-negative and anaerobic organisms.

Silver nitrate, 0.5% solution, is used infrequently. It is ineffective in treating established burn wound sepsis since it does not penetrate eschar and, in the presence of certain organisms, may produce methemoglobinemia. Nitrofurazone ointment (Furacin) is effective against staphylococci and is frequently substituted for silver sulfadiazine (Silvadene cream) when emergence of silver sulfadiazine–resistant staphylococci are noted in the burn wound.

The effectiveness of burn wound therapy is assessed by quantitative bacteriology, histologic examination of burn wound biopsy specimens, and the overall status of the patient. Some controversy continues regard-

TABLE 12–7.
Topical Antibacterial Agents*

	Silver Sulfadiazine Cream (Silvadene)	Mafenide Cream (Sulfamylon Burn Cream)	Silver Nitrate Soaks	Nitrofurazone Ointment (Furacin Ointment)
Form of treatment	Occlusive dressing	Exposure	Occlusive dressings	Occlusive
Concentration of active agent (%)	1	11.2	0.5	0.2
Advantages	Painless on application; wound readily visible when cream is applied without dressings; compatible with treatment of associated injuries; motion of involved joints is maintained	Penetrates eschar; wound readily visible; compatible with treatment of associated injuries; no gram-negative resistance identified; motion of involved joints is maintained	No hypersensitivity; painless except at time of dressing change; no gram-negative resistance; reduces heat loss from wound; most compatible with hypertonic resuscitation regimen	Broad-spectrum activity, especially effective against Silvadene-resistant staphylococci; relatively nontoxic to epithelial cells
Limitations	Poor penetration of eschar; bone marrow suppression with neutropenia; hypersensitivity (infrequent); resistance of many *Enterobacter cloacae* and some *Pseudomonas*	Painful for 20–30 min after application to second-degree burns; accentuates postburn hyperventilation; hypersensitivity noted in 7% of patients; delays spontaneous eschar separation	No penetration of eschar; marked transeschar loss of Na^+, K^+, Ca^{++}, and Cl^-; methemoglobinemia (rare); dressings limit motion of involved joints; discolors unburned skin of patient, skin of attending personnel, and any environmental objects in contact	No penetration; polyethylene glycol in base may produce renal impairment, increased BUN, anion gap, and metabolic acidosis

* Adapted from Print BA: *Curr Probl Surg* 1979; 16:5. Used by permission.

ing the reliability of swab techniques as opposed to burn wound biopsy methods in longitudinal bacteriologic assessment of the burn wound. It is essential, however, that the bacteriologic flora of the burn unit be carefully evaluated and followed. This permits a more enlightened approach in the selection of topical antibacterials and systemic antibiotics when wounds or systemic complications dictate their use. Continuous bacteriologic surveillance and the use of agar well diffusion studies to assess the susceptibility of bacterial isolates to topical antibacterial agents is of great importance.

The absolute number of bacteria is of far greater clinical importance than the mere presence of bacteria in the burn wound. Thus, burn wound sepsis has been defined, in numerical terms, as the presence of greater than 10^5 bacteria per gram of tissue in the burn wound. The presence of a solitary septic focus in the burn wound, however, may not itself be productive of systemic disease. However, when systemic signs of sepsis develop, prompt, effective intervention is imperative. The differentiation between gram-positive and gram-negative sepsis can be reasonably achieved from a number of clinical parameters, including the rapidity of onset of symptoms, fever, the presence or absence of hypotension, oliguria, leukocytosis, and the mental status of the patient. Examination of the burn wound on a daily or twice-daily basis is essential. Close observation of the burn wound may reveal septic foci or areas of changing or deteriorating burn eschar. Prompt institution of local and systemic therapy is imperative because waiting for the results of blood cultures may greatly delay the institution of appropriate therapy. In addition, positive blood cultures are obtained in only about 50% of patients with sepsis. An additional aid to diagnosis of sepsis may be the blood glucose level. Gram-negative sepsis is generally associated with a hypoglycemic state (less than 100 mg/L), whereas gram-positive sepsis is accompanied by hyperglycemia (more than 135 mg/L).

Hemodynamic support, institution of systemic antibiotic therapy, local wound management, and elimination of septic foci are mainstays of treatment. A knowledge of the bacterial ecology of the burn unit is of great value. The maintenance of satisfactory nutrition, aggressive wound management, and ventilatory and hemodynamic support are requisites in the care of these patients. It is important to differentiate between sepsis arising from the burn wound itself and sepsis emanating from other sources such as septic thrombophlebitis, bacterial endocarditis, meningitis, urinary tract infection, sinusitis, acalculous cholecystitis, pneumonitis, pancreatitis, or intra-abdominal abscesses.

SURGICAL MANAGEMENT OF BURN WOUNDS

The ultimate goal of burn care remains closure of the burn wound by elimination of devitalized tissue and coverage with autologous skin. Debridement of nonviable burn tissue may be accomplished in several ways. Conservative management of the burn wound in anticipation of spontaneous eschar separation has generally been replaced by a more aggressive surgical approach to the burn wound. This may be achieved by layered ("tangential") excision of the burn wound, excision to fascia, early enzymatic debridement, or in selected cases, amputation.

The timing of burn wound debridement is important, and numerous factors must be considered. These include the overall physiologic status of the patient, local wound factors, the quality and availability of skin graft donor sites, the presence or absence of inhalation injury, the involvement of priority or special areas such as the hands, face, feet, or perineum, as well as burn center hospital factors. The availability of the operating room and the presence of a skilled and experienced burn team along with experienced anesthesia personnel are important considerations.

Patients who have sustained sizable body surface area burns generally undergo aggressive surgical debridement and early wound closure in an attempt to eliminate necrotic tissue and achieve rapid closure of the burn wound, thus minimizing septic complications. Deep partial-thickness and full-thickness injuries are best managed by excisional therapy. Although early excision of the burn wound has not appreciably shortened hospital stays of patients with major thermal injuries, it nonetheless appears to have had a major impact on burn morbidity and mortality. In those patients with less than 20% total body surface area burns, early excision and grafting have resulted in decreased hospital stay. In extensive burn injuries, early excision and grafting permit reharvesting of donor sites at an earlier time.

Our policy is to limit the extent of excision to less than the loss of one total blood volume or 2 hours of operating room time in major burn injuries. Excision should not exceed more than 20% of the total body surface area per operation. Control of hemorrhage is essential and can be aided by the use of topical epinephrine spray, pressure dressings, and the use of tourniquets whenever possible. Large vessels should be ligated or electrocoagulated. If tourniquets are employed, it is helpful to not exsanguinate the extremity prior to initiating layer excision because the blood remaining within the dermal vessels may be helpful in distinguishing viable from nonviable tissues. Wound coverage, permanent or temporary, is imperative at the time of surgery.

Priority areas for excision are dictated by the depth and extent of injury. Functional and cosmetic areas receive priority. In major burns, however, functional areas may be addressed first only if the mortality risk resulting from the burn wound is not great. If the risk of mortality is significant, then early reduction in the size of the open wound can be achieved through burn wound excision and grafting. In burns of critical size, the prime concern should be maximal reduction in the size of the open wound. Excision of the deepest burn wound should be carried out first. Excision of the burn wound should not be carried out if closure of the burn wound cannot be accomplished. Sheet grafts are employed for the face, neck, hands, and antecubital and popliteal areas. Meshed autografts not exceeding a 3 to 1 ratio can be employed in other areas. Exceeding the 3 to 1 ratio generally results in poor functional and cosmetic results along with delayed wound healing. Fresh cadaver or frozen cadaver allografts or the semisynthetic skin substitute Biobrane are excellent temporary substitutes if sufficient donor sites for autograft coverage are unavailable.

Patient selection and preparation are of critical importance in achieving a successful outcome. The excision is usually performed within 5 days following the injury. A skilled and experienced anesthesia team and nursing staff are necessary to minimize operative risk. It is incumbent upon the anesthesiologist that the patient's temperature, fluid volume, and respiratory and metabolic parameters be carefully monitored and maintained.

Theoretical advantages of early excision include the amelioration of burn hypermetabolism and immunosuppression as well as improved functional and cosmetic results. The disadvantages of early excision of the burn wound include cardiac and respiratory instability and major blood loss.

Closure of the burn wound is an essential component of early surgical treatment. Since complete closure of the burn wound by an autograft is often not possible in a single operation with significant body surface area burns, familiarity with alternative methods of wound closure is imperative. Wounds cannot be left open because of the potential for desiccation and infection. In addition, the deleterious consequences of increased evaporative loss, protein loss, and metabolic alterations must be considered. Biological dressings such as cadaver homograft, either fresh or frozen, or porcine xenograft may be used. Likewise, the biosynthetic skin substitute Biobrane has been useful. The use of sheets of autologous keratinocytes is of limited value in the treatment of freshly excised burn wounds since the "take" of this material is unpredictable, the resulting cover is inferior to that of autografted skin, and the time for generation of sufficient cells precludes availability after early excision. No skin substitute, biological or biosynthetic, should be applied to a wound that is incompletely debrided.

PAIN MANAGEMENT

Pain following thermal injury has been shown to have wide and frequent fluctuations; therefore, no single consistently effective method of management has been described. The present analgesic practices in burn patients, especially for debridement and dressing changes, have serious deficiencies. Wide variations in dosing practices and routes of administration are the rule for burned patients. In one study, children were four to five times more likely than adults to receive no analgesia for dressing changes despite the fact that the intensity and extent of pain were judged to be the same for both groups. At rest, burn patients experience a relatively low level of pain when compared with periods of wound manipulation. Wound manipulation and dressing changes are accompanied by excruciating pain, and the analgesia provided is generally insufficient to achieve even a moderate reduction in pain. Furthermore, the severity of pain is often unrelated to the extent or degree of burn injury. Third-degree burns may be "anesthetic" immediately after injury, but within a short time the pain may become intense. Although it is well accepted that there is a need for improved methods of pain control in burned patients, little data exist regarding the means by which effective pain control can be achieved. Techniques for pain management during painful procedures range from hypnosis to general anesthesia. Nonetheless, some type of pharmacologic intervention is fundamental to pain control in burn patients.

Hypnosis

At the present time, no firm conclusions can be made about the efficacy of this modality in burn patients.

Anesthetic Agents

The use of general anesthetic agents has been advocated for pain-producing procedures in burn patients. However, repeated exposure to these agents increases the potential for toxicity or tolerance and requires the presence of an anesthetist or anesthesiologist. In addition, the necessity for discontinuing nutrition support prior to implementation of an anesthetic agent disrupts metabolic support in these patients.

Narcotic Agents

Because of the availability and multiple routes of administration, narcotic agents have gained nearly universal acceptance for pain control in burn patients. Oral agents are frequently employed but are generally ineffective in controlling severe postoperative pain or pain associated with burn debridement and dressing changes. Morphine and meperidine (Demerol) are the most widely used narcotic agents in both pediatric and adult burn patients. The intravenous or intramuscular routes are most often employed; however, even with intravenous administration, the onset of analgesic action and time to achieve the peak effect of these agents is relatively slow. Adequate time must be provided before initiation of wound manipulation. The long duration of action of Demerol may result in oversedation with possible respiratory depression. Repeated large doses of Demerol over long periods of time may result in accumulation of the toxic metabolite normeperidine, which may provoke convulsions. Milder symptoms such as agitation frequently appear long before the more severe responses such as twitching, seizures, and tremor. Short-acting narcotics such as Fentanyl have significant advantages when used to relieve discomfort. The rapidity of onset allows for dose adjustment and the short duration of action prevents prolonged sedation. In general, the use of short-acting narcotics is preferable to the usual analgesics when a procedure is expected to be exceptionally painful. The use of patient-controlled anesthesia or continuous infusion methods employing morphine may be preferable to the usual "as-needed" dosing. For patients on respirators, continuous morphine infusion with supplementation before painful therapeutic procedures should be satisfactory. In patients who are able to communicate the severity of their pain, baseline pain can generally be controlled by the use of oral analgesics. The use of transcutaneous electrical nerve stimulation as an adjunct to pain management may be helpful in selected patients.

METABOLIC SUPPORT OF BURN PATIENTS

Major thermal injury results in a hypermetabolic response that is directly proportional to the severity of the injury. Baseline energy expenditures and requirements may be increased as much as 2.5 to 3 times above normal in patients with wounds exceeding 30% of the total body surface area. This increased energy expenditure is mediated by the neurohumoral axis in response to stress and represents a normal host reaction to major wounding. This results in marked catabolism and a failure to replenish energy stores with rapid weight loss and potentially fatal consequences. Thus, nutrition support should be initiated as early as possible, preferably 24 to 48 hours following injury. An assessment of the nutritional needs of the patient and maintenance of those needs by appropriate intake coupled with continual monitoring is essential (Table 12–8). The use of indirect calorimetry on a routine basis to monitor the appropriate level of metabolic support is helpful. The enteral route is preferred since initiation and maintenance of enteral feeding mechanisms maintain the intestinal villi and augment immunoglobulin production. The use of central lines and total parenteral nutrition should be avoided if possible because of a high frequency of septic complications as well as the recent demonstration that paren-

TABLE 12–8.
Nutritional Requirement by Age*

	BMR†			Protein (g/kg/day)§	
Age (yr)	kcal/kg/day‡	kcal/m^2/hr‡	Growth ‡ (kcal/kg/day)	1974	1980
0–1	60	53	31	2.0–3.5	2.0–2.2
1–3	57	51	29	2.5–3.0	1.8
3–6	52	50	24	3.0	1.5
6–9	48	47	16	2.8	1.2
9–12	44	43	12	2.0	1.0
12–15	37	42	8	1.7	1.0
15–18	31	40	3	1.5	0.9
18–20	27	39	0	1.0	0.8
20–30	27	36	0	1.0	0.8
30–40	27	36	0	1.0	0.8
40–50	27	35	0	1.0	0.8
50–60	27	33	0	1.0	0.8
60–70	27	33	0	1.0	0.8
70+	27	32	0	1.0	0.8

Nutritional formulas

Curreri
Adult: 25 kcal × wt (kg) + 40 kcal × % TBSAB†
Child: 60–90 kcal × wt (kg) + 35 kcal × % TBSAB
UCSD†
1.4 kcal (BMR × m^2 × 24 hr) + wt (growth + 0.6 TBSAB)
Harris-Benedict equation
Male: BMR (kcal) = 66 + (13.7 × wt [kg]) + (5 × Ht [cm] − 6.8 × age)
Female: BMR (kcal) = 665 + (9.6 × wt [kg]) + (1.7 × Ht[cm]) − (4.7 × age)

* From Boswick JA Jr (ed): *The Art and Science of Burn Care.* Rockville, Md., Aspen Publishers Inc. 1986. Used by permission.
† BMR = basal metabolic rate; TBSAB = total body surface area burn; UCSD = University of California, San Diego.
‡ The basal and growth requirements for ages 12 to 18 years may be too low.
§ Protein requirements from recommended daily allowances by the National Research Council for 1974 and 1980.

teral feeding fails to restore immunocompetence in burn patients.

The use of jejunostomy tube feedings for patients with burns exceeding 60% of the total body surface area may be helpful. Nasogastric tube feedings may be interrupted frequently because of intermittent bouts of sepsis or the necessity for multiple surgical procedures. As a result, nutrition support frequently lags considerably, thus making nutritional goals impossible to realize. Jejunostomy tube feeding permits continuous enteral feeding by means of elemental diets.

A number of formulas have been developed to estimate caloric requirements. The Curreri formula (24-hour caloric requirement = 25 × wt [kg] + 40 × percent burn) is most frequently employed, with adjustments made based on indirect calorimetry results. Prognostic nutritional indices should be obtained on all major burn patients by employing serum transferrin levels, recall-antigen skin testing, anthropomorphic measurements, and total lymphocyte counts. A dietician should be an integral part of the burn team to ensure close monitoring of the patient's nutritional status.

IMMUNE CONSEQUENCES

Following thermal injury, there is a marked alteration in the immune response since the burn injury directly affects the complex interaction of numerous components of this physiologic response. It is not clear whether the alteration in immune function following thermal injury is truly a deficiency disease, is caused by circulating toxins, or is a combination of both. Nevertheless, the end result is an overstimulation of several immune system components, namely, suppressor T cells, complement activation, as well as a depression of other components, including T-helper and T-killer cells and polymorphonuclear leukocytes. The reduction in antibody activity is the result of inadequate T-lymphocyte stimulation of B lymphocytes, and the resultant deficiency states prevent adequate toxin neutralization, bacteriolysis in the presence of complement, and opsonization of bacteria. Additional defects in antibody reduction result in altered complement activation and active white cell function.

HIGH-VOLTAGE ELECTRICAL INJURIES

In the United States, nearly 1,000 people die every year as a result of electrical injuries. About 3% of the total number of burns treated in burn centers annually are the result of electrical injury.

Electrical injuries are classified as either low voltage or high voltage. Low-voltage injuries (less than 1,000 V) most commonly occur around the home. They vary from oral commissure burns to electrocution. High-voltage injuries (greater than 1,000 V) are more common in the work setting, especially near high-voltage transmission lines or high-voltage equipment. Patterns of injury with high-voltage current include severe soft-tissue injury, thermal injury by ignition of clothing, fractures, occult internal injuries, central nervous system trauma, or death. High-voltage electrical injuries result in significant morbidity. Major amputations are required in 25% to 60% of patients treated. Although the cutaneous surface area burned may be small, instances of ignition of clothing may result in extensive body surface area burns. Mortality rates range from as low as 3% to as high as 15%.

A consistent pattern of injury has been identified. Epidemiologic studies reveal a seasonal peak in the spring, with nearly two thirds of accidents occurring on the job. Young males less than 30 years of age are the most common victims. Accidents involving females are extremely uncommon. The majority of individuals who are injured are the major breadwinners in the family, and the dominant upper extremity is the most commonly injured part. Lower extremities are frequently injured, but these injuries are most often the result of exit wounding. High-voltage electrical injuries are seldom accompanied by extensive cutaneous burn injuries.

Pathophysiology

In the United States, nearly all industrial and domestic electricity is alternating current (ac). Direct current (dc) is, however, available and encountered in many situations. At voltages of less than 1,000, ac is far more devastating than dc. However, above 1,000 V, ac and dc are equally dangerous. Ohm's law provides the relationship between voltage, current, and resistance: $I = E/R$ (I = current in amperes; E = voltage in volts; and R is the resistance in ohms).

Joule's law defines the relationship between current and heat production: $J = I^2RT$, where J is the number of joules of heat produced, I represents the current in amperes, R is the resistance in ohms, and T is the time in seconds. By this equation, it is the current flow, or amperes, that is the most significant variable in this equation (Table 12–9).

Electroporation has recently been described as another potential cause of high-voltage electrical injury. Electroporation is believed to occur when strong electrical forces drive water molecules into the defects of a bilaminar lipid membrane and cause these

TABLE 12–9.
Effects of Low-Frequency Electrical Current

Current (mamp)	Physiologic Effect
1–2	Sensory perception
5	Painful stimulus
10–15	Sustained muscular contraction
30–100	Tetany of respiratory muscles
	Ventricular fibrillation
1,000	Sustained myocardial contractions
5,000	Deep conduction injury
10,000	Massive irreversible CNS damage

pores to enlarge. Progressive enlargement of the pores results in membrane rupture. This event requires less than 100 μs and may explain the appearance of the rhabdomyolysis and neurolysis that are commonly associated with high-voltage electrical injuries. Evidence for this phenomenon occurring as a pathophysiologic mechanism to explain high-voltage electrical injury is mounting since not all the events that characterize high-voltage electrical injury can be explained by tissue heating alone. Whereas the changes associated with tissue heating, cell destruction, and coagulation necrosis are irreversible, electroporation damage may be amenable to therapeutic manipulation to preserve or salvage skeletal muscle and neural structures.

Injuries may occur by a number of mechanisms: direct contact, arcing to the grounded victim, ignition of clothing by the intense heat of the arc flash, falls, or severe muscular contractions. When an individual comes in contact with a voltage source, the primary resistance to current flow is generated by the skin. As skin resistance is overcome, the current flows through the tissues of the body and finally exits through the skin at a different site as it flows to a grounding source. However, many variables determine the degree of resistance of the skin. They include humidity, site of skin contact, the presence or absence of moisture on the skin, and atmospheric condition. It was thought that once current entered the deeper tissues, it flowed differently in different tissues according to their varying resistance. Although some investigators have confirmed these observations, others have shown that current flows nearly uniformly through all tissues once the resistance of the skin has been overcome. It is generally accepted, however, that bone heats to a very high temperature and retains this heat for prolonged periods of time. Because of the slow dissipation of heat and conduction into adjacent tissues, the greatest damage in an extremity is deep, in proximity to bone. However, clinical findings may not always agree with this general observation. Theoretically, nerves should conduct electrical impulses well, but they sustain severe injury with only slight temperature increases above 45°C.

Another important concept is that the cross-sectional area is an important determinant of the degree of injury. High current flow in small cross-sectional areas will generate greater heat and consequently more severe injury to the extremity than were it to flow through a larger cross-sectional area. At points of contact, both entrance and exit, where current density is greatest, the severity of skin injury is extreme. Entrance and exit wounds are leathery and depressed and frequently appear to be the result of an explosive or implosive charge. Intense coagulation necrosis is present. With severe injury in the upper extremity, the wrist is characteristically flexed as a result of coagulation necrosis of the flexor forearm musculature. The pathway of current flow is of great significance, for it may cause injury to any tissue or structure within its path. A high index of suspicion is necessary to diagnose occult intrathoracic or intra-abdominal injuries. Cervical spine or more caudal spinal fractures may be present, and peripheral nerve involvement is common.

Arcing injuries are much less common than contact or conduction injuries. However, under appropriate atmospheric conditions, arcing to a grounded victim may occur as far as 10 ft away. In addition, local arcs may have occurred in the skin of flexed joints and produce very deep, localized lesions. The temperature of an arc flash may range from 2,000°C to as high as 20,000°C. The resulting tissue damage is generally severe. Electrical injury is frequently associated with the "nonrelease phenomenon." When a patient grabs a high-tension source, the forearm muscles go into a state of fixed contraction, and the victim is unable to free himself from the current source. A patient may escape from this current source by being rendered unconscious and falling away from the source. This often results in skeletal or internal injuries.

Specific Clinical Effects and Injuries

The effects of electrical injury may be acute or chronic. The onset of symptoms may be manifested immediately following injury or may develop insidiously over months (and perhaps years) following the initial injury.

Musculoskeletal Injuries

Patients sustaining electrical injuries may have variable degrees of cutaneous and muscle injuries. These may involve only a small area of the body or may encompass significant areas of the total body surface area as well as multiple extremities. The severity and extent of damage are related to the numerous, previously outlined factors.

Cardiac

The most acute and potentially most lethal effect of electrical injury is ventricular fibrillation, or asystole. Nearly one third of patients sustaining electrical injuries demonstrate electrocardiographic changes, including the entire array of bundle-branch blocks as well as arrhythmias. The specific etiology of these electrocardiographic findings includes direct myocardial injury, injury to the conducting system of the heart, spasm of coronary arteries, and arteritis of the coronary vessels. Acute myocardial infarction and direct injury to the myocardium occasionally occur.

Nervous System

Neurologic sequelae following high-voltage electrical injuries are extremely common. These may involve the central, autonomic, and peripheral nervous systems. High-voltage electrical injury may induce acute cerebral or brain-stem injury, which is immediately fatal. A common finding in electrical injury is loss of consciousness of varying length. This is generally not associated with respiratory paralysis, and recovery is the rule. However, in a small percentage of patients, permanent central nervous system disorders may result, including hemiplegia, with or without aphasia, brain-stem dysfunction, cerebellar ataxia, and visual disturbances. These may develop slowly and not become apparent for many months.

Further central nervous system damage may involve the spinal cord. Acute manifestations may include paraplegia or parasthesias, quadriplegia or quadraparesis, pain, and paresthesias. Delayed manifestations of spinal cord injury resembling transverse myelitis (Panse's syndrome) may develop. This syndrome is characterized by the development of motor signs days or months following the injury, including gait disturbances, muscle imbalance, bladder dysfunction, or impotence. Progression of the syndrome may evolve into frank quadriplegia, hemiplegia, or paralysis. Recovery following the development of this syndrome is unusual. The most likely mechanism of spinal cord injury is progressive damage to neurons as a result of either direct physiologic changes or secondary ischemia with obliteration of nutrient vessels to the spinal cord.

Peripheral nerve injuries are more frequent. These are seen in both the acute and chronic setting and result either from direct electrical interruption of Schwann cells with resulting axonal disruption or from progressive vascular obliteration with nerve fibrosis. Additional mechanisms of peripheral injury include scarring and perineural fibrosis. The autonomic nervous system may show significant abnormalities, including causalgia and causalgia-like symptoms as well as vasomotor instability.

Pulmonary

Although respiratory arrest involving high-voltage electrical injury may produce immediate death, pulmonary conditions may develop in the immediate postinjury period or later in the patient's course. Direct electrical contact to the chest wall may result in severe chest wall injuries with musculoskeletal damage, pleural involvement, as well as injury to the lung parenchyma. Pneumothorax, hydrothorax, empyema, lung abscess, and post-traumatic respiratory distress syndromes may be the result of direct chest wall injuries.

Gastrointestinal

Electrical injury to the abdominal wall may result in variable degrees of injury. Disruption of the integrity of the abdominal wall may result in evisceration. Infrequently, intra-abdominal viscera may sustain injury. A high index of suspicion is necessary in patients with evidence of abdominal wall involvement. Occult intra-abdominal visceral involvement may result in an acute abdominal catastrophe. Perforation of the bowel may be seen acutely or as long as 2 to 3 weeks following injury.

Bowel fistulas, paralytic ileus, or gastric and duodenal ulcers may occur. Gallbladder pathology is frequent. The gallbladder shows either necrosis or perforation, and the incidence of cholelithiasis following high-voltage electrical injury is high. Pancreatitis and hepatic necrosis in association with acute coagulopathies have also been described.

Vascular

Vascular lesions predominate following high-voltage electrical injuries. Direct damage and subsequent obliteration, endarteritis, and necrosis of both major arteries and nutrient vessels constitute the primary mechanisms of injury. In addition, the development of massive delayed hemorrhage is a major threat following such injuries. Although the major arteries may be profoundly affected, the most substantive injuries are at the nutrient artery level and are most responsible for the broad array of organ and tissue damage that accompanies electrical injury.

Ophthalmologic

Electrical injury may produce a wide array of eye injuries, including injury to the globe and selected lesions of the optic nerve, cornea, and fundus. The arc flash may produce retinopathy, but the most common sequela of high-voltage electrical injury is the development of cataracts. These may be unilateral or bilateral and may develop as early as 3 weeks or as late as 3 years following such injury. The potential for cataract development is directly related to the likelihood of current passage through the head.

Clinical Management of High-Voltage Electrical Injuries

A complete and accurate evaluation of the condition of the patient following high-voltage electrical injury is essential for the preservation of life and limb. Establishment of the airway and maintenance of the circulation are of foremost importance. If endotracheal intubation is necessary, the possibility of cervical spine injury should not be overlooked. Following emergency stabilization, a careful history of the injury, the medical status of the patient, and a general physical examination must be performed. Thoracic and abdominal evaluation, electrocardiograms, and appropriate radiologic tests should be carried out. Concurrent with other stabilization procedures, a large-bore intravenous catheter and Foley catheter should be inserted. Vital signs must be monitored carefully, and the patient should undergo frequent evaluations and continuous electrocardiographic monitoring. Laboratory analysis should include hemoglobin, hematocrit, electrolyte, blood urea nitrogen (BUN), creatinine, and cardiac isoenzyme determinations, liver function tests, and urinalysis for hemochromogens. Fluid therapy should proceed to restore the intravascular volume and replace obligatory fluid losses into the area of electrical injury. Lactated Ringer's solution is employed as the resuscitation fluid at infusion rates that will maintain urinary outputs of 75 to 100 cc/hr. In the presence of hemochromogens, urinary output should be maintained at or slightly above 100 cc/hr until hemoglobinuria or myoglobinuria is no longer present. Mannitol (12.5 g/hr) should be administered to promote an osmotic diuresis. In addition, alkalinization of the urine by the addition of sodium bicarbonate to the intravenous solution may diminish the likelihood of tubular precipitation of hemochromogens and the subsequent development of acute renal failure. Monitoring of urine pH is helpful, and urine pH in excess of 6 should be the goal.

An assessment of the extent and severity of the injury must be performed. The calculation of the total body surface area of a cutaneous burn is highly inaccurate in estimating the total volume of tissue loss or injury. Palpation of all involved extremities is essential. Direct compartment measurement to assess the presence or development of compartment syndrome is essential. Prompt surgical intervention with fasciotomy and decompression of neurovascular structures is frequently necessary. An initial neurologic assessment should be performed, and the patient should be reevaluated frequently.

Initial wound care should consist of careful cleansing of the wounds and fasciotomy when indicated by the presence of coolness, pallor, paresthesias, or pulselessness or by direct compartment pressure evidence of incipient compartment syndrome. Prompt decompression of neurovascular structures may result in limb salvage and provide diagnostic and prognostic information. Mafenide (Sulfamylon) cream (11.2%) is the topical antibacterial of choice because of its ability to penetrate eschar and devitalized tissue. Systemic antibiotic prophylaxis should be instituted until all devitalized tissue has been debrided.

Aggressive management of the wound is fundamental to successful management of high-voltage electrical injuries. Successive debridements initiated in the acute postinjury phase achieve removal of necrotic tissue, prevent sepsis, and prepare the wound for earlier closure. The timing of initial surgical intervention depends on a number of factors, including the general condition of the patient and the status and extent of the wound. Prompt performance of escharotomy and fasciotomy can reduce secondary ischemic necrosis while providing a better assessment of the extent and severity of injury to the deeper structures. Frozen section assessment of questionable areas and marginally viable tissues may be helpful. When total loss of essential structures of a limb is obvious, early amputation by the "guillotine" method is indicated. The open stump is then amenable to delayed primary closure. Serial repeated debridements are necessary in most cases in order to achieve excision of all devitalized tissues. The patient may require a return to the operating room every 2 or 3 days to accomplish this goal. The wound should not be closed until all devitalized tissue has been removed. The use of radioisotope scanning may be helpful in selected cases to assess the presence of nonviable tissue.

Wound coverage is generally accomplished by the use of split-thickness skin grafts. However, when muscle, tendon, and nerves are exposed, the initial use of biological dressings to prevent desiccation and infection followed by flap coverage may be necessary to preserve these structures. The type of flap coverage required will be dictated by a number of factors. Local tissues in the form of muscle or myocutaneous or fasciocutaneous flaps are frequently unavailable because of damage to these tissues by the electrical injury. Therefore, free tissue transfer may be required for coverage of exposed vital structures. It is imperative that the microvascular anastomosis be performed at a site of undamaged recipient vessels beyond the "zone of injury" lest thrombosis result in flap failure. Pedicled groin flaps are often useful for coverage of the hand, wrist, or forearm areas.

Amputation is common following high-voltage electrical injury. A high percentage of patients (35% to 50%) require one or more amputations. The types of amputation may be relatively minor or may result in the loss of one or more limbs. Resultant disabilities require prolonged and extensive rehabilitation and prosthetic fitting. Generally, the patients are unable to return to the work force, and long-term consequences are severe. The most common amputations involve the dominant upper extremity, while the majority of exit wounds are found in the lower extremities. Objectives of amputation in high-voltage electrical injury include the following:

1. Removal of devitalized tissue to prevent infection and obtain earlier wound closure
2. Control of invasive sepsis (occasionally an emergency)
3. Removal of a functionless or painful limb
4. Functional improvement in an amputation revision

The level of amputation is primarily determined by the nature and extent of the electrical injury. Although preservation of the length and functional considerations should be kept in mind, these are frequently not applicable because of the extent and nature of the injuries. The timing of amputation is dictated by the condition of the patient and the severity of injury to the extremity. Primary closure at the time of amputation is seldom done. Wound closure is most frequently obtained by the use of meshed split-thickness skin grafts, although the use of local flaps is often preferable, especially when covering the ends of bone in an amputation stump. Problems following amputation include skin breakdown, improper prosthesis fitting, joint pain and stiffness, and psychological resistance to the wearing or use of prostheses.

Reconstructive surgery is frequently required following high-voltage electrical injury. The primary goals of reconstruction are the restoration of form and function. The choice of reconstructive methods is specific to the individual patient and is dictated by the severity and location of the injuries, the patients' needs and desires, and the abilities of the treating surgeon.

CHEMICAL INJURIES

Chemical injuries are uncommon. Domestic or laboratory accidents and criminal assaults account for most cases. Chemical injuries often involve only small percentages of the total body surface area but may produce significant morbidity. Lethal chemical injuries are usually the result of industrial accidents or military conflicts.

The mechanism of injury is a combination of chemical and thermal components. The most destructive of chemical injuries is that caused by phosphorus, which melts at body temperature. The vast majority of chemical injuries are the result of an exothermic reaction along with denaturation of protein, protein precipitation, and alkalinization. Histologic examination of chemically injured tissue reveals severe edema of skin and subcutaneous tissue, vacuolization of the nuclei of cells of the skin, separation of epidermis from the dermis, severe disorganization of the cellular architecture of the dermis, and severe disruption or fusion of dermal collagen bundles. The severity of chemical injuries depends on the duration of the exposure as well as the type and concentration of the offending chemical agent (Table 12–10).

Acid Burns

The distribution and severity of acid burns depend on a number of factors. These include the type of agent, its concentration, the duration of exposure, and the type of initial treatment rendered. Spill burns or splatter burns are most common, with contact being spotty and in the form of droplets or small rivulets that stream down the body. The resultant injuries are generally small; however, tissue destruction is generally quite severe.

Industrial accidents often result in varying degrees of immersion and are therefore far more serious than those caused by domestic or laboratory accidents. Such injuries are frequently lethal. Acid burns produce extremely painful wounds, and the pain is persistent. The longevity of pain is a consequence of continued chemical reaction.

The appearance of chemical wounds is variable and may range from mild erythema to superficial graying of the skin or to a yellowish brown or black eschar that is characteristic of deep lesions (Table 12–11). Superficial wounds are characterized by a soft, pliable texture, whereas deeper wounds result in leathery consistency of the skin. Acid burns may be accompanied by systemic complications that generally are not significant, except in the case of hydrofluoric acid, which may produce alterations in the clotting mechanism, or formic acid burns, which may result in renal or hepatic dysfunction. Industrial acid burns, however, are often accompanied by severe systemic dysfunction as well as injury to the

TABLE 12–10.
Histology—Acid and Alkali Burns

The epidermis may appear intact but is not
Cytoplasmic edema
Epidermal perinuclear vacuolization with elongated pyknotic nuclei
Dermal-epidermal separation
Collagen banding and loss of collagen
Intercellular edema with separation and irregularity of cells of sebaceous and sweat glands
Endothelial thickening and thrombosis of deep dermal capillaries

TABLE 12–11.
Pathophysiology of Chemical Injury

Agent	Mechanism of Action	Appearance	Texture
Acid burns			
Sulfuric Nitric Hydrochloric Trichloroacetic Phenol	Exothermic reaction, cellular dehydration, and protein precipitation	Gray, yellow, brown, or black depending on duration of exposure	Soft to leathery eschar depending on duration of exposure
Hydrofluoric	Same as in other acids plus liquefaction and decalcification	Erythema with central necrosis	Painful, leathery eschar
Alkali burns			
Potassium hydroxide Sodium hydroxide Lime	Exothermic reaction, hygroscopic cellular dehydration with saponification of fat and protein precipitation	Erythema with bullae	Painful, "soapy" slick eschar
Ammonia	Same as other bases plus laryngeal and pulmonary edema	Gray, yellow, brown, or black, often very deep	Soft to leathery depending on duration of exposure
Phosphorus	Thermal effect, melts at body temperature, ignites at 34°C, acid effect of H_2PO_4	Gray or blue green, glows in the dark	Depressed, leathery eschar

tracheal bronchial tree that results in acute respiratory distress or progressive respiratory dysfunction.

The treatment of acid burns is most effective when instituted immediately following exposure. Prompt initiation of first aid is the most important element in definitive therapy, for it reduces the duration of exposure and the concentration of the agent. Copious irrigation with water should be initiated as quickly as possible following chemical injury. Simple dilution of the agent is extremely effective in reducing the depth and severity of injury. Wound lavage for as little as 2 hours or as long as 24 hours has been recommended. Although specific antidotes may be available in the industrial setting, attempts to neutralize chemicals frequently result in more severe tissue injury because of generation of heat via an exothermic reaction. Therefore, copious irrigation with water is considered the best and most effective initial therapy for chemical injuries. In-hospital treatment is dictated by the extent and severity of the injury. Most often it requires removal of devitalized tissue, provision of adequate analgesia, and general support in fluid resuscitation as with thermal injuries. Following initial care of these patients, the treatment of acid burns is generally the same as that provided for thermal injuries.

Alkali Burns

The circumstances of the injury, the appearance and distribution (see Table 12–11), as well as the treatment of alkali burns are virtually the same as that of acid burns (Table 12–12). Specifically, burns resulting from anhydrous ammonia are common in the agricultural setting and are often deep and painful. They are frequently associated with severe injuries to the eyes and tracheal bronchial tree. Specific attention to these areas is imperative. However, removal of the offending substance from the skin as quickly as possible following exposure along with copious irrigation of the eyes and skin is imperative in order to prevent extensive and irreversible damage.

RADIATION INJURIES

Radiation injury is the end result of cellular damage by ionizing radiation. The extent of injury is determined by the dosage of

TABLE 12–12.
Management of Chemical Burns

Agent	Cleansing	Neutralization	Debridement
Acid burns			
Sulfuric	Water	Sodium bicarbonate solution	Debride loose, nonviable tissue
Nitric			
Hydrochloric			
Trichloroacetic			
Phenol	Ethyl alcohol	Sodium bicarbonate solution	Debride loose, nonviable tissue
Hydrofluoric	Water	Same as other acids plus magnesium oxide, glycerin paste, local injection, calcium gluconate	Debride loose, nonviable tissue
Alkali burns			
Potassium hydroxide			
Sodium hydroxide	Water	0.5–5.0% acetic acid or 5.0% ammonium chloride	Debride loose, nonviable tissue
Lime	Brush off powder	0.5%–5.0% acetic acid or 5.0% ammonium chloride	Debride loose, nonviable tissue
Phosphorus	Water	Copper sulfate soaks	Debride and remove particles of phosphorus

radiation as well as the importance of the injured or damaged cellular molecular structures to the overall function of the cell. The primary injury is to cellular DNA. Following radiation injury, histologic and clinical changes can be observed in tissues.

The ability of cells to repair themselves and return to normal activity depends on the dose of radiation received as well as the type and number of surviving cells. Radiation injuries may be local or systemic. The local effects of radiation injury may be categorized as acute, subacute, or chronic. The systemic effects of radiation injury are generally described as radiation sickness and are divided into three specific stages: the prodromal, latent, and main phases.

Local Effects

Acute radiation injury is most often the result of accidental exposure to high doses of radiation over a relatively short period of time. This exposure results in an injury to the skin and local tissues that frequently resembles a thermal burn. The evolution of these injuries, however, is considerably different from that seen with thermal burns, for radiation injuries are slow to evolve and are of significantly greater depth. Erythema is generally observed within minutes following exposure but may recur in a cyclic fashion. Edema, severe pain, and itching may accompany the erythema. These symptoms are followed by scaling, flaking, blistering, and weeping of the skin with ultimate sloughing and skin ulceration. The underlying tissue may undergo partial or complete necrosis. Histologic examination of the microvasculature of the region reveals obliterative endarteritis and chronic vasculitis. These changes are responsible for further development of tissue ischemia, secondary bacterial invasion, and ultimate tissue necrosis. *Subacute radiation injury* is the result of repeated administration of low-dose radiation over an extended period of time. The cumulative results are injuries characterized by inflammation. However, tissue ulceration and necrosis generally do not occur. Edema, erythema, and pain may be present but subside with time. These changes are frequently seen following therapeutic radiation. The ultimate result is the development of thickened skin and subcutaneous tissue with hyperpigmentation. Histologic examination of such tissues reveals marked fibrosis of connective tissue as well as perivascular fibrosis.

Chronic radiation injury is also the result of repeated exposures to low-dose radiation over prolonged periods of time. Thus the mechanism is essentially the same as that seen with subacute radiation injury but involves lower doses and longer periods of exposure. Such injuries are most common in workers who are exposed to ionizing radiation as an occupational hazard. The end result of these injuries may be malignant transformation of skin, subcutaneous tissue, and bone. The vascular changes are of greatest significance, and chronic ischemia of the involved tissue is the end result of these injuries.

Systemic Effects

Total-body irradiation produces radiation sickness. The *prodromal phase* is characterized by severe gastrointestinal symptoms, including anorexia, nausea, vomiting, and diarrhea. The *latent phase* represents the time necessary for destruction or loss of cells that have been irreparably damaged by radiation. This period may last for hours or weeks. The rapidity of onset of this phase depends on the magnitude of radiation and the particular cellular type that is involved. The *main phase,* or final phase, of systemic radiation injury becomes evident as the loss of cells during the latent phase becomes clinically apparent. The degree of the main or final phase depends on the organ system involved. Severe radiation damage to the cardiovascular or nervous system will produce death within a short period of time, whereas irreparable injury to the gastrointestinal system or bone marrow will result in fatal consequences within days or weeks.

Treatment

The treatment of radiation injuries is, for the most part, conservative. Since radiation injury has been described as permanent, continuous, and progressive, the extent of injury may not be readily apparent at the outset. The primary clinical feature of such injuries is pain, which generally requires hospitalization and large doses of narcotic analgesics. The use of topical antimicrobial creams and steroid creams may reduce erythema and aid in controlling pain. When radiation injuries involve the hands, splinting in the position of function is important. Range-of-motion exercises and hydrotherapy should be carried out if possible to preserve function. Surgery is generally withheld until the wound has entered the chronic phase and the total extent of tissue destruction or damage can be clearly appreciated. The use of topical antimicrobial agents to prevent infection of these wounds is an essential component of care. Debridement of devitalized tissue and wound coverage by split-thickness skin grafts or vascularized flaps when indicated are the mainstays of wound therapy. The treatment of patients who have sustained an acute radiation injury is primarily supportive until the extent of injury has been clearly defined and definitive treatment can be undertaken.

COLD INJURIES

Frostbite and hypothermia constitute the two major groups of cold injuries. Frostbite is the result of exposure to low environmental temperatures and the formation of ice crystals within living tissues. Tissue freezing begins with the formation of tiny particles of ice in the extracellular space and continues with the formation of more ice crystals as water is drawn from surrounding cells into the extracellular space. The resultant ice crystal growth mechanically compresses surrounding cells and results in rupture of cell membranes. This cellular disruption may occur during either the freezing or thawing phases. Perhaps the most serious effect of extracellular ice crystal formation is the cellular dehydration that produces loss of intracellular water and subsequent destruction of intracellular structures. The second major pathophysiologic component is vascular impairment. This results from both mechanical compression of vessels as well as direct endothelial injury that induces thrombus formation, hemoconcentration, and increased blood viscosity with sludging. In addition, increased sympathetic tone may produce marked vasoconstriction, stasis, and shunting of blood.

Frostbite may be classified as superficial or deep. This classification system replaces earlier attempts to describe injuries as first-, second-, third-, or fourth-degree frostbite. In superficial frostbite, the injury is limited to the skin, whereas in deep frostbite injuries, subcutaneous structures are also damaged. Numerous factors have been shown to have an influence on the severity of frostbite injury. These include the ambient temperature, duration of exposure, moisture, humidity, wind velocity, stress, fatigue, type of protective clothing, and immobility. Preexisting occlusive arterial disease, cigarette smoking, or previous frostbite may also predispose to the development of cold injuries. Fatigue, the presence of coexisting injuries, and alcohol intoxication also contribute to these injuries.

The initial management of acute frostbite injury should entail examination of the entire patient as well as the frozen part. Important steps in initial evaluation and treatment include an accurate determination of core body temperature with appropriate treatment of hypothermia. Associated injuries, malnutrition, or shock must be evaluated and treated. The frostbitten part should be carefully examined, and specific treatment should then be undertaken. This includes rapid rewarming of the frozen part in a 40 to 44°C water bath, sedation, and provision of adequate analgesia. Warming of the frozen part should continue until evidence of circulatory return is present. In the situation of deep frostbite, however, this may not be evident. Elevation of the injured part to control edema, splinting, and topical antimicrobials should be applied. Tetanus prophylaxis should be provided, and systemic antibiotic therapy should be initiated during the edema phase.

Although systemic anticoagulation has been shown to be of value in experimental animal studies, the efficacy of such treatment in humans has not been demonstrated. The use of antisludging agents such as low–molecular-weight dextran has been studied extensively, but the results are inconclusive. The use of antithromboxane drugs such as aspirin has been shown to be of value, and topical thromboxane inhibitors such as aloe vera have also been demonstrated to be useful in diminishing the degree of tissue loss. Wound care should be directed toward prevention of infection and physiotherapy instituted to maintain active range of motion as part of the therapeutic regimen. The use of radioisotope scanning to determine the viability of questionable areas, especially in the extremities, may hasten the decision to provide vascularized tissue cover or to proceed with amputation. Premature amputation should be avoided.

Closure of wounds should be accomplished by the most appropriate means. In case of amputation, sufficient bone shortening should be carried out to permit skin closure while maintaining optimal length. Split-thickness skin grafts and local or distant flaps may be required. With deep frostbite, loss of the affected part (either subtotal or total) is the rule. Long-term consequences of such injuries include a predilection to future frostbite injury, vasospastic syndromes in the extremities, intrinsic muscle atrophy in the hand, cold hypersensitivity, and cosmetic and functional sequelae.

BURN REHABILITATION AND RECONSTRUCTION

Burn reconstruction and rehabilitation begin at the initiation of care. As the ability to manage critically injured burn patients has improved and the size of lethal burn injury has been pushed further up the scale of magnitude, the challenge confronting caretakers has become more complicated. Successful management of burn patients is no longer measured by survival. Instead, the criteria for success must be expanded to encompass the reconstructive and total rehabilitation needs of burn patients.

Even survivors of relatively small burn injuries may experience prolonged difficulties, both physical and emotional. These include scarring, wound breakdown, contractures, limitations of motion, chronic pain, itching, sleeplessness, sexual dysfunction, alteration of body image, depression, anger, withdrawal, and reduced endurance.

Therefore, discharge from the burn center with a closed wound represents little more than a singular event in the continuation of the long and arduous recovery from burn injury. An appreciation of this problem and its magnitude and implications is fundamental to the development of a philosophy for the reconstruction and rehabilitation of burn patients.

The principal goals of burn reconstruction and rehabilitation are the restoration of form and function along with reintegration of the individual with society and daily life. Successful rehabilitation commences at the time of initial evaluation and care. The primary goal should be the provision of care so comprehensive and so effective that further reconstruction is avoided.

A number of factors during both the inpatient and outpatient phases will have a strong influence on the ultimate outcome. These include early institution of proper positioning and splinting, range-of-motion exercises, early ambulation, and exercises to maintain strength, endurance, and mobility. Early debridement and closure of burn wounds, splinting in the antideformity position, edema control, prevention of skin graft loss, and institution of anticontracture regimens are essential elements in this process. Prompt institution of pressure therapy to modulate hypertrophic scars and aggressive management of progressive contractures that interfere with function are imperative. Therefore, careful and frequent patient examination and an assessment of patient needs are necessary. Likewise, the provision of psychosocial support and the inclusion of the patient as a willing participant in the rehabilitative program are key components in the process.

Surgical reconstruction can be categorized as urgent, essential, or desirable. *Urgent* procedures are necessitated by specific problems arising during the acute period and are generally directed toward coverage of exposed joints, eyes, neurovascular or tendinous structures, and bone. *Essential* procedures are performed to restore function. These may involve any region of the body where function has been adversely affected by the burn injury. *Desirable* procedures are intended to restore a more normal appearance or to optimize function. Because of their goal, these procedures are frequently both challenging and frustrating since most reconstructions are inadequate in completely restoring the preinjury appearance of the patient. In addition, these reconstructions require significant planning and preparation to attain the intended results.

The specific reconstructive needs will vary from one anatomic location to another. Careful examination of the patient along with an appreciation of aesthetic and functional alterations subsequent to burn injury will serve as a foundation for treatment. Additionally, the wishes of the patient and the observations of other burn team members are important components in formulating a list of priorities from which will evolve a surgical plan. (For reconstruction of specific structures, please refer to the appropriate chapters in this text.)

SUGGESTED READING

Boswick JA Jr (ed): *The Art and Science of Burn Care.* Rockville, Md, Aspen Publications, 1987.

Heimbach DM, Engrave LH: *Surgical Management of the Burn Wound.* New York, Raven Press, 1984.

Martyn JAJ: *Acute Management of the Burned Patient.* Philadelphia, WB Saunders, 1990.

Moylan JA, Alexander LG: Diagnosis and treatment of inhalation injury. *World J Surg* 1978; 2:185–191.

Chapter 13

Congenital, Aesthetic, and Functional Problems

Joseph G. Bauer, M.D.
Fritz E. Barton, Jr., M.D.

CONTENTS

Congenital disorders
Cutaneous aging
Actinic damage
Generalized skin disorders
Lipodystrophy
Cutaneous inflammatory processes

CHAPTER OBJECTIVE

At the end of this chapter the resident is familiar with common congenital disorders and generalized disease processes of the skin and with the physiology of aging and successfully undertakes plastic surgical treatments of these processes and disorders.

LEARNER OBJECTIVES

On completion of this chapter the resident

1. **Knows the basic physiology of the aging process of the skin.**
2. **Understands the basic physiologic processes of sun exposure effects on the skin.**
3. **Recognizes common inflammatory disorders of the skin such as impetigo, cellulitis, lymphangitis, hidradenitis suppurativa, and necrotizing fasciitis.**
4. Demonstrates knowledge of the common congenital disorders of the skin, including xeroderma pigmentosa, Ehlers-Danlos syndrome, basal cell nevus syndrome, albinism, etc.
5. Understands the basic principles of medical management and surgical treatment of common congenital disorders of the skin.
6. Is familiar with common nonsurgical methods and agents for treatment of the aging process of skin.
7. Knows the principles of prevention of sun exposure effects and is familiar with pharmacologic agents for prevention of sun exposure and the details of their prescription and use.
8. Demonstrates knowledge of common generalized dermatologic disorders such as scleroderma, dermatomyositis, and lupus erythematosus.
9. Is familiar with basic principles of medical treatment of generalized skin disorders.
10. Has detailed knowledge of surgical aspects of the treatment of patients with generalized skin disorders such as scleroderma and lupus erythematosus.
11. Understands the physiology of lipodystrophy and basic principles of fat metabolism.
12. Is familiar with medical management and surgical treatment of inflammatory disorders of the skin.
13. Recognizes processes of localized lipodystrophy such as Romberg's disease and is familiar with surgical and ancillary methods for treatment.

■ CLINICAL PRACTICE ACTIVITIES

During the course of the training program, the resident

1. Performs surgery on patients with congenital skin disorders.
2. Utilizes pharmacologic agents for treatment of aging skin.
3. Recommends pharmacologic agents for prevention of sun exposure; instructs patients in use of the agents and in general principles of skin protection from sun.
4. Evaluates and treats patients with bacterial, viral, and fungal infections of the skin such as cellulitis, lymphangitis, necrotizing fasciitis, and gas gangrene.
5. Performs surgical extirpation and reconstruction for hidradenitis suppurativa of the axilla and other areas of the body.
6. Performs reconstructive procedures for patients with localized lipodystrophy such as Romberg's disease.
7. *Performs surgical procedures on patients with generalized dermatologic disorders such as scleroderma and lupus erythematosus.*

CONGENITAL DISORDERS

Congenital skin disorders include those that are manifested as premature aging as well as others that predispose the skin to malignant transformation. Rare congenital disorders that are manifested as premature aging include Ehlers-Danlos syndrome, cutis laxa, pseudoxanthoma elasticum, progeria, and Werner syndrome.

Ehlers-Danlos syndrome is an inheritable disorder characterized by joint laxity; thin, friable, hyperextensible skin; subcutaneous tumors; and subcutaneous hemorrhage. Ocular and intestinal pathology may also be present. The basic underlying pathology shows abnormal collagen fasciculation and cross-linking that results in collagen with a markedly diminished tensile strength. Elective surgical intervention is not recommended in affected individuals because the marked vascular fragility and relative lack of adjacent tissue stroma for tamponade result in excessive hemorrhage and poor wound healing.

Cutis laxa is characterized by skin that is minimally elastic, nonfriable, and redundant. Three types have been described: a dominantly inherited form that affects only the dermis; a recessive form that is accompanied by pulmonary emphysema, cardiomegaly, great-vessel aneurysmal dilatation, and bowel and bladder diverticula; and an X-linked form that shows some systemic as well as the cutaneous manifestations. The primary histopathologic feature is dermal elastic fiber degeneration. Wound healing occurs in a relatively normal manner; consequently, surgical skin contouring procedures are possible and often beneficial.

Pseudoxanthoma elasticum is characterized by skin that appears thickened, leathery, and redundant, with associated yellow plaques and papules. Ocular and vascular involvement is also seen. Four subtypes based on method of inheritance are recognized. The basic histopathologic defect appears to be elastic fiber degeneration and fragmentation. In the absence of significant vascular and ocular disease, plastic surgery may be beneficial.

Progeria (Hutchinson-Gilford syndrome) is manifested as growth retardation beginning in the first year of life, scalp alopecia, craniofacial disproportion, and atrophic, dry, shiny skin. Systemically there is a loss of subcutaneous fat, arteriosclerosis, and cardiac disease. Affected patients do not reach sexual maturity. The underlying pathologic defect as well as the mode of inheritance is unknown. The short life expectancy of affected patients precludes most elective plastic surgery.

Werner syndrome (adult progeria) is characterized by growth retardation, alopecia, indurated patches of scleroderma-like skin, pigmentation changes, and an aged facies. Other findings include cataracts, diabetes mellitus, osteoporosis, muscle atrophy, arteriosclerosis, and various neoplasms. A chromosomal abnormality inherited as an autosomal recessive trait is responsible. Plastic surgical procedures are not recommended in affected patients because the atrophic skin and microangiopathic vascular characteristics portend a poor surgical result.

Congenital disorders that predispose the skin to malignant transformation include albinism, basal cell nevus syndrome, and xeroderma pigmentosum. Albinism is an inherited disorder characterized by hypomelanosis of the hair, eyes, and skin. Loss of the natural photoprotective effect of melanin places affected individuals at risk for the development of skin cancers. Solar avoidance and the liberal use of sunscreens are indicated.

The basal cell nevus syndrome (Gorlin's syndrome) is characterized by multiple cutaneous basal cell carcinomas, jaw cysts, and palmar and plantar pits. Other findings may include a widened nasal root, hypertelorism, frontal bossing, calcification of the falx cerebri, and neurologic abnormalities. The syndrome is transmitted as an autosomal dominant trait. The skin lesions, which may number in the hundreds, usually undergo malignant transformation during puberty. The behavior of the lesion is similar to other epidermoid skin cancers and should be treated accordingly.

Xeroderma pigmentosum is a rare systemic disorder characterized by intolerance of the integument and eyes to ultraviolet (UV) radiation. It is transmitted as an incomplete sex-linked recessive gene. The cutaneous manifestations of this disorder are seen early in life, with persistent erythema, freckling, pigmentary changes, premature skin aging, and the appearance of skin cancers. The underlying pathology is that of a defect in the DNA repair mechanism for UV radiation–induced damage. Death is the result of metastatic disease. Treatment is aimed at absolute solar radiation avoidance and protection, aggressive control of skin cancers, and oral retinoid therapy.

CUTANEOUS AGING

The aging process of the integument is characterized primarily by atrophy. The stratum corneum undergoes little change in thickness, but there is a reduction in dermoepidermal papillae. There is also a reduction in the number of melanocytes and Langerhans' cells. The most significant cutaneous changes are seen in the dermis, especially in the superficial layers. The three primary components, i.e., glycosaminoglycan gel, elastic fibers, and collagen—are affected. Specifically, the total quantity of glycosaminoglycans and proteoglycans has been demonstrated to decrease with age. Elastic fibers, which are responsible for maintaining collagen orientation, physiologic recoil, and laxity, undergo intrinsic degenerative changes. This results in a compromising functional alteration and loss of elastic tissue. Dermal collagen, which accounts for 70% to 80% of the dry weight of the skin, also decreases with aging. Much of this loss occurs in the reticular dermis, with an average decrease in dermal thickness of 6% per decade of life.

Type I collagen, usually found in a ratio of 6:1 with type III collagen, decreases disproportionately faster than type III. This may be because of impaired type I synthesis. Skin appendages are also affected by the aging process. There is a decrease in the number of pacinian and Meissner's corpuscles, which results in impaired pressure and touch sensation. Sebaceous gland hypertrophy with relative preservation of density is also seen.

Nonsurgical methods to control or reverse the cutaneous manifestations of aging include topical retinoids and cutaneous peeling agents. Tretinoin (Retin-A), a topical form of *trans*-retinoic acid, is a vitamin A derivative. It has been used in the management of acne vulgaris, actinic keratoses, and sun-damaged skin. This agent is thought to exert its hormone-like effect at the level of the nuclear DNA and, like all vitamin A derivatives, is known to be a potent teratogen. Retin-A causes an increase in epithelial turnover that is manifested histologically as the recreation of an essentially normal epidermis. The dermis becomes substantially widened, with the deposition of type III collagen in the most superficial aspects of the papillary dermis. Small blood vessel density is also increased.

Clinical results of treatment with Retin-A depend on the patient's complexion, the treatment area, and the regimen. More darkly pigmented individuals seem more tolerant of the agent's irritative effects. Results in facial skin are superior to those seen in the extremities. The treatment regimen should be individualized, but an initial period of treatment of 2 to 4 months is usually required before results are evident.

For skin "rejuvenation" a variety of cutaneous peeling agents are currently available. These agents can instill a freshened quality to the skin without altering color and texture or can alter the quality of damaged skin by modulating deep wrinkles and scars. While random epidermal shedding is a normal physiologic function caused by the upward migration of cells from the basal layer of the epidermis, a peeling agent functions by causing a uniform level of skin destruction that is subsequently replaced by an even layer derived from deep tissue.

Peels can be categorized by depth of effect. Light peels affect the upper epidermis and result in a new layer of skin with a freshened appearance. Medium peels affect the entire epidermis and the upper dermal tissues. It is this effect on the dermis and its subsequent fibroplasia that cause the skin to tighten and lessen the depth of wrinkles and scars. Deep peels affect the deeper layer of the dermis. Deeper peels are more likely to cause pigmentary changes and a thinning of the epidermis, thus imparting a shiny or translucent quality to the skin, and producing skin pore prominence secondary to excessive tightening.

The marked degree of fibroplasia and collagen deposition stimulated by these peels can cause a dramatic improvement in skin wrinkles and scars. The degree of beneficial cosmetic result is usually a reflection of the peel depth. Consequently, a variety of different peeling agents may achieve the same tissue response if their level of cellular destruction is similar.

The histologic effects of chemical peels are similar to those seen in dermabrasion. The peeling agent causes selective destruction of the epidermis and a portion of the dermis. Epithelial regeneration occurs from the remaining pilosebaceous units. A zone of fibroplasia (Grenz zone) occurs at the dermal-epidermal junction. This forces the older damaged dermis deeper and in theory tightens the skin, with resultant reduced wrinkle and scar depth.

The pigmentary changes seen with chemical peels are the result of melanocyte destruction and disruption in the epidermal basal layer. This pigmentary change is reversible as long as the deeper hair follicles still exist to serve as a source of melanocytes for their subsequent migration up into the basal cell layer.

The selection of a particular peeling agent and its concentration depends on the cutaneous abnormality that exists and the depth at which it resides. The more common agents used for chemical peels include phenol, trichloroacetic acid, resorcinol, salicylic acid, lactic acid, and α-hydroxy acids.

The classic "chemical peel" utilizes phenol (carbolic acid) as a potent keratocoagulant in high concentrations. The phenol is usually utilized as a saponified suspension with croton oil and liquid soap. While its beneficial effects can be dramatic, its risks include cardiac arrhythmias, which result from systemic absorption.

Trichloroacetic acid (TCA) can be used in three concentration ranges (unlike phenol) to yield a light, medium, or deep peel. It is poorly absorbed systemically and is regarded as less toxic than phenol.

Jessner's solution, which is a combination of the keratolytics resorcinol, salicylic acid, and lactic acid, is a superficial peeling agent. Its effect is primarily on the stratum corneum, although in successive applications it has a deeper effect. This mixture has been popularized as an adjunct to more potent agents because of its initial potentiating effect on the stratum corneum.

α-Hydroxy acids are superficial peeling agents and as a result are useful in freshening the skin or as a preliminary treatment adjunct.

ACTINIC DAMAGE

The effects of solar radiation on the skin cause it to behave in a markedly different way from aging skin that has been sun protected. While atrophy is the hallmark of normal aging skin, sun-damaged skin is thicker. Skin ground substance is increased, and type III immature collagen becomes dominant. Elastosis (i.e., thickened, degraded elastic fibers) is also seen. In combination, these histologic changes impart a characteristic "actinic" quality to the skin. Sun-damaged skin appears coarse, wrinkled, telangiectatic, mottled, and lax. These changes are accentuated by cigarette smoking.

The electromagnetic radiation wavelengths responsible for actinic damage lie in the UV range. While the earth's ozone layer effectively absorbs damaging solar radiation below 290 nm, most UVB (290 to 315 nm) and a majority of UVA (315 to 400 nm) waves are transmitted. UVB radiation is the most carcinogenic and is felt to be responsible for most of the actinic cutaneous changes. UVA has also been shown to cause actinic damage when delivered in doses 100 to 1,000 times that of UVB. This level of radiation can be measured in normal sunlight, under fluorescent lighting, and in tanning booths (changes characteristic of dermal elastosis can be seen after as few as 150 tanning sessions).

Most topical sunscreens, while protective against UVB radiation, provide no UVA benefit. Furthermore, it has been shown that infrared radiation accelerates the dermal damage caused by UV radiation.

Two major classes of topical agents are available to protect the skin against UV radiation: reflective and absorptive agents. Reflective agents such as zinc oxide and titanium dioxide are opaque creams that effectively reflect a majority of the UV spectrum. These agents are very visible, thus somewhat limiting their cosmetic usefulness.

Absorptive agents such as para-aminobenzoic acid (PABA) or its esters benzophenones, cinnamates, and butylmethoxydibenzoylmethane (Parsol 1789) exert their effects by selective wavelength absorption. PABA binds to cutaneous proteins after penetrating the stratum corneum. Its effect is primarily in the UVB waveband. Benzophenones offer a wider spectrum of absorption. Cinnamates also have a wider spectrum of absorption than PABA but bind poorly to the stratum corneum. Parsol 1789 offers excellent UVA absorption but poor UVB coverage, which makes it an effective "combination" agent.

The topical sunscreen agents are rated and compared by their sun protective factor (SPF). This is a measure of the amount of UVB necessary to cause a minimal erythematous reaction in normal and protected skin. In usual outdoor conditions, SPF 15 is the highest factor needed, although recent experimental evidence suggests that further protective effects can be seen with higher SPF formulations. The vehicle in which the absorptive agent is contained will also affect the SPF, as well as its water resistance.

Systemic photoprotective and tanning compounds include β-carotene and canthaxanthine. β-Carotene has been shown to offer no universal photoprotectant effect in that its peak of UV absorption is outside the UVB spectrum. It can be used in persons sensitive to UVA, such as patients who have erythropoietic protoporphyria. Canthaxanthine, the "tanning" pill, is a naturally occurring red-orange pigment. Oral ingestion causes adipose pigment accumulation and results in golden coloration in the skin. Retinal changes associated with this drug prompted the Food and Drug Administration to issue an alert warning of the danger of these preparations.

GENERALIZED SKIN DISORDERS

A diffuse group of generalized disorders may exhibit cutaneous manifestations. Included in this group are scleroderma, dermatomyositis, and lupus erythematosus. These disorders share the underlying features of vasculitis and multisystem involvement as a portion of their pathophysiology.

Scleroderma is a connective tissue disease of unknown etiology. It is characterized by fibrosis secondary to fibroplasia and thickening of collagenous tissues, elastic fiber fragmentation and thickening, and arterial intimal thickening. It occurs more frequently in women, with an onset in the third through sixth decades. Systemic manifestations may also affect the heart, lungs, kidneys, central nervous system, and gastrointestinal tract. The skin of the hands, fingers, and forearms is affected early. These changes consist of a thickening of the integument, with the skin assuming a shiny, nearly translucent appearance. Joint range of motion becomes limited, and forearm musculature may develop a woody induration. Finger cold intolerance is an early finding, with gradual progression to numbness and possible pain at rest if the degree of tissue ischemia is severe. This may progress to fingertip atrophy, ulceration, and in severe cases, gangrene or amputation.

Treatment is conservative. At present there is no way to halt the progression of this disease, although systemic steroids may slow disease progression. Calcium channel blockers have been used with mixed success in treating some aspects of distal extremity ischemia. Sympathectomy is rarely of value, although some success has been reported with sympathectomy at the digital level. Amputation is often necessary once gangrene is established.

Dermatomyositis is an inflammatory condition marked by a cutaneous inflammation that produces a characteristic rash. It occurs in an area of polymyositis, which is an inflammatory disease of voluntary muscle marked by lymphocyte infiltration, muscle fiber damage, and degeneration. The etiology of the disorder is unknown, although it has been postulated to be either the result of an antecedent viral infection or an autoimmune process. The cutaneous manifestations may occur in any temporal order in relation to the muscle symptoms. The manifestations, which may be localized or diffuse, include erythema, eczematoid dermatitis, and maculopapular eruptions. The distribution of lesions includes facial, chest, articular, and periungual areas. Perioral and periocular edema is commonly seen in the more severe forms of the disorder. Occasionally, ulceration and subcutaneous calcification occur. An underlying malignancy should be excluded in patients past the sixth decade.

The diagnosis of dermatomyositis is based on clinical findings, electromyographic (EMG) studies, elevation of serum creatine kinase levels, and diagnostic muscle biopsy findings. Treatment is primarily conservative. Corticosteroids are the mainstay of treatment, while immunosuppressive agents are reserved for more fulminant disease. It should be noted, however, that the cutaneous lesions are often resistant to treatment. The overall mortality rates for patients with this disorder are approximately four times that of the general population, with death often attributed to cardiac, renal, or pulmonary complications.

Systemic lupus erythematosus is another inflammatory disorder of unknown etiology. Antibodies directed against cellular nuclear antigens as well as specific cell lines and tissue are common. It has been postulated that this disorder may also result from an antecedent viral infection or from some other autoimmune process.

The pathologic cutaneous findings include facial erythema and edema (butterfly rash) with progression to localized telangiectasias and skin atrophy. These eruptions are more common in the areas of solar exposure. Patchy alopecia may also occur. Dermal vasculitis, manifested as digital infarcts, may be seen. Other findings include oral and nasal mucosal ulceration, purpura, hives, Raynaud's phenomenon, and discoid changes marked by hyperkeratosis. Systemic manifestations may affect the kidneys, central nervous system, heart, and lungs. Histologically, the findings correlate with clinical stage. Specifically, tissue edema, red blood cell extravasation, perivascular to diffuse dermal inflammation, and epidermal hyperkeratosis are seen.

The diagnosis of systemic lupus erythematosus is based on the presence of a constellation of clinical and laboratory findings, the most important of which is the presence of antinuclear antibodies. Treatment is primarily conservative, with corticosteroids the cornerstone of therapy. Antimalarial compounds, cytotoxic and immunosuppressive drugs, and plasmapheresis have been used with mixed success. UV light exposure should be avoided, especially in patients with active or recurrent skin lesions.

LIPODYSTROPHY

Lipodystrophy, or defective fat metabolism, is characterized by a nearly total lack of subcutaneous adipose tissue. It may be of three different types: generalized (congenital), localized (Romberg's disease), or progressive. The latter type is manifested by loss of subcutaneous tissue from the upper part of the torso, with an increase in pelvic adipose tissue.

Adipocytes, or mature fat cells, are responsible for fat storage and synthesis and are consequently an effective energy reservoir as well as thermal insulator. White adipose tissue constitutes a majority of human adipose tissue. It is this subtype that is associated with lipid metabolism. Brown adipose tissue is important for newborn thermoregulation, but its role in adults is less clear.

The distribution of adipose tissue depends on sex, age, and race. Women exhibit a *gynoid* pattern of deposition, with accumulation of fat in the lower portion of the trunk, hips, buttocks, and upper part of the thighs. Men exhibit an *android* pattern of fat deposition (uniform about the trunk). Women have a higher proportion of body fat than men do. Adipose distribution is also age dependent. A newborn has one fifth the fat stores found in an average adult. Truncal adiposity increases with age, as does its internalization. Adipose stores in the extremities shift from a subcutaneous location to intermuscular and intramuscular sites. Racial differences are also apparent. Blacks exhibit increased adipose accumulation in the buttocks, which is further accentuated by lumbar lordosis, when compared with other races.

In the torso and lower extremities, there are both deep and superficial subcutaneous tissue compartments. The superficial layer contains multiple small, dense compartments, whereas the deep layer is less well organized, with looser fat pockets. This deeper layer is most evident in the periumbilical, paralumbar, and gluteal-thigh regions.

Suction-assisted lipectomy allows the selective removal of adipose tissue deposits. This technique utilizes a vacuum delivered through a cannula placed subcutaneously to effect its result. While the basic technique is simple, an ideal aesthetic result depends on proper patient selection, surgical judgment, meticulous attention to detail, and the ability to manage large volume shifts. Proper patient selection is paramount.

Suction-assisted lipectomy is effective for minimal to moderate deposits refractory to body conditioning and dieting. The adipose tissue should be located in the subcutaneous plane and underlie skin of sufficient elastic quality to allow for proper redraping. Good muscle tone and the absence of a panniculus are also important. A blunt-tipped liposuction cannula should be used and maneuvered through at least two separate incisions to allow for cross-tunneling and uniform tissue contouring. Recognition of the procedure's end point is also important. This is demonstrated by the volume of tissue removed, the surface appearance, the appearance of blood mixed with the adipose extract, and the change in consistency experienced with cannula passage. Postprocedure compression garments should be worn for at least 10 days.

Large volume shifts accompany suction lipectomy. There is an approximate 1% drop in patient hematocrit for each 150 cc of fat removed. This should be replaced with crystalloid solution at a 3:1 ratio, with consideration for blood transfusion when greater than 1,500 cc of fat is removed. For a more detailed description of suction lipectomy, see Chapter 5.

Localized lipodystrophy such as Romberg's disease or hemifacial atrophy is a form of regional adipose tissue deficiency. The etiology of this disorder is unknown, although current evidence supports the original theory postulated by Romberg that this is a form of vasomotor trophoneuritis. The sympathetic nervous system is probably the final common pathway. No genetic predisposition has been found. Women are affected slightly more frequently than men.

The onset of symptoms is typically before the third decade and is heralded by the selective unilateral atrophy of subcutaneous tissue. Elastic fibers are relatively spared. There is a loss of adnexal structures and thinning of the stratum granulosum. Epidermal keratoses are also seen and impart a leathery texture to the skin. Underlying muscle function is impaired both directly by selective muscle fiber atrophy and indirectly by the constrictive effect of the overlying integument. The osteocartilaginous skeleton may also be affected.

The course of the disease is usually self-limited, with atrophic cessation occurring after 2 to 10 years. Therapy directed toward restoration of form and function is usually withheld until the disease has been quiescent for at least 1 year. As with other types of lipodystrophy, it is the anatomic location that dictates the disease pathology. Specifically, unaffected adipose tissue will atrophy when transplanted into an affected site, while affected adipose tissue will hypertrophy when transferred away from the area of pathology.

Skeletal restoration, when necessary, is a prerequisite to soft-tissue reconstruction. While onlay autogenous bone grafting remains the standard, synthetic mesh, ceramics, and cadaveric cartilage have been used with mixed success. A variety of methods has been employed for soft-tissue reconstruction. Free fat or dermal fat grafts have been employed but have high resorption rates. Synthetic materials such as injectable silicone resist absorption but are associated with inflammation and extrusion. Consequently, vascularized free tissue transfer has become the reconstructive method of choice. While the greater omentum is commonly selected because of the variable contour correction it can achieve, other tissues such as the parascapular region have been utilized.

CUTANEOUS INFLAMMATORY PROCESSES

A number of bacterial, viral, and fungal skin disorders may be manifested as a cutaneous inflammatory process. The bacterial skin disorders include impetigo, lymphangitis, necrotizing fasciitis, gas gangrene, and synergistic gangrene.

Impetigo is a superficial cutaneous infection characterized by a series of intraepithelial abscesses. The lesions appear as small pustules that may coalesce and are intensely pruritic. Impetigo is caused by hemolytic streptococci with or without *Staphylococcus aureus.* It occurs more commonly in children in warmer climates. In adults it may complicate an eczematous dermatitis. Complications include hemorrhagic abscesses and nephritis. Treatment entails local wound care and appropriate systemic antibiotic therapy. Topical antibiotics are reserved for very localized disease.

Lymphangitis is an inflammatory process affecting the lymphatic pathway, often visualized as cutaneous erythematous streaking. While the causative organism may vary, it is commonly associated with streptococcal infections. This inflammatory process and its frequent association with lymphadenitis represent a normal host defensive response to a distal infection. The majority of patients respond to appropriate antibiotic therapy, local wound care, rest, and elevation.

Necrotizing fasciitis is a rapidly invasive fascial infectious process usually caused by multiple pathogens, including streptococci, staphylococci, gram-negative bacteria, and anaerobes. It is characterized by skin necrosis caused by thrombosis of the cutaneous perforator vessels. It tends to begin in a localized area and progresses along the relatively avascular fascial planes. With progression, the overlying skin becomes devascularized. This is manifested as hemorrhagic bullae, necrosis, tissue edema, and inflammation in an area smaller than that of fascial involvement. The fascia assumes a dull gray, edematous appearance. Myonecrosis may also be present.

Treatment involves maintenance of adequate volume support, debridement of nonviable tissue, and antibiotic coverage. Penicillin and gentamicin are usually begun initially, with further selection guided by culture results. Debridement should remove all nonviable tissue, but where overlying skin or underlying muscle is viable, attempts should be made at preservation. This may require multiple "access" incisions and multiple operative debridements.

Gas gangrene (diffuse clostridial myositis) represents an advanced form of clostridial infection. A number of clostridial species infect humans, and all of them are saprophytes. The spore form of this organism requires conditions of low oxygen such as that seen with tissue ischemia, muscle injury, severe edema, and foreign bodies, to convert into its anaerobic vegetative form. This form synthesizes a number of enzymes such as lecithinase, collagenase, hyaluronidase, lipase, protease, and hemolysin that destroy local tissue and promote further invasion.

Gas gangrene is a rapidly progressive process usually evident within 3 days of the precipitating event. It is manifested by local pain, edema, and a brown-tinged, suppurative exudate. The cutaneous edema, hemorrhagic discoloration, and necrosis are more localized than the underlying inflammatory process. Crepitus and fever are variable, but toxemia and delirium can be common findings. The diagnosis is based on the clinical appearance of the wound and the presence of large gram-positive rods in the tissue or exudate.

Treatment is primarily surgical and should be directed toward wide debridement and open drainage. Initial amputation should be avoided if possible, but serial debridements are often indicated. Penicillin therapy should be given concurrently. Hyperbaric oxygen may limit the degree of invasion, but surgical intervention is required to eliminate the disease focus.

Meleney's progressive synergistic gangrene is caused by microaerophilic or anaerobic streptococci along with staphylococci or gram-negative organisms. It may begin in a surgical wound, ostomy site, or area of local trauma and appears as a central, small, painful, ulcerated region surrounded by an area of necrotic skin. This is further surrounded by a violaceous region blending into an area of tissue erythema. Surgical debridement is the mainstay of therapy, along with penicillin coverage.

Hidradenitis suppurativa is a chronic infectious process involving the apocrine sweat glands with extension into the subcutaneous tissue and fascia. It occurs in those cutaneous regions where this glandular type predominates, specifically, the axilla, groin, perineum, and the circumanal and circumareolar areas. The disease begins as a localized subcutaneous indurative process that progresses to suppuration with surrounding cellulitis. Pain is often intense. Incision and drainage are required at this stage, along with improved hygiene and antibiotic therapy. This may be curative early in the course of the disease.

In chronic cases, more aggressive surgical intervention is necessary, with radical surgical excision of the involved area and appropriate closure. Mild forms of the disease can be controlled with oral tetracycline, while reports of control of the chronic form have been noted with long-term oral isotretinoin therapy.

Common viral disorders of the skin include verrucae and herpetic whitlow. Verrucae (common warts) are caused by the human papillomavirus. They occur in up to 20% of the population, with a peak incidence in the second decade. The lesions appear as elevated, round, roughened extrusions that contain multiple keratinized finger-like projections. They occur mainly in unprotected areas and are transmitted by person-to-person contact or by autoinoculation.

Treatment by electrodesiccation, cryotherapy, or topical bichloroacetic acid is effective, although healing is prolonged. Spontaneous resolution does occur. Surgical excision is not recommended because of the tendency for wound autoinoculation.

Herpetic whitlow is caused by the herpes simplex virus and is manifested as an exquisitely painful fingertip lesion with minimal edema and induration. This precedes the development of multiple small vesicles that contain clear fluid. The infectious process is self-limited, although topical acyclovir has been shown to decrease the severity and duration of symptoms.

Dermatophytosis is a chronic fungal infection of the skin, hair, or nails. It is caused by a variety of fungal species referred to as dermatophytes. They have a propensity for the body's keratinized structures and remain confined to this area. The manifestations vary with the site of involvement and the fungal species. Common findings include cutaneous scaling, fissuring, alopecia, and localized inflammation. Treatment includes the use of topical antifungal preparations such as clotrimazole or miconazole and oral agents such as griseofulvin for severe infections.

SUGGESTED READING

Barton FE: The aging face: Rhytidectomy and adjunctive procedures. *Selected Readings Plast Surg* 1991; 6:19.

Markman B: Anatomy and physiology of adipose tissue. *Clin Plast Surg* 1989; 16:235–244.

Seropian DM: Chemosurgical peel, in Riley WB (ed): *Instructional Courses,* vol 1. St Louis, Mosby–Year Book, 1988, pp 3–33.

Sohn SA, Cochran TC: The aging face and total facial rejuvenation. *Adv Plast Reconstr Surg* 1992; 8:103–127.

Zarem HA, Lowe NJ: Benign growths and generalized skin disorders, in Smith JW, Aston SJ (eds): *Grabb and Smith's Plastic Surgery,* ed 4. Boston, Little, Brown, 1991, pp 819–850.

PART IV

Plastic Surgery of the Head and Neck

Chapter 14

Anatomy/Physiology/Embryology

Edward Ricciardelli, M.D.
John A. Persing, M.D.

CONTENTS

NOTE: The material in this chapter is frequently covered during the prerequisite training period of many plastic surgery residents. This chapter should serve as a valuable review of important material in such cases. For residents who have not mastered this material, this chapter is essential.

CHAPTER OBJECTIVE

At the end of this chapter the resident is thoroughly familiar with the anatomy, physiology, and embryology of the head and neck and applies this knowledge to the medical and surgical management of disorders and processes in this anatomic area.

LEARNER OBJECTIVES

On completion of the unit, the resident

1. **Knows the anatomy of the skull, including suture lines, foramina, and structures exiting foramina, and is familiar with the anatomy and functions of the cranial nerves.**
2. **Knows the anatomy of the facial bones and their ostia and bony relationships.**
3. **Has special knowledge of the vascular structures of the skull, head, and neck.**
4. **Knows the anatomy of the eye, including bony structures, the eyelids, the extraocular muscles, the innervation of the eye and adnexal structures, the vascular supply, and the lacrimal apparatus.**
5. **Knows the anatomy of the ear, including common measurements of the ear, relationships of the ear to other structures, and the vascular and sensory supply.**
6. **Knows the anatomy of the nose and septum, including bones and cartilages and nerve and vascular supply.**
7. **Is familiar with the physiology of the nose with particular reference to airflow and airway obstruction.**
8. **Knows the anatomy of the oropharynx, including muscular structures, lymphatic drainage, and contiguous neurovascular structures.**

9. **Is familiar with the physiology of the oropharynx, including palatal function, speech, and swallowing.**
10. **Knows the anatomy and function of facial structures, including facial muscles, fascial layers, and salivary glands.**
11. **Is familiar with the general principles of embryology of the head and neck, with special reference to the development of the facial structures, including the lip, palate, and ear.**
12. Is familiar with general aspects of the physiology of the eye and the function of the lacrimal apparatus.
13. Knows the basic anatomy of the dental structures and the temporomandibular joint.
14. Knows the anatomy of the neck structures, including the thyroid gland, larynx, muscles, and vascular and nerve supply.
15. Is familiar with cephalometric analysis of facial structures and other forms of facial analysis.

■ CLINICAL PRACTICE ACTIVITIES

During the course of the training program, the resident

1. **Applies knowledge of head and neck anatomy in a variety of clinical settings.**
2. Performs cadaver dissection of the head and neck.
3. Analyzes and utilizes cephalometric studies.

OVERVIEW OF HEAD AND NECK EMBRYOLOGY

The specific prenatal events leading to the differentiation of individual head and neck structures must be studied within the context of overall embryologic development. Head and neck embryology involves an intricate interaction of cellular proliferation, migration, resorption, and growth.

The branchial apparatus plays an essential role in the development of the head and neck. The branchial or pharyngeal arches develop during the fourth week of fetal life. There are six branchial arches, and each arch is characterized by its own skeletal, muscular, nervous, and arterial components (Table 14–1). The arches are derived from mesodermal tissue that gives rise to the musculature of the head and neck (Fig 14–1). The neural crest cells give rise to the skeletal components of the face. The first pharyngeal arch, called the mandibular

TABLE 14–1.
Major Skull Foramina

Cranial Fossa	Foramen	Contents
Anterior	Anterior ethmoidal	Anterior ethmoid artery and nerve
	Posterior ethmoid and nerve	Posterior ethmoid artery
	Cribriform plate	Olfactory nerve
Middle	Optic canal	Optic nerve Ophthalmic artery
	Superior orbital fissure	Cranial nerves III, IV, V_1, VI Ophthalmic veins
	Foramen rotundum	V_2 (maxillary nerve)
	Foramen ovale	V_3 (mandibular nerve)
	Foramen spinosum	Middle meningeal artery
	Foramen lacerum	Internal carotid artery (roof) Sympathetic and venous plexi
Posterior	Foramen magnum	Spinal cord Vertebral arteries Spinal arteries
	Jugular foramen	Internal jugular vein Cranial nerves IX, X, XI
	Hypoglossal canal	Cranial nerve XII

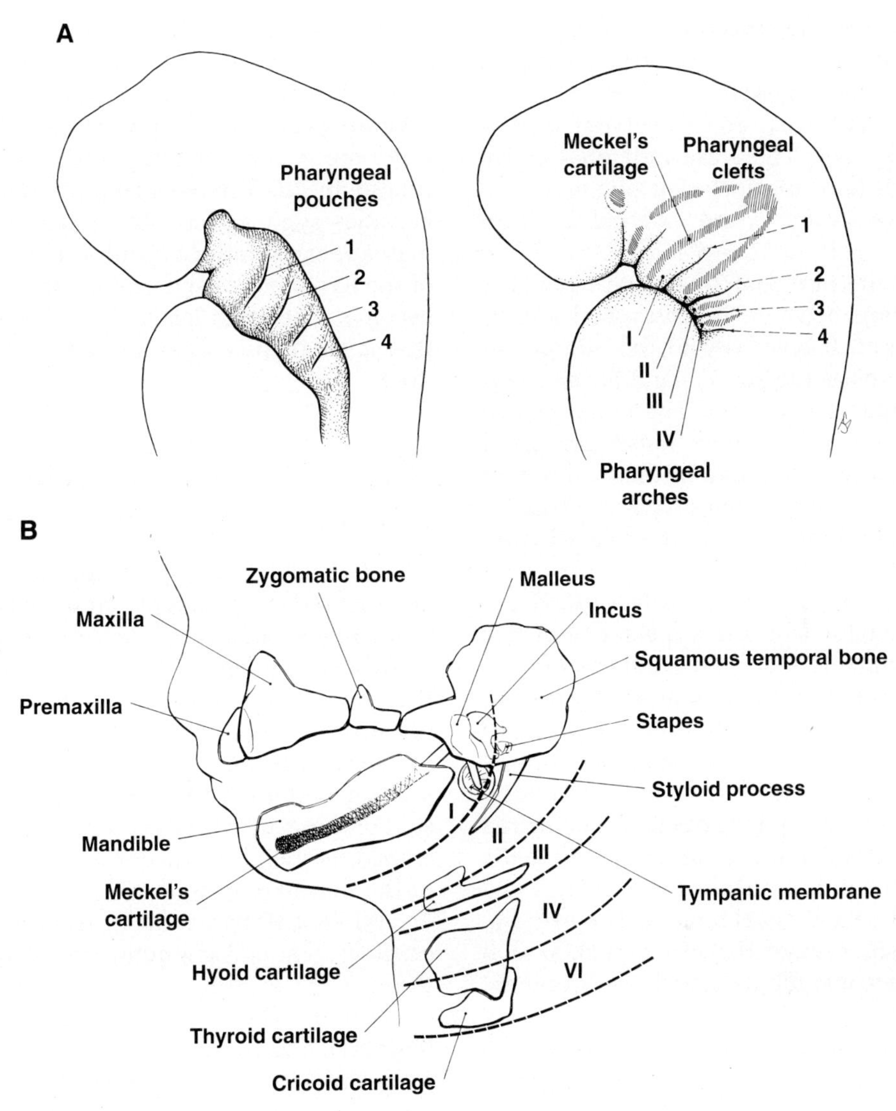

FIG 14–1.
Pharyngeal arches and clefts **(A)** and their adult derivatives **(B).**

arch or Meckel's cartilage, gives rise to the mandible, maxilla, zygoma, and squamous portion of the temporal bone. The incus and malleus of the middle ear are also derived from the first pharyngeal arch. The mesenchyme of the first arch forms the muscles of mastication, as well as the anterior belly of the digastric muscle, the mylohyoid, the tensor tympani, and the tensor palatani. The innervation of these muscles is derived from the trigeminal nerve. The second arch (hyoid arch or Reichert's cartilage) gives rise to the stapes, the stylohyoid ligament, and portions of the hyoid bone. The muscles of the second arch are the muscles of facial expression, as well as the posterior digastric muscle, the stapedius, and the stylohyoid muscle. These muscles are innervated by the facial nerve. The third arch produces portions of the hyoid bone. The muscles of the third arch are limited to the stylopharyngeal muscles. The nerve of the third arch is the glossopharyngeal nerve. The fourth through the sixth pharyngeal arches give rise to the cartilage of the larynx, with the fourth contributing the thyroid cartilage and the sixth contributing the cricoid cartilage. The musculature of these arches involves the intrinsic and extrinsic musculature of the larynx as well as the constrictors of the pharynx. These muscles are innervated by the laryngeal branches of the vagus nerve.

Each pharyngeal arch is separated by a pharyngeal cleft. There are four pharyngeal clefts, with only the first cleft giving rise to a definitive structure, the external auditory canal.

There are also four pharyngeal pouches that develop between the branchial arches. The first pouch gives rise to the middle ear cavity as well as the eustachian tube and part of the tympanic membrane. The second pouch develops into the palatine tonsil. The third pouch forms the thymus and the parathyroid glands. The fourth pouch also contributes to the development of the parathyroid glands.

Early in the fourth week, facial development is heralded by the appearance of five facial prominences or local swellings of mesenchymal tissue. Each of these facial processes serves as an active growth center for the facial skeleton. The frontonasal prominence appears just cranial to the stomodeum and contributes to nasal and cranial development. The paired maxillary prominences form just lateral to the stomodeum and contribute to nasal, lip, maxillary, and palatal development. The mandibular prominences of the first branchial arch contribute to mandibular and lip development (Fig 14–2).

The thyroid gland originates from epithelial proliferation at the base of the tongue at the foramen cecum. The thyroid tissue then descends to the level of the laryngeal cartilage, where it reaches its final position during the seventh week of development. During migration, the gland remains connected to the tongue by the thyroglossal duct, which later becomes solid and is obliterated. This duct may appear anterior or within the substance of the hyoid bone itself. Failure of this duct to become obliterated leads to the formation of thyroglossal duct cysts or remnants of the duct.

SKULL AND CRANIAL BASE

Embryology

The skeletal components of the calvarium are derived from neural crest cells, which ultimately form mesenchymal tissue, which in turn forms cartilage and bone. The majority of the cranial base is formed by endochondral ossification. Important areas for growth are the spheno-occipital synchondrosis, the nasal septum, and the frontonasal complex. Expansion of these areas leads to lengthening of the cranial base and protrusion and lengthening of the maxillary complex.

While the basicranium is formed from cartilage (chondrocranium), the majority of the calvaria is formed by intramembranous ossification. The frontal, parietal, squamous temporal, and portions of the occipital bones are formed by direct ossification.

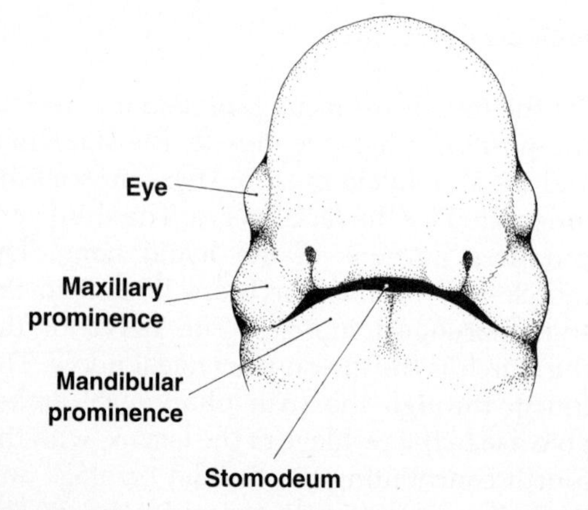

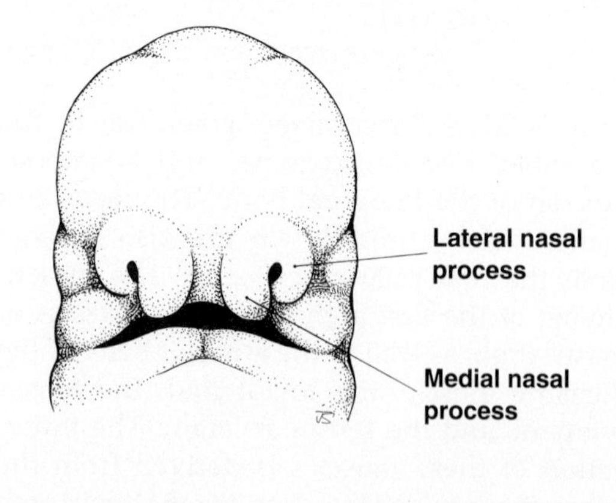

FIG 14–2.
The facial prominences associated with facial, lip, and palatal development. Four-week **(A)** and 5-week **(B)** embryos.

Anatomy

The cranium is composed of the calvaria, or roof, and the cranial base. The anterior portion of the calvaria consists of the frontal bone. In development and in the young child, the frontal bone consists of two halves that articulate in the midline at the metopic suture. The frontal bone articulates posteriorly with the parietal bones bilaterally at the coronal suture. Anteromedially, the frontal bone articulates with the two nasal bones and the frontal processes of the maxillary bones at the frontonasal suture. Inferolaterally, the frontal bone articulates with the zygoma at the frontozygomatic suture. The frontal bone itself forms the forehead and roof of the orbit. Immediately behind the glabella lie the frontal sinuses. The orbital roof forms part of the anterior cranial fossa floor.

The paired parietal bones join at the midline at the sagittal suture. Laterally, they articulate with the squamous portion of the temporal bones at the squamous suture. Posteriorly, the lambdoid suture is formed by the articulation of the parietal bones with the occipital bone. The occipital bone forms part of the floor of the posterior cranial fossa and surrounds the foramen magnum through which exit the spinal cord and vertebral and spinal arteries.

The sphenoid bone lies at the cranial base and is made up of two lesser and two greater wings and the pterygoid processes. The lesser wings of the sphenoid project inferolaterally to encircle the optic nerve, thus forming the optic canal. The lesser wings also form the superior border of the superior orbital fissure. The greater wings of the sphenoid form the inferior border of the superior orbital fissure through which exit cranial nerves III, IV, V_1, and VI and the ophthalmic veins. The pterygoid processes project inferiorly and consist of medial and lateral plates. They form the posterior boundaries of the pterygomaxillary fossa. The hamulus is a small process projecting from the medial pterygoid plate around which run the tensor and levator palati muscles to the soft palate. The sphenoid bone also contains the foramen rotundum, which transmits the maxillary or second division of the trigeminal nerve, and the foramen ovale, which transmits the mandibular or third division of the trigeminal nerve (see Table 14–1).

The temporal bones consist of a lateral squamous portion that forms the lateral aspect of the cranial vault. The petrous and tympanic portions of the temporal bones house the otic and vestibular apparatus. The mastoid and styloid processes also originate from the temporal bone. The petrous apex of the temporal bone forms a portion of the floor of the middle cranial fossa along with the greater wing of the sphenoid bone.

THE EYE

Embryology

The initial event in the differentiation of the eye occurs early in the fourth week of development with the formation of outpocketings of the forebrain called the optic vesicles. The optic vesicles subsequently invaginate to form the optic cups. Initially the optic cups are vascularized by the hyaloid artery. During the seventh week of development the mouth of the optic cup forms a round opening called the choroid fissure, which later forms the pupil.

The lens itself is formed as the optic vesicles induce the surface ectoderm to form the primitive lens placode. Retinal formation is heralded by the appearance of pigment granules called the pigment layer of the retina. There is differentiation of the posterior optic cup cells into light receptor elements, or rods and cones. The iris is formed from the anterior inner layer of the optic cup, which also gives rise to the ciliary body.

At the end of the fifth week, the optic vesicle is surrounded by mesenchymal tissue that differentiates into the choroid layer as well as the sclera. The mesenchymal tissue overlying the anterior aspect of the eye forms the anterior chamber, which splits the mesenchyme into an inner and outer layer. The outer layer is continuous with the sclera and forms the cornea.

The optic nerve connects the eye to the brain. Initially the optic cup is connected by the optic stalk. The nerve fibers of the retina are found in the optic stalk. Eventually the optic stalk becomes the optic nerve, which contains in its center the hyaloid artery. This artery later becomes the central artery of the retina. The optic nerve is surrounded by a continuation of the dura mater, which is a continuation of the choroid and sclera anteriorly.

The bony orbits form by a condensation of mesenchyme derived from the maxillary processes below and the lateral nasal processes above. The lateral and inferior walls are formed from the maxillary processes, which give rise to the zygoma and parts of the maxilla. The medial walls develop from the lateral nasal processes, which form the frontal process of the maxilla and the nasal, lacrimal, and ethmoid bones. Posteriorly the orbital apex is formed by the ossification of the sphenoid bones during basicranial development.

The eyelids are formed during the second month of fetal development as folds in the surface ectoderm above and below the eye. The upper lid is developed from the frontonasal process, while the lower lid is formed from the maxillary processes. The outer layer of ectoderm forms the epidermis, while the inside of the fold becomes the conjunctiva. The tarsal plate and muscular tissues of the eyelids are formed from an ingrowth of mesoderm. The eyelid folds fuse during the third fetal month and remain fused until the end of the fifth month when they separate. The lacrimal apparatus is derived from a solid row of ectodermal cells buried beneath the maxillary and lateral nasal processes. Through a process of canalization of the nasolacrimal duct, canaliculi in the lacrimal sac are formed.

The extraocular muscles are formed from a condensation of mesoderm associated with the optic vessicle. The individual muscles are independently formed by the seventh week of development. After development of the four recti and two obliques, the levator palpebrae superioris is formed from the separation of fibers from the superior rectus muscle.

Anatomy

Bony Orbit

The bony orbit of the eye is composed of seven bones: the frontal, maxillary, zygomatic, lacrimal, ethmoidal, palatine, and sphenoid bones (Fig 14–3). The orbit is roughly a

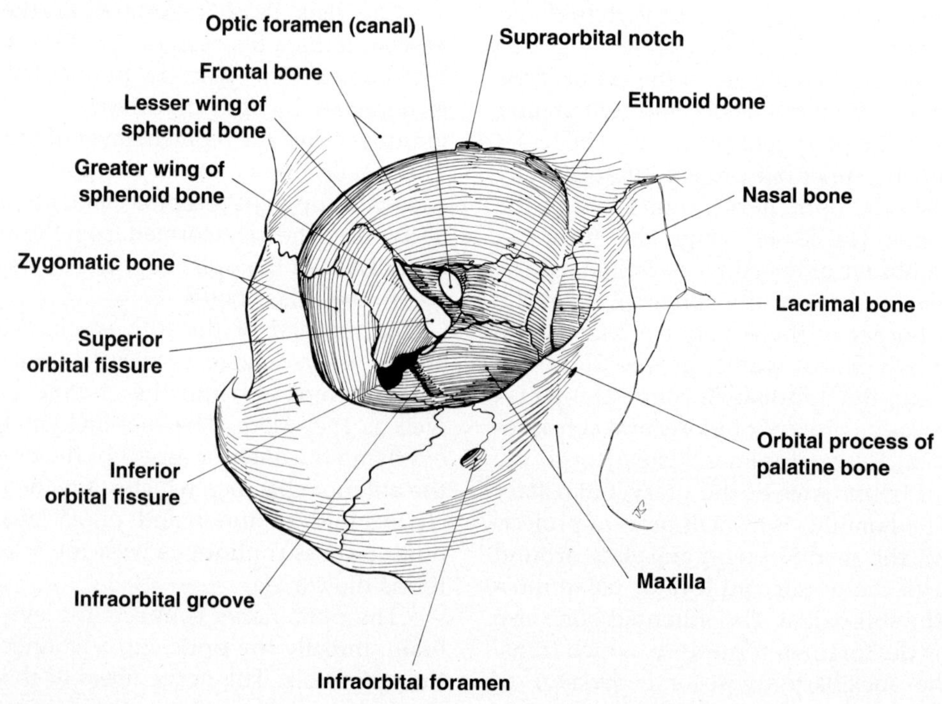

FIG 14–3.
Bony architecture of the orbit with associated foramina.

quadrangular pyramid with its apex directed medially and superiorly. Dimensions vary, but on average orbital volume is approximately 30 ml, and the depth of the orbit is approximately 40 mm. The average adult interorbital distance (dacryon to dacryon) is 25 mm.

The frontal, zygomatic, and maxillary bones form the orbital rim, proceeding superiorly to laterally. The superior rim formed by the frontal bone transmits the supratrochlear and supraorbital neurovascular structures through their respective foramina. The trochlea or pulley for the superior oblique muscle lies just within the superomedial rim. The medial rim is formed by the maxillary bones. The lateral orbital rim is formed by the frontal and zygomatic bones. Whitnall's tubercle lies approximately 10 mm within the orbit on the frontal process of the zygoma and provides attachment for the lateral canthal tendon.

The roof of the orbit is formed by the frontal bone separating the orbit from the frontal sinus anteriorly and the anterior and middle cranial fossae posteriorly.

The medial wall is the weakest component of the bony orbit, which accounts for its propensity to be injured in cases of blunt orbital trauma. It is made up mostly of the structurally weak lamina papyracea of the ethmoidal bone and the sphenoid, the maxillary, and the lacrimal bones. The lacrimal sac lies within the lacrimal fossa, which connects with the nasolacrimal duct inferiorly to the inferior meatus of the nose. The medial canthal tendon attaches to the periosteum of the medial orbital wall (lacrimal bone). The anterior and posterior ethmoid foramina traverse the medial wall of the orbit and are located approximately 6 and 12 mm from the medial orbital rim, respectively.

The maxillary and zygomatic bones form the floor of the orbit and separate it from the maxillary sinus antrum. The floor is structurally weak and is crossed by the infraorbital nerve, which exits at the infraorbital foramen of the maxillary bone approximately 10 mm below the inferior orbital rim.

The lateral wall is structurally strong since it is formed by the frontal process of the zygomatic bone anteriorly and the greater wing of the sphenoid bone posteriorly. At the orbital apex, separating the floor from the lateral wall of the orbit is the inferior orbital fissure, which transmits the infraorbital and zygomatic nerves, infraorbital artery, and inferior ophthalmic vein. It is contiguous with the infratemporal fossa. The superior orbital fissure separates the greater and lesser wings of the sphenoid and transmits cranial nerves III, IV, the ophthalmic branch of V, and VI, as well the ophthalmic veins and orbital artery. The optic foramen itself lies within the sphenoid bone and transmits the optic nerve, ophthalmic artery, and associated sympathetic nerves.

Eyelid and Adnexa

In primary gaze, the upper eyelid lies 1 to 2 mm below the superior limbus of the iris. It is composed of seven layers at the supratarsal or preseptal level: skin, orbicularis oculi muscle, orbital septum, fat pads, levator aponeurosis, Müller's muscle, and conjunctiva. The tarsal plate itself serves as the framework of the eyelids. It is a fibrocartilaginous plate approximately 12 mm in vertical height in the upper lid and 4 mm in the lower lid. At the pretarsal level the eyelids are separated into anterior (skin and orbicularis muscle) and posterior (tarsus and conjunctiva) lamellae.

The orbicularis muscle surrounds the palpebral fissure and has pretarsal, preseptal, and preorbital components overlying the tarsus, orbital septum, and orbital rim, respectively (Fig 14–4). The superficial heads of the upper and lower pretarsal muscles join to form the anterior limb of the medial canthal tendon. The deep heads (also known as Horner's muscle) join to insert behind the lacrimal sac to form the posterior limb of the medial canthal tendon. The lacrimal sac lies in the lacrimal fossa between the two limbs of the canthal tendon. The deep and superficial heads of the preseptal and pretarsal orbicularis muscle play important roles in the lacrimal pump system, which allows drainage of the lacrimal sac into the nasolacrimal drainage systems during eyelid closure by compressive actions on the sac. At the lateral canthus, the orbicularis inserts into Whitnall's tubercle, posterior to the lateral orbital rim on the frontal process of the zygoma.

The orbital septum is a continuation of orbital periosteum. It separates the extraor-

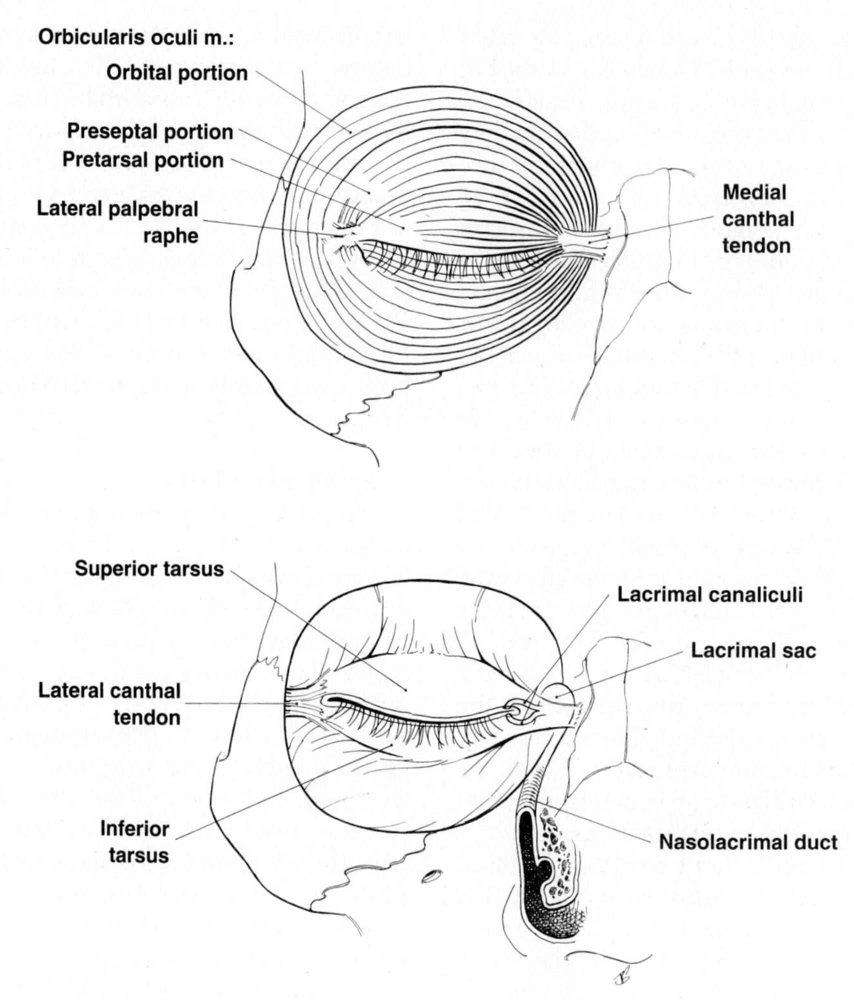

FIG 14–4.
Diagrammatic representation of the orbital, preseptal, and pretarsal portions of the orbicularis muscle.

bital from the intraorbital contents, confines the orbital fat, and serves as a barrier to infection. Deep to the septum and just above levator aponeurosis lies preaponeurotic fat. There are usually two fat compartments (medial and prelevator or central) in the upper lid from which fat is removed during blepharoplasty. The levator palpebrae superioris provides the principal elevation of the upper eyelid. The tenuous proximal muscle originates from the sphenoid bone and is crossed approximately 15 to 20 mm above the tarsal border by Whitnall's ligament. This ligament is a condensation of fascia that inserts into Whitnall's tubercle laterally and the medial orbital wall to redirect the horizontal action of the levator into a vertical pull. The levator then extends as a thickened anterior aponeurosis and a thinner posterior leaf, Müller's muscle. The anterior leaf inserts widely into the anterosuperior third of the tarsal plate. There is also a dermal insertion into the upper lid skin that forms the upper lid fold approximately 12 mm above the eyelid margin. This insertion is absent in the Asian eyelid. The posterior leaf, or Müller's muscle, inserts into the cephalic border of the tarsal plate. The levator aponeurosis is innervated by the third cranial nerve, while Müller's muscle receives sympathetic innervation.

In the lower eyelid the capsulopalpebral fascia is an extension of the inferior rectus sheath and is analogous to the levator aponeurosis in the upper lid. It splits around the inferior oblique muscle and proceeds anteriorly to fuse with the orbital septum. Lockwood's ligament is derived from the capsulopalpebral fascia and the inferior oblique fascia and serves to support the globe as a suspensory ligament.

The lacrimal gland lies in the superolateral aspect of the orbit and serves as a secretory gland that forms the tear film responsible for protection and lubrication of the globe. It is separated into a palapebral and orbital lobe by Whitnall's ligament and the levator aponeurosis. It receives its innervation from parasympathetic fibers that originate in the pons and travel via the greater superficial petrosal nerve on the floor of the middle cranial fossa. These fibers are joined by sympathetic fibers from the internal carotid artery to form the nerve of the vidian canal. These fibers synapse in the sphenopalatine ganglion. Postganglionic axons travel via the zygomatic, zygomaticotemporal, and lacrimal nerves to the gland. The tear film is drained through a system of canaliculi that originate in the superior and inferior puncta. The two canaliculi join to form a common canaliculus that enters the lacrimal sac located between the anterior and posterior lacrimal crest of the lacrimal bone. The lacrimal sac is drained during the act of blinking by the pumping action of the anterior and posterior limbs of the medial canthal tendon. The sac enters the nasolacrimal duct, which courses through the ethmoid bone to the inferior meatus of the nose.

The extraocular muscles consist of the inferior, superior, lateral, and medial rectus muscles as well as the superior and inferior oblique muscles. These muscles course anteriorly in the orbit and insert onto the globe to provide movement of the globe. The lateral rectus muscle receives its motor innervation from the abducens or sixth cranial nerve, while the superior oblique muscle receives innervation from the trochlear or fourth cranial nerve. All other extraocular muscles receive their motor innervation from the oculomotor or third cranial nerve. In all cases the innervation occurs in the posterior third of the muscle, with the exception of the inferior oblique muscle. The superior oblique muscle courses anteriorly and passes around a cartilaginous pulley formed by the trochlea and then proceeds posterolaterally to insert into the globe superiorly. The inferior oblique muscle originates in the maxilla and proceeds posterolaterally to insert into the globe inferiorly.

The blood supply to the orbit is derived from the internal and external carotid arteries. From the external carotid artery are derived the infraorbital artery, the transverse facial artery, the zygomaticofacial artery, and other branches of the superficial temporal and maxillary arteries. From the internal carotid artery arises the ophthalmic artery. It runs with the optic nerve and enters the orbit through the optic foramen. It gives off the important central retinal artery (blood supply to the retina) and more distally the anterior and posterior ethmoid arteries, which course through the orbit to the nasal cavity. The supratrochlear and dorsal nasal arteries provide blood supply to the forehead and face and are terminal branches of the ophthalmic artery. The venous drainage of the orbit is a continuation of the venous drainage from the face and runs posteriorly to drain into the superior and inferior ophthalmic venous system. This valveless system eventually drains to the pterygoid plexus and cavernous sinus. The sensory innervation of the cornea and surrounding eyelid and facial skin is derived from the ophthalmic and maxillary branches of the trigeminal or fifth cranial nerve. The ophthalmic branch enters the orbit through the superior orbital fissure and gives off the nasociliary, frontal, and lacrimal nerves. The maxillary nerve exits the middle cranial fossa via the foramen rotundum. It gives off as one of its branches the infraorbital nerve, which lies in the floor of the infraorbital groove and exits via the infraorbital foramen a few millimeters below the infraorbital rim. This nerve provides sensation to the midface. Parasympathetic innervation to the globe is derived from the ciliary ganglion via the short ciliary nerves. The orbicularis oculi muscle derives its innervation from the facial or seventh cranial nerve.

THE EAR

Embryology

Embryologically, the auricle and external auditory canal develop separately from the inner ear, which is composed of the cochlea and vestibular end organs. The temporal events in the fetal development of the ear can be understood if one recalls the parallel phylogenetic development of the ear, where vestibular function appears first (in early fishes) and specialized sound transmission appears later (in amphibians, birds, and mammals). Similarly, in embryologic development of the ear, the inner ear (the cochlea and vestibular end organs) begins to form early in development and is fully differentiated by 12 weeks of fetal life. In contrast, the external ear develops later, with the canalization of the external auditory canal shortly before birth. This relationship has implications when dealing with congenital deformities of the external ear where middle and inner ear anomalies may or may not be present, depending on the stage of developmental arrest.

The inner ear first appears as an ectodermal thickening on the lateral aspect of the developing head, the otic placode, which eventually invaginates and encysts to form the otocyst. From the otocyst develops the cochlea, the semicircular canals, and their associated neurosensory epithelium. The protective otic capsule of the petrous portion of the temporal bone develops from surrounding mesenchyme endochondrally. Only the petrous portion of the temporal bone is endochondral in origin. The remainder of the temporal bone is of membranous bone origin.

The sound-conducting structures of the middle ear, the ossicles and associated muscles and ligaments, are derived from the mesenchyme of both the first (Meckel's or mandibular cartilage) and second (Reichert's or hyoid cartilage) branchial arches. The middle ear cleft itself arises primarily as an expansion of the first pharyngeal pouch during the third week of fetal development. The first pouch expands laterally to meet the medially expanding ectoderm of the first branchial groove to form the trilaminar (all three embryologic layers) tympanic membrane.

The auricle is derived from the first and second branchial arches. Beginning at approximately the 6th week of development, condensation of arch mesenchyme forms six hillocks that coalesce to form the auricle (Fig 14–5). The root of the helix and antihelix are derived from the second arch. The tragus is derived from the mandibular cartilage or first arch. The auricle assumes an adult configuration by the 20th week and continues its postnatal growth until around the age of 9 years. The auricle has reached 85% of its growth by the age of 3 years. The initial ventromedial orientation of the pinna changes to a dorsolat-

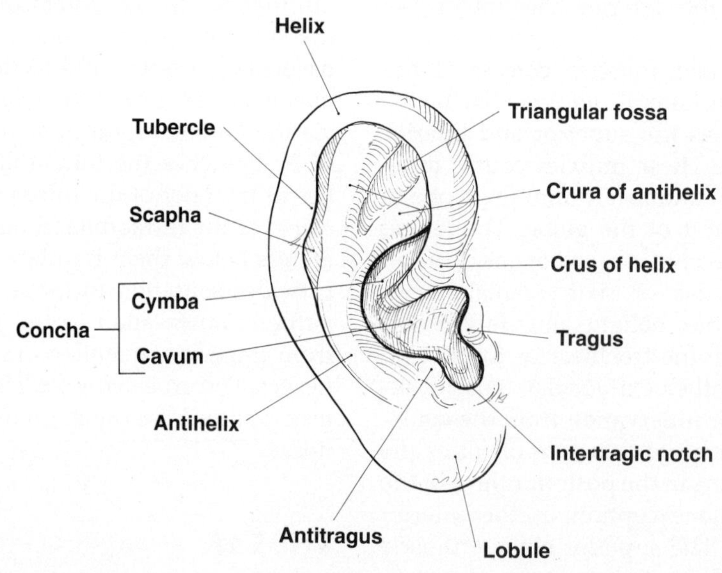

FIG 14–5.
External landmarks of the auricle. The auricle is derived embryologically from six hillocks, demonstrated in the figure.

eral orientation on the skull during the second month of development because of mandibular growth.

The external auditory canal begins to form at approximately the eighth week of gestation. It arises as a medial ingrowth of ectoderm that eventually forms the lateral third or cartilaginous portion of the canal. A core of epithelium at the medial boundary of the invagination eventually meets the endoderm of the first pharyngeal pouch. This core of epithelium remains until shortly before birth, when it is resorbed. Failure of the core to reepithelialize results in meatal atresia. This resorption occurs well after the differentiation of the inner ear, middle ear, and auricle, so meatal atresia may be associated with a normal pinna.

Anatomy

Auricle

The auricle or pinna is composed of an elastic cartilage framework covered by perichondrium and a thin skin envelope with a scant subcutaneous layer posteriorly. The topography of the auricle is highlighted by four main cartilaginous convolutions: the helix, antihelix, tragus, and antitragus. The auricle is attached to the skull by the cartilaginous extension of the concha, which is continuous with the cartilaginous external auditory canal. The anterior, superior, and posterior auricular ligaments as well as six intrinsic auricular muscles also provide attachment of the pinna to the temporal bone.

The spatial relationships of the auricle on the skull are important for surgeons dealing with reconstruction of traumatic or congenital deformities of the ear. The dimensions of the pinna are such that the width is approximately 55% of its height. The protrusion of the ear, measured by the conchomastoid angle, is approximately 20 to 30 degrees, which places the helix at about 15 to 20 mm from the skull. Auricular protrusion is primarily determined by the antihelix. Absence or attenuation of the antihelix, particularly the posterior crus, results in the "lop-ear" deformity (prominent ears). Three measurements of auricular position have been described: the axis, level, and distance in degrees of inclination posteriorly, from a line drawn nearly parallel to the axis of the nasal dorsum. The level of the ear should correspond to the level of the brow superiorly and the base of the columella inferiorly. The position of the ear on the face and skull should be approximately one ear length posterior to the lateral orbital rim.

Sensory innervation of the auricle is from cervical nerves C2 and C3 as the lesser occipital and greater auricular nerves, which provide sensation to the mastoid skin as well as the skin of the posterior and lateral auricle. The fifth, seventh, and tenth cranial nerves also lend innervation to the pinna and external meatus as the auriculotemporal, auricular, and Arnold's nerves, respectively.

Blood supply is derived from branches of the external carotid artery. The postauricular artery courses along the mastoid posteriorly, as does the occipital artery. Anteriorly, the superficial temporal artery lends blood supply to the pinna.

NOSE AND PARANASAL SINUSES

Embryology

Sinonasal differentiation occurs within the global events of midfacial development and growth. As a result, congenital nasal anomalies occurring secondarily to arrest in development or a failure of differentiation are often associated with midfacial, lip, or oral cavity deformities.

Nose

At approximately the fourth gestational week, the nasal placode develops as a thickening of surface ectoderm just superior to the primordial stomodeum at the frontonasal process. The nasal placode eventually deepens to form the nasal pit, which then forms the nasal vestibule and posterior choanae. The nasal septum is formed by intervening mesenchyme between the invaginating nasal pits. At the sixth fetal week, the ectoderm of the deepening nasal pit joins the ectoderm of the oral cavity roof to form the buccopharyngeal membrane. This membrane ruptures to form the choanae or posterior nasal cavity. Failure of the membrane to rupture leads to choanal atresia or stenosis.

Surrounding the nasal placode early in nasal development are the lateral and medial nasal swellings. Between 6 and 8 weeks, the medial nasal swellings fuse and then join the maxillary facial ectodermal swellings. Along with maxillary swellings, they fuse with the medial lateral cartilage, premaxilla, and the primary palate. It is clear that failure of the medial swelling to fuse or maintain the union of the maxillary swellings will result in nasal as well as associated facial clefts.

The lateral nasal swellings do not participate in the formation of the lip. Rather, they differentiate into the paired nasal bones, the upper lateral cartilages, and the lateral crus of the lower lateral cartilages. By 2 months of gestation the nasal cavity has completely developed. The nostrils themselves remain closed until the sixth month, when they canalize to form a patent nasal cavity.

Paranasal Sinuses

The paranasal sinuses arise initially as outpockets of the lateral nasal cavity. The maxillary, anterior ethmoid, and frontal sinus diverticula arise from within the middle meatus above the inferior turbinate, thus determining the position of the respective ostia in the adult. The posterior ethmoid sinus and sphenoid sinus diverticula arise from the superior and supreme meati, respectively.

The ethmoid sinuses are the first to develop in humans. They are well formed at birth, and their development is complete by the age of 14 years. They may pneumatize into the maxillary, nasal, frontal, sphenoid, or lacrimal bones. The maxillary and frontal sinuses are rudimentary at birth. The maxillary sinus slowly expands until around the age of 10 years, while the frontal sinus is not fully formed until 20 years of age. Four percent of the population has aplastic frontal sinuses. Hypoplasia of the maxillary sinuses is more common. The sphenoid sinus is not present until 3 years of age. It has completed development by approximately the age of 12 years.

Anatomy

The nasal pyramid is composed of a superior bony and inferior cartilaginous skeleton. The bony vault consists of thin, paired nasal bones that abut the frontal process of the maxilla laterally and the nasal process of the frontal bone superiorly. The hyaline cartilaginous vault is composed of two lower lateral cartilages, two upper lateral cartilages, a quadrangular septal cartilage, and several sesamoid cartilages. The lower lateral cartilages provide an important element of nasal tip support through their medial crura, which lie caudal to the nasal septum at the columella. The lateral crus of the lower lateral cartilages provides contour to the nasal alae and also plays a role in maintaining nostril patency during periods of high inspiratory nasal airflow. The paired upper lateral cartilages join the dorsal aspect of the septum medially and the nasal bones superiorly to provide structural support to the nasal tip and nasal vestibule (Fig 14–6). Patients who have lost architectural support from the upper lateral cartilages from trauma or congenital or iatrogenic causes may suffer from nasal vault collapse with associated high nasal airflow resistance and nasal obstruction. In addition, an aesthetically unpleasing "pinched" or excessively narrowed appearance of the nasal pyramid will result.

The muscles of the external nose are divided into superior and inferior groups. The superior group of muscles consists of the procerus, which appears anatomically as a continuation of the frontalis muscle, and the corrugator supercilii muscles. These are innervated by the temporal branch of the facial nerve and are responsible for glabellar furrowing (procerus) and vertical frown lines (corrugator). The lower group of muscles consists of the levator labii superioris and alar fibers of the nasalis, which dilate the nasal apertures, and the transverse fibers of the nasalis, which serve as constrictors. The depressor septi nasi muscle passes from the maxilla to the septum and alae and serves to depress the nasal tip. The lower group is innervated by the buccal branch of the facial nerve.

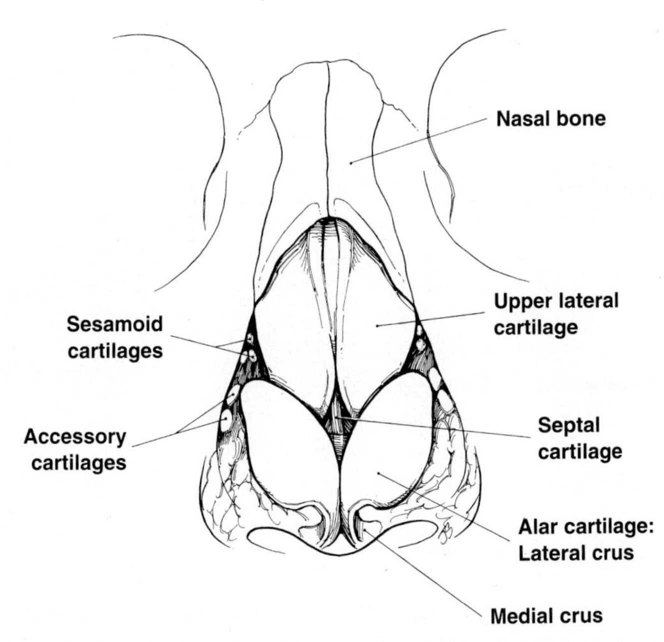

FIG 14–6.
Bony and cartilaginous framework of the external nasal skeleton. Approximal a third of the nasal pyramid is composed of the paired nasal bones, and the distal two thirds are composed of the upper and lower lateral cartilages. Both the upper and lower lateral cartilages articulate with the septum in the midline.

The intranasal anatomy of the lateral nasal walls ideally suits the physiologic roles of olfaction and air humidification, warming, and purification. Each nasal cavity has inferior, middle, and superior turbinates that divide the lateral wall into the inferior, middle, superior, and supreme meati. The paranasal sinus ostia drain into the lateral wall such that the maxillary, frontal, and anterior ethmoid cells drain into the middle meatus. The posterior ethmoid cells drain into the superior meatus, and the sphenoid sinus drains into the supreme meatus. The nasolacrimal duct drains into the inferior meatus. The turbinates are composed of a thin shelf of bone, mucoperiosteum, and a rich submucosal venous plexus. The physiologic role of the turbinates is to increase the overall surface area of the intranasal mucous membrane and to create airflow turbulence. In this way, inspired air is maximally warmed and humidified. Through a thick blanket of mucous and ciliary activity, the mucosa also allows first-line clearance of particulate matter. The airflow stream across the turbinates causes a parabolic flow into the superior nasal vault preferentially, thus maximizing flow across sensory olfactory epithelium. Furthermore, airflow resistance is partly modified by the autonomic regulation of the submucosal venous plexus, which engorges and congests several times per day in a regular nasal cycle. Turbinate size and thus airflow resistance are modified in response to a host of intrinsic and external factors that affect autonomic outflow.

The nasal septum is composed of a large, anteriorly situated quadrangular cartilage that joins the medial crus of the lower lateral cartilages caudally (Fig 14–7). Posterosuperiorly, the cartilaginous septum abuts the perpendicular plate of the ethmoid bone. Inferiorly, the vomer articulates with the ethmoid posteriorly and the quadrangular cartilage anteriorly. The maxillary crest and the palatine bone contribute to the septum along its floor. The quadrangular septum is prone to injury in cases of blunt facial trauma and often buckles and contributes to posttraumatic nasal obstruction. It may also play a central role in midfacial development and growth in the

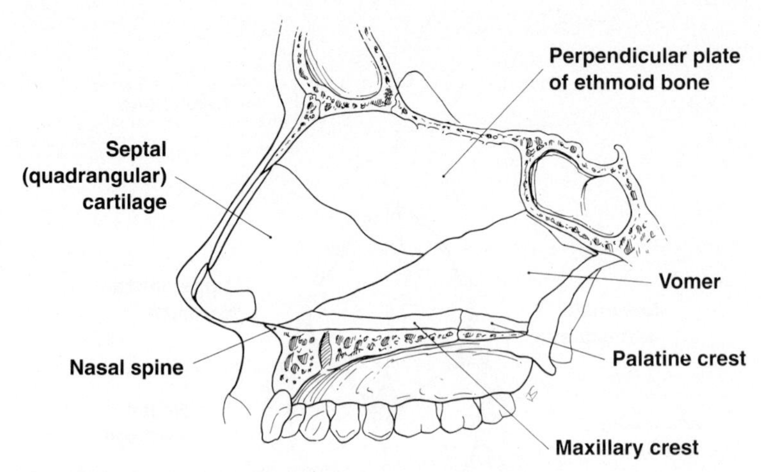

FIG 14–7.
The nasal septum consisting of the quadrilateral cartilage, the perpendicular plate of the ethmoid, the vomer, and the maxillary and palatine crests.

child and as such could be the cause of midfacial growth disturbances in cases of childhood injury or surgical removal.

The nasal blood supply is derived from both external and internal carotid arteries. The anterior and posterior ethmoidal arteries are branches of the ophthalmic artery from the internal carotid system and enter the nasal cavity medially via the orbit at the level of the cribriform plate. The ethmoidal vessels supply the roof of the nasal vault as well as the anterior lateral and septal mucosa. Persistent epistaxis from high in the nasal vault often originates from the ethmoidal vessels. The sphenopalatine artery, which is a terminal branch of the internal maxillary artery, supplies the posteroinferior lateral nasal wall and septum. The superior labial artery from the facial artery and the greater palatine vessels also lend blood supply to the nose.

The venous drainage of the nose parallels the arterial supply, with the sphenopalatine veins draining posteriorly into the pterygoid plexus and thereby into the cavernous sinus. The ethmoidal veins drain through the superior ophthalmic veins. Of special importance is the fact that the venous system of the nose and midface are valveless. This allows infections of the nose and paranasal sinuses to progress retrogradely to the orbital and cavernous sinus systems with resultant periorbital and orbital cellulitis, abscess, or cavernous sinus thrombosis.

Innervation of the external nose is supplied by the external nasal nerve (nasal tip) and infratrochlear nerves via the ophthalmic branch of the trigeminal nerve. The infraorbital nerve, derived from the maxillary branch of the trigeminal nerve, also provides sensation to the external nose (lateral caudal portion of the nose). The nasal cavity is innervated by the anterior and posterior ethmoidal nerves anteriorly and superiorly and from branches of the sphenopalatine nerve posteriorly. The sympathetic and parasympathetic supply is carried through the nerve of the pterygoid canal. The nasal cavity plays a role in pulmonary reflexes through its innervation. Clinical and experimental evidence demonstrates altered pulmonary vascular resistance in response to intranasal stimulation, which can occur during nasal anesthesia, packing, or surgery.

ORAL CAVITY, OROPHARYNX, AND SALIVARY GLANDS

Embryology

Within the primitive stomodeum, the tongue, palate, and teeth are formed. The tongue is derived from the first, second, and part of the fourth pharyngeal arches. At approximately 4 weeks of development the lateral lingual swellings and one medial swelling, the tuberculum impar, fuse to form the anterior two thirds of the tongue. Being derived from the first pharyngeal arch, the anterior two thirds of the tongue receives its somatic sensory innervation from the mandibular branch of the trigeminal nerve. Separated from the anterior two thirds of the tongue by the circumvallate papillae, the posterior third of the tongue is derived from the second, third, and part of the fourth pharyngeal arches. The sensory innervation for the posterior third of the tongue is supplied by the glossopharyngeal nerve and vagus nerve, which are the nerves of the third and fourth pharyngeal arches, respectively. The motor innervation of the tongue musculature is derived from the hypoglossal or 12th cranial nerve.

Within the migratory events of the five facial prominences during facial development, the palate itself is formed by the medial migration of the maxillary and medial nasal swellings. The merging of the two medial nasal swellings deep within the facial substance forms the intermaxillary segment. The inner maxillary segment gives rise to the primary palate as well as the philtrum of the upper lip. The secondary palate is formed from the more lateral maxillary prominences. Around the sixth week of development, the palatine shelves form and fuse in the midline to form a secondary palate. The palatine shelves lie in a vertical plane initially and then descend to arrive at a final horizontal orientation later in development. The right palatine shelf descends embryologically before the left palatine shelf. This may have implications regarding the clinical observation that cleft palates arise more frequently on the left side than on the right. Inferiorly, the palatal shelves fuse with the primary palate to form the incisive foramen, which marks the border between the secondary and primary palates. At the same time the nasal septum, derived from the frontonasal process, grows downward to meet the palate.

The teeth arise around the sixth week of development from the basal layer of oral epithelium, which gives rise to the dental lamina. The dental lamina gives rise to the ectodermal components of the teeth, which include the enamel (formed by ameloblasts). The mesenchymal derivatives arise from the dental papillae. The dental papillae eventually differentiate into the dentin, which arises from odontoblasts. They also give rise to the pulp of the tooth. The cementum is formed from mesenchymal tissue at the root of the tooth. The first or deciduous teeth appear approximately 6 to 24 months after birth. The definitive or permanent teeth appear later but are formed during the third month of development.

The salivary glands arise as epithelial buds from within the stomodeum. The parotid gland is of ectodermal origin and appears at approximately the sixth week of development. These buds migrate toward the preauricular sulcus and eventually grow to incorporate the facial nerve and lymph nodes. The submandibular gland appears at approximately the sixth week of development, and the sublingual gland appears during the eighth fetal week. The submandibular gland buds elongate to traverse the mylohyoid muscle and eventually are located in the submandibular triangle. Unlike the parotid gland where lymph nodes lie within the substance of the gland, the submandibular gland capsule is formed early, so no lymph nodes lie within its capsule. The sublingual gland forms multiple buds that appear in the floor of the mouth and eventually form multiple sublingual ducts.

Anatomy and Physiology

The oral cavity is bounded by the lips anteriorly, the junction of the hard and soft palates superiorly, and the lingual circumvallate papillae inferiorly. Lateral margins are formed by the cheeks and the anterior tonsillar pillars bilaterally.

The teeth consist of two central and two lateral incisors, two canines, four premolars, and six molars on both the upper and lower jaws. The crown is that part of the tooth above the gingiva. That part below the gingiva is the root of the tooth. Externally, the crown is covered by enamel, and the root is covered by cementum. The inner layer of the tooth is made of dentin. The interior of the tooth is the pulp. Each tooth is held in place (to the alveolus) by the periodontal ligament.

The lips and cheeks, which bound the oral vestibule, attach to the mandible and maxilla at the gingivobuccal and gingivolabial sulci. Posteriorly, the cheeks attach to the anterior edge of the mandibular angle in an area called the retromolar trigone. The lips consist of four layers: skin, muscle, submucous glands, and mucosa. The muscles of the cheek and lips are the buccinator and orbicularis oris, respectively. They are innervated by the facial nerve. The muscles of mastication are innervated by the trigeminal nerve.

Histologically, the lips are composed of keratinized squamous epithelium anterior to and nonkeratinized squamous epithelium posterior to the vermilion wet line.

The floor of the mouth is a muscular diaphragm composed of the mylohyoid and stylohyoid muscles laterally and the geniohyoid and genioglossus muscles medially. Below the mylohyoid muscle lies the submandibular gland, whereas the sublingual salivary gland lies submucosally in the floor of the mouth.

The hard palate forms the roof of the oral cavity. It is formed by the palatine processes of the maxilla and the horizontal plates of the palatine bones. Posterior to the upper central incisor teeth lies the incisive foramen. Through this foramen are transmitted the nasopalatine nerves and arteries. These vessels anastomose with the sphenopalatine arteries of the nose. Anterior to the incisive foramen lies the premaxillary portion of the maxilla, also known as the primary palate. Posterior to the incisive foramen lies the horizontal palatine process of the maxilla, otherwise known as the secondary palate. Directly medial to the third molar tooth lies the greater palatine foramen through which are transmitted the greater palatine vessels and nerves. The hard palate is covered by mucosa that is closely adherent to the underlying periosteum. Deep to the mucosa lie the palatine glands that secrete mucus. There is no muscle under the hard palate. The soft palate forms the roof of the oropharynx and is made up of five muscles. The levator veli palatini consists of paired muscles that arise from the posteromedial eustachian tube and insert at the junction of the hard and soft palates at the palatine aponeurosis. The function of these muscles is to elevate the palate. The tensor veli palatini muscles originate at the base of the skull anterolaterally and the lateral side of the eustachian tube. They then hook around the hamulus of the medial pterygoid plate and insert into the palatine aponeurosis. The tensor veli palatini muscles tighten the soft palate and open the eustachian tube during the act of swallowing. The palatoglossus muscle arises from the palate and inserts into the side of the tongue. It underlies the mucosa of the anterior tonsillar pillar. The palatopharyngeus muscle arises from the posterior border of the hard palate at the palatine aponeurosis and inserts into the posterior border of the thyroid cartilage and the side of the pharynx. It underlies the mucosa of the posterior tonsilar pillar. Together these muscles help to close the oropharyngeal inlet. Finally, the uvula assists in closing the nasopharynx during swallowing. These muscles are innervated through the pharyngeal plexus by the ninth and tenth cranial nerves, except for the tensor veli palatini, which is innervated by the trigeminal or fifth cranial nerve. Blood supply to the palate is derived from the greater palatine artery as well as the lesser palatine artery. The sensory innervation is derived from the greater and lesser palatine nerves and the nasopalatine nerve.

The tongue is composed of three intrinsic and six extrinsic muscles that control its movement. These muscles are innervated by the hypoglossal or 12th cranial nerve, with the exception of the stylohyoid muscle, which is innervated by the facial nerve, and the palatoglossus muscle, which is innervated by the vagus or 10th cranial nerve. The anterior two thirds of the tongue receives sensory innervation from the trigeminal nerve. Special taste fibers are supplied by the facial nerve via the chorda tympani nerve. The posterior third of the tongue receives its sensory innervation from the 9th and 10th cranial nerves.

The structures of the oral cavity perform the functions of mastication, taste, deglutition, and speech. Mastication is accomplished through the coordinated movements of the muscles of mastication, which are innervated by the mandibular division of the trigeminal or fifth cranial nerve. Muscles of the face, including the buccinator and orbicularis oris muscles as well as the tongue, also contribute to the chewing mechanism. The masseter, temporal, and medial pterygoid muscles all function to close the mouth. The posterior temporalis muscle also produces a lateral movement of the jaw. The mylohyoid, digastric, and the lateral pterygoid muscles open the jaw. Contraction of the lateral pterygoids protrudes the jaw, while the posterior temporal and geniohyoid muscles act as mandible retractors. Following mechanical grinding of food through the act of mastication, deglutition follows with a transfer of food from the mouth to the stomach. The initial oral or buccal phase of swallowing involves movement of the food bolus posteriorly to the oropharynx through the movements of the tongue, cheeks, and lips. In addition, the soft palate contacts the posterior of the pharynx at the level of the upper edge of the superior constrictor known as Passavant's ridge to prevent nasopharyngeal reflux. After the voluntary oral phase, the reflexive pharyngeal phase of swallowing is initiated by the food bolus, which is propelled distally by the pharyngeal constrictors. The swallowing mechanism is coordinated at the swallowing center in the medulla and involves multiple cranial nerves for the innervation of intrinsic and extrinsic tongue muscles as well as the pharyngeal constrictors, the muscles of mastication, and the muscles of facial expression.

The neurosensory receptor cells for taste are located on the tongue. The chorda tympani nerve supplies the special sensation of taste to the anterior two thirds of the tongue, whereas the glossopharyngeal and vagus nerves supply taste to the posterior third of the tongue. The taste buds are located on the dorsum of the tongue surface and detect salty, sour, sweet, and bitter tastes. Each taste bud preferentially detects a particular taste. The alterations in taste result from different stimulation frequencies as well as different patterns of nerve fiber excitation. Central mechanisms also play a role in the perception of taste.

The anatomy and physiology of the salivary glands are also related to the functions of the oral cavity. The parotid gland is the largest of the salivary glands and is located lateral to the mandibular ramus. The gland has a well-developed fibrous capsule and is divided somewhat artificially into a larger superficial lobe and smaller deep lobe by the facial nerve that runs through the substance of the gland. On the medial aspect of the gland is the styloid process as well as the internal carotid artery, internal jugular vein, and cranial nerves IX, X, and XII. Superiorly the gland is limited by the zygomatic arch, and inferiorly the gland may extend to or below the angle of the mandible. Posteriorly it is bounded by the mastoid process of the temporal bone and the digastric muscle. The deep lobe of the gland is intimately related to the superior constrictor muscle of the hypopharynx as well as to the carotid sheath structures.

This accounts for the clinical finding that tumors of the deep lobe of the parotid gland will often appear as parapharyngeal masses. The parotid duct (or Stensen's duct) courses anteriorly along the surface of the masseter muscle and ends in the buccal mucosa at a point immediately adjacent to the second maxillary molar tooth. Other structures that are immediately associated with the gland are the auriculotemporal nerve and the posterior facial or retromandibular vein. The parotid gland receives its parasympathetic innervation from the inferior salivatory nucleus of the brain stem, which sends its preganglionic parasympathetic nerve fibers to the otic ganglion via the lesser petrosal nerve. Here the parasympathetic fibers synapse with the cell bodies of the second-order neurons, which send their fibers to the parotid gland via the auriculotemporal branch of the trigeminal nerve. Following parotidectomy, regenerating parasympathetic fibers may aberrantly reinnervate dermal sweat glands and result in "gustatory sweating." This phenomenon of facial sweating during eating is termed Frey's syndrome.

The submandibular gland also has superficial and deep lobes that are separated by the mylohyoid muscle. Its salivary duct, or Wharton's duct, travels between the hyoglossal and mylohyoid muscles to enter in the floor of the mouth on either side of the frenulum of the tongue. The sublingual gland lies in the sublingual space of the floor of the mouth between the mylohyoid and hyoglossal muscles. Several sublingual gland ducts enter the floor of the mouth. The submandibular and sublingual glands receive their innervation from the superior salivatory nucleus, where preganglionic parasympathetic fibers travel with the chorda tympani branch of the seventh cranial nerve to synapse in the submandibular ganglion. Postganglionic parasympathetic fibers then travel to the submandibular and sublingual glands to provide secretomotor innervation.

Saliva plays an important role in the physiology of the oral cavity. The total daily production of saliva is approximately 1,500 mL. The electrolyte composition of saliva depends on the salivary flow rate, with the concentrations of sodium chloride, bicarbonate, and calcium increasing with increasing rates of flow. Saliva also contains a variety of enzymes such as amylase, lysozyme, and hydrolase to assist in digestion. In addition, concentrations of IgA are high in saliva. Several other polypeptides including epidermal growth factor, nerve growth factor, and kallikreins are present. Saliva also plays an important role in maintaining tooth integrity. This is evidenced by the fact that after head and neck irradiation a subsequent decrease in salivary flow results in an increased incidence of dental caries.

FACE AND NECK

The general embryology of the face and neck is reviewed in the discussion of the branchial apparatus.

Anatomy

The muscles of facial expression are responsible for the movement of the forehead, brows, cheeks, lips, ears, and scalp. Motor innervation to these muscles is supplied by the facial nerve.

The facial nerve exits the stylomastoid foramen and courses anteriorly through the substance of the parotid gland. It then branches into cervicofacial and temporofacial divisions within the substance of the gland. The main branches of the facial nerve are the temporal, zygomatic, buccal, mandibular, and cervical branches. Variable connections exist between the separate branches of the facial nerve (Fig 14–8). The muscles of facial expression are innervated at their deep aspect by the branches of the facial nerve. The marginal mandibular nerve courses immediately deep to the platysma muscle approximately 2 cm below the lower border of the mandible. The temporal branch of the facial nerve passes over the zygomatic arch and becomes superficial as it approaches the lateral aspect of the orbit.

The superficial musculoaponeurotic system (SMAS) is a fascial layer in the parotid and cheek areas that is separate and superficial to the parotomasseteric fascia. It extends into and is continuous with the fibers of the frontalis muscle superiorly and the platysma muscle inferiorly. Anteriorly, it is attenuated and inserts into the dermis of the cheek skin. The motor branches of the facial nerve lie deep to the SMAS, as do the main facial arteries and veins. The SMAS plays a role in transmitting the actions of the facial musculature in facial expression and plays a role in dermatochalasis, which occurs as part of the aging process.

Cutaneous sensory innervation is supplied by branches of the trigeminal nerve as well as the cervical nerves. If a line is projected from the pogonion (chin) to the vertex of the skull, the trigeminal nerve will supply innervation to the skin lying anterior to this line, while the cervical nerves provide innervation to the skin posterior to this line. Major branches that are of special importance are the supratrochlear and supraorbital nerves, which supply innervation to the forehead region, the infraorbital and zygomaticofacial nerves, which supply innervation to the infraorbital and malar areas, and the auriculotemporal and mental nerves, which supply innervation to the temporomandibular areas. Blood supply to the face is derived predominantly from branches of the external carotid artery via the facial artery, superficial temporal artery, and terminal branches of the

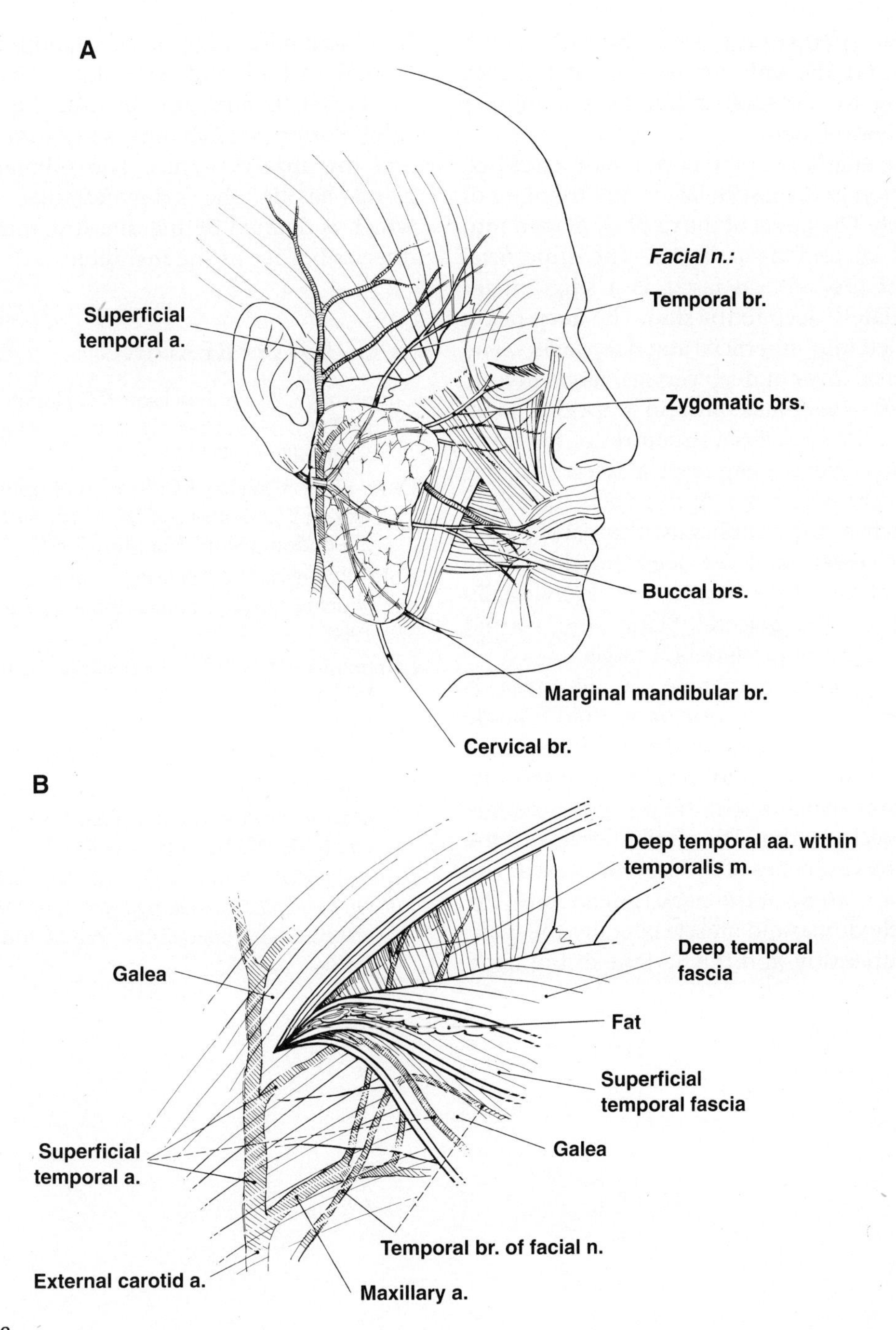

FIG 14–8.
A, the facial nerve is shown exiting the stylomastoid foramen, 1 cm deep to the tympanomastoid suture. The nerve divides into five main branches within the substance of the parotid gland. **B**, fascial relationships in the temporal area.

internal maxillary artery system. The internal carotid artery supplies portions of the face via the supraorbital and supratrochlear arteries, which are branches of the ophthalmic artery. Venous drainage generally parallels the arterial supply of the face. Lymphatic drainage of the face follows regional patterns, with the scalp draining primarily to the occipital, periparotid, and parotid lymph nodes and the anterior portion of the face draining to the submandibular and jugular chain lymph nodes.

The anatomy of the neck is best described in relation to the fascial layers and triangles of the neck. The fascia of the neck is divided into superficial and deep layers. The superficial layer of the cervical fascia is a single layer immediately deep to the skin. The deep fascia is divided into superficial and deep layers. The superficial layer of deep cervical fascia invests the sternocleidomastoid and trapezius muscles and the superficial structures of the neck. The deep layer of deep cervical fascia encircles the visceral structures of the neck, including the trachea and esophagus, the parotid and jugular vessels, and the deep muscles of the neck. These three layers are individually known as the visceral fascia, the carotid sheath, and the prevertebral fascia.

The posterior triangle of the neck is defined by the sternocleidomastoid muscle anteriorly, the anterior border of the trapezius muscle posteriorly, and the clavicle inferiorly. Important structures in the posterior triangle of the neck are the 11th cranial nerve and the cutaneous branches of the cervical plexus. The anterior triangle of the neck is defined by the sternocleidomastoid muscle laterally, the mandible superiorly, and the midline of the neck. It is subdivided into the submandibular, submental, carotid, and muscular triangles. The carotid sheath structures include the common carotid artery, cranial nerves IX, X, XI, and XII, and the ansa cervicalis. The submandibular gland lies in the submandibular triangle, which is defined by the digastric muscle and inferior border of the mandible.

SUGGESTED READING

Cummings CW, Frederickson JM, Harker LA, et al: Ear & skull base. *Otolaryngol Head Neck Surg* 1986; 4:2555–2569.

Duke-Elder S, Wybar KC: System of ophthalmology, in *The Anatomy of the Visual System,* vol 2. London, Henry Kimpton, 1961.

Kohn R: *Textbook of Ophthalmic Plastic & Reconstructive Surgery.* Philadelphia, Lea & Febiger, 1988.

Langman J (ed): *Medical Embryology.* Baltimore, Williams & Wilkins, 1981.

Lee KJ (ed): *Text Book of Otolaryngology and Head and Neck Surgery.* New York, Elsevier, 1989.

McCarthy JG (ed): *Cleft Lip and Palate and Craniofacial Anomalies,* vol 4, in *Plastic Surgery.* Philadelphia, WB Saunders, 1990.

Paparella MM, Shumrick DA, Gluckman JL, et al: *Otology and Neur-Otology,* vol 2, in *Otolaryngology,* ed 3. Philadelphia, WB Saunders, 1991.

Chapter 15

Congenital Disorders

Scott P. Bartlett, M.D.
Jack Yu, M.D.

CONTENTS

CHAPTER OBJECTIVE

At the end of this chapter the resident is thoroughly familiar with the anatomy, embryology and principles of the treatment of congenital disorders of the head and neck (with special focus on cleft lip and palate) and has successfully undertaken comprehensive management of these disorders.

LEARNER OBJECTIVES

On completion of this chapter the resident

1. **Demonstrates intimate knowledge of the common congenital disorders of the head and neck, including cleft lip and palate, craniofacial syndromes, vascular malformations, and auricular abnormalities.**
2. Understands the basic principles of the surgical and nonsurgical management of common congenital disorders of the head and neck.
3. Demonstrates broad general knowledge of less common congenital disorders of the head and neck.
4. Comprehends the etiology, genetics, embryology, and anatomy as related to these congenital disorders.
5. Is familiar with the radiographic and special diagnostic studies necessary to

fully evaluate these anomalies as well as the specialty care that may be required for each anomaly.
6. Is familiar with craniofacial growth and development and the effect of particular anomalies or their treatment on such development.
7. Is able to formulate a definitive short- and long-term treatment plan for patients with common congenital disorders and choose the most appropriate surgical or nonsurgical modality.
8. Is familiar with the organization of specialty clinics (cleft palate clinic, craniofacial clinic), including the coordination of all special services in the evaluation of the patient.

■ CLINICAL PRACTICE ACTIVITIES

During the course of the training program, the resident

1. **Participates in the surgical planning for patients with common congenital disorders of the head and neck, including cleft lip and palate.**
2. **Performs primary and secondary surgery on patients with common congenital disorders of the head and neck (cleft lip and palate, auricular abnormalities, etc.)**
3. Recognizes and coordinates nonsurgical treatment of congenital head and neck disorders and provides pre- and postoperative care for such problems.
4. Participates in multidisciplinary evaluation and treatment programs for patients with congenital disorders of the head and neck (e.g., cleft palate clinic, craniofacial anomaly clinic).
5. Provides perioperative care and participates in surgical treatment of patients with major craniofacial anomalies such as telorbitism and Crouzon's disease.

CLEFT LIP

Etiology and Genetics

The lip and primary palate formation in human facial morphogenesis occurs between 4 and 6 weeks of embryogenesis. Nasal placodes, which first appear in the fourth week, divide the frontal process into medial nasal and lateral nasal processes. The maxillary processes undergo rapid growth during the fifth week and unite with each other as well as with the medial nasal process to form the primary palate. The secondary palate forms by the fusion of palatal shelves after they assume a horizontal orientation. The growth of the developing mandible, which allows the tongue to "drop out of the way," is important in changing the palatal shelves from a vertical orientation to this more horizontal one. In palatal shelf fusion, a communicating channel linking the nasal cavity to the oral cavity exists and is known as the nasopalatine canal; this will become the incisive foramen marking the junction of primary and secondary palate. A similar groove is left when the medial nasal process is fused with the maxillary process, i.e., the nasomaxillary groove, which will become the nasolacrimal ridge and eventually the nasolacrimal duct system.

The etiology of cleft lip and palate is not clear, although population and laboratory investigations now suggest a single major autosomal recessive gene. This gene may be located very close to the region of the major histocompatibility complex and determines the susceptibility of the individual to environmental factors. Some well-known teratogens that can predictably produce cleft lip and palate in mice include dexamethasone (Decadron), phenytoin (Dilantin), and phenobarbital. It is also felt that cleft lip with or without cleft palate is different in pathogenesis from isolated cleft palate. In cleft lip the palate defect is secondary to the lip defect. The general population incidence for cleft lip and palate is 1 in 700; it is lower in blacks and higher in Orientals. The cleft palate incidence is 1 in 2,500 with a male-to-female ratio of 1:2. If there is a first- or second-degree relative affected, the risk increases to 5%; with two first- and/or second-degree relatives affected, the risk is 15% to 20%.

Anatomy and Classification

A normal upper lip (Fig 15–1) consists of the Cupid's bow with the tubercle below and the philtrum above, which has a central dimple bordered by two lateral curvilinear pillars leading to the columella. The vermilion is the everted, protruding oral mucosa. The junction of the mucosa and skin, i.e., the mucocutaneous junction or white roll, plays an important role in cleft lip repair. At birth, the vertical length of upper lip measured from the peak of the Cupid's bow to the base of the columella is 10 mm and increases to 13 mm at 3 months. The average adult upper lip has a vertical upper lip length of 17 mm.

In cleft lip deformity (Fig 15–1), the Cupid's bow is incomplete, with one pillar missing and cephalad rotation of the lip elements. Additionally, there is a deficiency of muscle (orbicularis oris) with an abnormal intradermal insertion at the cleft edge, and the lower lateral nasal cartilage on the cleft side is flattened, twisted, and frequently associated with a hypoplastic bony foundation.

The earliest classification method was developed by Davis and Richie in 1922, and all clefts were divided into three groups: prealveolar, postalveolar, and clefts of both primary and secondary palates. The most functional classification of cleft lip and palate, based on embryology, was published in 1971 by Kernahan, who used a striped Y logo schematic with the junction of the two arms and the stem of the Y representing the incisive foramen. Both arms of the Y are divided into three parts representing the lips, alveolus, and hard palate anterior to the incisive foramen. The stem of the Y contains three squares numbered 7, 8, and 9, which represent the secondary hard palate, the hard and soft palate, and the soft palate only. Overt clefting is recorded by stippling the appropriate square and submucosal clefting by cross-hatching.

Primary Surgical Treatment

The goals of surgical treatment reflect the technique available. The very first repairs

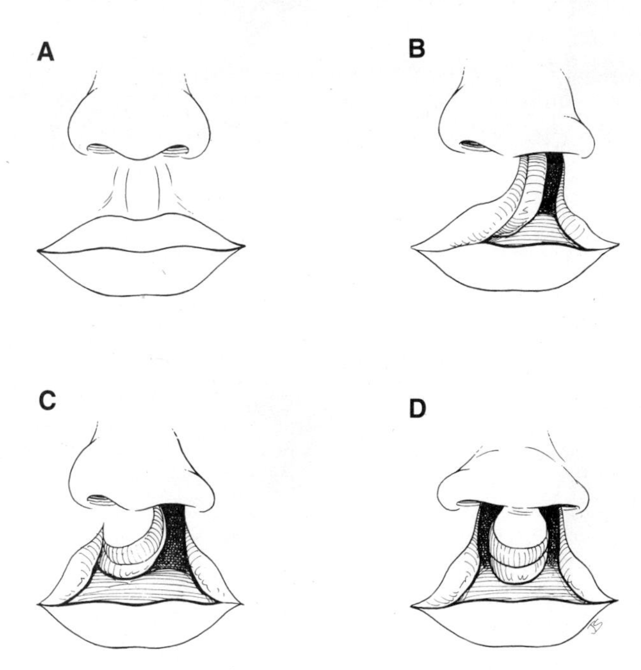

FIG 15–1.
Normal and cleft lip anatomy. **A,** normal lip. **B,** complete unilateral cleft of the lip and palate. **C,** bilateral cleft lip, incomplete on the right, complete on the left. **D,** bilateral complete cleft lip and alveolus.

focused primarily on coverage. The edges of the cleft lip were incised in a straight line fashion followed by simple closure without attempting to repair the orbicularis oris. This method could not achieve a symmetrical lip because of the deficiency in vertical lip height on the cleft side. It was not until the late 19th century that curved incisions were used by Rose and Thompson. These curved incisions, when closed in a straight fashion, extended the vertical lip length to match the noncleft side. However, the continuous scar was obvious, and lip notching was still common. To break up this linear scar, triangular flaps were devised by Mirault; these were later modified by Blair, Brown, and McDowell. The first technique to recreate a normal-appearing Cupid's bow was LeMesurier's quadrilateral flap. Tennison and Randall in the late 1950s popularized the Z-plasty repair with a triangular flap (Fig 15–2,A). The normal landmarks were identified first: philtral dimple, peak of the Cupid's bow on the normal side, peak bordering the cleft side, and base of the columella on the normal and cleft side. Based on the difference in vertical lip heights between the normal and cleft side, an equilateral triangular flap was designed with each side equal to that difference. The misdirected orbicularis oris fibers were reoriented in a more normal, horizontal direction. During this same period, Millard developed the rotation-advancement flap repair (Fig 15–2,B). This method was unique in that the entire existing

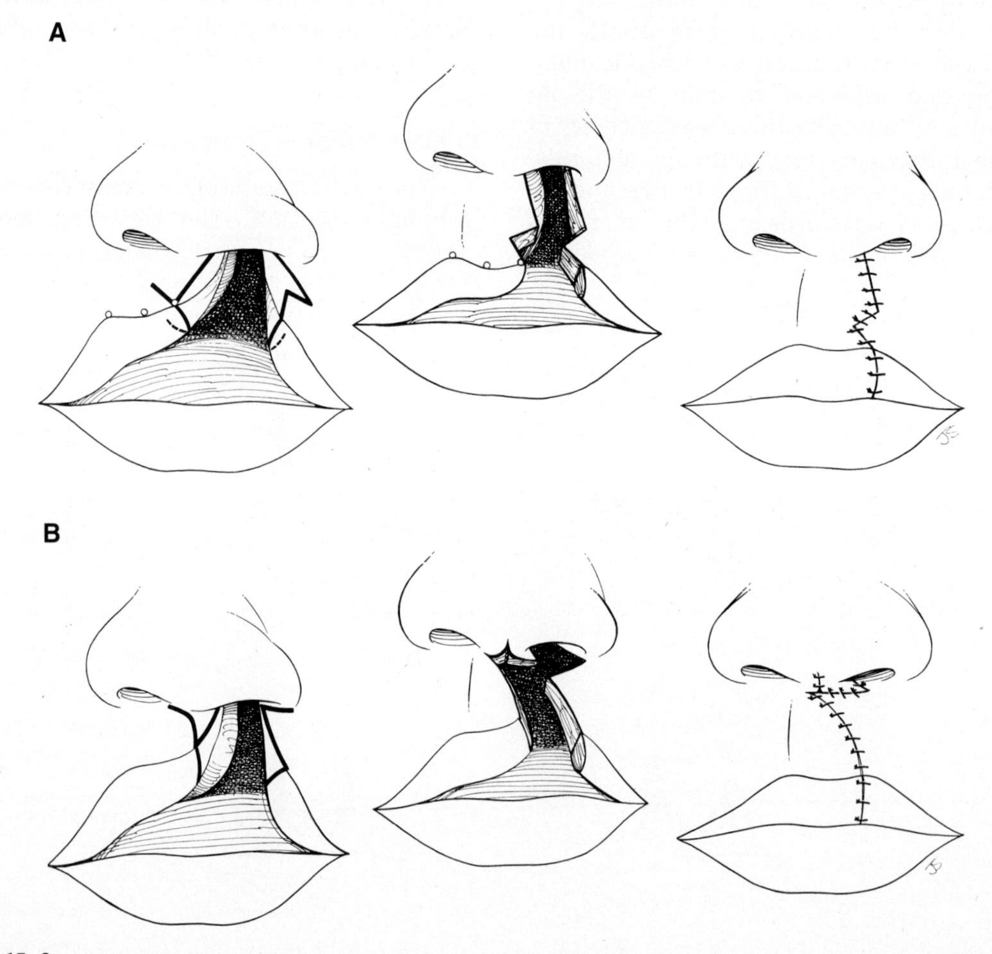

FIG 15–2.
Most commonly employed methods of cleft lip repair. **A,** Randall-Tennison triangular flap method. **B,** Millard rotation-advancement method.

Cupid's bow was rotated down into position with advancement of tissue from the cleft side into the defect created by the rotation. A gentle curve recreating the philtral pillar with a more normal-appearing, longer columella could be achieved.

Other Surgical Procedures

Lip Adhesion

In the very wide unilateral or bilateral complete cleft lip deformity, lip adhesion can be performed prior to definitive repair. This allows molding of the premaxilla into a more posterior, normal position and converts a wide complete cleft lip into an incomplete one. The associated veloplasty or palatoplasty can be performed at the same time that definitive lip repair is carried out.

Cleft Nasal Surgery

The nasal deformity associated with cleft lip is the most difficult problem to correct. The abnormalities on the cleft side include lengthening of the lower lateral cartilage, drooping of the nostril rim, caudal rotation of the nasal ala, an oblique ridge in the vestibule, and shortening of the nasal lining. Surgical correction is achieved by hemirhinoplasty involving wide dissection with repositioning and reshaping of the lower lateral cartilage.

CLEFT PALATE AND VELOPHARYNGEAL INCOMPETENCE

Anatomy

The human palate has two major parts: the primary and secondary palate. The primary palate forms the premaxilla, while the palatine processes of the maxilla and the horizontal plates of the palatine bones, together with the soft palate, form the secondary palate. The palatine processes of the maxilla fuse at the midline to form the median palatine suture; they unite anteriorly with the primary palate and posteriorly with the horizontal plates of the palatine bone to form the transverse palatine suture. The premaxilla contains the central and lateral incisors. The soft palate is posterior to the horizontal plates of the palatine bones. There are five pairs of extrinsic muscles that together with the superior constrictor, the muscular uvula, and the hard palate provide normal velopharyngeal function. The five paired extrinsic muscles are the tensor veli palatini, levator veli palatini, salpingopharyngeus, palatoglossus, and palatopharyngeus. The major elevators of the soft palate are the levator veli palatini and the palatopharyngeus. The major depressor is the tensor veli palatini. All the extrinsic muscles are innervated by the pharyngeal plexus supplied by glossopharyngeal, vagal, and spinal accessory nerves, except the tensor veli palatini, which is supplied by the mandibular division of the trigeminal nerve.

Cleft palate can be either unilateral or bilateral, and it can involve either the primary or the secondary palate or both. Since the primary palate is a central structure, cleft palate involving the primary palate is associated with malalignment of other midline structures such as nasal cartilages and the perpendicular plate of the vomer. The cleft itself is located laterally, between the lateral incisor and canine, and extends posteromedially toward the incisive canal. Secondary palate clefting is in the midline because embryologically the cleft forms as a result of incomplete palatal shelf fusion. The abnormalities of the cleft side include foreshortening of the palatal shelf anteroposteriorly with hypoplasia of the palatine aponeurosis and the extrinsic muscles. These muscle fibers have a more anterior insertion and run parallel to the cleft. The end functional result is an inability to completely seal off the nasopharynx from the oropharynx during speech or deglutition, which is known as *velopharyngeal incompetence* (VPI).

Diagnosis

In addition to the standard oral examination, evaluation of the velopharynx requires specialized visualization of the soft palate and the pharyngeal wall both at rest as well as during speech and deglutition. Currently there are two methods to provide this imaging: fluoroscopy and nasopharyngoscopy. In the fluoroscopic examination, the images are recorded with a high-resolution video camera in posteroanterior, lateral, and oblique projections following instillation of a small amount of radiopaque contrast material into the nasopharynx and oropharynx. This is known as multiview videofluoroscopy and gives a two-dimensional representation of a tubular structure. Nasopharyngoscopy is performed with a flexible 3-mm fiber-optic nasopharyngoscope, which allows direct visual inspection of the velum and pharynx. The objective of the examination is to establish the diagnosis, to document the presence and the extent of VPI, and to allow postoperative follow-up of these patients.

Surgical Treatment of Cleft Palate

The goal of surgical treatment of a cleft palate is to achieve normal glottal, velar, and pharyngeal articulation during speech and deglutition. Currently three types of repair are commonly employed: the von Langenbeck repair, the V-Y Veau-Wardill-Kilner repair, and the Furlow palatoplasty (Fig 15–3). The von Langenbeck repair utilizes lateral relaxing incisions to allow primary repair of the cleft following elevation of the palatal mucoperiosteum as a bipedicle flap. There is no reorientation of the muscle fibers of the tensor and levator veli palatini, and the length of the palate is not increased with this

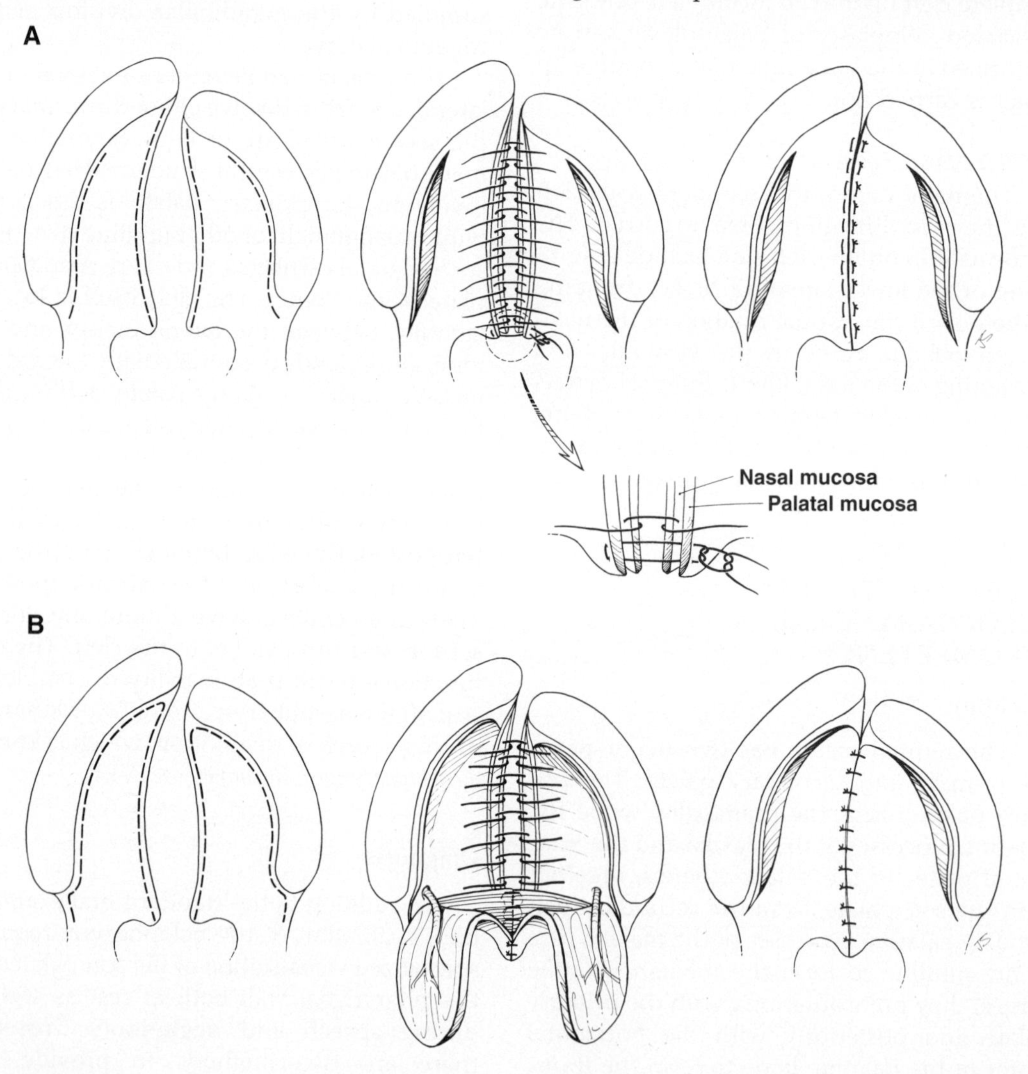

FIG 15–3.
Methods of palate repair. **A,** von Langenbeck. **B,** Wardill-Kilner pushback.

repair. The V-Y Veau-Wardill-Kilner repair attempts to lengthen the palate by the pushback technique. The mucoperiosteum is mobilized anteriorly off the hard palate and advanced in a V-Y fashion to close the defect.

The Furlow palatoplasty utilizes two Z-plasties termed "double opposing" by Furlow and "double reversing" by Randall. The repair elevates the palatal mucosa in layers and, with the dual Z-plasty, achieves a multilayered closure of the defect while at the same time reorients the muscle fibers in a more physiologic, horizontal position.

VPI may be due to a poorly functioning velum following palate repair, an unrecognized submucous cleft, or incompetence of the velum secondary to neuromuscular dysfunction. Following standard palate repair, up to 30% of patients experience VPI manifested as hypernasal resonance, nasal emission, and nasal regurgitation. Treatment most commonly consists of a superiorly or inferiorly based posterior pharyngeal flap inset into the palate to reduce the size of the nasal port (and hence nasal emission) or a pharyngoplasty.

C

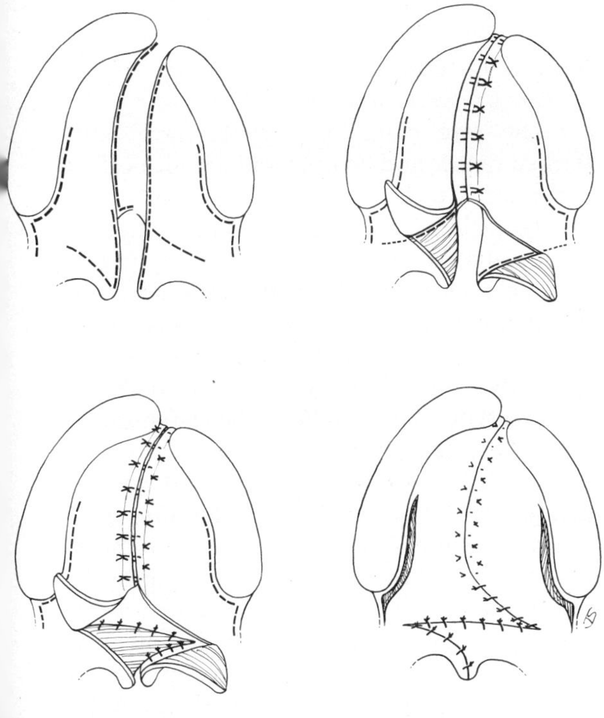

FIG 15–3 (cont.).
Methods of palate repair. **C,** Furlow double Z-plasty.

CRANIOFACIAL ANOMALIES

Craniofacial anomalies are characterized as a congenital, developmental, or acquired deformity of the cranial and/or facial skeleton often accompanied by a wide variety of soft-tissue anomalies. It has been estimated that approximately 1,200 persons are born annually in the United States with these anomalies. These anomalies run the gamut from mild deformity to severe impairment, including mental retardation, visual deficiency, and disorders of breathing, deglutition, and occlusion. In addition to the functional impairment, it is the attendant cosmetic deformity, with its often profound impact on the individual and his family, that demands attention.

Embryology

The fourth to eighth weeks of gestation mark the period of greatest change in the facial region of the developing embryo. Beginning in the fourth week, the frontonasal prominence, surrounded by the primitive forebrain above and the stomodeum centrally and defined laterally by the nasal and optic placodes, makes its appearance. Over the subsequent fifth through eighth weeks, through the processes of merging and fusing and bolstered by the forceful migration of neuroectoderm, the primitive face becomes evident. Clearly, any process that arrests or interferes with growth during this critical period will have a profound influence. Although there is a wealth of information available regarding human embryogenesis, knowledge concerning processes that lead to malfunction is limited. Even though genetic factors, specific teratogens, etc., have been implicated in at least 65% of congenital anomalies, the cause of specific deformities is unknown.

TABLE 15–1.
Classification of Craniofacial Anomalies

I. Clefts
  Centric
  Acentric (Tessier system)
II. Synostoses
  Symmetrical
  Asymmetrical
III. Atrophy/hypoplasia
IV. Neoplasia, hypertrophy, hyperplasia
V. Unclassified

Classification

Although multiple classification systems have been put forth for defining these anomalies, many are incomplete and others cumbersome; the system proposed by the Committee on Nomenclature and Classification of Craniofacial Anomalies of the American Cleft Palate Association serves best (Table 15–1).

Clinical Evaluation

Since multiple organ systems may also be involved and associated with craniofacial deformity, it is essential that multiple specialties be involved in the care of these patients. Over the past several decades this has evolved into a craniofacial team that should include a plastic surgeon, neurosurgeon, anesthesiologist, ophthalmologist, otolaryngologist, geneticist, pediatrician, physical anthropologist, orthodontist, pedodontist, psychiatrist, radiologist, and speech therapist. Each patient with a complex anomaly should be evaluated, not only with a complete physical examination but also with multiple diagnostic tests and radiographs. When contemplating surgery on these patients the surgeon may wish to obtain life-sized photographs, cephalometric studies, computerized tomograms, and magnetic resonance images.

Surgical Planning and General Operative Technique

Prior to embarking upon corrective surgery, each patient should have an extensive evaluation, the extent of which depends on the deformity. This evaluation should include a classification of the deformity, the diagnosis and treatment of any concomitant malformation, and a definition of the functionally important associated conditions. Based on the location of the deformity and the surgery required for its correction, different surgical approaches may be required. For the upper orbits and forehead, a transcoronal approach is utilized. If the lower orbits and nasal region require treatment, then a coronal incision combined with lower lid incisions is mandated. Treatment of the maxilla is best approached through an upper buccal sulcus incision, while mandibular deformities are primarily treated through a lower buccal approach. Following exposure, any osteotomies required are completed, fixation and bone grafting are performed, and soft-tissue redraping is accomplished. Fixation of osteotomies may take the form of plate or wire osteosynthesis. It is unclear at this time whether or not plate osteosynthesis is the preferred method or, in fact, whether it is contraindicated because of its potential growth-limiting effects.

Specific Deformities

Rare Craniofacial Clefts

The rare craniofacial clefts have been termed *centric* and *acentric* and are also called orbitofacial clefts or oro-ocular clefts and medial facial clefts. The best classification of these clefts is that of Tessier (Fig 15–4). In this classification system the cleft position is numbered, much like the spokes of a wheel, with the orbit as the central point of reference. Typically, when designating a cleft, both the facial cleft number and the ocular cleft number are utilized (e.g., cleft 5-9).

As with the more common cleft lip and palate, repair of a rare cleft requires that normal anatomic relationships be reestablished. It is therefore essential to provide mucosal lining, bony support, and soft-tissue coverage. Mucosal lining is provided by turning in the cleft edges where necessary. Subsequent bony malpositions are addressed by osteotomy and repositioning, while overlying soft-tissue deformities are managed by a combination of Z-plasty, rotation-advancement

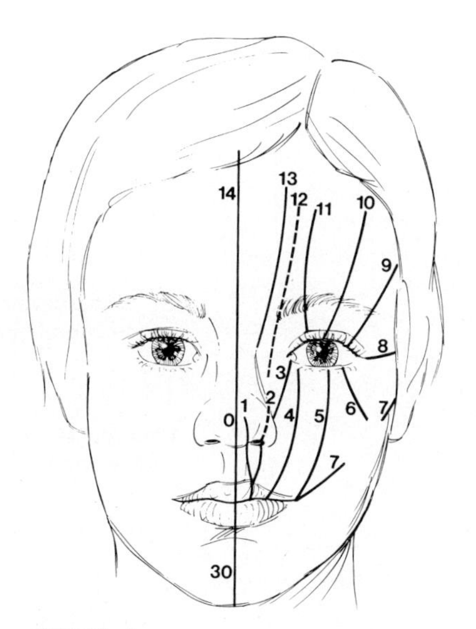

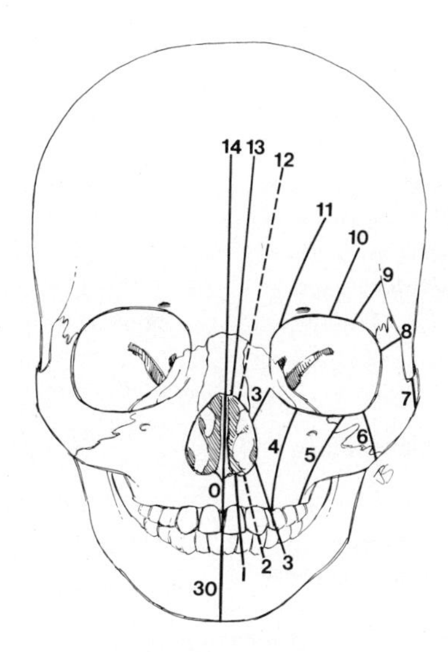

FIG 15–4.
The Tessier classification of rare craniofacial clefts.

flaps, and the like. Treatment is generally begun in infancy to optimize speech development and to provide eye protection, although major bony shifts are frequently delayed until 5 years of age or later.

It is convenient to consider the *Treacher Collins syndrome,* or mandibulofacial dysostosis, one of the clefting deformities because it is not infrequently associated with lateral facial clefts. This deformity is inherited as an autosomal dominant trait with variable penetrance and thus may display minimal to severe deformity. Manifestations include absent or poorly developed supraorbital, lateral, and inferolateral orbital rims, aplastic zygomas, a hypoplastic posteriorly short mandible, downward-sloping palpebral fissures, lateral canthal dystopia, and lower eyelid pseudocolobomas with medial lower eyelash deficiency. Associated deformities include minimally deformed ears to severe microtia, macrostomia, and cleft palate. Mental status is generally normal.

Management of these deformities is complex. For malar midface deficiency, a bone graft and/or synthetic materials may be utilized. Bone grafting can take the form of nonvascularized or vascularized bone, and it is not unusual for several grafting procedures to be required. For canthal and lid malposition, no absolutely satisfactory method is available, and combinations of Z-plasty, upper lid-to-lower lid transposition flaps, and canthopexies have been attempted. The auricular deformities can be managed with prostheses or total ear reconstruction (see below). Mandibular and midface hypoplasia may require Le Forte or mandibular osteotomies to level and align the occlusion.

Craniofacial Microsomia

Hemifacial microsomia (first and second branchial arch syndrome, otomandibular-auricular deformity, otomandibular dysostosis) is also conveniently placed in the clefting category because it may be manifested by lateral orofacial clefts. This deformity is second in frequency only to cleft lip and palate and occurs in 1 to 3,500 to 1 in 5,600 live births. Most cases are sporadic, although occasional family clustering has been documented. The etiology is unknown, but experimental studies have shown that early damage to the differentiating tissues in the ear region may lead to this deformity. Manifestations include ear malformations ranging from prominence to complete aplasia, orbital dystopias (primarily inferior and lateral displacement), maxillary hypoplasia, and mandibular deformity (Fig 15–5). The mandibular deformity is typically thought to be the hallmark of the disease and ranges in severity from minimal hypoplasia to complete absence of the ascending mandible

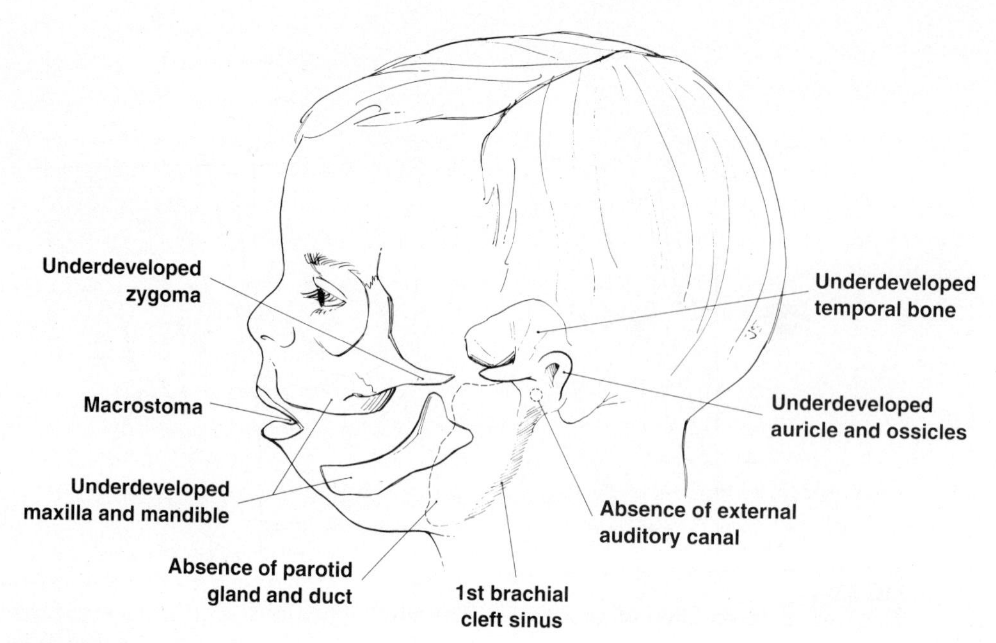

FIG 15–5.
Pathologic anatomy of the first and second branchial arch syndrome (hemifacial microsomia).

and temporomandibular joint apparatus. These deformities, in concert with the maxillary hypoplasia, lead to dental malocclusion with a shift of the dentition to the affected side, cross bite, open bite, and an upward occlusal cant. Although this deformity is primarily manifested as a unilateral disease, bilateral involvement may be evident in 10% of patients.

Treatment of the mandibular and maxillary deformity varies with the severity of the hypoplasia. For a patient with mild deformity, contour restoration with bone grafts or cartilage is suitable. In more severe deformity, maxillary and mandibular osteotomies to level, align, and reposition these segments may be required. When the ascending ramus and glenoid are missing, complete reconstruction with carved costal cartilage grafts is required. Orbital deformities are treated by osteotomy and repositioning.

Timing of the treatment of craniofacial microsomia is debatable. Early treatment (4 to 5 years of age) during the stage of mixed dentition or treatment following the completion of facial growth in adolescence have both been advocated. At this point, there are no clear data to suggest one treatment time as clearly superior to the other. In addition to bony osteotomies and repositioning, treatment may include augmentation of deficient soft tissue in the form of free tissue transfer or nonvascularized dermis grafts. The auricular deformity is managed as below.

Craniosynostosis (Craniofacial Dysostosis, Craniostenosis, Craniofacial Synostosis, Premature Synostosis of the Cranial Sutures)

The hallmark of this second major group of craniofacial syndromes is premature closure of one or more cranial sutures leading to abnormalities of the calvarium, cranial base, and orbits. Although the etiology is unknown and it is uncertain as to whether the synostosis is a primary or secondary event, certain pathologic consequences of this sutural fusion are evident. Following premature closure, brain expansion is limited in a direction perpendicular to the suture. Accordingly, there is a compensatory overexpansion of the cranium at the sites where sutures remain open. The resultant skull shape forms the basis of a subclassification system (Fig 15–6). A skull shape that is short from front to back and wide in the transverse dimension is termed *brachycephaly;* one in which the skull is elongated in the anteroposterior dimension and narrowed in the transverse dimension is termed *scaphocephaly;* one that is asymmetrical and retruded on one side, front or back, is termed *plagiocephalic;* and one that is keel-like and pointed in the forehead is termed *trigonocephalic.* In addition to these nonsyndromic descriptions, certain syndromic synostoses occur. The most common of these are Apert's and Crouzon's syndromes. Apert's syndrome is characterized by a turribrachycephalic skull, midface hypoplasia, class III malocclusion, orbital hypertelorism, and the associated clinical findings of acne, syndactyly of the hands and feet, and occasional cleft palate. This deformity is autosomal dominant in transmission, although most cases are sporadic. Crouzon's syndrome is also characterized by a tower skull with occasional orbital hypertelorism and exorbitism, midface hypoplasia, and class III malocclusion with a beak nose and high arched palate. This condition is also autosomal dominant, although, again, most cases are sporadic. Other syndromic craniosynostoses include Pfeiffer's syndrome, Carpenter's syndrome, and Saethre-Chotzen syndrome. Each of the latter three have some associated digital abnormality.

Functional abnormalities are most often associated with the more severe syndromic synostoses. These include associated deformities, intracranial hypertension secondary to synostosis, abnormalities of speech and hearing, dental malocclusion, strabismus, and other anomalies of the visual axis and ocular adnexae.

The earliest treatments of the craniosynostoses involved simple craniectomy. This gave only modest results, and therefore the more

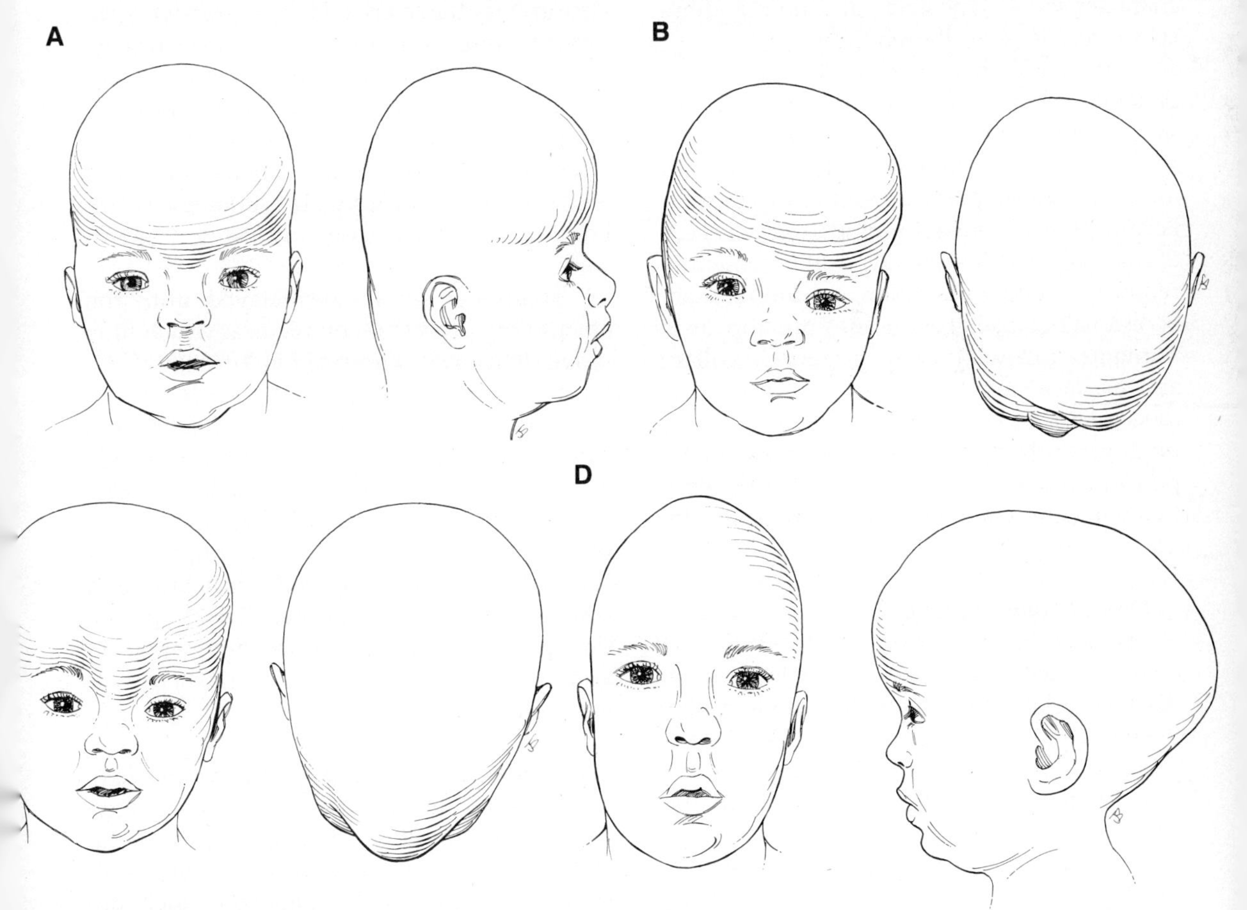

FIG 15–6.
Morphologic expression of craniosynostosis. **A,** turribrachycephaly. **B,** plagiocephaly. **C,** trigonocephaly. **D,** scaphocephaly.

aggressive and satisfying osteotomy and repositionings have gained favor. In general, osteotomies are performed to free, shape, and reposition abnormally situated segments. In those patients in whom the forehead and orbits are characterized by retrusion and exorbitism, this typically takes the form of osteotomy and repositioning of the supraorbital bar in concert with forehead advancement and reshaping. This can be done as either a unilateral or bilateral procedure, depending on the deformity. For those in whom midface deficiency and severe exorbitism is present, treatment takes the form of a Le Forte I/III procedure in which the entire midface is osteotomized and advanced forward. The extent of osteotomy and advancement is, of course, dependent on the severity of the deformity. Mandibular deformity is not characteristic of synostosis, and no mandibular surgery is typically required.

The timing of treatment is variable. In general, it has been found in nonsyndromic single-suture synostoses that treatment by suture release, osteotomy, and advancement in infancy gives satisfying and lasting results. For the more severe deformities, early surgery of this nature, although advocated, frequently requires a repeat operation on one or more occasions because growth does not appear to normalize following early surgery. Maxillary and midface surgery is usually performed at the earliest time during the stage of mixed dentition, although it is also recognized that if performed at this juncture, repeat osteotomy following the completion of growth in adolescence may be required.

Orbital Hypertelorism

Defined as lateralization of the entire orbit associated with an increase in the interorbital distance, orbital hypertelorism is not in itself a diagnosis but is a component of other disease processes that are themselves fit into the classification system. These include craniofacial clefts, craniosynostosis, frontonasal encephaloceles, and frontonasal dysplasia. As defined by Tessier in the adult, interorbital distances beyond 30 mm are considered pathologic. In first-degree orbital hypertelorism the interorbital distance is 30 to 34 mm; second degree, from 34 to 40 mm; and third degree, greater than 40 mm. Orbital hypertelorism is repaired by either the transcranial or extracranial route. For mild to moderate deformity, the extracranial route in which medial wall osteotomies and repositioning are performed is advocated. For more severe hypertelorism, a complete 360-degree orbital osteotomy, removal of midline excess bone and soft tissue, and medial translocation of the orbits is completed. Intervention for severe deformities is typically delayed until the child is older than 5 years of age, although earlier intervention may occasionally be necessitated.

Atrophy and Hypoplasia

Included in this third major diagnostic category are a wide variety of syndromes. *Romberg's syndrome* (progressive hemifacial atrophy) is characterized by progressive atrophy of the skin, muscle, bone, and cartilage that is confined to one side of the face. This disease typically begins in childhood, with the atrophy progressing over a 5- to 10-year interval before spontaneously ceasing and leaving a fixed atrophy. The etiology is unknown, with most cases occurring sporadically.

Treatment should be delayed until the atrophying process is complete, at which time tissue deficiency is replaced in kind. In effect, for bony or cartilaginous tissue deficiency, grafts are placed. For the soft-tissue deficiency, especially when severe, free tissue transfers are required. Dermis grafts and local tissue rearrangements may also be performed. *Binder's syndrome* (nasomaxillary hypoplasia) is characterized by a flattened nasal bridge, a shortened columella, and maxillary hypoplasia. Treatment consists of onlay augmentation and, if malocclusion is severe, maxillary advancement.

Hyperplasia, Hypertrophy, and Neoplasia

Included in this category are a large number of conditions that can cause facial enlargement. These include neurofibromatosis and vascular malformations, which are discussed elsewhere. *Fibrous dysplasia* of the craniofacial skeleton is an abnormal proliferation of fibro-osseous tissue, which can be either monostotic or polyostotic and is characterized by an insidious onset and slow progressive growth, typically ceasing in the third or fourth decade. Treatment involves either contour reduction or complete resection and bony reconstruction. *Benign hemihypertrophy* is a condition of unknown etiology in which one side of the face and/or body is enlarged in all elements. Treatment is usually less than satisfactory, and only if reduction of bone and soft tissue is possible without destruction of functioning tissue (i.e., the facial nerve).

Secondary Surgical Treatment

As in all craniofacial syndromes, secondary surgical treatment may be necessary when relapse occurs or, more frequently, when surgery is performed early and growth of the operated part does not keep pace with the remainder of the adjacent structures. Secondary surgical treatment may take the form of complete reoperative osteotomy and repositioning as described previously or the form of camouflage procedures such as soft-tissue rearrangements or bone grafting.

Nonsurgical Treatments

The goal of craniofacial surgery is to provide autogenous tissue whenever possible, and only rarely are prostheses required. Orthodontics is a critical part of presurgical and postsurgical management of those deformities requiring dental/facial osteotomies. Many of the patients with cleft lip and palate may also require speech therapy as part of their overall management. Psychological therapy is also very important because patients have been shown to respond favorably to psychological intervention when dealing with these deformities.

AURICULAR DEFORMITIES

The external ear arises embryologically from the first and second arches and is formed from the coalescence of six hillocks. When this fails to occur properly, various ear deformities may result, including anotia (total absence of the ear), microtia (nearly complete absence of the ear), cup ear or lop ear, and prominent ears. *Microtia* occurs once in 7,000 to once in 8,000 births, with right side predominance. It is estimated that 50% of patients with microtia have associated hemifacial microsomia. Total anotia, or ear absence, is unusual; in most instances there is, even with extreme microtia, a small lobular component that remains, although it may be misplaced.

Total ear reconstruction involves creating a new external ear from either autogenous or artificial materials. Most reconstructions utilize costal cartilage and are undertaken at 5 or 6 years of age. Prior to this time, rib cartilage is usually insufficient for adequate framework construction, and the age of 6 years is a frequent time for children to first experience peer pressure. The ear has reached 90% of its final size at this age, having achieved 85% of development by 3 years of age.

Two major types of ear reconstruction are available. A Silastic framework has been used in the past with some success. There is, however, a significantly higher incidence of extrusion with this implant material as compared with cartilage. The material of choice appears to be autologous costal cartilage. Reconstruction involves harvesting either the ipsilateral or typically the contralateral segments of ribs 6, 7, and 8. Ribs 6 and 7 are utilized to carve the base of the implant, while costal segment 8 is used to provide the helical framework. Although the stages of ear reconstruction may vary depending on the author, total ear reconstruction generally involves four stages: (1) placement of the cartilaginous framework, (2) transposition of the lobule to a more normal position relative to the framework, (3) elevation of the new ear from the overlying scalp and placement of a retroauricular skin graft, and (4) tragal construction.

A constricted cup or lop ear is characterized by folding over of the helix in concert with various constricting deformities of the scapha and triangular fossa. Depending on the degree of the deformity, various reconstructive options are available and vary from mere detachment of the folded helix and reattachment or trimming, various unfurling, refolding, and cartilage resuturing techniques, to partial removal of the deformed cartilage and replacement with contralateral concha or carved costal cartilage. These deformities represent some of the most challenging reconstructions.

Ear prominence is characterized by conchal excess with or without unfurling of the antihelical fold. The deformity arises during the later stages of embryogenesis when final folding and settling of the ear occur. Although multiple techniques have been described, each typically involves various combinations of (1) resecting excess conchal cartilage, (2) mobilizing and repositioning the enlarged concha in relation to the mastoid fascia and, (3) creating a neo-antihelical fold by various methods of scoring, weakening, and suture. Treatment of this deformity should also be delayed until 5 or 6 years of age to limit the adverse effects that subsequent growth might produce.

ABNORMALITIES OF THE EYELID

Colobomas are congenital clefts of the lower or upper eyelids. They are frequently associated with a diverse group of craniofacial syndromes, of which Treacher Collins syndrome is the most common. Anatomically there is a complete or incomplete cleft with an associated deficiency of that portion of the eyelid. Numerous techniques have been advocated for the correction of colobomas: (1) wedge resection and advancement of the lid margin with or without canthopexy or canthotomy, (2) correction by Z-plasty or a local flap, (3) transposition of the upper to the lower lid, and (4) various combinations of the above. Frequently, these procedures must be combined, and no treatment has proved completely reliable and satisfactory in all cases.

Congenital ptosis or blepharoptosis, i.e., drooping of the upper eyelid, is manifested as either a bilateral or a unilateral deformity with or without associated facial malformations. Milder forms of ptosis demand treatment for only cosmetic purposes, while in severe ptosis when vision is obscured either partially or completely, functional restoration is mandated. Various procedures have been described for ptosis correction, and the procedure of choice depends on the degree of deformity and the experience of the surgeon. In general, surgical options include (1) resection of the levator, (2) occipital frontal dynamic suspension, and (3) through-and-through resection of upper lid tissues with resuture in an anatomic position (Fasanell-Servat).

MISCELLANEOUS CONDITIONS OF THE HEAD AND NECK

Choanal Atresia

A newborn infant with congenital closure of the posterior nasal passage bilaterally will make respiratory efforts but will not be able to move air; severe respiratory distress will develop immediately after birth. Choanal atresia must be entertained as a possible diagnosis for early postpartum upper airway obstruction. The baby can be made to breathe by induction of crying with insertion of an oral airway. In unilateral choanal atresia, a useful test is to hold a wisp of cotton below the nostrils—no movement will be noted on the atretic side. Another test is to insert a red rubber nasogastric tube. The definitive treatment is transpalatal choanal-plasty, which is ideally performed at the age of 4 to 5 years.

Congenital Tumors—Benign

The incidence of benign neoplasms in newborns and infants is 10%, the great majority of them being facial hamartomas (hemangioma, lymphangioma, and neurofibroma). *Hemangiomas* are the most common and appear as blanchable red, blue, or purple cutaneous lesions. The clinical course of hemangiomas is variable, although spontaneous regression following a period of rapid growth is the rule. They may, however, enlarge at an alarming rate, ulcerate, and cause functional and developmental problems. Systemic steroids have been advocated, but the treatment of hemangiomas is usually observation, with surgical ablation reserved for selected cases. This can be done with either laser or conventional surgical excision, usually in multiple stages.

Lymphangiomas are neoplastic malformations of the lymphatics and occur in the head and neck in 70% of the cases. Clinically, they are soft, raised masses with finger-like projections and no clear encapsulation. Most lymphangiomas have mixed histology—cystic, capillary, and hemangiomatous. If the cystic component predominates, the lesions are termed *cystic hygroma*. The presentation is usually a diffuse cervical swelling that can extend from the base of the tongue to the superior mediastinum and can cause stridor and respiratory distress. The lesions enlarge slowly, but progressively and on occasion may undergo spontaneous regression. Surgical excision is the preferred treatment, with total extirpation of the involved abnormal lymphatic tissue if possible.

Diffuse systemic neurofibromatosis is more commonly found in infancy than an isolated neurofibroma is. This is also known as von Recklinghausen's disease, an autosomal dominant condition with a prevalence of 0.04%. Clinically one finds multiple well-encapsulated neurofibromas, polyostotic fibrous dysplasia, café au lait spots, and axillary freckles. This is a difficult condition to treat; excision is usually compromised, recurrence is common, and significant disfigurement is the rule.

Dermoid cysts are common soft-tissue lesions in the pediatric population and appear as firm, nodular lesions with attachment to the deeper tissues but not the overlying skin. They are typically located at the lateral aspect of the supraorbital ridge, nasal dorsum, or midline of the neck. Nasal dermoid cysts can involve the nasal septum and more central structures such as the cribriform plate, paranasal sinuses, meninges, and cerebrum. They should be excised to establish the histologic diagnosis and to remove the pressure/mass effect on the underlying developing structures. The extirpation of centrally located dermoid cysts must be undertaken only after a thorough workup and preparation for possible craniotomy. More laterally located lesions usually require only simple excision.

Congenital Tumors—Malignant

Malignancy is distinctively rare before the age of 1 year. From 1 to 5 years, the incidence increases to 1 in 5,000 births, with leukemias, retinoblastomas, and central nervous system lesions making up the majority. From the ages of 5 to 10 years the incidence drops to 1 in 10,000; the majority of these are rhabdomyosarcomas and lymphosarcomas.

Cystic Lesions

Cystic lesions can occur laterally or in the midline. Those lesions located near the midline must be approached with special caution because they may represent developmental defects that have communication with the central nervous system. A detailed history and careful examination with attention to the exact location, depth, texture, mobility, and color together with appropriate magnetic resonance and/or computed tomographic imaging facilitate an accurate diagnosis and treatment.

Thyroglossal Duct Cyst/Sinus

During the third week of fetal life, the thyroid gland first appears as a median endodermal thickening at the level of the second branchial arch. This thickening will develop into a diverticulum known as the thyroid diverticulum, which descends in the anterior midline of the neck to settle in the lower cervical region. The origin, just posterior to the tuberculum impar, is the foramen cecum at the base of the tongue; the tract that is usually obliterated is the thyroglossal duct. Thyroglossal duct cysts are located in the midline of the neck with no attachment of the overlying skin. The cystic mass will move in concert with the thyroid gland during deglutition. The epithelial tract passes through the central portion of the hyoid bone to end near the base of the tongue. Surgical treatment is complete excision with resection of the central portion of the hyoid bone.

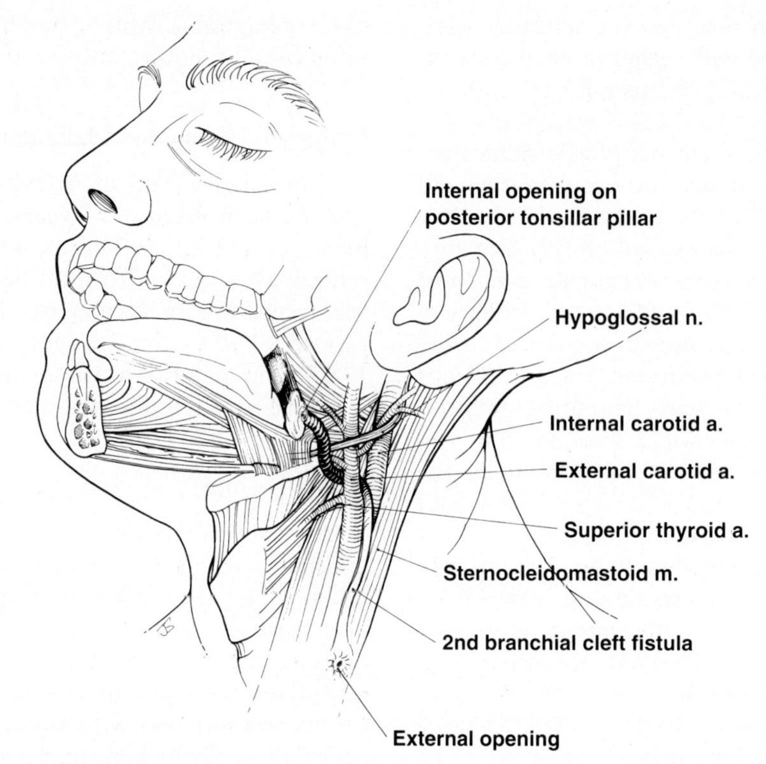

FIG 15–7.
Pathologic anatomy of branchial remnants.

First Branchial Cleft Lesions

A first branchial arch fistula (Fig 15–7) is much less commonly seen than second arch lesions. The upper opening is typically located within the external auditory canal, with the lower opening inferior to the mandible, at the level of the hyoid. The presentation is often that of a retromandibular, retroauricular swelling. Complete surgical excision is the treatment of choice. The cervicofacial trunk of the seventh cranial nerve is in close association with this fistula and must be avoided at the time of fistulectomy.

Second Branchial Cleft Sinuses and Fistulas

The second branchial arch (Fig 15–7) is the most commonly involved arch in congenital branchial cleft lesions. In general, 25% of these lesions are bilateral; cysts are more common than sinuses or fistulas. A cyst is an epithelial-lined, fluid-containing cavity; if there is an opening—either externally or internally—it is called a sinus, and if both an external and internal opening exists, it is called a fistula.

The external opening of a second branchial cleft sinus is at the junction of the middle and lower thirds of the sternocleidomastoid muscle along its anterior border. Occasional ectopic auricular cartilage is found flanking the opening. In the case of a second branchial cleft fistula, the internal opening is along the anterior surface of the posterior tonsillar pillar. The fistulous tract is lined in the lower part with stratified squamous epithelium and in the upper part with columnar epithelium; it penetrates the platysma muscle, passes between the internal and external carotid arteries, and stays lateral to the internal laryngeal and hypoglossal nerve. During the terminal portion of its course, it passes superficial to the glossopharyngeal nerve, through the superior constrictor to enter the palatopharyngeus muscle, eventually to exit on the anterior surface of posterior tonsilar pillar. The treatment of a second branchial cleft sinus or fistula is surgical excision.

Ranula and Other Salivary Retention Cysts

Blockage of a minor salivary duct can lead to retention phenomenon, which can be manifested as a soft-tissue lesion deep within the substance of the lip or, if the location is very superficial, as a vesicular lesion. A *ranula* is a retention cyst along the lateral floor of the mouth and results from blockage of either the sublingual or submandibular gland. It is reasonable to observe these lesions for a brief period of time because they can establish spontaneous drainage. Should the lesion persist or the diagnosis be uncertain, excision or marsupialization can be performed through an intraoral approach.

Pierre Robin Sequence

This is a series of related anomalous conditions starting with micrognathia and retrognathia, which produce glossoptosis, which in turn causes inspiratory obstruction. Pierre Robin in 1923 reported his observations; the combination of upper airway obstruction resulting from retrognathia or micrognathia plus related glossoptosis now carries his name. The etiology of retrognathia is not clear but is thought to be related to intrauterine pressure with a failure to straighten the cephalic angle. As a result, the developing tongue cannot caudally transpose to allow the palatal shelves to rotate down to a horizontal position. This nicely accounts for the increased incidence of cleft palate and high arched palate that is seen in Pierre Robin sequence. Care of these patients centers on nutrition and airway protection via prone positioning early in life. Should conservative therapy fail, surgical intervention may be needed to secure the tongue in a more anterior position, such as is accomplished in the Routledge-Randall tongue-lip adhesion or transmandibular K-wire fixation of the tongue base. If these procedures are unsuccessful, tracheostomy is performed until mandibular growth occurs and the glossoptosis disappears.

SUGGESTED READING

Furnas DW (ed): Reconstructive surgery for deformities of the ear. *Clin Plast Surg* 1990; 17:193–419.

Kernahan DA, Thomson HG, Bauer BS: *Symposium on Pediatric Plastic Surgery.* St Louis, Mosby–Year Book, 1982.

Millard DR: *Cleft Craft. The Evolution of Its Surgery,* vol 1–3. Boston, Little, Brown, 1976.

Mulliken JB, Young AE: *Vascular Birthmarks—Hemangiomas and Malformations.* Philadelphia, WB Saunders, 1988.

Whitaker LA, Bartlett SP: Craniofacial anomalies in Jurkiewicz MJ, Krizek TJ, Mathes SJ, et al (eds): *Plastic Surgery Principles and Practice.* St Louis, Mosby–Year Book, 1990, p 99.

Chapter 16

Benign and Malignant Tumors

Jeffrey D. Wagner, M.D.
Riley S. Rees, M.D.

CONTENTS

NOTE: The material in this chapter is frequently covered during the prerequisite training period of many plastic surgery residents. This chapter should serve as a valuable review of important material in such cases. For residents who have not mastered this material previously, this chapter is essential.

CHAPTER OBJECTIVE

At the end of this chapter the resident recognizes the gross and histologic features of all common benign and malignant tumors of the head and neck, understands the biological behavior and treatment options for these lesions, and performs complete management of such lesions including diagnosis, surgery, and nonsurgical therapy.

LEARNER OBJECTIVES

On completion of this chapter the resident

1. **Knows the lymphatic drainage pattern of the head and neck structures and its relationship to the management of malignant tumors.**
2. **Understands the methods for diagnosis and the options for treatment of squamous cell carcinoma of the head and neck, particularly the oropharynx.**
3. **Understands the methods for diag-**

nosis and the options for treatment of benign and malignant processes of the salivary glands.

4. **Is familiar with the treatment of other benign processes of the head and neck such as rhinophyma.**
5. Is familiar with diagnostic techniques for head and neck tumors, including radiographic methods (e.g., sialogram, MRI scan, etc.) and fine-needle aspiration.
6. Knows the TNM staging system for tumors of the head and neck; knows the histologic features and biological behavior of these lesions.
7. Is familiar with the diagnosis and treatment of benign and malignant tumors of specific head and neck structures, including the eyelid, lacrimal apparatus, nasal cavity, and paranasal sinuses.
8. Is familiar with the diagnosis and treatment of benign and malignant tumors of bony and dental origin.
9. Knows the general principles and techniques of radiation therapy and chemotherapy for head and neck malignancies.
10. Is familiar with the treatment of other neoplastic processes of the head and neck such as tumors of vascular origin. (For benign and malignant lesions of the skin of the head and neck, see Chapter 11.)

CLINICAL PRACTICE ACTIVITIES

During the course of the training program, the resident

1. **Evaluates and treats patients with benign processes of the head and neck structures.**
2. Evaluates and treats patients with malignant tumors of the head and neck structures.
3. Participates in extirpative surgery for oropharyngeal tumors, including radical neck dissection.
4. Participates in extirpative surgery for salivary gland lesions.
5. Evaluates and treats patients with head and neck tumors of vascular and lymphatic origin.
6. Evaluates and treats patients with rhinophyma and other benign processes.
7. Evaluates and treats patients with inflammatory and infectious processes of the head and neck.

UPPER DIGESTIVE TRACT EPIDERMOID CARCINOMA

Carcinoma of the head and neck is a category of malignancies for which all the goals of medical oncology can be achieved. Since most of these cancers can be easily visualized, the goal of early detection can be realized. Because 80% to 90% of cases are induced by known chemical carcinogens, an opportunity exists for prevention through education and regulation. Individuals at high risk can be identified and screened. Once a histologic diagnosis is established, the extent of the tumor can be determined by clinical staging, and treatment plans can be formulated in most cases without expensive diagnostic studies. However, despite these theoretical advantages, the results of treatment of these cancers have been disappointing, with combined cure rates in the 40% to 50% range.

Ninety-five percent of all upper aerodigestive tract carcinomas are squamous cell carcinomas. As a collective group, head and neck carcinomas make up approximately 4.5% of all malignancies, with about 40,000 new cases diagnosed each year. The sex ratio is 3:1, male to female, but the incidence is increasing among women because of an increase in tobacco usage. The most commonly affected age groups are 45 to 70 years.

Anatomy

For the purposes of classification and staging, neoplasms of this area are separated by anatomic location—oral cavity, nasopharynx, oropharynx, hypopharynx, larynx, and paranasal sinuses (Fig 16–1). The most common sites of disease are the oral cavity and the

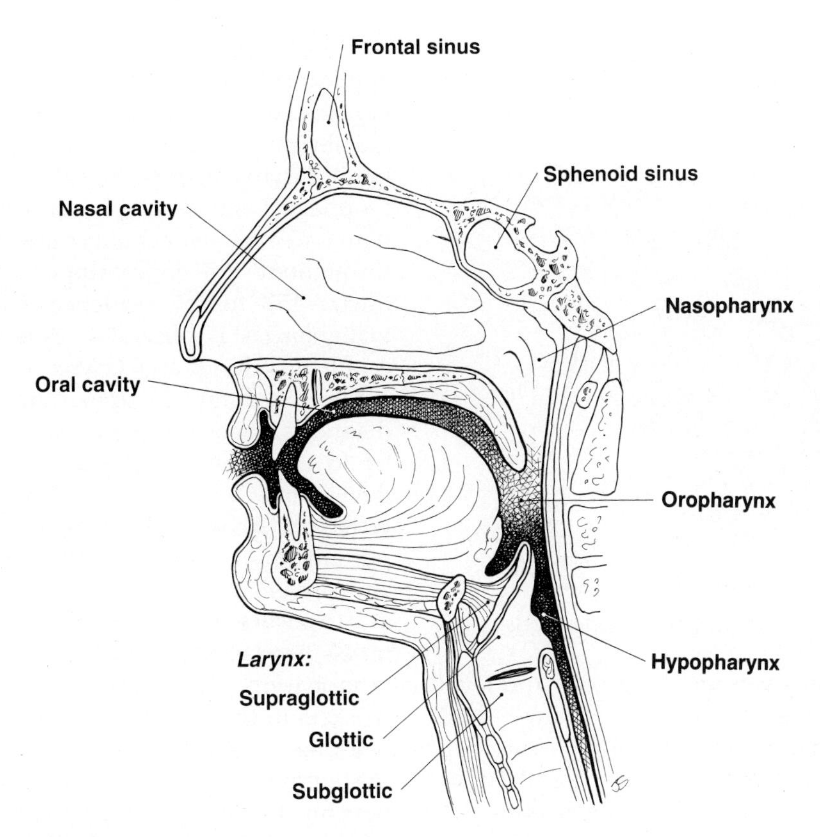

FIG 16–1.
Anatomic subsites of the head and neck.

oropharynx, which account for nearly 50% of all cases, followed by the larynx, which accounts for about 30%.

The oral cavity encompasses the area anteriorly from the vermilion border of the lips to its posterior limit, which is an imaginary vertical plane from the junction of the hard and soft palates to the circumvallate papilla of the tongue. This area includes the lips, buccal mucosa, anterior two thirds of the tongue, floor of the mouth, alveolar ridges, hard palate, and retromolar trigone.

The oropharynx extends the remainder of the way posteriorly and includes the soft palate, anterior tonsillar pillar, tonsils, tonsillar fossa, base of the tongue (posterior third), and the lateral and upper posterior pharyngeal walls.

The nasopharynx includes the superior vault above the level of the soft palate. It includes the eustachian tubes and Rosenmüllers' fossa and is immediately adjacent to the skull base.

The hypopharynx includes areas caudad to the base of the tongue and posterior to the larynx. It consists of the pyriform sinuses, postcricoid area, and lower posterior pharyngeal wall down to the level of the cricopharyngeus.

For the purposes of classification the larynx is subdivided into three areas: the supraglottic area, including the epiglottis, aryepiglottic folds, ventricular walls, and false cords; the glottis, which is limited to the true cords and anterior and posterior commissures; and the subglottic area, which is the remainder of the larynx below the level of the true cords.

A thorough understanding the lymphatic drainage of the head and neck is mandatory for the management of patients with head and neck cancer. Lymph node groups are classified into five major levels: level I is the submandibular nodes, level II contains the upper jugular or subdigastric nodes, level III represents the midjugular lymph node groups,

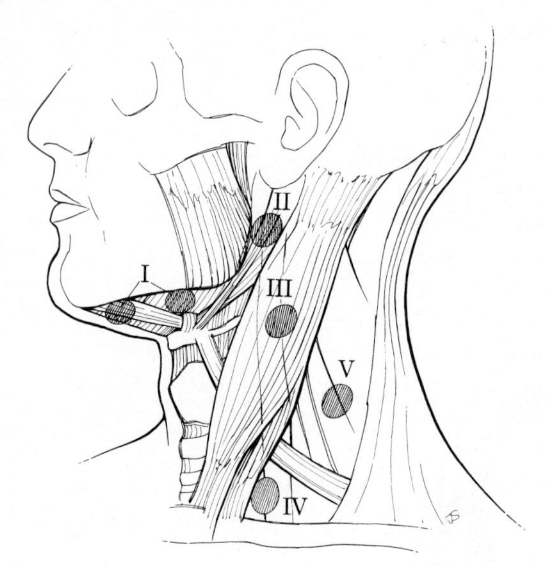

FIG 16–2.
Classification of cervical lymph node levels.

level IV is the lower jugular group, and level V contains posterior cervical triangle and supraclavicular groups (Fig 16–2). Tumors of the various anatomic sites have predilections for certain levels of lymphatic metastasis.

Pathophysiology

Effective management of aerodigestive cancers requires an understanding of known etiologic associations. Although the exact cause of these tumors is not known, ample evidence suggests that repeated exposure of the upper aerodigestive tract mucosa to a variety of carcinogens leads to their development. The most frequently observed irritants are tobacco and alcohol.

Tobacco abuse is associated with 90% of all cases of head and neck cancer. A history of alcohol abuse is noted in 75% of all cases of head and neck cancer. Tobacco smoke is convincingly related to laryngeal and oral cancers, and topical tobacco is associated with greatly increased risks of oral carcinomas. Alcohol abuse is a more significant risk factor than tobacco for hypopharyngeal and upper esophageal cancers. Isolating the differential effects of smoking from alcohol is difficult because many patients abuse both substances. Substance abuse also contributes significant comorbidity in this population.

The concept of "field cancerization" is applicable to head and neck squamous malignancies, i.e., exposure to carcinogens makes all membranes at higher risk. This includes oral, nasal, laryngeal, pharyngeal, bronchial, and esophageal mucosae. Widespread premalignant and malignant changes are often noticed throughout the entire upper aerodigestive tract. A 15% to 20% incidence of synchronous malignancies is observed, especially in the esophagus, lung, and larynx. Because many patients continue to smoke and drink after diagnosis, metachronous lesions develop in up to 40%. The risk of a second malignancy developing is up to six times higher in refractory smokers. This observation has important implications for evaluation, therapy, and surveillance.

Exposure to occupational hazardous materials has been implicated in cancers of the nasopharynx and paranasal sinuses among workers in the nickel, chromium, and woodworking industries. In the Far East, the Epstein-Barr virus has a strong, constant relationship to nasopharyngeal cancer. Chronic mechanical trauma to the oral mucosa such as poor dental hygiene, malfitting dentures, or broken teeth has been associated with oral cancers. Previous radiation exposure is associated with a slightly increased risk for mucosal carcinomas but is more strongly associated with thyroid and salivary gland malignancies. The Plummer-Vinson syndrome has been associated with carcinomas of the tongue and hypopharynx. The incidence of epithelial cancers is increased in immunosuppressed organ transplant patients, with an estimated risk of 20 to 30 times the expected rates, thus suggesting an important role for the immune surveillance system in preventing this group of cancers.

Clinical Behavior

The majority of head and neck squamous cell primary tumors are characterized by slow infiltrative or exophytic growth. These tumors arise from mucosal surfaces. Some tumors are diagnosed early because their location leads to a multitude of symptoms. In many cases, however, diagnosis is delayed because symptoms do not occur or go unnoticed until a large primary tumor develops. In such a patient, cervical metastases may be the initial manifestation. Regional lymphatic metastases occur in predictable anatomic patterns and are present in up to 50% of cases. Systemic metastases are much less common, rarely occurring without advanced primary tumors or cervical nodal involvement. They are present in fewer than 10% of cases initially but may develop in the course of treatment in up to 30% of cases. The most common site of distant metastatic disease is the lung, followed by bone and liver. Nonetheless, the most common pattern of failure after therapy is local or regional recurrence, with 75% of all treatment failures occurring above the level of the clavicles.

Clinical Evaluation

History

Cancers of the head and neck have a variety of local symptoms, frequently reflecting their location. A mass in the mouth or a sore tongue may be the first sign of oral carcinoma. A nonhealing sore in the mouth should be considered malignant until proved otherwise. Poorly fitting dentures or loose teeth may be related to cancers of the gingiva or palate. Trismus is a sign of advanced mandibular, masseteric, or skull base involvement. Hoarseness and coughing are the most frequent signs of laryngeal carcinoma, although referred otalgia may be the only symptom. Inspiratory stridor, dyspnea, and wheezing are signs of advanced upper airway obstructions. Dyspnea or aspiration pneumonia may occur with large posterior tumors of the tongue, hypopharynx, or supraglottic larynx. A bloody nasal discharge or recurrent sinusitis may provide clues to the presence of nasopharyngeal or sinus carcinomas. The proximity of the nasopharyngeal mucosa at the base of the skull makes cranial nerve dysfunction a frequent manifestation of these tumors. An isolated neck mass may be the initial symptom and commonly occurs with tumors of silent primary areas such as the nasopharynx and hypopharynx. Symptoms of weight loss, dyspnea, anorexia, and bony pain should be sought as clues to the presence of possible distant metastatic disease.

Clinical Examination

Examination of the upper aerodigestive tract is essential in the primary evaluation of patients with head and neck cancer. Inspection *and* palpation of the oral cavity are of utmost importance. Exophytic growths are quickly identified visually because they are friable and bleed easily. However, endophytic masses, common in areas such as the base of the tongue, are easily missed unless palpation is performed. The size, location, ulceration, depth of invasion, and fixation of the primary tumor are noted. Initial photographs should be taken, and multiple biopsies are indicated. Any mucosal lesion present for more than 2 weeks should undergo biopsy.

Special mention should be made of premalignant lesions frequently seen in these patients. Leukoplakia is a white patch of oral mucosa that cannot be wiped away. It represents hyperkeratosis resulting from chronic irritation. The incidence of premalignant transformation in leukoplakia is 3% to 5%. Leukoplakia that persists should undergo biopsy or be excised. Erythroplasia is a red, velvety patch on the mucosa and is characterized by severe dysplasia or carcinoma in situ in up to 90% of patients. All such lesions should be excised.

Occasionally, small lesions are not readily seen but become more visually discrete upon the direct application of 1% toluidine blue. This principle can also be applied by using a mouthwash technique. The size of the lesion may be underestimated when using this method in infiltrative tumors that do not involve the overlying mucosa. Oral rinse exfoliative cytology can also be performed. This study may help diagnose small cancers but has a 10% to 15% false negative rate and is therefore useful only when positive. Direct biopsy of the mass remains the standard diagnostic method.

Physical examination of the nasopharynx, larynx, and hypopharynx is mandatory and can be facilitated by using a head mirror and dental mirror or a nasal fiberoptic endoscope. The nasopharynx can be examined either by turning the dental mirror upward or by fiberoptic nasoendoscopy. The endolarynx and hypopharynx are well visualized by either technique. The practitioner should be familiar with and capable of performing both techniques because they are complementary.

Palpation of the cervical lymph nodes throughout the neck completes the head and neck examination. Notes are made of the size, number, and presence of fixation of any enlarged lymph nodes. Diagnostic fine-needle aspiration of enlarged cervical nodes with an unknown primary tumor should be considered at the initial office visit.

Examination Under Anesthesia

Examination under anesthesia (EUA) is necessary for diagnosis, accurate staging, and biopsies of tumors of the larynx and most tumors of the posterior oral cavity and pharynx. Bimanual palpation, inspection, direct laryngoscopy, and pharyngoscopy are always performed for these tumors prior to definitive therapy.

Because of the significant incidence of synchronous tumors, many surgeons have advocated panendoscopy (bronchoscopy, laryngoscopy, and esophagoscopy) for all patients with head and neck malignancies. Subsequent clinical studies have shown that bronchoscopy is of low yield in the presence of normal chest x-ray findings. In addition, most esophageal lesions are likely to be associated with dysphagia and are usually located in the cervical esophagus. The use of directed cervical esophagoscopy and bronchoscopy with washings in selected patients is therefore a reasonable approach.

Staging Workup

Laboratory/Radiograph

Because head and neck cancers rarely give rise to hematogenous metastases before regional nodal metastases are evident, only patients with N2 or N3 disease require extensive staging studies. Evaluation is otherwise guided by the presence of examination findings and symptoms such as bone pain, jaundice, and dyspnea. The minimum staging workup required is a plain-film chest radiograph and liver enzyme panel, particularly alkaline phosphatase. Liver imaging is valuable only in patients with abnormal enzyme profiles or advanced locoregional disease. There are currently no specific tumor markers for most head and neck cancers. A possible exception is nasopharyngeal carcinoma, where elevated titers of anti–Epstein-Barr virus IgA and IgG can be used for surveillance.

Additional radiologic studies are indicated in some patients. Plain films of the skull and mandible plus panorex and cervical spine films have been used to evaluate bony invasion in large tumors involving these areas, but these have been largely replaced with computed axial tomographic (CAT) scanning of the face and neck. CAT scans are sensitive for bone invasion, soft-tissue infiltration, and adenopathy. This technique should be used in the staging evaluation of advanced primary tumors with extensive cervical nodal metastases and in cases of nasopharyngeal carcinoma. Magnetic resonance imaging (MRI) has even higher resolution than CAT scanning and appears to be promising for soft-tissue evaluation of tumors of the nasopharynx and skull base. Barium contrast studies of the pharynx and esophagus are useful in patients with dysphagia or unexplained weight loss. Sinus films, laryngography, and tomographic studies have largely been replaced by CAT and MRI scans. Bone scans are done only if the patient has an elevated alkaline phosphate level, advanced local disease, or complaints of bone pain.

Staging Classification

The classification of head and neck cancers is a clinical staging system. It is based on examination findings and is assigned once the diagnosis is proved by biopsy and after the tumor extent is quantified by all available preoperative studies but *before* definitive treatment is begun. The accepted staging system is the TNM staging system, popularized by the American Joint Committee of Cancer Staging and Results Reporting (AJC). This was most recently revised in 1988.

Primary. The T classification of the primary tumor depends on the site, size, and

TABLE 16–1.
Primary Tumor (T) Classification for the Oral Cavity

Tis	In situ
T1	Tumor ≤ 2 cm in diameter
T2	Tumor > 2 cm ≤ 4 cm in diameter
T3	Tumor > 4 cm in diameter
T4	Tumor invades adjacent bone, skeletal muscle, sinus, or skin

extent of invasion into surrounding tissues. Tumors of the oral cavity and oropharynx are classified by the measured size of the lesion (Table 16–1). Tumors of other areas are classified according to anatomic extension.

Cervical Lymph Nodes. The N stage is determined by the size, number, and distribution of cervical lymph nodes believed to be clinically positive. The previous determination of fixed or mobile nodes is not applicable in the current staging system (Table 16–2).

Metastases. The assignment of the M stage is either M1 if there are systemic metastases or M0 if none are present.

Stage Grouping

Four clinical stages represent the increases in severity of disease (Fig 16–3) and are reflected by decreasing cure rates. Prognosis is correlated both with the stage and with the site of primary (see individual tumor sites).

Therapy

Therapy for head and neck cancers is extremely complex. The most frequently seen patients have poor oral hygiene and generally take poor care of their health. Multiple comor-

TABLE 16–2.
Metastatic Cervical Lymph Node (N) Classification

N0	No clinically positive nodes
N1	Single ipsilateral node, ≤ 3 cm in diameter
N2	
N2a	Single ipsilateral node, 3–6 cm in diameter
N2b	Multiple ipsilateral nodes, none > 6 cm in diameter
N2c	Bilateral or contralateral nodes, none > 6 cm in diameter
N3	Metastases in any lymph node > 6 cm in diameter

Stage I	T1 N0 M0
Stage II	T2 N0 M0
Stage III	T3 N0 M0
	T1 or T2 or T3, N1 M0
Stage IV	Any T4
	Any T, N2, or N3, M0
	Any T, any N, M1

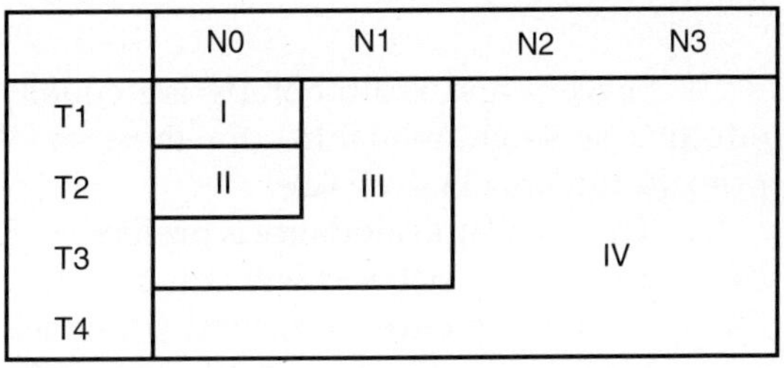

	N0	N1	N2	N3
T1	I	III	IV	IV
T2	II	III	IV	IV
T3	III	III	IV	IV
T4	IV	IV	IV	IV

FIG 16–3.
Stage groupings.

bid factors such as poor nutrition, hypertension, chronic obstructive pulmonary disease (COPD), cirrhosis, diabetes, and substance abuse complicate the decision-making process as well as the postoperative course of those patients who undergo treatment. Noncompliance is a significant problem in this population. While many patients are initially seen with advanced tumors and have little hope for cure, palliation for pain, infection, and odor are worthwhile goals.

Cooperative multidisciplinary joint consultations prior to treatment and in posttherapy clinics are essential. The head and neck cancer team includes the primary care physician, head and neck surgeon, radiation and medical oncologists, dentist, pathologist, nutritionist, speech pathologist, rehabilitation expert, prosthetist, and social worker. The goals are eradication of malignancy, maintenance of function, and socially acceptable cosmesis. Each of these factors is considered in the formulation of an individualized treatment program for the patient.

There are presently three modalities commonly employed in therapy for head and neck cancers: surgery, radiotherapy, and chemotherapy. Both surgery and radiotherapy are potentially curative as primary therapeutic modalities for both the primary and regional metastases. Chemotherapy alone has not proved curative but is frequently used as palliation and is being investigated in organ preservation protocols.

Although treatment planning for head and neck cancers considers therapy for both the primary and cervical metastases, it is useful to consider them separately. General principles guiding treatment planning are as follows:

1. Surgery and radiotherapy are equally effective as single modalities for most small primary tumors (T1 and T2).
2. The use of one modality is preferable to two because many patients will require future therapy for recurrence or second primaries.
3. Small primaries (T1 and T2) are usually best treated by a single modality, the choice of which depends on tumor location, presence of metastatic disease, and patient factors such as compliance or comorbidity.
4. Large primaries (T3 and T4) are usually best treated by combined modalities, the approach again depending on tumor and patient factors.
5. Clinically positive necks are treated for cure or control.
6. Clinically negative necks at high risk for subclinical metastases are treated prophylactically.

Treatment of the Primary

Surgery. Extirpative surgery as therapy for head and neck cancer has several advantages. It allows an accurate determination of the extent of the lesion and its spread. It is usually well tolerated, even if extensive. Large tumors are readily ablated. The disadvantages of surgery are that microscopic foci of tumor near margins and subclinical disease may remain and produce later recurrence. In addition, function and cosmesis may be adversely affected.

All gross disease should be removed en bloc with clear margins confirmed by frozen section. Gross free margins should be at least 1 and preferably 2 cm since margins less than 0.5 cm are associated with an 80% local recurrence rate. Surgical resection is *required* for tumors that invade bone, large tumors (T3 or T4), tumors associated with overt cervical metastases, and residual disease after primary radiotherapy. Surgery is favored over radiotherapy for patients who are likely to be noncompliant. A variety of surgical approaches is available, including peroral, lip splitting, tongue splitting, mandibulotomy, and apron or visor flaps with pull-through resections combined with neck dissections.

Radiotherapy. Radiotherapy for head and neck cancers has two major advantages. First, no tissue is removed, so a good cosmetic result is usually obtained. Second, radiotherapy covers a wide area and eradicates microscopic tumor cells at some distance from the lesion. The major disadvantage is that large lesions with hypoxic portions respond poorly. In addition, radiotherapy injures surrounding tissue and reduces tolerance to toxicants such as traumatization by dentures, heat, cold, and tobacco. Some types of tumors such as adenocarcinoma tend to be radioresistant. Radiotherapy is therefore most effective for squamous cell T1 or T2 primaries without bone or cartilage invasion. Radiotherapy is also used as primary therapy for nasopharyngeal carcinomas. Typical dosing schedules are 150 to 200 rad/day over a period of 6 to 12 weeks for a total of 5,000 to 7,000 rads, depending on the tumor size and location. Adjuvant radiotherapy is required for gross residual postoperative disease, close margins, large primaries (T3 or T4), or any primary with extensive nodal metastases (N2 or N3). Radiotherapy is favored over surgery for small tumors where extirpation is particularly disabling, such as the larynx, base of the tongue, or the hypopharynx.

Combination therapy is preferred over single-modality therapy for T3 and T4 tumors in order to achieve maximal control of the malignancy. No randomized prospective trial has demonstrated a survival advantage for this combined approach vs. single-modality therapy. The order of applied treatments is based largely upon institutional preference. One approach is preoperative radiotherapy (usually 5,000 rads) followed by radical surgery possibly with a smaller dose of postoperative radiotherapy. The more common approach combines radical surgery with immediate flap reconstruction, followed by 6,000 to

7,000 rads of postoperative radiotherapy started within 6 weeks of surgery. This approach allows higher doses of radiotherapy to be given and has demonstrated lower complication rates than preoperative radiotherapy.

Treatment of Cervical Metastases

Since failure in head and neck cancer therapy is usually locoregional, treatment programs must also address the regional lymphatics. Some form of therapy should be planned for any N(+) neck, as well as for those patients with N0 necks who have a greater than 15% probability of subclinical metastases. This includes head and neck tumors at all sites except for T3 or smaller tumors of the lip and T1 or possibly well-differentiated T2 lesions of the oral cavity and glottic larynx. Cervical metastases are clinically present in 30% of patients at the time of presentation, and subclinical metastases are present in another 20%. Nodal metastases are the single most important predictor of survival because they predict an increased risk for distant metastases. An increased risk of cervical nodal involvement is predicted by increasing size of the primary, posterior tumor location, tumor thickness greater than 2 mm, anaplastic cellular differentiation, the presence of perineural or perivascular invasion, and a high tumor mitotic index. Among patients with cervical metastases, the prognosis is influenced by the size and number of involved nodes (bilateral or contralateral nodes) and by extracapsular tumor invasion.

Both surgery and radiotherapy are useful modalities for the management of cervical metastases. Treatment of cervical lymphatic metastases may alter the natural history of the disease by improving regional control but has never been clearly demonstrated to improve survival.

Surgery. Surgical therapy for cervical metastases consists of neck dissection with cervical lymphadenectomy. The classic radical neck dissection (RND) as described by Crile in 1906 is a complete cervical lymphadenectomy from the clavicle to the base of the skull that removes the sternocleidomastoid muscle, internal jugular vein, cranial nerve XI, and the submandibular gland. It is the standard of therapy to which all subsequent forms of neck dissection must be compared. RND carries significant functional morbidity primarily because of the sacrifice of cranial nerve XI and trapezius function. In addition, bilateral simultaneous RND should not be performed because of the high incidence of severe facial edema and elevated intracranial pressure.

Modifications of the classic RND have been popularized by various surgeons over the past several decades, who have retained combinations of the above-mentioned nonlymphatic structures in an effort to decrease the morbidity of the operation. The combined use of surgery and radiotherapy has led some centers to use neck dissections that remove only gross disease or only those nodal groups that are at highest risk of containing metastases. There are no randomized prospective trials comparing RND with modified forms of neck dissection. Several retrospective and nonrandomized studies show no survival difference provided that all gross tumor is excised. The consensus among surgeons favors RND for gross disease in the neck, especially N2 or N3, and reserves modified neck dissections for N0 or, in rare instances, N1 necks. Surgical therapy for neck disease is required for extensive gross disease and for residual or recurrent disease after primary radiotherapy when primary tumor control is achieved. Salvage neck dissection is contraindicated if control of the primary tumor cannot be achieved. Surgery is also favored when the primary is treated via excision.

Lymphadenectomy is effective as the sole therapeutic modality only if a single node less than 3 cm in size (N1) without extracapsular invasion exists. Recurrence after neck dissection alone is high (40% to 50%) in N2 or N3 necks or if extracapsular invasion is found. In these situations adjunctive radiotherapy is employed.

Radiotherapy. Radiotherapy for cervical metastases is used to eliminate minimal or microscopic disease. As noted above, adjuvant radiotherapy is useful to decrease the failure rate in those patients undergoing lymphadenectomy for N2 or N3 disease and in those patients with extranodal spread. It may be useful as the sole treatment modality for N1 necks and in some series yields control rates similar to surgery. Elective nodal irradiation of high-risk N0 necks is a reasonable therapeutic approach when the primary is being treated with radiotherapy alone. Employed in this manner, radiotherapy can reduce the risk of appearance of neck metastases to less than 5%.

Special mention should be made of the management of patients with cervical lymphadenopathy of unknown origin. A number of studies have demonstrated that approximately 85% of cases of cervical lymphadenopathy in adults are due to metastatic malignancy. Of these, approximately 85% are from head and neck cancers. Isolated cervical metastases may be the sole initial symptom in up to one third of head and neck cancers. The location of metastases gives important clues to the origin of the primary site.

The approach to a patient with suspected metastatic carcinoma to cervical nodal basins begins with a thorough head and neck examination. Occult tumors are often missed in the scalp, nasopharynx, base of the tongue, hypopharynx, and supraglottic larynx, and these sites deserve careful examination. Examination of nodal areas in the groin and axilla must be done to rule out systemic lymphoma. Chest radiography is routinely performed to rule out lung tumors and mediastinal adenopathy.

If the initial head and neck examination does not yield the primary tumor site, fine-needle biopsy of the neck mass should be the next step. This should be performed at the time of the initial office visit. Fine-needle aspiration is 95% accurate in diagnosing metastatic squamous carcinoma. Only suspected lymphomas and nondiagnostic results require open biopsy procedures.

If the primary is still unlocated, a computed tomographic (CT) scan of the head and neck will define areas of lymphadenopathy and will visualize silent areas such as the nasopharynx. The patient should thereafter be taken to the operating room for EUA. If a primary tumor is still not seen, directed biopsies of the most likely sites such as the base of the tongue and the nasopharynx are done.

If still no primary is discovered, the neck should be considered for definitive therapy. The node should be excised and the diagnosis confirmed by frozen section. The incision should be placed in an appropriate position for a neck dissection, which is performed at this point if the diagnosis of metastatic squamous cell carcinoma is confirmed. If the diagnosis cannot be confirmed or if lymphoma is still a possibility, neck dissection is postponed until final pathology results are available.

Therapy for metastatic squamous cell carcinoma of the neck of unknown primary is worthwhile. After neck dissection, high-dose radiotherapy is given to both the neck and possible occult sites. This approach yields 80% local control and up to a 50% survival rate in patients in whom the primary is controlled. The primary tumor is eventually discovered after therapy in approximately 25% of patients. The prognosis is worse for this subset.

Chemotherapy. Despite extensive investigations, chemotherapy in the management of head and neck malignancies has been disappointing. Although several active agents have been identified and response rates have been good, to date randomized trials have not demonstrated a survival advantage for any chemotherapeutic regimen.

Chemotherapy has traditionally been used as adjuvant therapy for stage III and stage IV tumors. Response rates of 30% to 50% have been demonstrated to single agents, the most useful being methotrexate, cisplatin, 5-fluorouracil, and bleomycin. Better responses have been achieved with combination regimens, but when used as adjuvant therapy, chemotherapy has significant toxicity in already malnourished postoperative patients. In addition, the agents have a limited duration of response. Most clinicians consider adjuvant chemotherapy to be palliative.

The most exciting investigations into chemotherapy recently are in the area of induction therapy. Induction therapy has several advantages over adjuvant treatment, including better patient tolerance and better tumor response. Additional cycles are associated with improved response rates, but cessation of therapy is almost always followed by recurrence. Several early uncontrolled trials suggested a survival advantage for responders. However, more recent controlled prospective trials have not demonstrated a survival advantage when compared with conventional surgery and radiotherapy. Recent investigations substituting induction chemotherapy for radical surgical resection in advanced laryngeal cancers followed by high-dose radiotherapy for responders suggest that although survival is unaltered, a significant percentage of these patients may be able to avoid surgery altogether and retain speech. Results of these trials are promising but should be regarded as preliminary. Studies are under way to investigate similar protocols in other head and neck locations.

Carcinoma of Various Sites

Lips

Ninety-five percent of lip cancers are squamous cell carcinomas, which are well-differentiated low-grade tumors. Over 90% of these tumors occur on the lower lips, while the remainder are equally divided between the upper lip and commissures. Most patients are men aged 60 years or older. There is very high correlation with ultraviolet light exposure; the correlation with tobacco use is less clear. Primary lymphatic drainage is to the submental and submandibular areas, although the upper lip and commissures may also drain to the parotid nodes. Cervical metastases are unusual except in the largest tumors and in the most undifferentiated primaries.

Surgical excision with lip shaving is the preferred treatment for lip cancer. Radiotherapy does not yield superior cosmetic results and may increase the likelihood of secondary tumors. Defects from excision of less than one third of the lip can usually be closed primarily. Defects of one third to two thirds of the lip are easily managed with lip advancement flaps. Total lip excisions can be reconstructed with cheek advancement flaps, although distant flaps such as the pectoralis major or free tissue transfers may be necessary. Because neck metastases are not common, elective neck dissection is not indicated for most tumors in N0 necks but should be considered for T3 or T4 lesions, especially if recurrent or poorly differentiated. Dissection must include the suprahyoid area and should be bilateral if the tumor is in the midline. The prognosis is the best for any site in the head and neck, with initial therapeutic successes in 75% to 80% of patients.

Oral Cavity and Oropharynx

The oral cavity and oropharynx are the most common sites for head and neck squamous cell carcinomas. Most anterior floor of the mouth lesions are well or moderately differentiated, while the posterior lesions tend to be poorly differentiated or undifferentiated. Widespread premalignant mucosal changes are often seen in conjunction with the primary. Strong associations with alcohol and tobacco abuse have been demonstrated.

Primary lymphatic drainage from the oral cavity is to the ipsilateral submental and submandibular (level I) and high jugular nodes (level II). Oropharynx tumors spread to the ipsilateral level II and III nodes, often bilaterally.

T1 and most T2 tumors of the oral cavity and oropharynx can be treated with either surgery or radiotherapy for the primary. Morbidity after excision is low for small anterior lesions and is favored in patients who are noncompliant because they will not stop smoking or reliably submit to follow-up. Radiotherapy is favored for small posterior lesions where functional morbidity is higher, such as the base of the tongue and the tonsil, with surgery reserved for failures. Larger primaries are managed with combined therapy, usually surgery followed by radiotherapy. Marginal en bloc mandibular resection is satisfactory for tumor adherent to the periosteum, but segmental resection is required for frank bone invasion. For patients requiring resection of large posterior tumors, laryngectomy may be indicated to achieve clear margins and prevent aspiration. Reconstruction with pedicled musculocutaneous or composite free flaps is often necessary.

Lymphatic spread occurs in a significant percentage of patients. Concomitant treatment of the ipsilateral portion of the neck is indicated in all tumors except T1N0 tumors of the oral cavity. Cure rates are favorable for small anterior lesions (90%) and worse (15% to 30%) for larger and posterior lesions.

Nasopharynx

Nasopharyngeal carcinoma is a common malignancy in certain parts of the world, particularly in the Far East, where there is a fairly constant relationship with the Epstein-Barr virus. An increased incidence is also found among workers in the nickel, chromium, and woodworking industries. Most tumors are poorly differentiated squamous cell carcinomas, although up to 30% may be lymphomas, adenocarcinomas, or sarcomas. The primaries are often very small, and staging is therefore based upon involvement of adjacent structures. Initial symptoms are usually subtle, and an asymptomatic neck mass alone is present in 35% to 50% of cases. Other symptoms are tinnitus, otitis media, epistaxis, headache, and cranial nerve dysfunction. Diagnosis is usually made from directed biopsies during EUA of a patient with a metastatic cervical lymph node with no known primary. CT or MRI scanning is an important part of the staging evaluation.

Surgical margins are unobtainable in tumors of the nasopharynx. Therefore, primary therapy for these tumors is confined to high-dose radiotherapy. Radiation treatment of both sides of the necks is indicated since bilateral metastatic rates are 50% to 90%. Neck dissection is reserved for those patients demonstrating a cure at the primary site with residual neck disease. Prognosis is poor because most tumors are seen in late stages. In addition, systemic metastases may be present in up to 25%. Five-year survival rates range from 50% to 70% for T1 and T2 lesions and 5% to 15% for T3 and T4 lesions.

Hypopharynx

The hypopharynx is a relatively silent area, with most tumors initially seen in advanced stages. Ninety-five percent of tumors are poorly differentiated squamous cell carcinoma. Dysphagia is the most common initial symptom, and a history of alcohol abuse is a constant finding. Invasion of the larynx is common and makes aspiration frequent. Cervical lymphatic metastasis is seen in 70% to 80% of patients and is the sole initially encountered symptom in one third of the cases. EUA and CT scanning are essential parts of the staging evaluation.

Therapy for hypopharyngeal carcinoma is usually combined surgical and radiotherapy. Selected T1 lesions may be treated by radiotherapy alone, but a combined surgical and radiotherapy approach will be required for T2 lesions and larger. Selected small T2 lesions may be excised with partial pharyngectomy, but most tumors will require partial or total laryngopharyngectomy. All postcricoid tumors or those invading the apex of the pyriform sinus will require total laryngectomy to prevent subsequent aspiration. Conservation laryngectomy is not possible in most instances. Reconstruction of the pharynx and cervical esophagus often requires myocutaneous flaps, gastric pull-up, or free jejunal interposition. Adjuvant radiotherapy is employed in all cases. The 5-year survival rate for hypopharyngeal carcinoma treated with combined therapy is 15% to 50% and depends on the presence of lymphadenopathy.

Nasal Cavity, Paranasal Sinuses

Tumors of the nasal cavity and paranasal sinuses are rare and constitute only 3% of all head and neck tumors. The etiology is usually undetermined but is associated with inhaled wood dust and arsenicals. Eighty percent of all tumors occur in the maxillary sinuses, and most of the remainder are in the ethmoids. The primary tumors are usually locally destructive and are manifested by local pain, swelling, sinusitis, or bleeding. Proptosis and loose teeth may occur with advanced lesions. CT scanning in the coronal and axial planes should be performed in all patients and can be used to direct the biopsy through the nose or through a Caldwell-Luc approach. First-echelon lymphatic drainage is to level I cervical nodes, but metastases are unusual.

Therapy is surgical resection of the maxilla and postoperative radiotherapy. Orbital exenteration is performed for tumors extending through the orbital periosteum. Cervical lymphadenectomy is performed for positive neck nodes. The N0 neck is included in the postoperative radiation fields. Five-year survival rates are 20% to 50%. Reconstruction of the oral-nasal defect is by maxillary prosthesis.

Larynx

Cancers of the larynx are subclassified according to anatomic sites: supraglottic, glottic, and subglottic locations. Tumors of the glottis are most common, followed by supraglottic tumors. Subglottic tumors are rare. Laryngeal carcinomas are usually well-differentiated squamous cell carcinomas and are typically diagnosed after a history of hoarseness in a middle-aged smoker. Glottic tumors produce early hoarseness and are usually discovered early in contrast to supraglottic lesions, which produce fewer symptoms. Both indirect and direct laryngoscopy are necessary to stage and perform a biopsy on the tumor. Diagnostic imaging, especially fine-cut CT scans, will demonstrate cartilage invasion and help assess the extent of the tumor. Staging at the various subsites is according to local tumor extension (Table 16–3).

Lymphatic drainage is to lymph nodes at levels III or IV. The glottic region has relatively sparse lymphatics, which is the reason that T1 and T2 lesions of the true cords rarely metastasize (only 1% to 10%), while T3 and T4 lesions have higher metastatic rates (25% to 50%). The supraglottic larynx has a rich lymphatic drainage pattern, and cervical nodal metastases are found more frequently. Subglottic tumors may metastasize to paratracheal nodes in the mediastinum. For this reason, all tumors of the larynx except T1 and well-differentiated T2 tumors of the true glottis should have some form of therapy directed to the cervical lymph nodes.

Therapy for laryngeal carcinomas depends on the stage, site, and patient factors. For tumors of the glottic larynx, T1 lesions are usually treated with radiotherapy, with a 90% cure rate. T2 lesions may be treated similarly, but the cure rates with radiotherapy alone are only about 60%. Vertical hemilaryngectomy is curative in 80% of cases of T1 and T2 lesions. T3 and T4 tumors of the glottis and all subglottic tumors require total laryngectomy, ipsilateral neck dissection, and adjuvant radiotherapy. Survival rates are in the 40% to 50% range for larger tumors.

Stage I and II supraglottic tumors may be treated with radiotherapy alone or with horizontal partial laryngectomy to preserve the

TABLE 16–3.
Primary Tumor (T) Classification of the Larynx

Supraglottis	
Tis	Carcinoma in situ
T1	Tumor confined to site of origin with normal vocal cord mobility
T2	Extension to an adjacent supraglottic subsite or the glottis with normal vocal cord mobility
T3	Limited to larynx with vocal cord fixation or invades the postcricoid area, pre-epiglottic space, or medial wall of the pyriform sinus
T4	Extends beyond larynx with soft-tissue invasion or cartilage destruction
Glottis	
Tis	Carcinoma in situ
T1	Confined to vocal cord(s) with normal mobility
1a	Single cord } May involve the anterior or posterior commissures
1b	Both cords } May involve the anterior or posterior commissures
T2	Extends to supraglottis or subglottis with normal or impaired vocal cord mobility
T3	Confined to larynx with vocal cord fixation
T4	Extends beyond larynx with soft-tissue invasion or cartilage destruction
Subglottis	
Tis	Carcinoma in situ
T1	Confined to subglottis
T2	Extends to glottis with normal or impaired cord mobility
T3	Confined to larynx with vocal cord fixation
T4	Extends beyond larynx with soft-tissue invasion or cartilage destruction

voice. Because of the risk of aspiration, only patients with good pulmonary function and performance status are candidates for this procedure. T3 and T4 tumors require total laryngectomy, neck dissection, and postoperative radiotherapy. Local recurrence rates are high, especially if the tongue base is invaded. Survival is worse for supraglottic tumors, with control rates ranging from 80% for T1 lesions to 10% to 20% for advanced disease.

SALIVARY GLAND TUMORS

The salivary glands are responsible for a wide variety of benign and malignant disorders that frequently require surgical treatment. There are three pairs of major salivary glands: the parotid, submandibular, and sublingual glands. There are also several hundred minor salivary glands located in the mucous membranes of the tongue, lips, cheeks, and palate.

Anatomy

The paired parotid glands lie just anterior to and below the ear and are the largest of the major salivary glands at a weight of around 25 g each. Each is a unilobular gland that is pierced by branches of the facial nerve. There are no clear anatomic planes between the so-called superficial and deep lobes. The duct of the parotid gland is Stensen's duct, which is about 7 cm long; it begins at the anterior aspect of the gland, crosses the masseter muscle, passes medially to pierce the buccinator muscle, and enters the mouth opposite the second maxillary molar.

The submandibular glands are about 3 to 4 cm in size and lie in the submandibular triangle on the hyoglossus muscle superficial to the lingual and hypoglossal nerves. Parasympathetic fibers reach the gland by way of the lingual nerve and corda tympani to the submandibular ganglion. Drainage is via Wharton's duct, which is about 5 cm long, lies on the hyoglossus muscle, and courses anteriorly between the lingual and hypoglossal nerves to enter the floor of the mouth.

The sublingual gland is the smallest of the three major glands with a weight of about 2 g. It lies in a submucosal pocket in the anterior part of the floor of the mouth. It is usually drained by several small ducts, each of which enter the mouth separately. Tumors of the sublingual gland are extremely rare.

Inflammatory Disorders of the Salivary Glands

Acute sialadenitis usually occurs during periods of relative dehydration and poor oral hygiene in debilitated patients, in diabetic patients, and in the elderly. These conditions allow retrograde passage of oral flora into Stensen's or Wharton's ducts. The parotid is more commonly involved than the submandibular gland. Bilateral involvement is seen in up to 20% of cases.

Diagnosis is made easily with findings of fever, painful swelling, induration, and tenderness over the involved gland. Purulent drainage may be expressed from the duct orifice. Management consists of rehydration, intravenous antibiotics, improved oral hygiene, and gland massage. A short course of steroids may lessen the inflammation. Surgical drainage is rarely required.

Chronic sialadenitis is initially seen as a series of recurrent, intermittent or persistent mild salivary swellings with a reduction in salivary output, often after a bout of acute suppurative sialadenitis. The pathophysiology is stricture of the ductal system. Occasionally patients with chronic sialadenitis may show symptoms of Sjögren's syndrome, which consists of keratoconjunctivitis sicca, parotid swelling, xerostomia, and polyarthritis.

Indications for surgical treatment of chronic sialadenitis depend upon the severity of symptoms. Medical management should be tried first. Surgical therapy consisting of total resection of the salivary gland is reserved for intractable symptoms.

Salivary Neoplasms

Although parotid neoplasms account for only 3% of all tumors of the head and neck region, they produce a wide variety of lesions peculiar to this tissue. Eighty percent of tumors occur in the parotid gland, and 80% of these are benign. The vast majority of the remainder of salivary neoplasms are found in the submandibular gland, but only 50% of these are benign. The only known risk factor for salivary tumors is prior radiation exposure. Those tumors are seen in adults between their third and fifth decades.

Evaluation of Parotid Masses

The most common manifestation is a painless mass in the parotid area. Facial nerve paralysis is uncommon unless the tumor is malignant. Pain is not a good predictor of malignancy. All parotid masses should be considered neoplastic until proved otherwise. Preoperative evaluation with CT scans or fine-needle aspiration is helpful but rarely alters management. Examination should include evaluation of the cervical lymph nodes and a search for a primary skin cancer as a source of metastasis to the intraparotid nodes. The intraparotid nodes drain the upper and midface regions, anterior part of the scalp, and auricle. Tumors here may result in a secondary parotid mass.

Benign Neoplasms

Pleomorphic adenoma (benign mixed tumor) is the most common parotid neoplasm and accounts for 65% of all tumors. It is a firm, slowly growing, painless mass typically present for several years. These lesions are benign, but approximately 10% will eventually undergo malignant degeneration. The treatment is total excision via superficial parotidectomy with facial nerve sparing. These tumors are encapsulated but have pseudopod-like extensions. Enucleation is a poor operation because local recurrence rates are unacceptably high. With superficial parotidectomy, including a small cuff of normal parotid tissue, recurrence rates should be less than 5%.

Warthin's tumors, also called papillary cystadenoma lymphomatosum, are found only in the parotid gland. This tumor is thought to arise from heterotopic salivary tissue entrapped within parotid lymph nodes during embryogenesis. They occur between the ages of 40 and 70 years and have a distinct male predominance. About 10% are bilateral and may also be multifocal. A technetium 99 scan will demonstrate the presence of Warthin's tumor and locate an occult tumor on the contralateral side. Treatment is superficial parotidectomy. Recurrence rates are about 10%.

Malignant Parotid Neoplasms

Malignant tumors are much less common than benign tumors and account for fewer than 20% of parotid tumors and 50% of submandibular gland tumors. Facial nerve paralysis occurs with 15% of parotid malignancies and portends a poor prognosis. Minor salivary gland neoplasms are usually found on the palate and are malignant in 70% to 80% of cases.

Malignant salivary neoplasms display a diversity of histologic types. These tumors can be divided into low- and high-grade malignancies, with low-grade tumors behaving similar to benign tumors and high-grade malignancies acting like aggressive cancers. Low-grade tumors include low-grade mucoepidermoid carcinomas, adenoid-cystic carcinoma, and acinar cell carcinoma. These tumors rarely metastasize and generally have favorable prognoses. Adenocarcinomas, high-grade mucoepidermoid carcinomas, malignant mixed tumors, squamous cell carcinomas, and undifferentiated tumors are considered high-grade malignancies with a significant risk of cervical lymphatic metastases. These types of tumors have poor prognoses.

The definitive therapy for *all* salivary gland malignancies is surgical excision. There is no curative nonoperative therapy, and radiotherapy is reserved for adjunctive therapy. The extent of surgical therapy depends on the tumor's histologic grade, presence or likelihood of cervical metastases, and involvement of surrounding structures. The minimal treatment of parotid malignancy is total parotidectomy. The facial nerve should be spared unless it must be sacrificed to obtain clear margins. Radical parotidectomy sacrificing the facial nerve is performed only if the facial nerve is invaded with tumor. Immediate nerve grafting by using the great auricular nerve is important when the facial nerve is

TABLE 16–4.
Salivary Gland Tumor (T) Staging (Parotid, Submaxillary, and Sublingual)

T0	No evidence of primary tumor
T1	Tumor ≤2 cm in diameter
T2	Tumor > 2 cm ≤ 4 cm in diameter
T3	Tumor > 4 cm ≤ 6 cm in diameter
T4	Tumor > 6 cm in diameter
All categories subdivided	
a	No clinical involvement of skin, soft tissues, nerve, or bone
b	Clinical involvement of skin, soft tissues, nerve, or bone
Stage groupings	
I	T1a or T2a, N0, M0
II	T1b or T2b or T3a, N0, M0
III	T3b or T4a, N0, M0
	Any T (except T4b), N1, M0
IV	Any T4b
	Any T, N2 or N3, M0
	Any T, any N, M1

sacrificed. Lateral tarsorrhaphy may be performed concomitantly to prevent exposure keratoconjunctivitis. Massive tumors may also require resection of the mandible, skin, or masseter muscle. For submandibular and minor salivary gland carcinomas, en bloc total gland resection is done for both diagnosis and therapy. This may include resections of the floor of the mouth or palate to obtain clear margins.

Therapeutic neck dissections are done for tumors with N(+) necks. Elective neck dissections are reserved for histologic subtypes with a high risk of occult metastases. Adjunctive radiotherapy is employed for locally extensive tumors, high-grade malignancy, and positive margins. Staging of salivary gland tumors is illustrated in Table 16–4.

TUMORS OF THE JAW

Tumors of the bony jaws include a diverse variety of benign and malignant lesions. Cysts and tumors of the mandible and maxilla can be classified as odontogenic or nonodontogenic. Odontogenic tumors are those lesions composed of cells normally involved in tooth development. These may include cysts or actual tumors. Nonodontogenic tumors arise from tissues not associated with tooth development.

Odontogenic Cysts

These may be either developmental or inflammatory in nature. The most common developmental odontogenic cysts are dentigerous cysts and keratocysts. Dentigerous cysts (also called follicular cysts) constitute about 18% of all jaw cysts. They are usually radiolucent, asymptomatic, unilocular cysts encircling the crown of an unerupted tooth in the region of the third mandibular molar. They are caused by fluid accumulation around the enamel after the crown root of an unerupted tooth has formed and are lined by nonkeratinized stratified squamous epithelium. They may become infected, displace teeth, or cause mandibular erosion. Treatment is enucleation, and recurrence is unusual.

Keratocysts (primordial cysts) make up about 10% of odontogenic cysts. They develop from dental lamina rests and basal hamartomas of the overlying oral mucosa. They may be large and can be locally destructive. Keratocysts occur in the 20- to 50-year-old age range, are three times more likely in the mandible than the maxilla, and are usually located posteriorly. Presentation is usually swelling with drainage, but pain or paresthesia may also be present. The radiographic appearance is that of a unilocular or multilocular cyst with sclerotic margins. Treatment of smaller cysts is by aggressive curettage, but the recurrence rate may be as high as 30%. Larger cysts and recurrences are managed with segmental resection and reconstruction with bone grafting.

Odontogenic tumors may be of epithelial or mesenchymal origin. Most are benign but behave aggressively with local bone destruction and invasion of adjacent structures. Benign tumors include ameloblastic tumors (adamantinomas), ameloblastic fibrosis, hamartomas, and cementoblastomas. Therapy for these tumors consists of segmental or marginal mandibulectomy. Recurrence rates for ameloblastomas after segmental resection are 15% to 20%. Mandibular reconstruction is frequently necessary.

Malignant odontogenic tumors are unusual. This group includes malignant ameloblastomas and fibrosarcomas. Malignant ameloblastomas result from malignant transformation of a benign ameloblastoma. Treatment is radical excision. Adjuvant radiation and chemotherapy are generally used. Five-year survival rates are in the 30% range.

Nonodontogenic tumors are tumors of skeletal origin and are similar to those seen elsewhere in the skeleton. Benign tumors include osteomas, osteoid osteomas, fibrous dysplasia, giant-cell tumors, and aneurysmal bone cysts. Treatment is simple surgical removal, usually via aggressive curettage.

Malignant nonodontogenic tumors include osteosarcomas, chondrosarcomas, fibrosarcomas, Ewing's sarcoma, lymphomas, and malignant histiocytomas. Staging and management are similar to those occurring elsewhere in the skeleton.

TUMORS OF THE EXTERNAL EAR

Common tumors of the auricle are basal and squamous cell carcinomas and, less commonly, melanomas. Diagnosis of the lesion is made by biopsy, and excision is the treatment of choice. This may be a wedge or rim auriculectomy for smaller lesions, but margins must be at least 5 mm. Larger lesions and deep melanomas require total auriculectomy. If ear canal invasion is suspected, temporal bone resection may be indicated. Lymphatic drainage of the anterolateral auricle is to the parotid nodes; drainage of the posterior auricle and the postauricular area is to the occipital nodes. Superficial parotidectomy and cervical lymphadenectomy are indicated for clinically positive nodes. Adjuvant radiotherapy is recommended for close or positive surgical margins and recurrent disease. Reconstruction of external ear defects can be by a variety of techniques such as an auricular advancement procedure, circumferential reduction, and conchal flaps.

EYELID TUMORS

The most common tumors of the eyelids are basal and squamous cell carcinomas. Melanomas or adnexal cell tumors occur with some frequency. Therapy is excision with histologically confirmed clear margins; to this end Moh's micrographic surgical technique preserves important structures. Electrodesiccation and curettage are contraindicated with tumors of the eyelid structures. When clear margins have been ensured, wound management may be via primary skin grafts (from the opposite eyelid or postauricular area) or cheek advancement flaps for partial-thickness defects. Defects of the tarsus and full-thickness defects may be closed primarily if small (less than 25% of lid) but, if larger, will require reconstruction via lateral canthotomy, lid switch flaps, or lined cheek flaps. Small defects near the medial canthus can be allowed to close secondarily with good cosmetic results.

Lacrimal Tumors

The lacrimal gland is located in the upper outer quadrant of the orbit just behind the supraorbital ridge in the lacrimal fossa of the frontal bone. As with salivary disorders, many inflammatory and neoplastic conditions are similar in clinical presentation.

Tumors of the lacrimal gland are rare. Histologically, about 25% are benign granulomatous disorders, about 25% are benign mixed tumors, around 25% are lymphoid tumors, and approximately 25% are carcinomas. Dermoid cysts and benign adenomas constitute the remainder. Rarely, acute dacryoadenitis accompanies a systemic viral infection. This condition is seen almost exclusively in children and resembles an abscess in the lateral part of the upper eyelid. Treatment is with warm compresses and antibiotics, and the problem is usually self-limited. If suppuration supervenes, drainage is indicated through a transconjunctival or transcutaneous approach.

It is absolutely necessary to be certain of the tissue diagnosis of a lacrimal tumor prior to definitive surgery since orbital exenteration may be necessary for treatment. Evaluation of suspected orbital neoplasms begin with CT or MRI scans to evaluate for invasion of bone or orbital structures and intracranial extension. Diagnostic biopsy procedures must be planned carefully to prevent spread of a controllable lesion. Needle biopsy may be done, but the tract must be placed in the line of planned excision. If the mass is relatively confined to the lacrimal fossa, the entire gland, surrounding periosteum, and capsule are removed en bloc as the biopsy specimen. If the mass is very large or obviously spread beyond the lacrimal fossa, an incisional biopsy is done and permanent sections tested prior to definitive therapy.

Most disorders will be confined to the gland and are adequately treated by resection of the entire gland, capsule, and surrounding periosteum. Benign mixed tumors may rarely invade bone; if so, resection of the involved lateral orbital wall may be indicated. Lymphomatous lesions are managed with radiotherapy. Malignant epithelial tumors, usually adenoid cystic carcinoma, are highly aggressive lesions that are life-threatening by means of their proximity and spread to the intracranial fossa. Therapy is by wide excision of the gland as well as the lateral orbital wall and orbital roof along with orbital exenteration and postoperative radiotherapy.

OTHER BENIGN HEAD AND NECK TUMORS

Granular Cell Myoblastoma

Granular cell myoblastoma is a tumor of the tongue that arises from striated muscle cells. It is a rare tumor, most commonly seen as a firm solitary lesion and often initially mistaken for an infiltrative carcinoma. It is a benign tumor with no malignant potential. Complete excision is curative.

Hemangiomas

Hemangiomas of the head and neck are usually seen first in early childhood. These lesions may be cutaneous or deep and do not differ in pathology, histology, or natural history from similar lesions found elsewhere on the body. Most lesions arise shortly after birth, increase in size over the first 6 to 12 months, and then undergo spontaneous involution over several years with little or no residual scarring. Deeper lesions may occur without cutaneous involvement. A typical example is the parotid hemangioma, the most common parotid neoplasm of childhood. Exceptions to spontaneous involution are often deeper lesions and those that have a component of arteriovenous malformation.

Complications of hemangiomas include ulceration, bleeding, scarring, infection, tissue necrosis, and thrombocytopenia resulting from platelet sequestrations (Kasabach-Merritt syndrome). In addition, large lesions involving the oral cavity or pharynx may compromise the airway.

Therapy must be individualized for each patient. The best therapy for most lesions is watchful waiting. This may be tempered with a short course of systemic corticosteroids to help induce involution. Aggressive interventions such as embolization, radiotherapy, or resection are reserved for complications or those lesions that do not resolve by early adolescence and are associated with significant cosmetic deformities. Therapy for such lesions is difficult and produces cosmetically unsatisfactory results.

Cystic Hygromas

Cystic hygromas are seen in childhood. They occur as a result of sequestration or obstruction of developing lymphatic vessels in the neck. Most lesions occur posterior to the sternocleidomastoid muscle. The cysts are usually multilocular and may involve deep structures. Surgical excision offers the best chance for cure since these lesions do not usually spontaneously regress. Since they are benign disorders and because of their close proximity to adjacent nerves and vascular structures, radical ablative surgery is not indicated. Rather, if the lesion cannot be completely excised without jeopardizing important structures, partial excision is indicated even if serial resections are necessary for eventual control.

Mucous Cysts

Mucous cysts (mucoceles) are benign tumors of the oral cavity that are formed by a small (<2 cm) collection of extravasated mucus from the rupture of a minor salivary gland duct. They are usually located in the lower lip or the floor of the mouth. Surgical excision is the therapy of choice. Electrodesiccation is also usually curative.

Rhinophyma

Rhinophyma is a rare, benign, gradual enlargement of the nasal skin. At times the adjacent cheek tissues are also involved. This disorder is of unknown etiology but is often associated with acne rosacea and usually seen in elderly males. The disorder consists of dermal hypertrophy of the nasal skin with an increase in the number and size of sebaceous glands and an increase in dermal collagen, sometimes with an inflammatory cellular infiltrate. Therapy is indicated for cosmetic purposes. A reasonable contour can usually be restored by tangential excisional sculpting with sharp or dermabrasion techniques. The skin of the nose is resurfaced from sebaceous gland remnants.

Fibrous Dysplasia

This is an uncommon, nonneoplastic benign bone disease of unknown etiology. It results from abnormal activity of bone-forming mesenchyme with arrest of bone maturation in the woven bone stage and metaplastic fibro-osseous ossification. This results in an increasing mass of abnormal bone that causes progressive deformity.

Two patterns of fibrous dysplasia predominate: monostotic (80%) and polyostotic (20%). The commonly involved craniofacial bones are the frontal and sphenoid bones and the maxilla and mandible. The monostotic variety commonly involves only the jaws. The polyostotic variety often involves the skull base and may be associated with extraskeletal manifestations such as Albright's syndrome.

Monostotic craniofacial dysplasia is usually manifested as a unilateral progressive jaw asymmetry. The lesion may cross the midline or grow into the sinuses. The radiographic appearance is a ground glass or cystic lesion with poorly circumscribed margins. In polyostotic fibrous dysplasia, symptoms are varied and related to the tumor mass and location. They may include pain, swelling, headache, proptosis, orbital dystopia, and cranial nerve palsies. Both varieties may be self-limited, sometimes becoming quiescent after puberty, but the point of arrest is unpredictable. Malignant transformation is a rare occurrence (<1%) but should be suspected in a painful or rapidly growing lesion.

Therapy has evolved from conservative observation with occasional bone contouring procedures to the currently recommended total excision of involved bone with immediate reconstruction with bone grafts. Interestingly, the resected dysplastic bone may be recontoured and replaced as an autogenous bone graft. These grafts and conventional bone grafts seem to function similarly and have a lower potential for recurrence when compared with in situ contouring.

INFECTIONS OF THE HEAD AND NECK

Because of its rich vascularity and lymphatic drainage, the head and neck region is remarkably resistant to infection. However, because of unique anatomic relationships, established infections can be rapidly progressive and even fatal. The well-described fascial planes of the neck are routes of minimal resistance to the spread of infections of the upper aerodigestive tract and neck into the mediastinum. The emissary veins of the scalp communicate directly through the cranium with the dural sinuses and allow direct spread of scalp infections intracranially. Similarly, the paranasal triangle of the face communicates intracranially via the ophthalmic veins with the cavernous sinus. Infections here can result in the lethal complication of cavernous sinus thrombosis.

Infections of the head and neck are most commonly related to traumatic wounds or to surgical complications. Peritonsillar, salivary gland, and periodontal infections are also seen with some frequency. Infection rates for major head and neck operations where the oral mucosa is violated are 25% to 40%. Prophylactic antibiotic coverage with a 24-hour course of perioperative parenteral broad-spectrum anti-anaerobic antibiotics such as moxalactam, clindamycin, or metronidazole is recommended to improve this rate to less than 10%.

Cellulitis of the tissues of the face and neck is usually due to gram-positive organisms such as *Staphylococcus* and *Streptococcus*. Appropriate therapy consists of prompt initiation of penicillinase-resistant penicillin or a first-generation cephalosporin. Important oral cavity flora are the anaerobic *Streptococcus* and *Bacteroides* species. Bites and infections communicating with the upper aerodigestive tract therefore require broad-spectrum antibiotic therapy directed at anaerobes and gram-negative organisms, including clindamycin or metronidazole in combination with an extended-spectrum penicillin or cephalosporin. If an abscess is suspected or if necrotic tissue or a fistula is present, exploration and wide drainage with debridement and open packing of wounds is performed in the operating room. In the case of deep cervical infections or fistulas, therapy involves opening of involved tissue planes with wide drainage and may include proximal pharyngostomy diversion of oropharyngeal secretions or coverage of exposed carotid artery with muscle flaps. Cultures are taken, and antibiotic coverage is adjusted as indicated and continued for a 10- to 14-day course. Later, definitive treatment of uninfected controlled fistulas may include the use of muscle flaps.

SUGGESTED READING

Ariyan S: Cancer of the upper aerodigestive system, in McCarthy JG (ed): *Plastic Surgery,* vol 5. Philadelphia, WB Saunders, 1990, p 3412.

Beahrs OH: Surgical anatomy and technique of radical neck dissection. *Surg Clin North Am* 1977; 57:663.

Coleman JJ: Salivary gland disorders, in Jurkiewicz MJ, Krizek TJ, Mathes SJ, et al (eds): *Plastic Surgery Principles and Practice.* St Louis, Mosby–Year Book, 1990, p 379.

Jackson IT (ed): *Local Flaps in Head and Neck Reconstruction.* St Louis, Mosby–Year Book, 1985.

Jackson IT, Shaw K: Tumors of the craniofacial skeleton and jaws, in McCarthy JG (ed): *Plastic Surgery,* vol 5. Philadelphia, WB Saunders, 1990, p 3336.

Johns ME: Parotid cancer: A rational basis for treatment. *Head Neck Surg* 1980; 3:132.

Medina JE: A rational classification of neck dissections. *Otolaryngol Head Neck Surg* 1989; 100:169.

Woods JE: A technique for the rapid performance of parotidectomy with minimal risk. *Surg Gynecol Obstet* 1976; 142:87.

Chapter 17

Craniofacial Trauma

Steven R. Cohen, M.D.

CONTENTS

Gunshot wounds of the face
- Low-velocity gunshot wounds
- Intermediate- and high-velocity gunshot wounds to the face

Mandibular fractures
- Dentition
- Maxillomandibular fixation
- Acrylic dental splints in maintenance of maxillomandibular fixation
- Classification
- Physical examination of the mandible
- Roentgenographic diagnosis
- Temporomandibular joint
- Treatment of mandibular fractures
  - Class I fractures
  - Class II fractures
  - Class III fractures
  - Complex and comminuted mandibular fractures
- Damage to teeth

■ CHAPTER OBJECTIVE

At the end of this chapter, the resident is familiar with the mechanisms of traumatic injury of the head and neck structures, understands the diagnostic techniques and therapeutic options applicable to such problems, and performs complete management of complex soft tissue and bony injuries of the head and neck.

■ LEARNER OBJECTIVES

On completion of this chapter, the resident

1. **Knows the priorities involved in treating patients with multiple trauma, the timing of treatment of head and neck injuries, and the indications for endotracheal intubation and tracheostomy in such patients.**
2. **Knows an orderly, systematic approach to the physical examination of patients with facial trauma.**
3. **Knows the indications for specific diagnostic studies including conventional radiography, panorex films, tomograms, computer-assisted tomography, three-dimensional CT scan imaging, and magnetic resonance imaging.**
4. **Knows the biomedical properties of the facial skeleton and patterns of injury associated with facial trauma, including associated cervical and cranial trauma.**
5. **Understands the management of open facial injuries, including anesthesia, local wound care, principles of debridement, and biologic features that distinguish facial injuries from those in other locations.**
6. **Understands the concepts of primary bone healing, malunion, nonunion, and osteomyelitis.**
7. **Recognizes the indications for operative treatment of facial fractures.**
8. **Knows the advantages and disadvantages of various techniques for treatment of facial fractures including nonoperative treatment, closed reduction, mandibulomaxillary fixation, open reduction with and without fixation, wire fixation, compressive and noncompressive fixation, intraoral splints, and external fixation (including halo and bi-phasic techniques).**
9. **Understands specific treatment of maxillary, mandibular, orbital, nasoethmoid, frontal, zygoma and zygomatic arch fractures; the potential complications of such treatment (including malposition, deformity, malocclusion, etc.); and the management of these complications.**
10. **Is familiar with the operative incisions for the treatment of facial fractures.**
11. **Understands the neuroanatomy, cranial anatomy, and soft tissue relationships pertinent to the facial nerve.**
12. **Knows how to perform an examination of the facial nerve.**
13. **Understands techniques for treatment of acute injuries to the facial nerve.**
14. **Understands the anatomy of the parotid gland and options for treatment of parotid injuries.**

15. **Understands the etiology of enophthalmos and its treatment options.**
16. Understands the anatomy of the lacrimal apparatus and options for treatment of lacrimal injuries.

■ CLINICAL PRACTICE ACTIVITIES

During the course of the training program, the resident

1. **Treats patients with minor and major soft tissue injuries of the face, including injuries to the facial nerve, lacrimal apparatus, and parotid gland.**
2. Diagnoses and treats patients with closed and open fractures of the facial skeleton.
3. Operates on patients with fractures of the facial skeleton and performs closed reductions, open reductions, internal fixations, and bone grafting.
4. Manages patients postoperatively after surgical treatment of facial fractures.
5. Manages patients with nasal fractures including reduction and splinting.

Complex injuries involving the face not only jeopardize appearance but also compromise functions of the head and neck. The approach to complex facial injuries requires a thorough knowledge of masticatory function, normal occlusal relationships, and ocular and orbital anatomy; a knowledge of the terrain of the sinuses; an understanding of the structural pillars of the craniofacial skeleton; a firm comprehension of muscular origins, insertions, and direction of pull; and finally, a clear concept of three-dimensional skeletal anatomy. In concert with the above-mentioned principles, the plastic surgeon must have expertise and grounding in a variety of incisions and exposure techniques, harvesting of autogenous bone grafts, the use of wide subperiosteal dissection, and the numerous available rigid fixation devices that are used for skeletal stabilization.

The purpose of this chapter is to present in a practical format the requisites necessary for management of facial trauma.

INITIAL ASSESSMENT

Prior to specific treatment of facial trauma, the physician must determine whether the patient with facial injuries has been adequately evaluated for the presence of other significant or potentially life-threatening problems. Control of the airway must be established and bleeding stopped. Manson as well as others recommend a trauma protocol for systems evaluation should be followed in almost all cases. Failure to follow standard protocols may lead to permanent injury or even fatal error.

Head Injuries

Head injuries frequently accompany fractures of the face. The Glasgow Coma Scale is used to assess the patient's level of consciousness (Table 17–1). In a patient with head injury, stable blood pressure, and associated trauma of the face and skull, computed tomography (CT) of the head is indicated. If feasible, the skull and facial bones should be visualized.

The presence of coma does not contraindicate treatment of maxillofacial injuries. Those patients in coma in whom intracranial pressure (ICP) measures less than 15 mm Hg may be considered for early treatment of facial fractures. When necessary, anesthesia can be safely performed with ICP monitoring. Treatment of craniofacial injuries in patients with

TABLE 17–1.
Glasgow Coma Scale (GCS)*

I. Best Verbal Response	
None	1
Incomprehensible sound	2
Inappropriate words	3
Confused	4
Oriented	5
II. Eyes Open	
None	1
To pain	2
To speech	3
Spontaneously	4
III. Best Motor Response	
None	1
Abnormal extension	2

* From Manson PN: Facial injuries in plastic surgery, Philadelphia, 1990, WB Saunders. Used by permission.

ICP over 15 mm Hg should be temporarily delayed until the ICP is stabilized within the normal range and neurosurgical clearance has been obtained.

Cervical Spine Injuries

Injuries to the cervical spine frequently accompany significant trauma to the head and face. A cervical spine film through C7 should be obtained and reviewed prior to open reduction/internal fixation of facial fractures. Patients with fractured mandibles are especially susceptible. Until the entire spine is visualized radiographically, the patient should be presumed to have a cervical fracture.

EMERGENCY TREATMENT

In patients with facial trauma there are three life-threatening emergencies: respiratory obstruction, hemorrhage, and aspiration.

Respiratory Obstruction

Establishment of an airway is of prime importance in a patient with maxillofacial injuries. When doubt exists, immediate *endotracheal intubation* should be carried out. If intubation is impossible, *cricothyroidotomy* is the treatment of choice. Once the airway is established, bronchoscopy can be performed to determine the exact level of tracheal penetration, and the cricothyroidotomy site can be converted to a formal tracheostomy.

Tracheostomy

The physician should have a low threshold for performing elective tracheostomy in patients with panfacial injuries. Tracheostomy facilitates placement of maxillomandibular fixation (MMF) by clearing the oronasal area of obstructing tubes.

Indications for tracheostomy may include the following:

1. Unrelieved airway obstruction
2. Edema with compromise of the airway
3. Associated intracranial or chest injury
4. High spinal cord injuries
5. Anticipation of prolonged postoperative airway problems
6. MMF in comatose patients or those with significant chest injuries
7. Panfacial fractures
8. Severe facial burns
9. Concern about difficult reintubation

Control of Severe Hemorrhage

When severe nasopharyngeal hemorrhage occurs, it is usually from the *internal maxillary artery*. Anteroposterior nasal packing can be efficiently accomplished. Several techniques are useful, including the following:

1. Two 30- to 50-cc Foley catheters inserted into the pharynx, which is pulled to occlude the posterior nasopharyngeal opening. Vaseline gauze is packed into the recesses of each nasal cavity. Catheters are secured by a suture tied over the columella. Columellar necrosis must be avoided.
2. Special balloon occlusion devices with a round posterior balloon and a sausage-shaped anterior balloon are commercially available.

When hemorrhage is uncontrolled, selective arterial embolization should be considered.

ROENTGENOGRAPHIC DIAGNOSIS

Roentgenographic evaluation is indispensable in the management of a patient with head and face injuries. However, it does not replace clinical examination, the most sensitive indication of facial injury. Plain facial films may be of value in selected circumstances but have a limited role in a patient with complex facial injuries. Occasionally, plain facial films are used as screening tools. When utilized, the most valuable and the most often employed views of the face are the facial bone series, including the Caldwell, submentovertex, Waters, Towne, and lateral skull views. In most circumstances, CT scans should be obtained. For a complete discussion of the common types of plain facial films the reader is referred to Manson's chapter on facial trauma in *Plastic Surgery* edited by McCarthy.

Roentgenographic Positions for Standard Facial Films

A. Posteroanterior projection
   1. Oblique anterior view of upper facial bounds: the orbits, malar bones, and zygomatic arches
B. Caldwell position
   1. Posteroanterior projection
   2. Demonstrates frontal sinuses, frontal bone, anterior ethmoidal cells, and zygomatic frontal suture
   3. Orbital margins, lateral walls of maxillary sinuses, and mandibular rami also seen
C. Fronto-occipital projection
   1. Used when injuries prevent examination of facial bones with the patient in the prone or seated position
   2. Satisfactory view of orbits and lesser and greater wings of the sphenoid, frontal bone, frontal and ethmoidal sinuses, nasal septum, floor of the nose, hard palate, mandible, and upper and lower dental arches
D. Reverse Waters position
   1. Mento-occipital position
   2. Used when patient cannot be placed in the prone position
   3. Demonstrates fractures of the orbits, maxillary sinuses, and zygomatic arches
E. Lateroanterior projection (Fuchs position)
   1. Gives an oblique view of the zygomatic arch projected free of superimposed structures
F. Occlusal views of the hard palate
   1. Demonstrates fractures of the hard palate
   2. Oblique views to demonstrate fractures of the alveolar process and views of the teeth and upper quadrant of the maxilla
G. Submentovertex and verticosubmental positions for the base of the skull
   1. Axial projection of mandible, the coronoid and condyloid processes, and the mandibular rami
H. Occlusal views of the mandible
   1. Demonstrates displacement and anterior mandibular fractures
I. Oblique lateral views of the mandible
   1. Demonstrates fractures of the mandibular ramus, body, and symphyseal region
J. Temporomandibular joints (TMJs)
   1. Oblique anteroposterior and fronto-occipital views
      a. Oblique posterior view of the condyloid processes of the mandible and mandibular fossa
      b. Fractures in the region of TMJ with displacement medially or laterally detected in these views
   2. Lateral transcranial projection
      a. Oblique lateral views to demonstrate the TMJs in the open- or closed-mouth position
      b. Demonstrates fractures and dislocations of the mandibular condyle and condylar process
   3. Mayer view
      a. Superior and inferior views
      b. Demonstrates medial or lateral displacement

When evaluating craniofacial trauma, axial and in many cases coronal CT scans should be ordered. These can be reformatted in a variety of manners, and discussion with a skilled radiologist can be helpful. For fractures of the mandible the single best screening study is the Panorex. When this cannot be obtained, axial and coronal views on CT and/or a mandibular series with TMJ views can be ordered.

TREATMENT OF SOFT-TISSUE WOUNDS

Tetanus Prophylaxis

A. No history of immunization
   1. Hypertet (tetanus immune globulin), 250 units intramuscularly plus
   2. Tetanus toxoid, 0.50 mL

3. Two additional tetanus toxoid (0.50 mL) boosters at monthly intervals

B. Immunization greater than 5 years
   1. Tetanus toxoid, 0.50 mL

C. Contaminated wounds, patient not immunized within 2 years
   1. Tetanus toxoid, 0.50 mL

When the patient is seen late with extensive tissue edema, subcutaneous hematoma, and crushing or when the wound edges are badly contused and tissue is devitalized, it may be preferable to delay wound closure until conditions for primary healing are more favorable. Relative indications for delayed primary wound closure include a facial wound that has been open for greater than 24 hours and an extensive associated soft-tissue injury as mentioned above.

Abrasions

To prevent tattooing, local anesthesia should be given, and the wound should be scrubbed, usually within 24 hours of injury, to remove all embedded foreign material.

Facial Nerve Repair

The facial nerve is a structure of primary consideration when evaluating facial injuries (Fig 17–1). The facial nerve exits from the skull at the stylomastoid foramen to enter the parotid gland in its deep surface, inferior to the auditory meatus. From this point, the nerve gradually becomes superficial as it passes across the masseter muscle to innervate the muscles of facial expression. The main trunk, which measures approximately 4 mm in diameter, divides into two main branches: the temporofacial and the cervical facial. Beyond this point, branching of the nerve is accompanied by intercommunicating arborization to form five branches:

1. Temporal or frontal—lateral aspect of the brow and forehead
2. Zygomatico-orbital—palpebral fissure and orbit
3. Buccal—cheek and upper lip

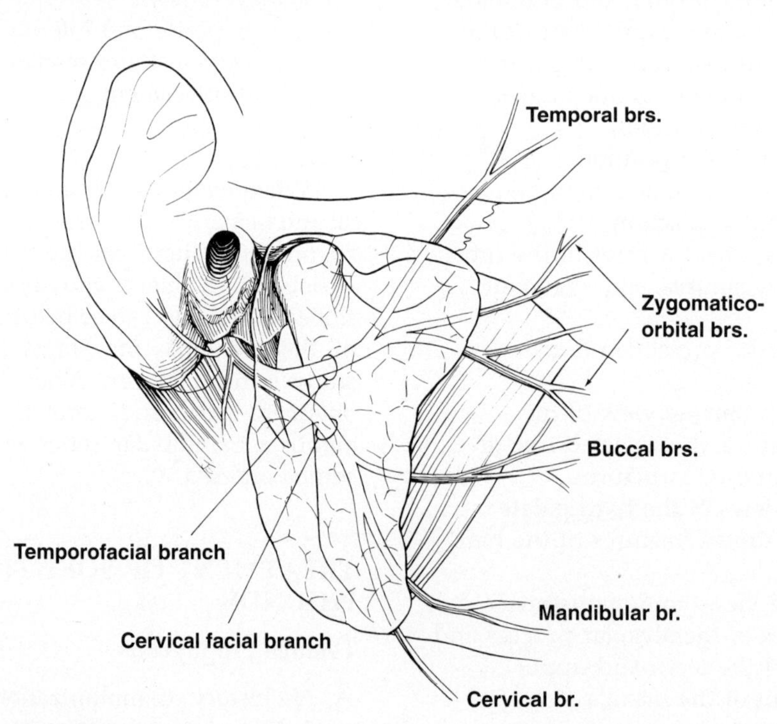

FIG 17–1.
Anatomy of the facial nerve

4. Mandibular—oral commissure
5. Cervical—platysma

It is often impractical and usually unnecessary to identify and suture the terminal branches of the facial nerve. In general, any identifiable branch of the facial nerve should be repaired. Manson suggests that anterior to a line perpendicular to the lateral canthus, nerve repair may not be necessary since the plexus of nerve fibers makes regeneration a common occurrence. Posterior to a perpendicular line at the lateral canthus, the branches of the facial nerve should be identified and repaired by using microsurgical techniques.

Any identifiable branch of the facial nerve should be repaired:

- Anterior to a line perpendicular to the lateral canthus, nerve repair is not necessary.
- Posterior to a perpendicular line at the lateral canthus, branches of the facial nerve should be identified and repaired with microsurgical techniques.

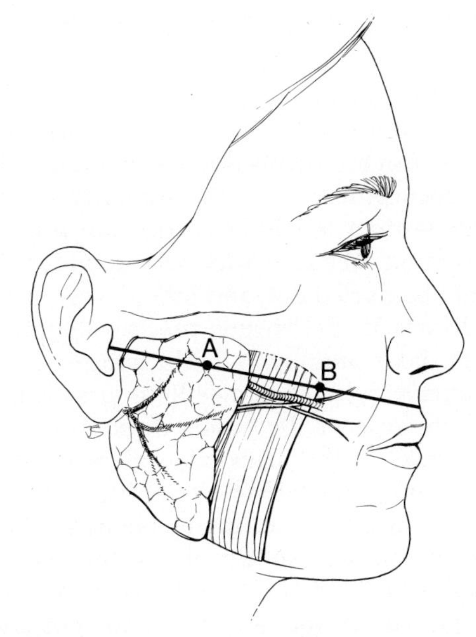

FIG 17–2.
The course of Stensen's duct from the parotid into the upper buccal area is deep to the middle third of a line drawn from the tragus of the ear to the midportion of the upper lip. The hilum of the gland is at approximately *point A,* and the opening of the duct in the mouth is opposite the second maxillary molar tooth deep to *point B.* The buccal branch of the facial nerve crosses Stensen's duct near *point B.*

Parotid Duct Lacerations

Relevant Anatomy

1. The course of Stensen's duct from the parotid to the upper buccal area is deep in the middle third of a line drawn from the tragus of the ear to the midportion of the upper lip (Fig 17–2).

2. The opening of the duct into the mouth is opposite the second maxillary molar.

Treatment

1. Injury to the duct is identified by gently dilating the orifice with small lacrimal dilators.
2. A Silastic tube or probe is inserted into the duct.
3. The duct is irrigated with saline through the catheter to identify complete or partial transection.
4. Once identified, Silastic catheter is threaded and the repair carried out with fine, absorbable suture.
5. Silastic tubing is anchored to the mucous membrane inside the mouth with a permanent suture—stent for 2 weeks.
6. Consider drainage for possible fistulization.
7. Persistent fluid accumulation is treated by intermittent aspiration and compression or reinsertion of the drain.

Laceration of the Lacrimal System

The lacrimal system should be considered injured with *any laceration at the region of the medial canthus.* If the canaliculus is severed, the ends are sutured over fine Silastic tubing by using microsurgical techniques. Late lacrimal duct obstruction is usually due to compression of the nasolacrimal duct following naso-orbital-ethmoid (NOE) trauma and is most commonly treated by dacryocystorhinostomy (DCR).

Injuries to the Soft Tissues of the Orbit

Superficial eyelid lacerations involving only the skin and orbicularis oculi can be closed primarily with careful approximation. A search for embedded foreign material and documentation of the integrity of the orbital septum should be carried out prior to performing repair. Minimal debridement should be carried out, and little tissue should be discarded. To ensure precise alignment of the lid margin, a 6-0 silk suture on an atraumatic ophthalmic needle is passed into the substance of the tarsus through one of the orifices of the meibomian glands, across the wound, and into the opposite tarsus to exit the lid margin at the meibomian orifice. Traction on this suture aligns the wound edges and lid margins. Additional sutures are placed at the anterior and posterior wound margins, tied, and left long. Upward traction on these three sutures maintains positioning, and the remaining sutures are placed. The pretarsal and muscle sutures are placed first, followed by skin closure (Fig 17–3).

Ophthalmologic consultation should be obtained for most injuries in and around the orbit. This should also be the case for simple zygomatic fractures. If an ophthalmologist is not available, visual function should be ascertained before any treatment is undertaken. Manson suggests that minimal examination should include the following:

1. Assessment of vision with Rosenbaum pocket cards
2. Determination of extraocular muscle function
3. Evaluation for diplopia
4. Funduscopic examination

Hyphema

Blunt trauma to the eye frequently causes bleeding. The presence of blood within the eye is called hyphema. Treatment varies from a conservative approach of bed rest to surgical intervention.

Lacerations of the Nose

Nose lacerations may be simple or complex (composite injury to the lining, cartilage/bone, skin).

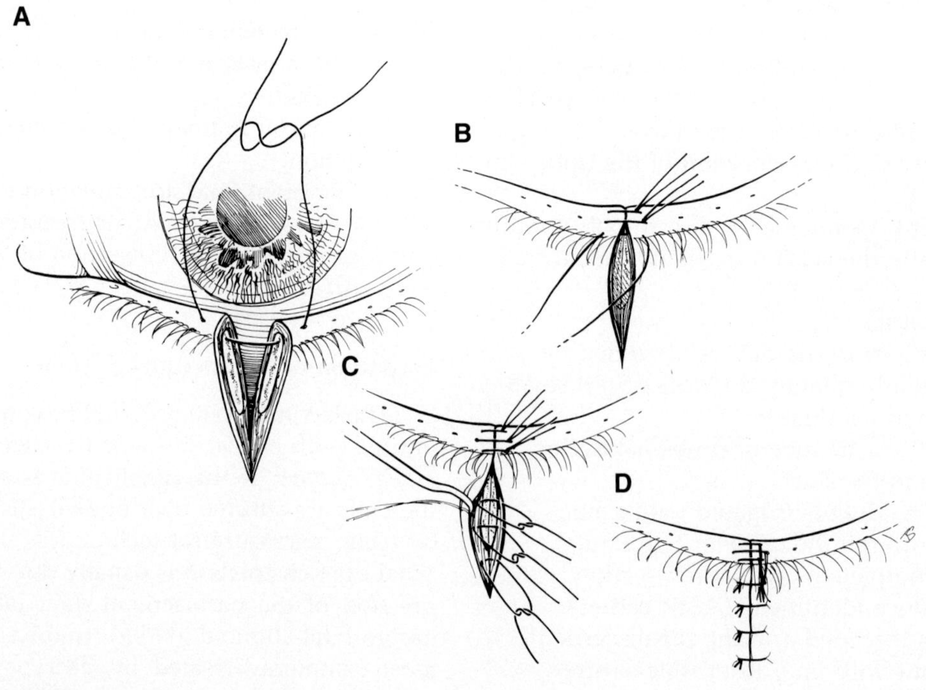

FIG 17–3.
Suture technique for primary eyelid closure.

Treatment

1. Cartilaginous and bony structures are reduced.
2. The intranasal lacerations are sutured or packed into position.
3. Avulsions near the tip and ala, if they involve cartilage and lining, are repaired by using the *avulsed segment as a composite graft* if available.
4. Full-thickness loss is treated by immediate, definitive vs. delayed soft-tissue reconstruction.

Laceration of the Lips

With full-thickness injuries to the lower lip that involve the underlying muscles, irregularity and puckering of the soft tissue, especially in the pogonial region, may persist. Each component of the lip should be repaired anatomically. Generally chromic suture is used for the vermilion and the mucosa. The muscle is repaired with polyglactin 910 (Vicryl). The first suture should be placed at the vermilion-cutaneous border. In addition, the wet-dry margin should also be realigned as a second reference point.

Injuries of the Ear

When simple lacerations occur, skin closure alone brings the cartilage into good position. Occasionally, the cartilage should be reapproximated first. A contoured dressing using Xeroform packing will prevent postoperative hematomas. Avulsion of small and moderate-sized segments of ear can be reconstructed with composite grafts or local flaps. With more complex injuries, consideration should be given to secondary reconstruction. Microsurgical reimplantation should be considered as the first option for total ear avulsion.

Extensive Soft-Tissue Loss

Rarely, high-velocity injuries require immediate restoration of adequate soft-tissue coverage following fixation of the underlying craniofacial skeleton. Whether the loss is small or large, one should always think ahead toward future reconstructions.

FACIAL FRACTURES

Nasal Fractures

It is important to differentiate subtle unilateral or bilateral NOE fractures from isolated nasal fractures since closed reduction alone will probably not prevent late telecanthus. Preinjury photographs should be checked to exclude pre-existing nasal deformity.

Diagnosis is usually made on physical examination. Mobility and crepitus on palpation with tenderness over the area of the fracture are present. Periorbital and nasal edema and ecchymosis may mark displacement. Roentgenograms are occasionally helpful in the diagnosis and treatment of nasal fractures and provide a legal record of injury. Manson recommends lateral low-density, soft-tissue roentgenograms as the best way to demonstrate fractures of the nasal dorsum.

The presence of a septal hematoma must be determined and drainage instituted to prevent septal necrosis and perforation. Most simple fractures can be managed on an outpatient basis. If edema does not prevent accurate palpation and visual inspection, closed reduction is carried out in the emergency department. The nose is packed with 4% cocaine, and an external nasal field block using lidocaine (Xylocaine) with epinephrine is performed. Nasal fractures in young children are best managed under general anesthesia. In situations where it is impossible to determine the extent of deformity, treatment should be deferred until the edema has subsided. Closed reduction should be accomplished within the first 2 weeks after injury.

Instrumentation for Reduction of Simple Nasal Fractures

1. Fiber-optic headlight
2. Intranasal specula of various sizes and lengths
3. Scalpel handle
4. Asch forceps
5. Walsham forceps
6. Plastic bandages and adhesive tape
7. Nasal splint
8. Tape

When nasal fractures are severely comminuted and the injury is more extensive with flattening of the nasal dorsum and saddle nose deformity, early bone grafting may be necessary. Open nasal fractures should be explored directly and fragments repositioned and wired into place or plated with microplates and screws to obtain accurate reduction.

Complications of Nasal Fractures

1. Subperichondral fibrosis with partial obstruction
2. Synechiae
3. Obstruction of the nasal vestibule from malunited fractures or scar contracture from loss of vestibular lining
4. Osteitis
5. Malunion of nasal fractures with residual deviation

Most commonly, closed nasal reduction leads to improvement but not total correction of lateral nasal deviation. In such cases, most surgeons wait 6 months prior to secondary closed or open rhinoplasty. This, however, depends on the severity of the deformity.

Zygomatic Fractures

Zygomatic fractures are one of the most common injuries of the facial skeleton. Failure to appreciate the complexity of these fractures has led to a relatively high incidence of posttraumatic deformity. It is critical to have an understanding of the three-dimensional anatomy of the zygoma and its intimate association with adjacent facial structures.

Surgical Anatomy

The zygoma articulates with the frontal, sphenoid, and temporal bones and the maxilla (Fig 17–4, A and B). The bone furnishes attachments for the masseter, temporalis, zygomaticus, and zygomatic head of the quadratus labii superioris muscles. The zygoma is the principal buttressing bone between the maxilla and cranium. The broad attachment of the masseter produces the major deforming force on the zygomatic body and arch when fractured.

Phillips and Gruss Classification of Zygomatic Fractures

1. Zygomatic body
   a. Intact
   b. Undisplaced
   c. Segmental
   d. Displaced
   e. Comminuted
2. Zygomatic arch
   a. Intact
   b. Undisplaced
   c. Segmental
   d. Displaced
      (I) Inferiorly with depression and/or telescoping
      (II) Laterally with outward bowing and/or telescoping
   e. Comminuted

Clinical Examination

Diagnosis of fractures of the zygoma may be suspected from a constellation of signs and symptoms (Fig 17–5):

1. Periorbital ecchymosis, edema, and hematoma
2. Subconjunctival and scleral ecchymosis
3. Lateral canthal ligament displacement with an anti-Mongoloid slant to the palpebral fissure
4. Retraction of the lower lid
5. Orbital dystopia secondary to fragmentation of the bony orbital floor with disruption of the continuity of suspensory ligaments of the globe and orbit
6. Unilateral epistaxis from fracture of the maxillary sinus
7. Pain on movement of the mouth and/or limitation of incisal opening because of direct mechanical interference with coronoid excursion
8. Sensation of malocclusion secondary to hypoesthesia or anesthesia of the maxillary teeth from injury to division II of the trigeminal nerve
9. Hypoesthesia or anesthesia of the ipsilateral upper lip, eyelid, medial portion of the cheek, and lateral aspect of the nose from injury to division II of the trigeminal nerve
10. Palpable step deformity of the inferior orbital rim and zygomatic frontal region
11. Posterior displacement of the malar eminence
12. Intraoral hematoma in the upper buccal sulcus

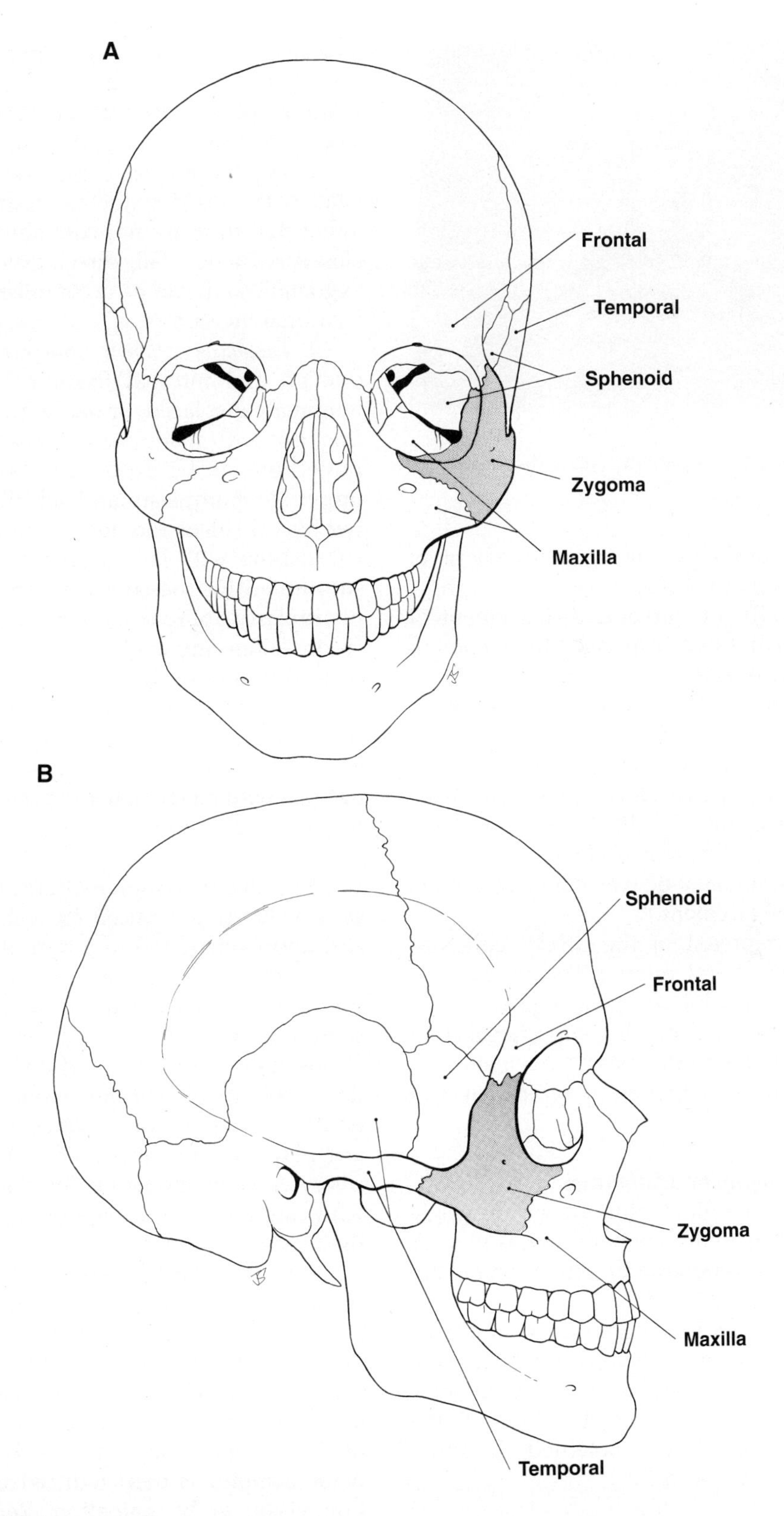

FIG 17–4.
A, frontal view showing the zygoma and its articulations. **B,** lateral view of the zygoma.

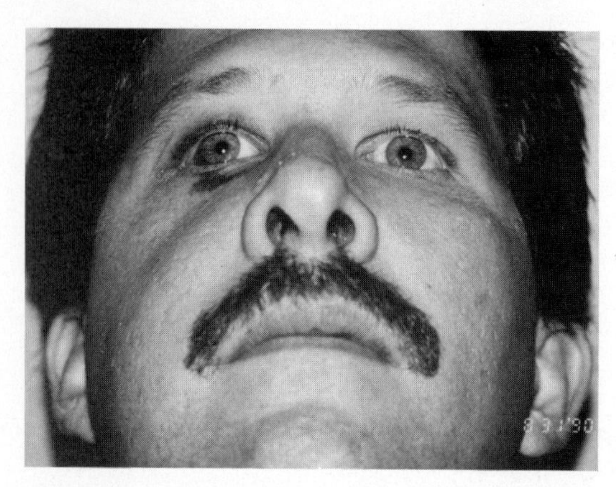

FIG 17–5.
Submental view of a patient with a displaced zygomatic fracture.

13. Enophthalmos from enlargement of the bony orbital volume
14. Inward or outward displacement of the zygomatic arch, especially if a comminuted fracture exists
15. Diplopia (extraocular muscle imbalance and diplopia are the result of muscle contusion or incarceration of soft tissues adjacent to the muscles. Deviation of the visual axis can account for diplopia. Downward displacement of the ocular globe must exceed 5 mm for diplopia to be reasonably attributed to globe displacement.)
16. Entrapment of the orbital contents, inferior rectus, and inferior oblique muscles producing limitation of upward gaze
17. Deepening of the supratarsal fold secondary to enophthalmos
18. Pain on palpation at typical sites of fracture

Roentgenographic Evaluation

1. The plain-film Waters view is the single best plain film; in the submentovertex view or Titterington position the zygomatic arches are well demonstrated.
2. A CT scan is required to demonstrate the intraorbital component accurately. Axial and coronal cuts should be included. Depression of the orbital floor may be observed. If a single radiologic study is obtained, the study of choice is a CT scan.

Surgical Treatment

1. *Nondisplaced zygomatic fractures without functional compromise*—no operation necessary. Patients should be followed for 3 to 6 months to ensure that late complications such as enophthalmos do not develop.
2. *Isolated zygomatic arch fractures*—managed with closed reduction techniques provided that they are not comminuted. Should closed reduction fail, direct exposure of the zygomatic arch can be accomplished through a coronal incision.
3. *Displaced zygomatic fractures*—open reduction and internal fixation. Undisplaced, minimally displaced, or moderately displaced fractures with maintenance of adequate arch projection can be exposed through a lateral upper blepharoplasty and subciliary and upper buccal sulcus incisions. A transconjunctival incision with lateral canthotomy may be substituted for the subciliary and upper blepharoplasty approach. (Transconjunctival incisions alone are seldom adequate for complete exposure of the inferior orbital rim and make exposure unnecessarily difficult.) Three-point fixation at the frontozygomatic suture, inferior orbital rim, and zygomatic maxillary buttress with metal plates and screws achieves the most stable result.

To prevent ectropion after subciliary incision, a skin flap is raised for a short distance and approximately 3 to 5 mm of muscle left superiorly. The incision is then carried through the muscle superficial to the orbital septum down to the inferior orbital rim. The periosteum is incised, and the rim, orbital floor, and orbital walls are exposed. Preservation of muscle provides better eyelid closure and may prevent subsequent ectropion. Subciliary incisions should be closed in two layers, with care taken to not inadvertently shorten the orbital septum.

It is important to expose the zygomaticosphenoid junction through the lateral upper blepharoplasty incision. With a small incision in the temporal hairline, an elevator can be passed below the superficial layer of the deep temporal fascia underneath the junction of the zygomatic arch and body. The zygomatic complex is then reduced under direction vision or by palpation. Reduction can then be confirmed by inspection of the inferior orbital rim, the zygomatic maxillary buttress, the fronto-zygomatic region, and most importantly the zygomaticosphenoid junction. Miniplates or microplates can be placed at the inferior orbital rim and at the frontozygomatic suture. A miniplate is then properly contoured and placed at the zygomaticomaxillary buttress. When comminution exists, fixation may be more of a problem but can usually be accomplished with a combination of microplates and miniplates.

Any defect of the anterior maxillary wall greater than 0.5 mm should be bone-grafted. The Tessier-Kawamoto technique takes, with an osteotome, a split-thickness cranial bone graft with the periosteum left intact. The periosteum allows the bone to curl up and controls the microfractures as the bone is elevated. This results in a smooth, slightly curved bone graft that is ideal for the orbital floor. Others prefer to take split-thickness cranial bone in the standard fashion and contour it by using bone benders. Autogenous rib or ilium can also be used. When extensive loss of the orbital floor is found, vitallium or titanium mesh can be inserted. Whether bone-grafting or placing a prosthetic material, it is necessary to identify the intact orbital floor posteriorly, which is usually located 35 to 38 mm behind the orbital rim.

Inorganic implants may also be used to restore the continuity of the orbital floor. The advantage of using an inorganic implant is that it is not necessary to retrieve autogenous material from a second site. Many materials have been employed, including Silastic, tantalum, stainless steel, Vitallium, methyl methacrylate, Teflon, and others. In long-term follow-up, patients with implants generally do well, with an incidence of late infection reported to be 1% to 2%. Currently, most craniofacial surgeons prefer autogenous material.

Complications of Zygomatic Fractures

The following complications of zygomatic fractures have been reported (Fig 17–6):

1. Nonunion
2. Malunion
3. Diplopia
4. Persistent infraorbital nerve anesthesia/hypoesthesia
5. Chronic maxillary sinusitis
6. Ectropion
7. Orbital dystopia
8. Fibrous ankylosis of the TMJ
9. Endopthalmos

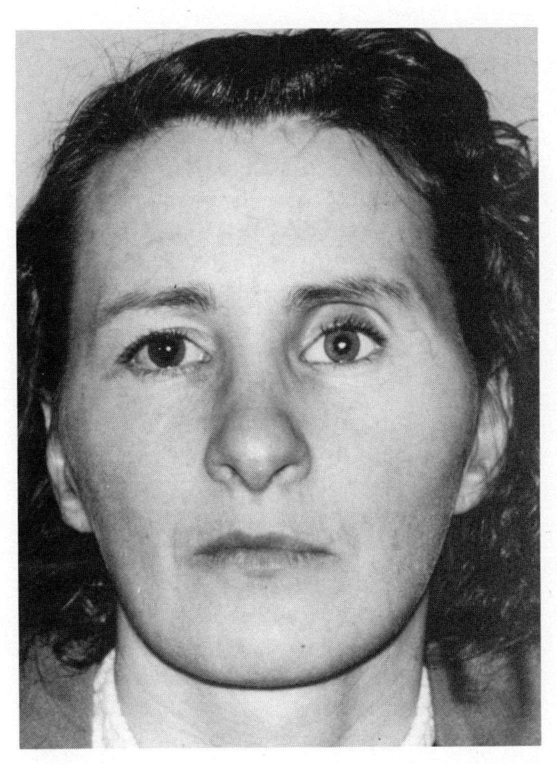

FIG 17–6.
Posttraumatic enophthalmos and malar displacement following repair of zygomatic fracture.

MAXILLARY FRACTURES

The classic patterns of midfacial-maxillary fractures occurring exactly in the lines of weaknesses of the face as originally described by Le Fort are rarely encountered in clinical practice. The great majority of maxillary fractures instead consist of combinations and permutations of Le Fort–type fractures. Injury patterns following high-speed motor vehicle accidents are often associated with comminution of the maxilla. The aim of treatment of maxillary fractures is to reestablish the normal anatomic position of the maxilla in relation to the cranial base above and the mandible below. Normal transverse, sagittal, and vertical dimensions must all be restored.

Anatomic Considerations

The midface consists of pneumatic cavities, or sinuses, that are reinforced by vertical and horizontal buttresses of bone. The importance of these structural pillars is to maintain the position of the maxilla in relation to the cranial base above and the mandible below. There are three principal maxillary buttresses (Fig 17–7):

1. The medial or *nasomaxillary buttress,* which extends from the anterior alveolus along the piriform aperture, the nasal process, and the maxilla to the frontocranial attachment
2. The lateral or *zygomaticomaxillary buttress,* which extends from the lateral maxillary alveolus to the zygomatic process of the frontal bone and laterally to the zygomatic arch
3. The posterior or *pterygomaxillary buttress,* which attaches to the maxilla posterior to the pterygoid plate of the sphenoid bone.

Manson Classification of Le Fort Fractures

The highest level in components of the fracture on each side
- Le Fort I:
  - Maxillary alveolus
  - Split palate
  - Alveolar tuberosity fracture
- Le Fort II:
  - Pyramidal fracture
- Le Fort III:
  - Craniofacial dysjunction
- Le Fort IV:
  - Frontobasilar fracture

Patterns of fragment, including the maxillary dentition "occlusal fragment"

Associated fractures:
- Mandible
- Naso-orbital-ethmoid
- Frontal sinus

Le Fort Classification of Facial Fractures

1. *Le Fort I fractures or transverse (Guerin) fractures* (Fig 17–8).—Fractures occur above the level of the apices of the teeth and include the entire alveolar process of the maxilla, the vault of the palate, and the pterygoid processes in a single block.

2. *Le Fort II (pyramidal) fractures.*—The fracture begins above the level of the apices of the teeth laterally and extends through the pterygoid plates in the same fashion as a Le Fort I fracture. Medially, it extends to involve a portion of the medial orbit extending across the nose to separate a pyramidally shaped

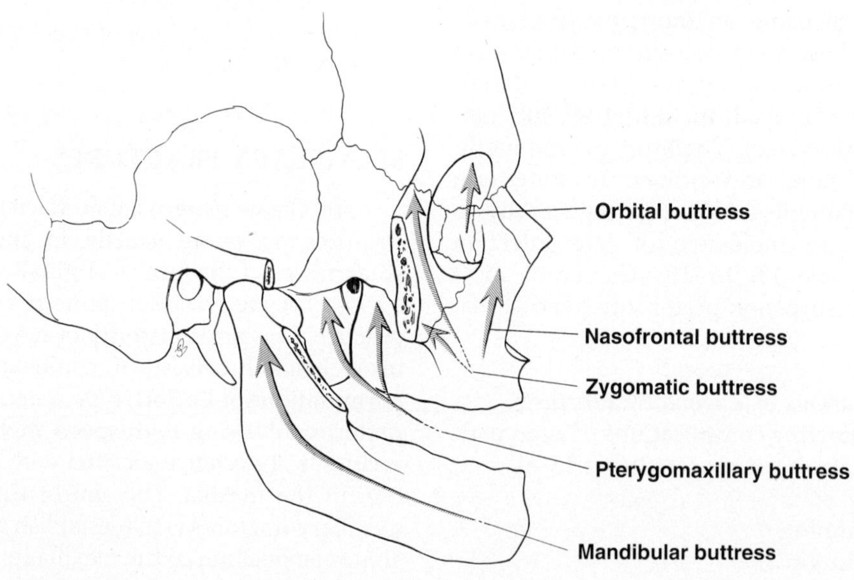

FIG 17–7.
The vertical buttresses of midfacial displacement.

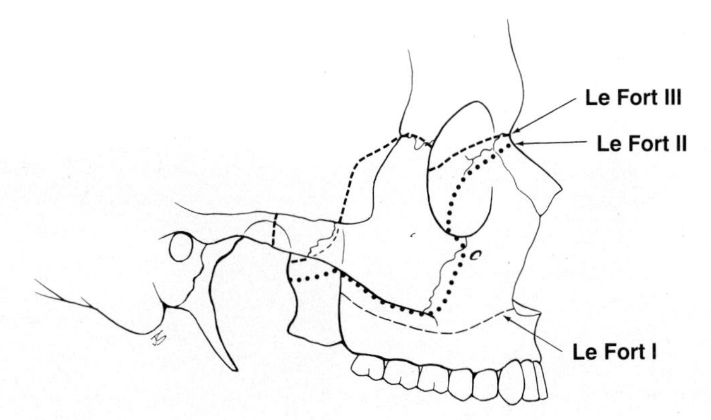

FIG 17–8.
Le Fort fractures.

maxillary segment from the superior cranial and midfacial structures. Damage to the ethmoidal area is routine in pyramidal fractures. Associated NOE fractures will frequently be present.

3. *Le Fort III fractures (craniofacial dysjunction).*—The fracture extends through the zygomaticofrontal sutures and the nasofrontal suture and across the floor of the orbits to effect a complete separation of the midface from the cranium.

Displacement after maxillary fractures is generally directed posteriorly and downward. The patient has an elongated, retruded appearance in the middle third of the facial skeleton with an anterior open bite. The pterygoid musculature aids the posterior and downward forces of maxillary displacement.

Clinical Evaluation

Although orbital signs will frequently be present in Le Fort II and III fractures, malocclusion with an anterior open bite is the hallmark of a fractured maxilla.

On palpation, step deformities may be present at the zygomaticofrontal regions bilaterally and at the nasofrontal junction if a Le Fort III fracture exists. Evidence of NOE trauma with telecanthus and loss of nasal projection will usually be present. An anterior open bite may be evident, and upon digital manipulation of the maxilla between the thumb and index finger, mobility of the maxilla will be found. By simultaneously manipulating the maxilla and palpating the nasofrontal region and zygomaticofrontal sutures the diagnosis of Le Fort II vs. III fractures can usually be distinguished.

Cerebrospinal rhinorrhea or otorrhea should be inspected for, especially in the presence of Le Fort II and III fractures where injuries to the anterior middle cranial fossa may be present. The palate should be inspected. Palatal mucosal lacerations may indicate that a sagittal fracture is present. Transverse relationships of the maxillary to the mandibular teeth may reveal collapse of the maxilla (Fig 17–9).

Roentgenographic Examination

Although plain films may be helpful in confirming facial fractures, in general carefully performed axial CT scans taken from the palate through the anterior cranial fossa will be diagnostic of the majority of Le Fort fractures. In concert with coronal views, virtually all Le Fort fractures should be detectable. In the presence of major midfacial trauma, mandibular fractures should be excluded. This can be accomplished by carrying the CT scan both axially and coronally through the mandible and/or ordering a Panorex. Any suspicious areas should be followed with more specific mandibular films or CT.

Surgical Treatment of Maxillary Fractures

The goal of Le Fort fracture treatment is reestablishment of midfacial height and projection.

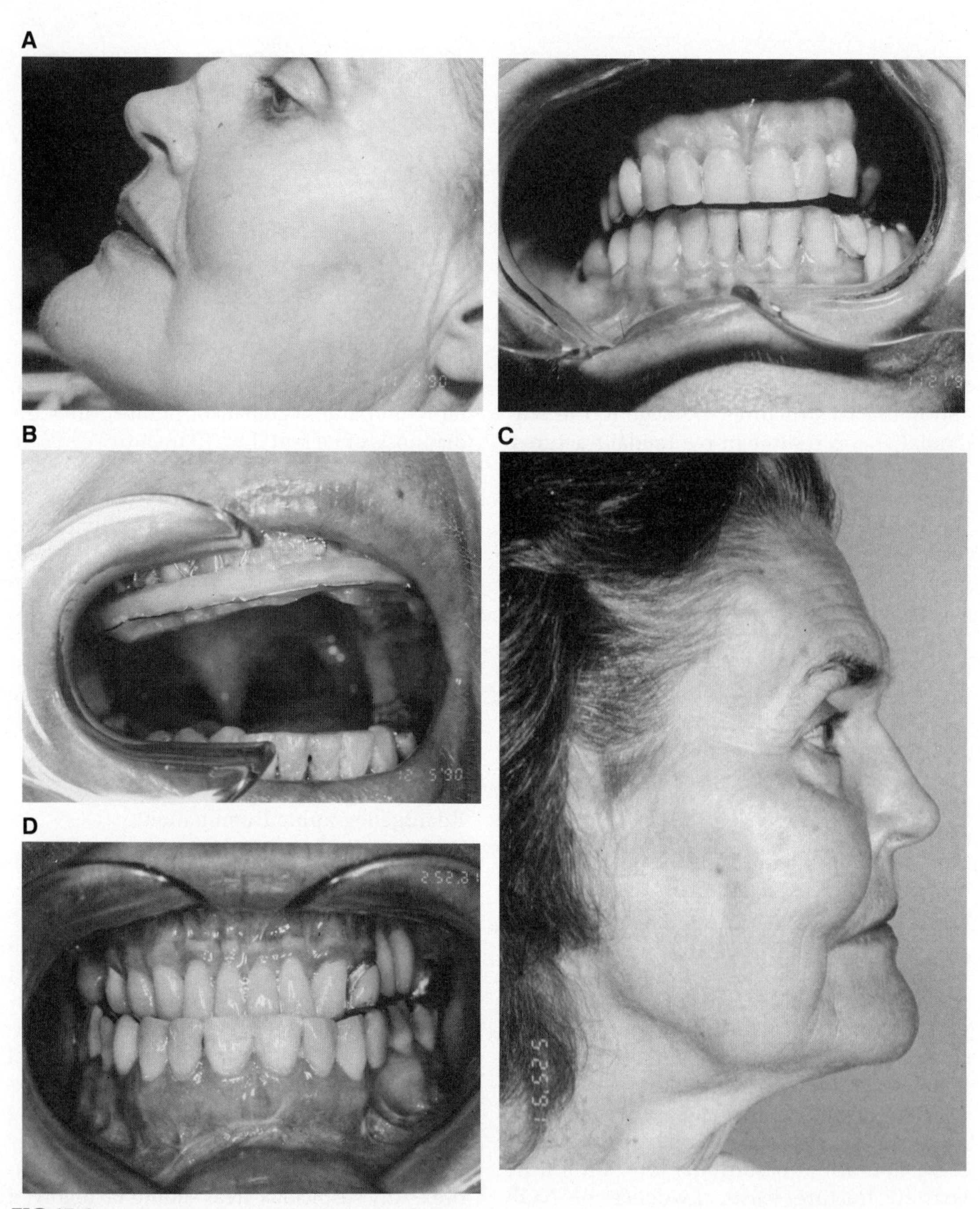

FIG 17–9.
A, patient with segmental Le Fort I and nasal fractures. **B,** treatment consisted of model surgery, fabrication of an occlusal dental splint, and open reduction/internal fixation of the maxilla and sagittal palatal fractures with plates and screws. **C,** postoperative appearance. **D,** postoperative occlusion.

Le Fort I

In a noncomminuted fracture, Erich arch bars are applied with 25-gauge wires to ligate them to the teeth. MMF is then accomplished by using either dental elastics or heavy-gauge wire. Following establishment of MMF, an upper buccal sulcus incision is made, and the maxilla is degloved. Each of the zygomatic and nasal maxillary buttresses are exposed. Comminuted fragments of the anterior wall and of the maxilla are left in place rather than removed. In an isolated Le Fort I fracture without an associated sagittal split of the palate, the inferior maxillary segment, coapted by MMF to the mandible, can be moved upward as a single unit and the condyles carefully seated in a posterosuperior position. The fracture segments are visualized, and with gentle vertical impaction, reduction is obtained. The least comminuted buttress is plated first, and then the assistant can release the chin while the remaining buttresses are rigidly stabilized. In general, four plates with two screws on either side of the fracture are utilized. Any osteotomy gaps larger than 0.5 mm are bone-grafted. The anterior maxillary wall is reduced and plated into position or, if missing, bone-grafted. It is essential to check occlusion after rigid fixation to ensure that the condyles are seated. Any occlusal discrepancies are corrected by removing and readapting the plates. MMF can be reestablished or discontinued depending on how comfortable the surgeon is with the rigidity of the bony fixation.

Fractures of the Palate

If palatal or alveolar fractures coexist with Le Fort I, II, or III fractures, a palatal-occlusal splint can be employed to position the tooth-bearing fragment accurately in apposition with the mandibular teeth. This prevents palatal rotation of the fractured maxillary segments, which is aggravated by the force of intermaxillary fixation. *If accurate reduction of a palatal fracture can be obtained manually, it is preferable to plate the palatal fracture through the mucosal laceration.* This improves stability but does not always obviate the need for a palatal-occlusal splint. It also ensures that the transverse facial dimensions are accurately set prior to reduction and fixation of mandibular fractures.

Le Fort II and III Fractures

Exposure for open reduction and internal fixation of Le Fort II and III fractures is similar. Coronal, upper buccal sulcus, and subciliary (or transconjunctival with lateral canthotomy) incisions are used for exposure. Occlusion is established by MMF. The order of treatment for Le Fort III fractures is to begin at the zygomatic arch. The arch is reduced bilaterally, and a fragmentation plate is secured on the posterior stable segments. Then, with a finger inside the lateral orbit, the body of the zygoma is grasped with a clamp and reduced so that there is no longer a stepoff at the zygomaticosphenoid fracture line. This area is palpated as well as visually inspected to ensure perfect reduction. Accurate reduction at the frontozygomatic fracture is also necessary. To establish the frontozygomatic region, 1.5- and 2.0-mm miniplates or newly available panfacial or microplus plates are used. Then, screws are placed in the zygomatic body into the previously placed fragmentation plate. Any comminuted segments of the zygomatic arch can be simply reduced and fixed with screws into the fragmentation plate. It is important to remember that the arch is straight and not "arched" throughout most of its length.

Next, through the upper buccal sulcus incision, the two jaws are moved as a single unit to reduce and plate the zygomaticomaxillary buttress if fractures at the Le Fort I level are present. Once facial height and width have been reestablished, attention can be turned to the more delicate NOE relations. The nasofrontal junction is reduced. Generally, a combination of microplates, panfacial or microplus and miniplates are used for stabilization. NOE fractures will be discussed in more detail later in this chapter. The medial canthi should not be stripped from the major fracture fragments if possible. The inferior orbital rim is then reduced and stabilized with a microplate, microplus, or panfacial plate.

For Le Fort II fractures, preinjury occlusion is again obtained first by MMF. Then, the nasofrontal area is inspected. Reduction can usually be accomplished and the first fixation plates fixed to the zygomaticomaxillary buttresses. Following this, the NOE complex can then be addressed.

When reduction of the midfacial segment is difficult, Row-Killey disimpaction forceps can be employed.

ORBITAL AND NASO-ORBITAL-ETHMOID FRACTURES

Anatomic Considerations

The bony orbit is described as a conical or pyramidally shaped structure. The widest diameter of the orbit is located just behind the orbital rim, approximately 1.5 cm within the orbital cavity. The orbital rim is an elliptically shaped structure, whereas the orbit immediately behind the rim is more circular. The medial wall has a quadrangular rather than a triangular configuration. The optic foramen lies on a medial and slightly superior plane in the apex of the orbit.

The orbits can be conceptualized in thirds from anterior to posterior. Anteriorly, the orbital rim consists of thick bone. The middle third is relatively thin, whereas again in the posterior third the bone thickens.

Fractures first occur at the weakest points in the floor and naso-orbital wall, i.e., in the convex portion of the orbital floor adjacent to the infraorbital nerve and in the medial (ethmoid) orbit. The optic foramen lies approximately 45 mm from the inferior orbital rim (Fig 17–10).

The globe is surrounded by orbital fat within the orbital cavity and occupies only the anterior half of the orbital cavity. The orbital cavity is separated by Tenon's capsule, a fascial structure subdividing the cavity into an anterior, or precapsular, segment, and a posterior, or retrocapsular, segment. Fine septal communications diffusely divide the extraocular fat into small compartments and provide ligamentous structures that attach to the bony orbital walls, to the extraocular muscles, and to Tenon's capsule. The orbital contents are maintained in position by the septum orbitale (orbital septum), a fascial structure inserting on the inner aspect of the orbital rim. The septum orbitale attaches to and blends with

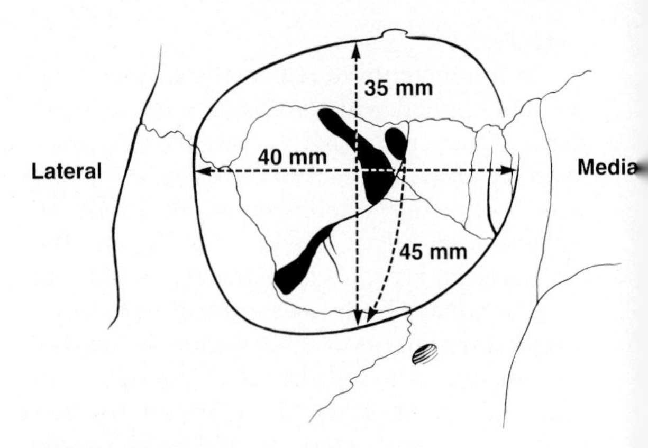

FIG 17–10.
Key measurements of orbital anatomy. Note that the optic foramen is 45 mm posterior and lateral to the inferior orbital rim.

the levator aponeurosis in the upper eyelid and is attached to the lower border of the tarsus in the lower eyelid.

The lamina papyracea is the largest component of the medial orbital wall and accounts for the structural weakness of this area. The lesser wing of the sphenoid and the optic foramen are posterior to the lamina papyracea. The optic foramen is located close to the posterior portion of the ethmoid sinus, not at the true apex of the orbit. In severe fractures involving the medial wall and its posterior portion, fractures may extend through the optic canal and produce blindness.

The anterior and posterior margins in the lacrimal groove form the respective lacrimal crests. The groove is continuous with the nasolacrimal duct at the junction of the floor and medial wall of the orbit. The lateral wall of the orbit is relatively stout in its anterior portion. It is formed by the greater wing of the sphenoid, the frontal process of the zygomatic bone, and the lesser wing of the sphenoid, lateral to the optic foramen. The superior orbital fissure is a cleft that runs outward, forward, and upward from the apex of the orbit between the roof and lateral wall. The fissure, which separates the greater and lesser wings of the sphenoid, allows passage of the three motor nerves to the extraocular muscles of the orbit: cranial nerves III, IV, and VI. The ophthalmic division of the trigeminal nerve also enters the orbit through this fissure.

Blowout Fractures of the Floor of the Orbit

A blowout fracture is caused by the application of traumatic force to the inferior orbital rim or the soft tissues of the orbit. It is usually accompanied by a sudden increase in intraorbital pressure. There are numerous controversies surrounding the exact mechanism of orbital blowout fractures.

Surgical Pathology and Enophthalmos

Diplopia. Extraocular muscle imbalance and subjective diplopia are the results of muscle contusion and/or incarceration of the soft tissue adjacent to the muscles. Deviation in the visual axes can account for diplopia. Contusion, which is the major cause, must be differentiated from entrapment of the soft-tissue structures in the area of the blowout fracture. Downward displacement of an ocular globe alone does not always result in double vision. It is thought that downward displacement must exceed 5 mm for diplopia to occur.

Enophthalmos. Enophthalmos is a major complication of orbital fractures (see Fig 17–6). The major cause is bony orbital enlargement with escape of orbital soft tissue into the enlarged cavity. The mechanism involves rupture of the periorbita and the fine ligaments connecting the orbital soft-tissue structures, thereby allowing soft-tissue displacement. This allows their displacement with remodeling of the shape of the soft-tissue contents into a spherical configuration.

Clinical Evaluation

In a typical blowout fracture, the patient is aware of double vision. This is usually present in the primary position and increases with upward gaze. *Ophthalmologic consultation is mandatory.* Once swelling and hemorrhage in the periorbital tissue subside, findings of enophthalmos with backward and downward displacement of the globe and deepening of the supratarsal sulcus may begin to appear. Globe injury or retinal detachment can accompany severe blunt trauma. Clinical evaluation of orbital injury should include a forced duction test or eyeball traction test, which provides a means of differentiating entrapment from contusion with a lack of muscle function.

Forced Duction Test

1. Local anesthetic is instilled into the conjunctival sac.
2. A forceps grasps the insertion of the inferior rectus at a point 7 mm inferior to the limbus.
3. The globe is then gently rotated upward and downward, medially and laterally, to confirm any resistance to motion.
4. Motion should be free and unencumbered unless entrapment has occurred.

Radiographic Evaluation of Orbital Fractures

Plain x-ray studies may suggest the presence of a fracture in the internal portion of the orbit, especially in the presence of blood in the maxillary sinus. However, CT scans are more reliable and are indicated for all cases. Axial and coronal CT scans are quite useful. Coronal CT may show extrusion of orbital contents into the maxillary sinus.

Surgical Treatment

Operative treatment of an orbital floor fracture is indicated for persistent entrapment or significant enophthalmos. Exploration of the orbital floor is performed through a subciliary or transconjunctival approach with lateral canthotomy. The objectives of treatment are to release the soft-tissue contents, accurately define the extent of the bony fracture, and reconstruct the floor and walls of the orbit in an anatomic position. In cases where entrapment has not occurred, if swelling limits the utility of clinical examination and CT does not indicate substantial extrusion of orbital contents, a "wait-and-see" attitude can be applied. If signs of enophthalmos then develop, surgery is indicated. This should usually be carried out within the first 2 weeks after injury.

It is important to have adequate lighting to dissect the orbital floor. Some authors also recommend loupe magnification. The intact floor should be located and traced around the edges of the blowout. In major blowout fractures, it is often only the palatine bone that remains as an intact ledge posteriorly. It is important to find the intact posterior ledge because bone grafts will need to be secured to prevent them from falling into the maxillary sinus. When linear fractures are present, the floor can often be reduced with a single wire or small microplate. With extensive comminuted fractures of the orbital floor, a custom implant of titanium or Vitallium can be used. Once anatomic reconstruction of the floor is accomplished, the cornea is examined to determine whether its anterior project is sufficient and symmetrical with the opposite side.

Fractures of the Orbital Roof

Fractures of the orbital roof generally occur in conjunction with fractures of the frontal bone, NOE complex, or zygoma. A combined craniofacial approach is required for proper neurosurgical exposure, repair of dural tears, and debridement of any damaged frontal lobe. Displacement of the orbital roof is generally downward and inward and produces a downward and forward displacement of the globe and orbital soft tissue. Proptosis is therefore often present. The superior orbital fissure syndrome (paralysis of cranial nerves III, IV, and VI) and the orbital apex syndrome (optic nerve involvement) may be present.

Naso-orbital-ethmoid Fractures

Fractures of the midface are frequently accompanied by fractures of the fronto-naso-ethmoid area and central midfacial skeleton. The bones of the middle third of the face are also in close anatomic proximity to the anterior cranial fossa and frontal lobes of the brain. Concomitant orbital floor and medial orbital wall blowout fractures are present, as are comminuted medial orbital roof fractures. Neurosurgical consultation is usually necessary.

Surgical Anatomy

The anterior and posterior ethmoidal foramina are situated along the upper border of the lamina papyracea and the frontal ethmoidal suture, where the orbital plate of the frontal bone and the lamina papyracea of the ethmoid are joined. The anterior ethmoidal foramen transmits the nasociliary nerve and the anterior ethmoidal vessel; the posterior ethmoidal foramen gives passage to the posterior ethmoidal vessels and nerves. The most medial posterior portion of the medial orbital wall is formed by the body of the sphenoid immediately in front of the optic foramen. In severe skeletal disruption of this area, the fracture line extends into the optic foramen and superior orbital fissure. This may result in blindness.

Intraorbital space designates the area between the orbits and the floor of the anterior cranial fossa. The intraorbital space is roughly pear shaped in transverse section, wider in the middle than in the posterior aspect.

The size of the frontal sinus varies greatly; it occupies most of the frontal bone or only a small portion of the lower central part.

The level of the cribriform plate is variable and should be individually identified on radiographic examination. The frontal sinus drains through the ethmoid, either as a distinct nasofrontal duct or by emptying into an anterior ethmoidal cell and then into the meatus.

Traumatic telecanthus is often present in patients with NOE fractures. The bony bridge of the nose is depressed and widened, and the eyes appear far apart as in hypertelorism. Traumatic telecanthus implies an increase in the distance between the medial canthi. In mild cases, unilateral or bilateral telecanthus may be the only sign distinguishing an NOE fracture from a nasal fracture.

Clinical Evaluation

The appearance of a patient who has suffered an NOE fracture is typical (Fig 17–11):

1. Flattened nose, loss of dorsal nasal projection
2. Telecanthus
3. Subconjunctival hemorrhage
4. History of or loss of consciousness
5. Cerebrospinal fluid (CSF) leak (CSF distinguished from blood by the "double-ring sign")

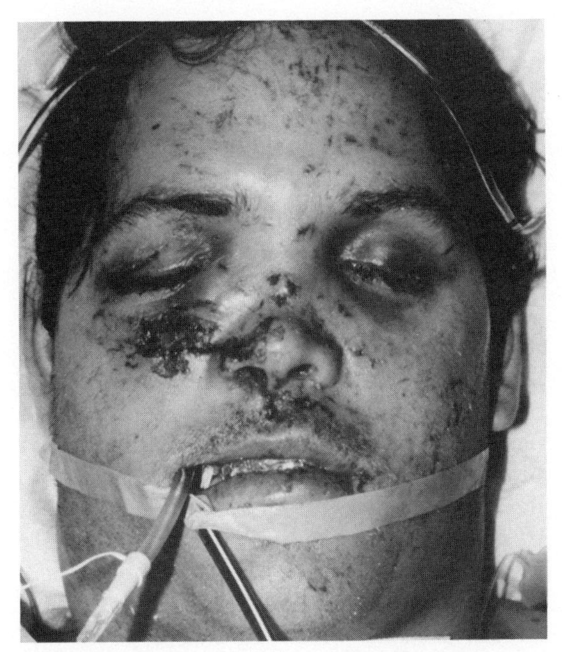

FIG 17–11.
Patient with naso-orbital-ethmoid fractures. Note the nasal collapse and traumatic telecanthus.

6. Mobile medial canthus on physical examination

Roentgenographic Examination
CT is essential and may reveal the following:

1. Air in the subdural or subarachnoid space or in the ventricle (may be an indication for neurosurgical intervention)
2. Air fluid level in the frontal sinus
3. Anterior and posterior wall of the frontal sinus evaluated
4. Fragmentation and/or buckled appearance of the cribriform plate (may be an indication for neurosurgical exploration)

The diagnosis of an NOE fracture on radiographs requires a minimum of four fractures that isolate the frontal process of the maxilla from adjacent bones:

1. Fracture of the nose
2. Fractures of the frontal process of the maxilla
3. Fractures of the medial orbital walls
4. Fractures of the nasofrontal region.

Surgical Treatment
Neurosurgical intervention may also be indicated in the presence of the following:

1. Coexistent depressed or open skull fracture
2. Brain injury (may require monitoring of ICP)

The surgical approach to NOE fractures is usually by a coronal incision. Occasionally an existing laceration may be utilized to provide direct exposure for reduction. However, these should not usually be extended, especially into the canthal area, because contractures of the scars will lead to a disappointing postoperative result. The medial canthal tendons bilaterally should be identified and their attachments preserved. Subperiosteal exposure includes the inferior rim of the orbit, the orbital floor, the medial orbit by dissecting behind the bone fragments, the orbital floor, and the nasofrontal region. An instrument placed intranasally may be helpful in elevating the fracture fragments and reducing them into position. Rarely, the canthi may be detached from the bone. More often, detachment of the canthi results from operative dissection. Should this occur, a separate incision may be needed over the canthal region and the canthus sutured with wire in preparation for transnasal canthopexy. The fragments bearing the medial canthi can usually be plated or wired to the frontal bone by using microplates or 1.5- or 2-mm miniplates. It is virtually impossible to achieve overreduction of an NOE fracture, especially at the level of the canthi. Indeed, overreduction may be preferred because it is impossible to stabilize the fractures posteriorly. In almost all circumstances, bone grafting is essential to restore nasal contour.

Complications
Complications of NOE fractures include the following:

1. Posttraumatic telecanthus
2. Nasal deformity

3. Enophthalmos (rarely)
4. Ocular globe injury
5. Blindness or loss of an eye (infrequently)
6. Lacrimal injuries (if transection of the canalicular system has occurred, it should be repaired over fine Silastic tubing)
7. True ptosis of the upper lid
8. Pseudoptosis resulting from enophthalmos
9. Canthal dystopia.

FRONTOBASILAR FRACTURES

When a frontal skull fracture occurs in concert with Le Fort fractures, it has often been labeled Le Fort IV. The dense structure of the frontal bone makes it the strongest bone of the face. Consequently, fractures in this region are less common, but often severe. Neurologic injuries should be excluded.

Fracture Patterns

A concise preoperative fracture classification was developed by Stanley (Table 17–2). Type I fractures rarely involve the ostia or ducts, even when the anterior table is severely depressed and the underlying intersinus septum is crushed. Depressed fractures are treated with open reduction and internal fixation with 1.5- or 2.0-mm miniplates or microplates. The sinus is irrigated free of blood and fragments, and severely lacerated or necrotic mucosa distant to the drainage orifice is removed prior to repositioning the fragments. When comminution of the anterior table is severe enough to preclude repositioning of fracture fragments, autogenous bone grafts are procured and rigidly fixed into position.

TABLE 17–2.
Classification of Frontal Sinus Fractures*

TYPE I
Anterior table fracture
Isolated to anterior table
Accompanied by supraorbital rim fracture
Accompanied by nasoethmoidal complex fracture
TYPE II
Anterior and posterior table fractures
Linear fractures
Transverse
Vertical
Comminuted fractures
Isolated to both tables
Accompanied by nasoethmoidal complex fracture

* From Stanley RB Jr.: Clin Plast Surg 16:115, 1989. Used by permission.

When anterior table fractures are accompanied by unilateral supraorbital rim fractures, the damage will generally involve direct injury to the mucosa and bone of 25% to 50% of the circumference of the orifice of the nasofrontal duct. The sinus should be explored and the orifice inspected closely to document patency. If a large ostium is patent in spite of injury, the fracture fragments are repositioned and the orifice left undisturbed. Patients must be followed for symptoms of frontal sinusitis. If the orifice is small and obviously occluded by bony fragments, the mucosa is stripped and the duct obliterated with properly conformed bone grafts.

When anterior table fractures are associated with naso-ethmoidal complex fractures, damage to the orifices are generally more severe. Usually, both sides of the frontal sinus must be obliterated. The material of choice for obliteration of the frontal sinus is varied, but the author prefers cancellous iliac bone. When type II fractures involve comminution of the anterior and posterior tables, consideration is given to cranialization by removal of the posterior table and frontal sinus. The anterior table is then reconstructed and the nasofrontal ducts obliterated with contoured bone grafts. When severe comminution of the anterior wall of the frontal sinus coexists with NOE fractures, exenteration of the sinus mucosa, removal of the sinus septa, and complete obliteration of the sinus with cancellous bone grafts and/or other material is indicated. The ducts are plugged with contoured bone grafts, and the anterior table is replaced or reconstructed with cortical bone.

PANFACIAL FRACTURES

The successful treatment of panfacial fractures requires an understanding of the component fracture patterns and an ability to relate them anatomically to the remaining stable elements of the skeleton. For an injury to be classified as panfacial it must involve the upper, middle, and lower portions of the face. Fractures of the NOE region, the zygomatic complex, the Le Fort midfacial area, and the mandible area are respective components of this complex facial dysjunction.

The approach to panfacial fractures requires an organized treatment plan. As with all facial trauma, other injuries are excluded, and airway, breathing, and circulation are addressed. Neurosurgical, intrathoracic, and intra-abdominal pathology take precedence and must be appropriately managed. Surgical management is initiated following the history, physical examination, and complete radiologic evaluation. CT is a mandatory component of the workup. CT scans are obtained from the cranium to the menton with axial and if possible coronal cuts. Not infrequently, tracheostomy will be necessary. Dental impressions are taken and dental splints fabricated if indicated to restore preinjury occlusion. Single-unit Erich arch bars are ligated to the upper and lower dental arch. MMF can then be accomplished. When sagittal fractures of the palate exist, they are rigidly stabilized with plates and screws if possible.

Establishment of maxillary and mandibular occlusal relationships will set the stage for reestablishment of facial width, projection, and height. Mandibular fractures are addressed first. Rigid fixation is used in the majority of cases. Once occlusion is reestablished, a coronal incision is made, and the zygoma and arch are built outward as previously described for Le Fort III fractures. With the zygoma properly positioned in reference to the zygomaticosphenoid junction, one can gently bring the maxilla into position and obtain excellent reduction. Setting the zygoma at its proper position ultimately determines the vertical height of the midfacial unit as well as the midfacial width.

Following fixation of maxillary fractures attention is turned to the more delicate NOE region. Again, the larger fracture fragments are stabilized at the nasofrontal junction. When frontobasilar fractures coexist, the frontal sinus is treated as previously described. The canthal-bearing segments are brought into position. Canthal reduction and fixation are usually accomplished both superiorly at the nasofrontal region and inferiorly at the medial aspects of the inferior orbital rims. Transcutaneous, transnasal wires are then placed and external bolsters applied. These *do not* aid in reduction or fixation but assist in soft-tissue redraping and resolution of edema. The orbital floor and walls are inspected and bone-grafted as necessary.

PEDIATRIC FACIAL TRAUMA

Facial injuries in children pose special problems in treatment and management. The maxillofacial skeleton is small in comparison to the size of the calvarium in the younger age group. In addition, the bone is soft and resilient with thin cortical plates and a greater proportion of cancellous bone. This translates into a high degree of elasticity and resistance to injury in the maxillofacial skeleton in children before 5 years of age.

Aside from nasal fractures, the most common facial bone fractured in children is the mandible. By 10 years of age the midfacial skeleton has almost reached adult proportions. The maxillofacial skeleton in this age group is thus more susceptible to injury by trauma.

The greater osteogenic potential of the periosteum in children and the rich vascularity of facial bones account for more rapid healing of fractured bony segments.

In general, the principles of treatment of facial bone fractures involving the maxillofacial skeleton in the adult can be applied to children, but technical modifications must be made because of the child's mixed dentition stage between the ages of 6 and 15 years. Stable fixation is somewhat more difficult to achieve in this age group and requires some degree of ingenuity and familiarity with dental appliances.

During the stages of mixed dentition, the bony portions of the mandible and the alveolar bony portions of the maxilla are occupied by the developing permanent dental follicles

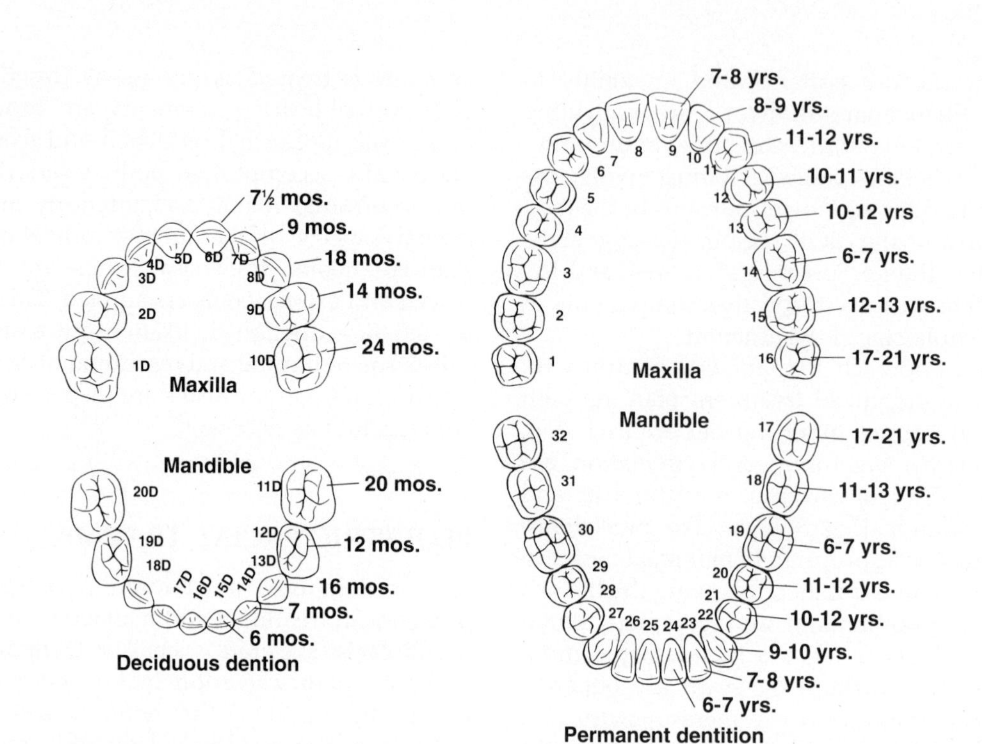

FIG 17–12.
Eruption schedules for deciduous dentition **(A)** and permanent dentition **(B)**.

in addition to the erupted deciduous teeth. The surgeon treating fractures in children must be familiar with the eruption schedules of both deciduous and permanent dentition (Fig 17–12).

Initial Injury Assessment

The physician must be adept in establishing an adequate airway in the younger age group. In general, it is better to intubate the patient than to perform tracheostomy. Tracheostomy should be used only as a last resort in young children. Because of the relatively high incidence of gastric dilatation in children with facial fractures and the possibility of aspiration, a nasogastric tube should be placed early as a prophylactic measure.

Alveolar Fractures

When alveolar fractures occur and teeth are dislodged, the fragments of bone can be molded into alignment, and the teeth will survive if adequately supported by an arch bar or fixation with an acrylic splint. If teeth are fractured and the alveolar structures hopelessly damaged, it is best to remove the teeth and suture the soft tissue over the retained injured bone. Bone fragments should not be dissected away from attached soft tissue. Even loose bone fragments, if covered with soft tissue, may survive as grafts.

Fractured crowns of teeth without exposure of the pulp should be protected by dental methods until they can be restored successfully. If the crown of a tooth is fractured and the dental pulp is exposed, the prognosis may be good if the tooth is capped or a partial pulpectomy is performed. Fracture of the root near the crown usually requires extraction. Sometimes retaining teeth, if only for a short period, may be useful in space maintenance until a prosthetic replacement can be fabricated.

Damage to permanent tooth buds may result in deformed tooth structures, false eruptions, or irregular arrangement of the erupting teeth. Dental injuries are divided into those that involve deciduous teeth and those that involve the permanent dentition. Between the ages of 1 and 2½ years, as children begin to walk, displacement of the upper incisors is the most common injury. When intrusion of the incisor into the premaxilla occurs, reeruption often takes place. In children older than 2½ or 3 years, calcific degeneration and pulp necrosis are common following reeruption. Total avulsion of deciduous teeth is less common than other forms of displacement but results in the greatest damage to the overlying permanent teeth. Because of the close proximity between the apices of the primary and the permanent teeth, trauma to the deciduous teeth may result in damage to the developing permanent dentition.

Subluxation of permanent teeth with the associated alveolar bone is treated by repositioning and splinting according to standard techniques. The teeth may become nonvital and require a later root canal. Dental follow-up is mandatory for all alveolar fractures.

In cases of complete avulsion of a permanent tooth, when the root is immature and the apex widely open, reimplantation within a few minutes of injury should be performed and the tooth stabilized. In such cases, pulp revitalization and revascularization as well as continued root formation may occur. Reimplantation of a complete avulsion when root formation is mature and the avulsion is over 30 minutes old generally leads to total resorption. The root resorption process, however, may be a slow process, and therefore reimplantation should still be considered. Reimplantation in such cases should include pulp removal, pulp space restoration, and splinting. Dental consultation is necessary.

Mandibular Fractures

In general, the principles of treating mandibular fractures are the same in children and adults. The bone fragments must be reduced to their preinjury position, occlusion reestablished, and stabilization provided until healing has occurred.

When rigid fixation techniques are utilized, direct wire fixation or plate and screw fixation with miniplates or microplates should be applied in a manner that avoids the developing teeth. Because of the position of the developing permanent teeth (i.e., lingual to the roots of the deciduous teeth), monocortical screws can often be safely placed.

Maxillomandibular Fixation in the Pediatric Patient

When the patient has a full complement of deciduous teeth, MMF can be accomplished with standard arch bars and circumdental wires. Generally, supplemental skeletal fixation wires that are placed around the mandible and/or suspended from the anterior nasal spine or piriform apertures lend stability to the arch bars and permit successful application of MMF.

Parasymphyseal/Symphyseal Fractures

Before eruption of the permanent or secondary dentition, the developing follicles occupy most of the body of the mandible. In order to avoid injury to the tooth buds of the permanent dentition, this anatomic characteristic must be accounted for when interosseous fixation is employed. Wires or a metal plate and screw fixation should be placed near the inferior border of the mandible. In younger children with primary dentition in whom rigid fixation cannot be utilized in spite of proper precautions, an impression of the mandible can be taken under anesthesia and an acrylic splint fabricated. After realignment of the fragments the splint can be placed over the mandibular arch, lined with softened dental compound, and maintained in position with circumferential wiring. Arch bars are not necessary for many cases of pediatric mandibular fractures, and combinations of circummandibular wiring and piriform or anterior nasal spine suspension wires with a third wire looped in between the two are often sufficient for immobilization.

At a later age, dentition may be adequate for MMF. During the mixed dentition period, particularly between the ages of 6 and 12 years, acrylic splints may still be necessary to supplement interdental fixation. In older children, Erich arch bars can be used. With the advent of microplate and 1.5-mm miniplate fixation, smaller plates and screws can be employed at the inferior border instead of wires to provide increased stability with a low risk of injury to the developing teeth. In young children it is seldom necessary to remove partially erupted or unerupted permanent dental follicles to obtain reduction. A small degree of inaccuracy will be tolerated, but as emphasized by Posnick and others, this is never an excuse for sloppiness.

Mandibular Body Fractures

Favorable muscle forces are generally present with mandibular body fractures, and closed reduction with MMF will often suffice. Because of the increased osteogenic potential of the mandible in younger children, union is often completed within 2 to 4 weeks. Thus, shorter time periods of MMF are satisfactory. In the very young or in situations of simple greenstick or nondisplaced fractures, a soft diet alone may provide adequate treatment. Miniplate or microplate and screw fixation may be necessary in selected cases.

Condylar Fractures

Condylar fractures in the child can be categorized as intracapsular or extracapsular. Fractures may be further classified as displaced or nondisplaced, open or closed. In addition, extracapsular fractures may be in the medial or lateral pole or be of the low or high condylar neck variety. High condylar neck fractures within the TMJ capsule are generally considered intracapsular. The attachment of the external pterygoid muscle in the condylar neck above the sigmoid notch accounts for the medial and forward dislocation of fractured (high) condylar head and neck segments. Extracapsular fractures are below the TMJ capsule and extend from the level of the sigmoid notch downward and backward below the neck of the condyle to the posterior aspect of the ascending ramus. Open reduction and fixation are not indicated in the majority of condylar fractures in children or adults. When deciduous or mixed dentition is present, adequate treatment involves immobilizing the jaws for a period of 2 weeks to maintain vertical height of the ramus. This is followed by gradual mobilization with opening and closing exercises. In some cases of unilateral subcondylar fractures with little displacement, minimal pain, and no deviation toward the fractured side on incisal opening, a liquid diet and analgesics can be considered. When this conservative type of treatment is pursued, it is important that patients be followed closely for evidence of occlusal deviation.

Children with bilateral subcondylar fractures should undergo MMF. Either an acrylic splint held by circummandibular wires or arch bars with both circummandibular and bilateral piriform and anterior nasal spine suspension wires can be used for a period of 2 weeks. These patients must be followed closely. After 2 weeks, they should be allowed to open and close their jaws gradually with a few simple intermaxillary elastics to maintain occlusion overnight and between meals. After 3 weeks the child's mandible can be released from maintenance fixation. Careful follow-up is necessary to ensure that fractures heal without complications. The following indications for exploration of condylar fractures in children have been proposed by Posnick:

1. Lateral displacement of the proximal fracture segment
2. The presence of a foreign body in the joint capsule
3. Fracture with dislocation into the mandible cranial fossa and clinical disability
4. An inability to open or close the mouth because of mechanical blockage of the fractured segments
5. A low condylar neck (ramus fracture with displacement and dislocation)

In children, bilateral condylar fractures, with or without midface fractures, are themselves not an absolute indication for open reduction and internal fixation unless the indications listed above are present. It is important to allow early controlled range of motion to limit the likelihood of TMJ ankylosis developing. In patients who are managed nonoperatively, after release of MMF it is critical that close follow-up be maintained to monitor occlusion and TMJ function. In younger children growth and development should also be followed by both a surgeon and orthodontist.

Frontobasilar Fractures, Fractures of the Cranial Vault and Supraorbital Rim

Fractures of the frontobasilar region in children are treated similar to those occurring in adults. The main difference is related to the age of the child and the relative development of the frontal sinus. The frontal sinus develops as evaginations from the nose during the second trimester of pregnancy. It can be distinguished from the ethmoid sinuses after 5 years of age. The sinus reaches adult size by late puberty. Thus, in younger children only small areas of the sinus are present, which makes obliteration more difficult. The nasofrontal ducts themselves should be plugged in order to prevent communication between the nose and the epidural space. Consideration should also be given to insertion of a galeal frontalis flap in this area.

In general, depressed skull fractures can be elevated and plated by using an available microsystem. When one is drilling through the thinner bones of the skull, if protection of the underlying dura cannot be afforded by placement of a malleable retractor, one should drill only through the outer table until "softening" is felt, which indicates that the diploic space has been entered. Generally, 3-mm screws are used in the younger age group.

NOE fractures are approached via a coronal incision for optimal exposure. Open reduction and internal fixation are indicated, and often microplates and screws can be utilized. As in the adult, the canthi should not be detached from their associated bony fragment. Instead, the fragments should be reduced and the medial canthi dragged along with them. Subciliary and/or transconjunctival incisions with lateral canthotomy incisions are necessary, and sometimes an upper buccal sulcus incision is needed to obtain adequate reduction. A fracture at the base of the frontal sinus always accompanies NOE injuries. These have not been routinely treated by frontal sinus manipulation. Late mucocele formation or nasofrontal duct obstruction is rare. It is important to let the family know that in the younger child who requires nasal bone grafting, growth may lag behind and require a secondary procedure to restore dorsal nasal projection. In addition, Ousterhout has reported growth deformities in children who had previously had midfacial trauma, and families should be appraised of the possibility of this occurring.

Zygomatic Fractures

Stabilization is similar to that in the adult, although caution must be applied in the application of any zygomaticomaxillary buttress plates because this may interfere with the developing dentition. In most situations, microplates should be considered for stabilizations at the frontozygomatic area, the inferior orbital rim, and possibly across the zygomaticomaxillary buttress in younger children. Again, autogenous tissues are preferred for bone grafting of the orbital floor, although linear cracks can be realigned without bone grafting. If the child is old enough, a split calvarial bone graft can be taken; otherwise rib is probably the preferred material because of its easy contouring.

Le Fort I, II, and III Fractures

Le Fort fractures generally occur in older children and adolescents and should be treated by open reduction and internal fixation to achieve anatomic restoration. In younger children, closed reduction in Le Fort I fractures may be considered if displacement is minimal. When Le Fort II and III fractures are present, however, a coronal incision should be made and stabilization obtained in the Le Fort III fracture at the zygomatic arch and zygomaticofrontal regions and at the nasal frontal junction. For Le Fort II fractures, rigid fixation can be safely applied at the nasal frontal junction even in young children but may need to be avoided in the maxillary component if the developing dentition is potentially jeopardized. In that circumstance, suspension wires and MMF can be considered. Orbital floors should be explored in Le Fort II and III fractures and bone grafting carried out as necessary. Acrylic dental splints may be necessary in cases where the application of arch bars is difficult.

GUNSHOT WOUNDS OF THE FACE

The surgical approach to severe facial trauma resulting from gunshot wounds presents a formidable challenge. Low-velocity gunshot wounds should be distinguished from intermediate- and high-velocity gunshot wounds to the face.

Low-Velocity Gunshot Wounds

In general, low velocity gunshot wounds involve little soft-tissue and bone loss and limited associated injury outside the path of the bullet. They may therefore be treated with immediate stabilization of bone and primary soft-tissue closure. Bone may need to be replaced. The patterns of low-velocity gunshot wounds of the face as outlined by Manson are as follows (Fig 17–13):

Lower portion of the face:
- Injuries involving the tongue and mandible.
- Usually limited bone loss
- Open reduction—internal fixation or closed reduction can generally be accomplished.
- If significant edema is present, tracheostomy should be considered.

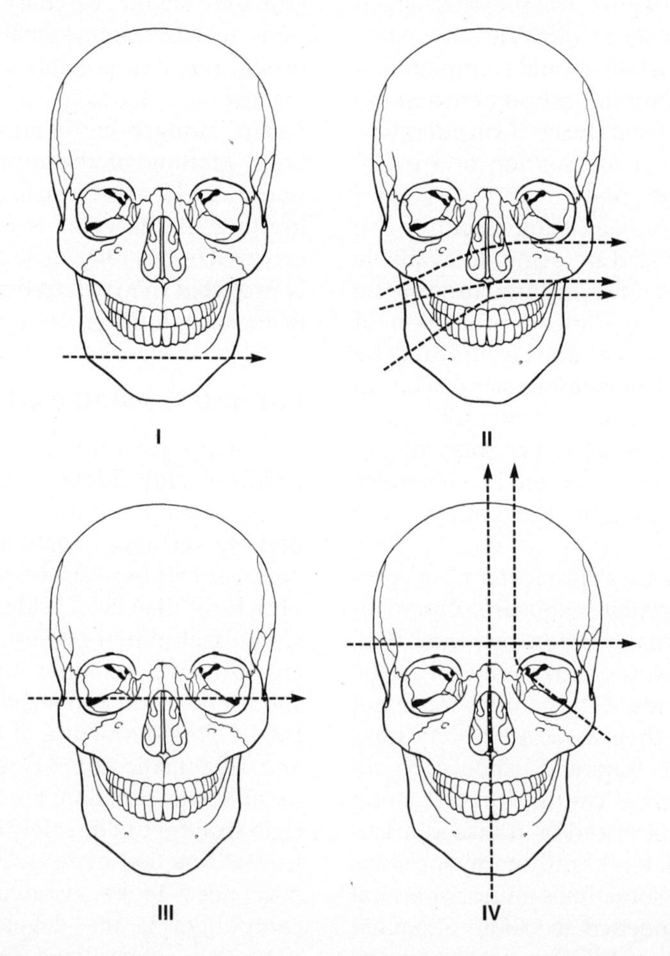

FIG 17–13.
Pattern I, lower facial wounds involve the mandibular area and tongue. *Pattern II,* involvement of the lower part of the midface and lower orbit constitute pattern II. *Pattern III,* involvement of both orbits and temporal mandibular joints. *Pattern IV,* involvement of the frontal bone and orbit. Adapted from Manson PN: Facial Injuries. In McCarthy JG, editor: *Plastic Surgery; Volume 2.*, Philadelphia, W.B. Saunders, 1990. Used by permission.

- Primary bone grafting only if a surgically clean wound is achieved.
- Soft-tissue coverage should be anticipated.

Midface:

- Injuries involving the maxilla, alveolus, sinuses, lower part of the nose, and zygoma.
- Palatal injuries may require local flaps.
- Immediate bone grafting and open reduction should be considered in most cases.

Orbital injuries:

- Orbits and nasal injuries.
- Usually treated by open reduction and immediate bone grafting.
- Damage to the globe is present in many cases.
- Ocular examination is imperative.
- The TMJs are frequently involved as exit wounds and are treated by open exploration with reduction or closed reduction, depending on the displacement.

Craniofacial:

- Intracranial involvement.
- Supraorbital, orbital, frontal bone, and frontal sinus structures injured.
- Neurosurgical intervention for dural tears and cerebral lacerations.

Intermediate- and High-Velocity Gunshot Wounds to the Face

The patterns of soft-tissue and bone loss in shotgun injuries as outlined by Manson is shown in Figure 17–14. Less loss is usually present than first suspected. Emphasis is placed on primary soft-tissue closure and stabilization of existing bone fragments with re-exploration for additional debridement at 48-hour intervals until the wound is controlled. It is critical that fractures be addressed and vertical, transverse, and sagittal proportions of the craniofacial skeleton be maintained. Maintenance of such proportions is necessary for future reconstructive and prosthodontic considerations.

Most authors advocate immediate wound care with conservative debridement of bone and soft tissue. Only small pieces of bone devoid of periosteum are removed. In less severe injuries immediate definitive repair of bone and soft tissue can be accomplished. In more severe injuries with extensive injury to or loss of bone and soft tissue, immediate debridement is followed by further "second-look" procedures. Within 7 to 10 days, delayed primary reconstruction with replacement of missing midfacial bone and soft tissue can be performed. Late repair involves scar revision, oral commissure creation, total nasal reconstruction utilizing forehead skin, and mandibular reconstruction. (See Part IV for the details of head and neck reconstruction.) As alluded to earlier, management depends on the anatomic location of the injury. Four specific patterns have been recognized:

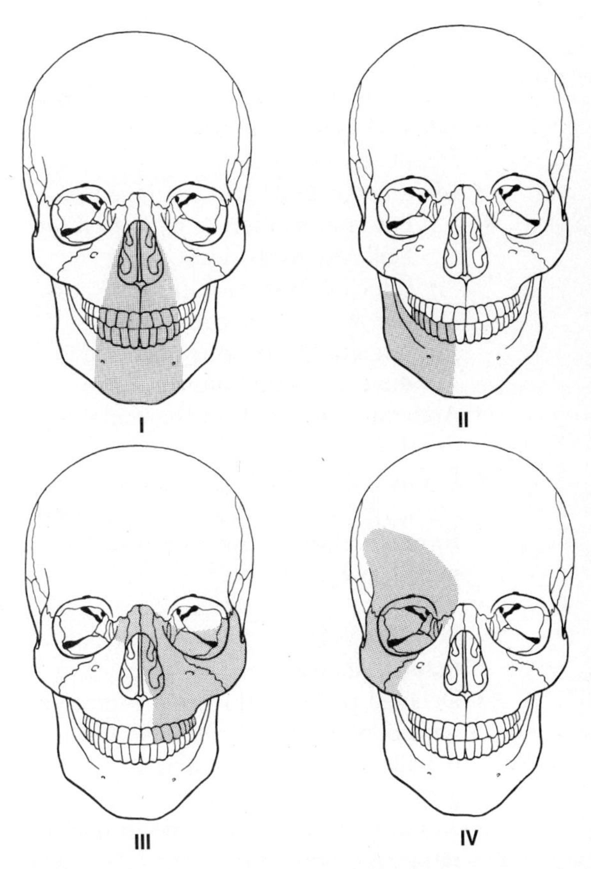

FIG 17–14.
Pattern I, central mandibular and midface soft-tissue and bone loss. *Pattern II,* lateral mandibular soft-tissue and bone loss. *Pattern III,* maxillary and orbital soft-tissue and bone loss. *Pattern IV,* orbital and cranial soft-tissue and bone loss. Adapted from Manson PN: Facial Injuries. In McCarthy JG, editor: *Plastic Surgery, Volume 2.,* Philadelphia, W.B. Saunders, 1990. Used by permission.

- **Central lower part of the face:**
  - Loss of the central portion of the mandible, maxilla, lips, and the nose.
  - Bilateral zygomatic fractures frequently coexist.
  - Mandibular bone loss managed by
    - External fixation (e.g., with a Joe Hall Morris device).
    - Internal fixation with plate and screw reconstruction of the remaining portions of the mandible in an anatomic position.
  - Arch bars are fixed on the remaining dentition.
  - Reduction of the zygomatic arch and zygomatic fractures will permit reconstruction of the zygomaticomaxillary buttresses.
  - Return to the operating room at 48-hour intervals for reassessment of tissue viability.
  - Delayed primary closure if required with bone grafting of the central maxilla, medial orbits, and nasal areas.
  - Not advised to perform definitive nasal reconstruction or lip reconstruction at the acute stage.
- **Lateral lower part of the face:**
  - Most frequently involved.
  - Loss of the lateral mandibular segment and surrounding soft tissue.
  - Injuries extend upward into the maxilla, lateral to the nose.
  - External fixation or reconstruction plate and screw fixation is used to open the mandibular bone gap.
  - Soft tissue is usually present for closure.
  - Facial nerve injuries are repaired primarily.
- **Midface:**
  - Delayed primary closure with bone grafting to the maxilla and orbital areas to provide an initial three-dimensional scaffold for midfacial support.
  - A free composite tissue flap should be considered.
  - Early consultation with a maxillofacial prosthodontist.
  - Arteriography may be indicated to define carotid artery integrity.
- **Craniofacial injuries:**
  - Characterized by intracranial involvement and thus carry a worse prognosis.
  - Primary reconstruction with open reduction, bone grafting, and sinus elimination.

MANDIBULAR FRACTURES

Dentition

It is imperative that the surgeon managing fractures of the craniofacial skeleton have knowledge of normal dentition and occlusion. The deciduous teeth begin to erupt at up to 5 to 6 months of age. The lower central incisors are generally first to be noted. By the age of 20 to 24 months, the child has a total of 20 teeth: 10 in the upper and 10 in the lower dental arch. At the age of 6 years, in addition to the temporary dentition the first permanent or 6-year molars erupt behind the second deciduous molars. At the age of 6 years the maxillary and mandibular central incisor teeth are replaced by the permanent teeth. At the age of 9 years, the permanent lateral incisors have erupted, and by 14 years of age all the deciduous teeth have usually been exfoliated and replaced by permanent teeth. When all permanent teeth have erupted, the adult has 32 permanent teeth. The teeth are numbered as indicated: maxillary dental arch, right to left, 1 to 16; mandibular dental arch, left to right, 17 to 32. The Angle classification of occlusion usually reflects the skeletal relationship between the maxilla and the mandible (Fig 17–15). The examining physician must be alert for abnormalities or deviations from normal. Missing teeth can produce a shift in dental relationships. The first step in identifying abnormal occlusal patterns is to count the teeth and identify those that are present and absent. Impressions and models may be obtained to allow a leisurely study of the dental relationships. The pre-existing occlusion is usually recognized. Wear facets indicate where the teeth habitually come together. A patient who had an Angle class III occlusal relationship before injury would be impossible to treat by attempting to force the teeth into a neutral position. Frequently, the patient can advise the physician about his preexisting occlusal pattern. Slight differences in occlusion will be immediately perceived by an awake and alert patient. Occasionally, information obtained from the patient's family, from old photographs, or from dentists or orthodontists who may have taken x-ray films or models will assist in documenting preinjury dental relationships.

Maxillomandibular Fixation

Although many techniques exist for MMF, the most common is the application of prefabricated arch bars. Generally Erich arch bars are ligated to the teeth with 24- to 26-gauge steel wires. If segments of teeth are missing or if the condition of the dentition is such that additional support is necessary, the arch bar may be stabilized by the use of an acrylic splint or supplemental wires. Increased stability of the maxillary arch bar can be obtained by suspension wires from the piriform aperture and/or anterior nasal spine. Increased stability of the mandibular arch bar can be obtained by circummandibular wires.

Mandibular fractures should be considered open, and all patients should be treated with antibiotics. Stabilization of mandibular fragments should be accomplished as soon after injury as possible. When surgery is delayed, Ivy loops can be placed on the teeth at the patient's bedside to establish temporary MMF. This measure will achieve (some) reduction of the fracture and allow the patient to be more comfortable prior to definitive repair, at which time the Ivy loops are replaced with arch bars. MMF can then be maintained with either dental elastics or heavy wires.

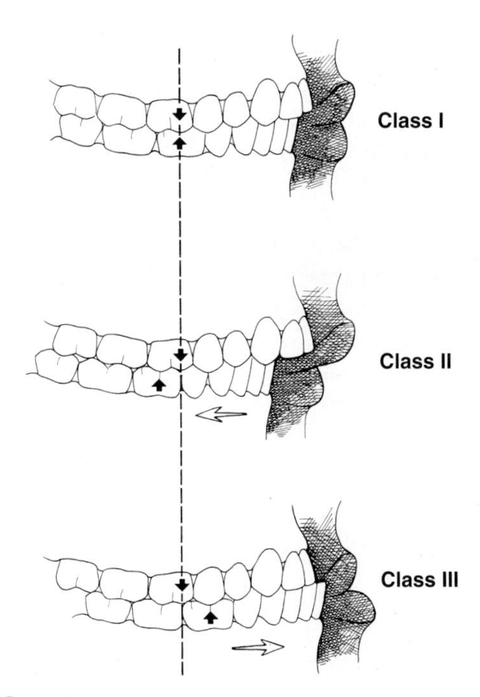

FIG 17–15.
The classification of occlusion includes three main types (after Angle). The classification is based on the position of the mesial buccal cusp of the maxillary first molar in relation to the mesial buccal groove of the mandibular first molar. The position of the cuspid teeth should also be noted. Subdivision of the three main classes are identified by differences in the mesial or lateral positioning of the teeth in the dental arches.

Acrylic Dental Splints in Maintenance of Maxillomandibular Fixation

A knowledge of acrylic splints and their fabrication is necessary to treat complex facial injuries involving the jaws (Fig 17–16). With edentulous or partially dentuous fractures, sagittal fractures of the palate, and complex

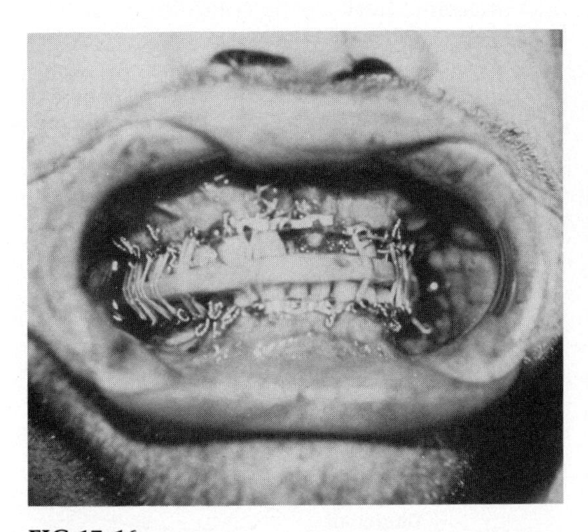

FIG 17–16.
Acrylic occlusal splint to key occlusion and establishment prior to fracture fixation.

mandibular and maxillary fractures, application of either a palatal or lingual splint or palatal-occlusal or lingual-occlusal splint may be helpful. The splint can be modified to include "occlusal stops," and a supplementary arch bar can be affixed directly to the splint with acrylic.

Classification

Mandibular fractures are classified by Manson and most authors according to their location, the condition of the teeth, the direction of the fracture, the favorability for treatment, the presence of a compound injury, and the characterization of the fracture pattern.

Location (Fig 17–17)

Parasymphyseal and symphyseal—fractures occurring between the mental foramina.

Mandibular body—fractures occurring from the cuspid tooth to the angle of the mandible.

Mandibular angle—fractures beyond the second molar. The angle is weak and is further weakened by the presence of uninterrupted third molar teeth.

Mandibular ramus—fractures between the angle of the mandible and the sigmoid notch.

Coronoid process

Subcondylar fractures—fractures below the anatomic neck of the condyle.

Alveolar fractures—fractures involving a segment of alveolar bone with or without attached teeth. Alveolar fractures may occur separately or in association with other fractures of the mandible.

Type of fracture

Greenstick

Simple

Compound—communication with the outside environment. All mandibular fractures should be considered to be compound.

Complex—fractures with multiple segments.

Comminuted—fractures with small fragments, some of which may be devitalized.

Impacted—fractures in which the bone ends are driven firmly together.

Severity of fractures

Simple—no contact with the outside environment.

Compound—direct communication between mucosa and/or skin with the potential for contamination.

Direction of fracture and favorability (Fig 17–18)

Horizontal.
- Favorable.
- Unfavorable.

Vertical.
- Favorable.
- Unfavorable.

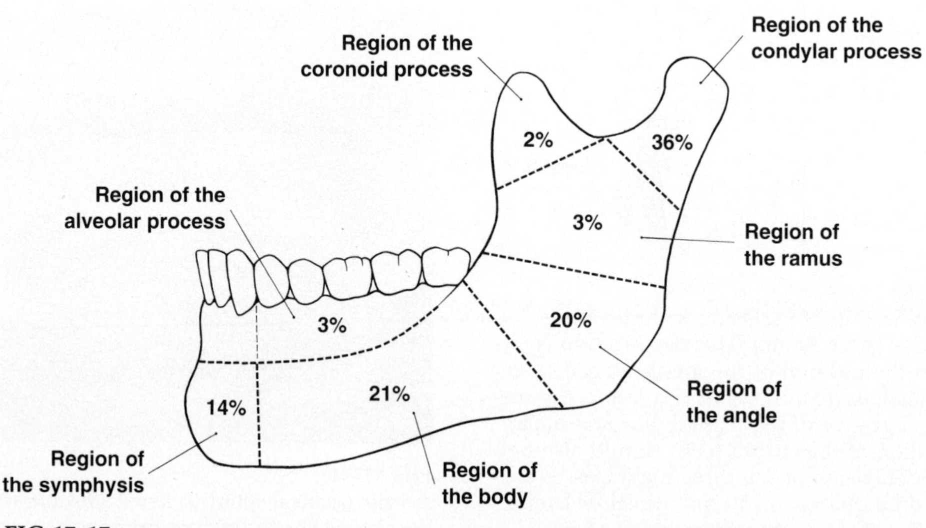

FIG 17–17.
Locations of mandibular fractures.

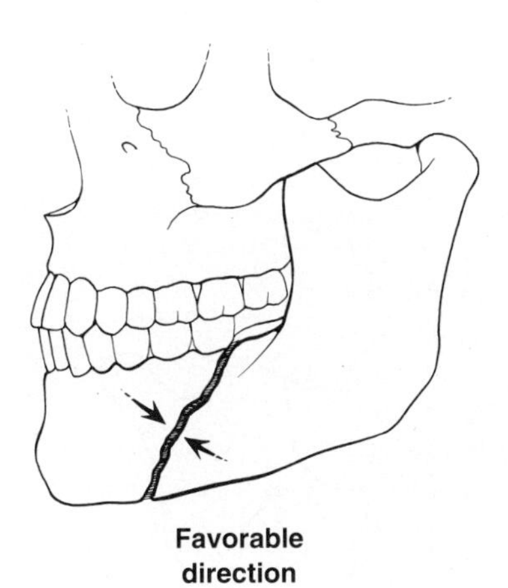

FIG 17–18.
Favorable and unfavorable directions of fracture lines.

Presence or absence of teeth and/or mandibular segments
Class 1—teeth present on both sides of the fracture line.
Class 2—teeth present on one side of the fracture line.
Class 3—fracture fragments contain no teeth.

Muscles influencing movement of the mandible. Muscular pull is an important variable in determining the degree and direction of displacement of fracture and mandibular segments. Reduction of fixation of mandibular fragments must overcome the forces of displacement.
Posterior group—muscles of mastication, including the temporalis, masseter, and the medial and lateral pterygoid muscles, move the mandible upward, forward, and medially (Fig 17–19).
Anterior or depressor group (Fig 17–20).
Group 1—the geniohyoid muscle elevates the hyoid and depresses the mandible.
Group 2—the genioglossus protrudes the tongue, elevates the hyoid, and depresses the mandible.
Group 3—the mylohyoid elevates the hyoid and depresses the mandible.
Group 4—the digastric elevates the hyoid and depresses the anterior portion of the mandible.

Physical Examination of the Mandible

The following clinical symptoms and signs may be indicative of a fracture of the mandible:

1. Pain
2. Numbness in the distribution of the mental nerve and ipsilateral teeth
3. Tenderness over the fracture site
4. Inability to open the mouth or bring teeth into proper occlusion
5. Excessive salivation
6. Edema and ecchymosis
7. Physical deformity
8. Abnormal mobility (in fractures of the condyle with displacement, the mandible shifts toward the involved side as the patient opens his mouth)
9. Crepitus

Roentgenographic Diagnosis

Following the clinical diagnosis, a Panorex film should be obtained. Specialized examination such as occlusal films, palatal films, and periapical views of the teeth are helpful in detecting fractures or in analyzing the degree of tooth-root injury. In complex panfacial fractures with associated fractures of the mandible, axial as well as coronal CT studies will reveal the majority of mandibular fractures. Axial CT alone will not diagnose all fractures of the mandibular ramus or condyle, but axial and coronal CT scans in combination may be used to dem-

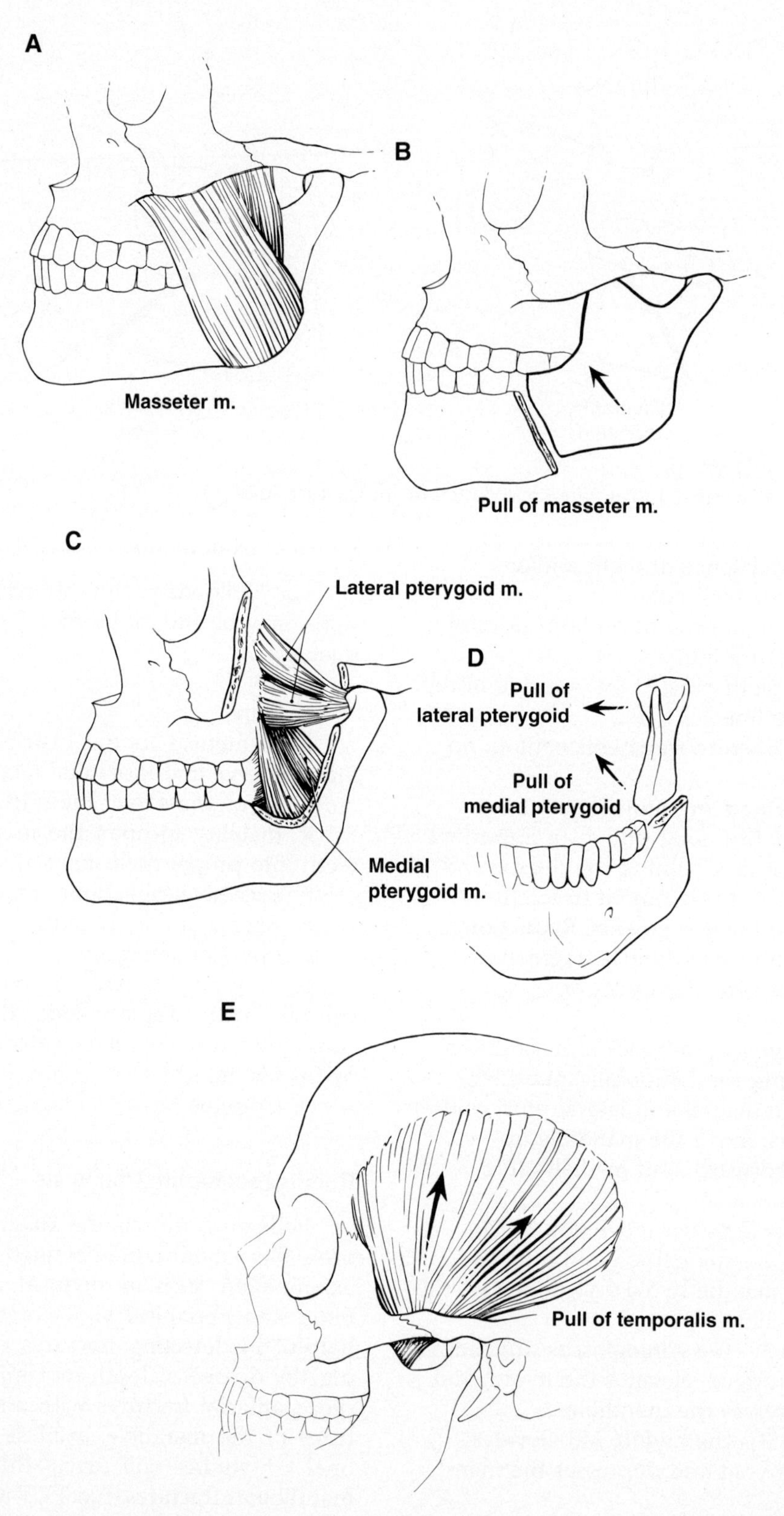

FIG 17–19.
A–E, the posterior group of muscles attached to the mandible. The overall force from activity of this group of muscles is movement of the mandible upward, forward, medially, or laterally.

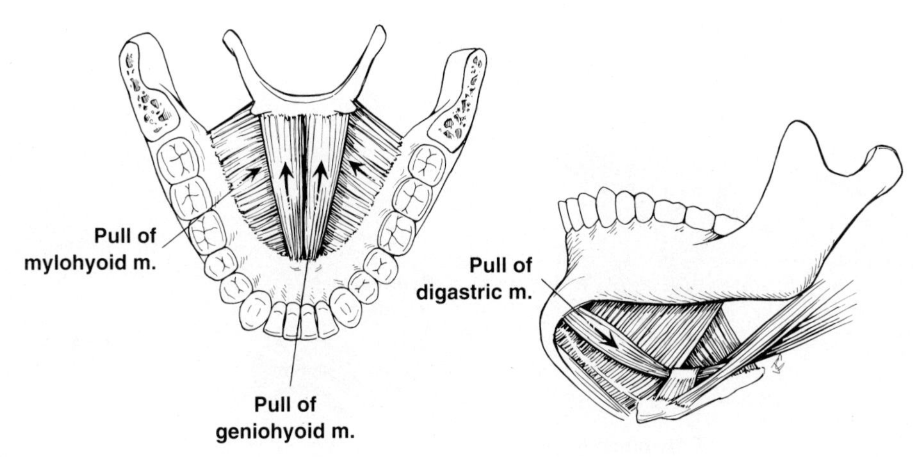

FIG 17–20.
The anterior or depressor group of muscles of mastication and the direction of pull and displacement of fragments.

onstrate the pathology of subcondylar fractures.

Temporomandibular Joint

The function and anatomy of the TMJ should be recalled when considering injuries to the mandibular condyle (Fig 17–21). The joint is a *ginglymoarthrodial joint* and thus has a hinge-like action as well as a gliding and rotating action. The joint is composed of the articular head of the condyle of the mandible and the glenoid fossa of the squamous portion of the temporal bone. The TMJ is a compound joint separated into two distinct chambers, one above and the other below an articular disk composed of fibrocartilage known as the meniscus. Movement of the articular disk is controlled by the attachment of the *lateral pterygoid muscle,* which inserts through the capsule of the joint into the inferior edge of the disk and by attachment of the disk to the posterior portion of the joint capsule.

Treatment of Mandibular Fractures

Restoration of function of the mandible and masticatory efficiency of the dentition must be accomplished in the treatment of mandibular fractures. Reduction of fractured segments into anatomic position and establishment of stable fixation to hold these segments until healing has occurred are the main principles of treatment. A more in depth discussion can be found in Manson's chapter on facial injuries in McCarthy's *Plastic Surgery.*

Class I Fractures

When teeth are present on both sides of the fracture, MMF for a period of 4 to 6 weeks may be all that is necessary. In practice, because many patients with mandibular fractures are noncompliant, open reduction and direct plate and screw fixation are employed. The techniques of rigid fixation are especially appealing because MMF is unnecessary, which permits intake of solid foods, better oral hygiene, and earlier return to work. (The author's preference is to use internal rigid fixation in the majority of mandibular fractures.)

Class II Fractures

When teeth are present on one side of the fracture and an edentulous fragment exists on the other, open reduction and plate and screw fixation are indicated. A lingual and/or lingual-occlusal splint with occlusal stops can be utilized to obtain stable MMF.

Class III Fractures

Fractures of the edentulous mandible represent less than 5% of mandibular fractures and are the most serious. Fractures occur through the portions of bone where atrophy is most advanced. The edentulous mandible is characterized by loss of the alveolar ridge. Atrophy of the bone may be minimal with

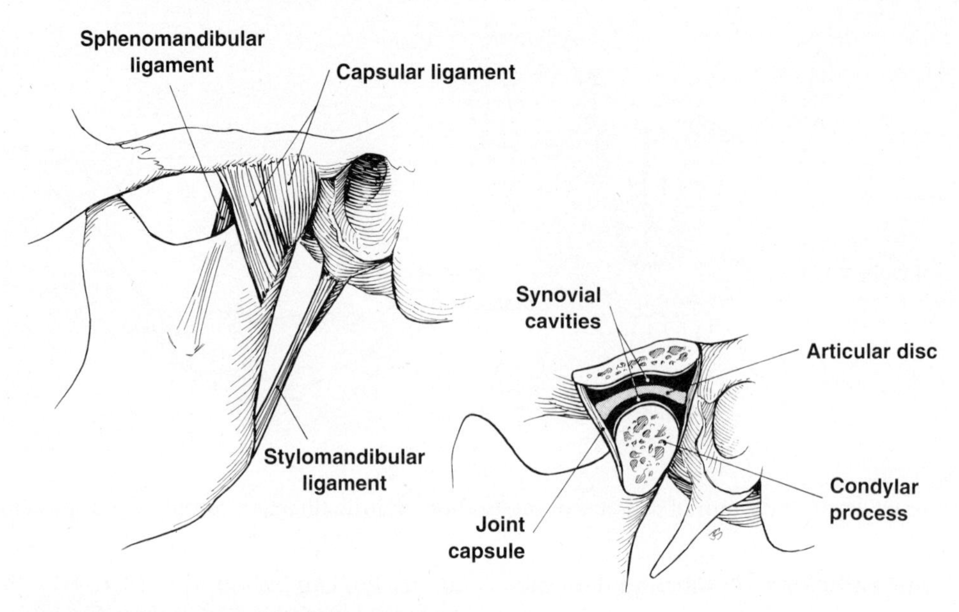

FIG 17–21.
Anatomy of the temporomandibular joint.

sufficient height of the mandibular body (>20 mm). In cases with moderate atrophy, the height of the mandibular body ranges from 10 to 20 mm. In cases in which the mandibular height is less than 10 mm, the atrophy is described as severe. Obwegser has found complications following fracture of the edentulous mandible directly parallel the extent of mandibular atrophy. Twenty percent of complications are seen in the 10- to 20-mm mandibular height group, while 80% of complications are experienced in cases demonstrating less than 10 mm. When open reduction of the edentulous mandible with less than 10 mm of height is required, consideration should be given to immediate bone grafting.

Intraoral appliances are quite useful in treating simple fractures of the edentulous mandible when displacement is minimal or absent. Either appropriately made splints or modification of the patient's own dentures by ligating arch bars to the teeth can be used to maintain stability. The splints and/or dentures are secured into position with circumferential or suspension wiring techniques. Open reduction may be necessary for comminuted or displaced fractures. The use of metallic plates and screws, generally with a reconstruction plate, is simple and direct and provides a mechanical advance over wiring techniques. Antibiotics should be employed.

Complex and Comminuted Mandibular Fractures

MMF is an essential part of complete fixation to ensure correct position of bony segments in segmental or comminuted fractures or in the bone gap in fractures with bone loss. The mandibular arch bar may have to be applied in segments to each cone fragment that contains teeth to facilitate fracture reduction and achieve correct occlusal repositioning. Splints ultimately will be necessary to bridge edentulous gaps by creating an occlusal stop where the arch bars are directly fixed with acrylic.

Tension banding of the upper mandibular border is generally accomplished by an arch bar. Occasionally, a miniplate and/or lag screw at the upper border of the mandible, especially posterior to the occlusion, may be necessary to create a tension band effect prior to final stabilization (Fig 17–22). Fracture reduction and stabilization are obtained following occlusal repositioning. *The most critical step is perfect reduction.* This is usually accomplished by a combination of MMF and interosseous wires. Occasionally, lag screws and miniplates might be necessary. Once contour is restored, final stabilization is accomplished by mandibular compression or reconstruction plates (Fig 17–22). In unstable or segmental fractures with good bone contact, a minimum of three screws in each lateral stable segment is preferable.

Maintaining adequate periosteal and soft-tissue attachments to bony segments may be difficult or impossible if the fragments are severely displaced and small. Smaller cortical cancellous segments can be discarded by bone grafting of gaps, and this should be performed at the primary procedure. Most commonly, iliac bone is used. Cancellous iliac bone can be packed into gaps and crevices quite easily. Larger segments of loss can be corrected with tricortical iliac bone, although frequently large losses are corrected on a delayed basis. Primary bone grafts in the mandible are less predictable and have higher rates of resorption and infection. Occasionally, primary bone grafting will be used to bridge a small gap or augment a thin, atrophic mandible after the plate has been applied. For larger gaps it may be wise to delay reconstruction. Sagittal splitting of the inner and outer cortex commonly occurs in association with segmental fractures. The obliquity of these fractures is ideally suited to lag screw fixation.

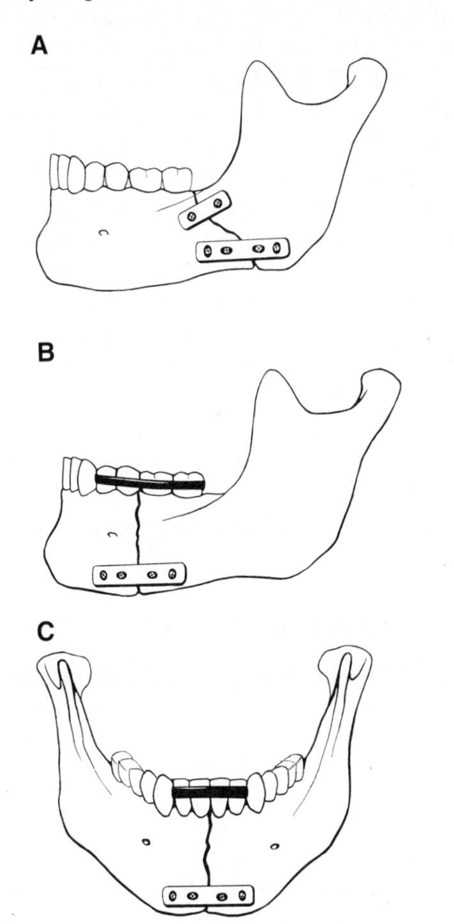

FIG 17–22.
Indications for different plate fixation techniques. **A,** at the angle of the mandible: compression tension band plate and stabilization plate. **B,** in the area of the lateral teeth: eccentric dynamic compression plate with an arch bar functioning as a tension band for a dentulous jaw. It can be used without an arch bar for the edentulous jaw. **C,** in the area of the front teeth: dynamic compression plate with an arch bar functioning as a tension band for the dentulous jaw. It can be used without an arch bar for the edentulous jaw. (From Spiessl B: *New Concepts in Maxillofacial Bone Surgery.* New York, Springer-Verlag, 1976. Used by permission.)

Specific Regions

Parasymphyseal/Symphyseal. The approach to the parasymphyseal and symphyseal regions is generally intraoral through a lower vestibular incision. Care must be taken to avoid injury to the mental nerves. When the nerve is identified and the fracture extends in close proximity, a vessel loop can be utilized for retraction of the nerve during fracture reduction and stabilization. When external wounds are present, these can be extended in the submental area if cosmetically acceptable.

Mandibular Body. Fractures of the mandibular body are also accessible via intraoral exposure. It is important to position the plate at the inferior border in order to prevent injury to the inferior alveolar nerve.

Mandibular Angle. Fractures in the mandibular angle are often posterior to the occlusion and difficult to approach intraorally. Occasionally simple fractures can be approached intraorally, and when nondisplaced, miniplates in the superior border functioning as tension bands, along with MMF, will suffice. However, in most cases it is preferable to make a Risdon incision and approach the fracture extraorally. Generally, a figure-of-8 wire is utilized at the inferior border to obtain reduction, and then a reconstruction plate is applied.

Mandibular Ramus. For ramal fractures that do not involve the low condylar neck, an open approach again is necessary, usually through a high Risdon or Hines incision. Plating can then be accomplished with a reconstruction plate and bicortical screws.

Subcondylar Fractures. Subcondylar fractures are generally managed by the application of MMF and closed reduction for a period of 2 to 3 weeks. MMF is then released and the patient encouraged to exercise the jaw. Dental elastics must be employed to resist vertical ramal shortening with a tendency toward anterior open bite. Patients are reevaluated on a weekly basis, and dental elastics are adjusted as indicated. Frequently, in the presence of unilateral subcondylar fractures, incisal opening will be restored with some deviation to the fractured side. Symptoms of TMJ pain are not infrequent, and referral to an orthodontist may be necessary for splint therapy. Careful follow-up is mandatory in order to determine whether further surgery will be necessary on the TMJ apparatus. Although subcondylar fractures can be managed in this way, some require open reduction. Manson, McCoy and other authors list indications for open reduction and internal fixation of subcondylar fractures include the following:

1. Inability to obtain adequate dental occlusion by closed reduction
2. Interference of mandibular movement by a displaced segment
3. Open facial wound with exposure of the condyle or a foreign body in the TMJ
4. Subcondylar fractures associated with panfacial fractures requiring reestablishment of the posterior vertical facial height
5. Subcondylar fractures in an edentulous patient where a splint is unavailable or impossible to use because of bone loss
6. Patients with medical conditions such as seizure disorders, substance abuse, neurologic injury, mental retardation, or psychiatric illness, where MMF may complicate the underlying condition
7. Fractures with unstable occlusions secondary to dentofacial deformities
8. Any other patient in whom early function is indicated for medical or dental reasons.

Damage to Teeth

Teeth in the line of the fractures should be retained if they offer any degree of stability to the bone fragments and if they have solid attachments. Once rigid fixation has been accomplished, the fractured teeth may then be removed either immediately or at the time of arch bar removal. Antibiotic therapy should be utilized to protect against infection. Third molars in the line of the fracture should be removed at the time of fracture reduction. Dental follow-up is mandatory following all fractures involving the occlusion. Apical views of the teeth and sensory simulation studies detect apical pathology or devitalization. Injured teeth may be amenable to root canal therapy and must be carefully observed for the development of periapical abscesses. In addition, it is our policy to refer all patients following mandibular fractures to an orthodontist for posttraumatic consultation.

SUGGESTED READING

Gruss JS, Phillips JH: Rigid Fixation of Zygomatic Fractures. In Yaremchuck, Gruss, Manson, editors: *Rigid Fixation of the Craniomaxillofacial Skeleton,* Boston, Butterworth-Heinemann, 1992.

Manson PN: Facial Injuries. In McCarthy JG, editor: *Plastic Surgery, Volume 2.,* Philadelphia, W.B. Saunders, 1990.

Manson PN, Hoopes JE, Su CT: Structural Pillars of the Facial Skeleton: An Approach to the Management of LeFort Fractures. *Plast Reconstr Surg* 66:54, 1980.

Paskert JP, Manson PN, Iliff NT: Nasoethmoid and Orbital Fractures. *Clin Plast Surg* 15:209, 1988.

Resnick JI, Kawamoto HK: Traumatic Enophthalmos. In Habal, Ariyan , editors: *Facial Fractures.* Toronto, B.C. Decker, 1989.

Stanley RB, Jr: Fractures of the Frontal Sinus. *Clin Plast Surg* 16:115, 1989.

Chapter 18

Aesthetic and Functional Problems

Elvin G. Zook, M.D.

CONTENTS

CHAPTER OBJECTIVE

At the end of this chapter the resident is familiar with aesthetic and functional problems of the head and neck, understands the principles of surgical treatment of such problems, and performs complete diagnostic and surgical management for a wide variety of aesthetic deformities of facial and allied structures.

LEARNER OBJECTIVES

On completion of this chapter, the resident

1. **Is familiar with the concepts of beauty and aesthetic principles of the facial structures.**
2. **Understands the principles and techniques of aesthetic rhinoplasty; recognizes the differences in approach between primary and secondary rhinoplasty.**
3. **Is familiar with diagnostic and therapeutic techniques in the management of nasal airway obstruction.**
4. **Is familiar with the application of aesthetic techniques to the cleft lip and nose.**
5. **Knows the complications of rhinoplasty and septoplasty and their prevention and treatment.**
6. **Recognizes the varying effects of aging and sun exposure on the facial skin and structures.**
7. **Is familiar with techniques of rhytidectomy, suction lipectomy, brow-lift, blepharoplasty, and other methods for treatment of the aging face.**
8. **Knows the complications of facial aesthetic surgery and their prevention and treatment.**
9. **Recognizes the various aesthetic deformities of the ear and knows the principles and techniques of surgical correction.**
10. **Is familiar with aesthetic and functional problems of the eyelid, including blepharochalasis and ptosis; knows the treatment techniques for these problems and their complications and prevention.**
11. **Is familiar with the diagnostic methods and treatment options for patients with facial palsy.**
12. Is familiar with the diagnostic principles and treatment techniques for alopecia and male pattern baldness.
13. Is familiar with the diagnostic methods and treatment techniques for the management of temporomandibular joint disorders.
14. **Knows the principles and techniques of orthognathic surgery.**
15. **Is familiar with other functional problems of the head and neck such as masseter hypertrophy.**
16. **Knows the various ancillary techniques for management of the aging face such as chemical peel, Retin A, dermabrasion, collagen injection, etc.**
17. **Knows the differential diagnosis and the management methods for facial atrophy.**

CLINICAL PRACTICE ACTIVITIES

During the course of the training program, the resident

1. **Evaluates patients with aging faces.**
2. **Performs surgical therapy for patients with aging faces, including rhytidectomy, brow-lift, etc.**
3. **Evaluates and treats patients with aesthetic problems of the eyelid; performs blepharoplasty.**
4. **Evaluates patients with nasal deformity and performs rhinoplasty and septal surgery.**
5. Performs ancillary procedures for the aging face such as chemical peeling, collagen injection, etc.
6. Evaluates and treats patients with functional problems of the eyelid such as ptosis.
7. Evaluates and treats patients with aesthetic problems of the ear; performs otoplasty.
8. Diagnoses and treats patients with facial palsy by using a variety of techniques.
9. Diagnoses and treats patients with facial atrophy.
10. *Evaluates and treats patients with alopecia and male pattern baldness.*
11. *Diagnoses and treats patients with temporomandibular joint disorders.*
12. *Evaluates patients for orthognathic surgery; participates in orthognathic surgical procedures.*
13. *Treats patients with other facial dis-*

orders such as masseter hypertrophy, facial hyperkinesia, etc.

INTRODUCTION

The old cliche "beauty is in the eye of the beholder" is true to a great extent. Many attempts have been made to qualitate and quantitate beauty by some use of proportions and relationships of various facial structures; for example, the width of one eye should be approximately equal to the distance between the eyes, the eyes should be in the exact center of the head, and the distance from the lateral edge of the orbit to the ear should equal the height of the ear.

Actual bony proportions may be measured and studied by using lateral cephalometric and computed tomographic (CT) radiographs. Soft-tissue proportions may be measured and studied by using life-size photographs. Recently, small-computer imaging techniques have been introduced to allow the surgeon to experiment with changes in facial relationships. A number of bony and soft-tissue landmarks have been utilized to analyze facial structure; these are discussed in more detail later in this chapter in the section on orthognathic surgery.

Unfortunately, attempts to define and produce beauty in terms of pure measurements do not always result in the actual achievement of this goal. We have all had the experience of seeing an attractive face whose individual features, when considered separately, do not meet the numerical criteria of perfection, but when viewed in combination, actually define beauty.

RHINOPLASTY

Rhinoplasty is one of the most difficult procedures to learn. Noses differ from the ideal in many ways. The most common cosmetic anatomic variations leading to surgery are the prominent dorsal hump, the wide dorsum and/or wide tip, the long nose, and the large nose. Traumatic nasal abnormalities usually have associated septal angulation, with or without nasal obstruction. The plan for each nasal procedure must take into consideration the shape and size of the patient's face and the patient's sex, age, and specific desires with regard to postoperative nasal appearance.

Anatomy

The nasal bones are roughly rectangular and are attached to the frontal bone at the glabella superiorly and to the medial aspect of the maxilla posteriorly (Fig 18–1). The upper lateral cartilages are also roughly rectangular and at their upper border lie beneath the distal edge of the nasal bones. The lateral crus of the alar (or lower lateral) cartilage is somewhat elliptically shaped and is continuous medially with the medial crus of the alar cartilage, which extends into the columella. There are several small cartilages between the inferior border of the upper lateral cartilage and the superior border of the lateral crus of the alar cartilage. Anteriorly, the nasal bones are joined to each other, as are the upper lateral cartilages. There is a varying amount of fat between the two medial crura, which are *not* attached to each other. If the lateral crus of the alar cartilage is excessively convex or large, the

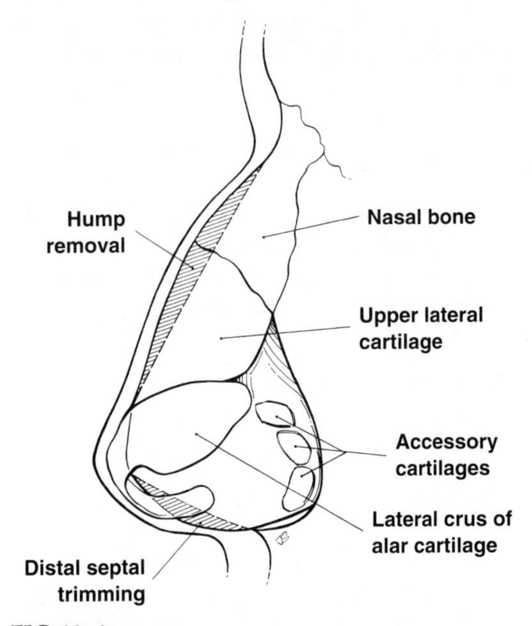

FIG 18–1.
The lateral anatomy of the nose showing a level of hump removal and distal septal trimming.

nasal tip will be large and/or bulbous in appearance. If there is fat between domes of the alar cartilages and the medial crus, the tip may appear bifid or widened.

A crooked nose (usually secondary to trauma) frequently has nasal septal deformities that must be corrected to allow straightening of the outer framework of the nose. (See the discussion on airway obstruction below.)

Planning the Procedure

It is essential to learn what the patient thinks is wrong with the appearance of the nose and to compare this with the anatomic abnormalities. The surgeon must then determine whether the changes desired by the patient are both aesthetically reasonable and surgically possible. If the patient is requesting a change that is not possible, the surgeon must discuss this with the patient. In this interaction the surgeon should point out other recommendations for change; between them, a plan should be established that will satisfy both. It is better not to operate on a patient than have an unhappy patient. (For additional discussion of patient selection for surgery, see Chapter 6.)

As part of planning, the surgeon must determine which of the following steps in a rhinoplasty are applicable to the particular patient: (1) exposure—"open" vs. "closed," (2) sculpting the nasal dorsum, (3) reshaping the tip, (4) revising the septum, (5) infracture, and (6) excision of "alar wedges." Not every patient requires all these steps. (Details of these various steps will be addressed in the section entitled "Surgical Procedure.")

Preoperative Preparation

Each surgeon should establish a technique and sequence for performing rhinoplasty. Rhinoplasties may be done with local anesthesia, which when combined with sedation, avoids endotracheal intubation as well as possible hemorrhage secondary to increased blood pressure during emergence from general anesthesia. Adequate preoperative sedation and the use of intraoperative intravenous medications such as midazolam (Versed), diazepam (Valium), etc., will relax the patient and make the application of the local anesthetic less painful. Topical application of cocaine or a mixture of tetracaine (Pontocaine) and epinephrine is also usually used, primarily for vasoconstriction. Infraorbital nerve blocks, infiltration of the glabella, or infiltration in the area of the nasal spine and beneath the alae with local anesthetic solution will provide adequate anesthesia. Following blocks, the dorsum of the nose is infiltrated subcutaneously with the epinephrine-containing solution for bleeding control.

Surgical Approaches

Until recently rhinoplasty has been done primarily through incisions between the upper and lower lateral cartilages ("intercartilaginous incisions") on each side that were carried downward between the septum and columella ("transfixion incision"). In this approach, the superior borders of the alar cartilages are trimmed after downward eversion. A variation of this technique is a "bucket-handle" incision, where the intercartilaginous and transfixion incisions are made along with a rim incision at the border of the vibrissae. This bipedicle flap of mucoperichondrium and cartilage is freed and brought out of the nose for alterations to be made (Fig 18–2). With both of these approaches, orientation is difficult to learn since trimming of the cartilages is carried out with less than ideal visualization and the cartilages are not in their normal positions.

More recently, the use of "open" rhinoplasty with an incision across the columella has allowed visualization of the nasal cartilages, bone, and septum in their normal positions. Some surgeons feel that this "open" approach allows a better result in difficult rhinoplasties particularly for less experienced surgeons, but leaves a visible scar. Both the "open" and "closed" approaches have great popularity.

The nose is primarily skin and fat covering a cartilaginous (lower) and bony (upper) framework. The congenital dorsal "hump" consists of approximately 50% nasal bone and 50% nasal cartilage (see Fig 18–1). To remove

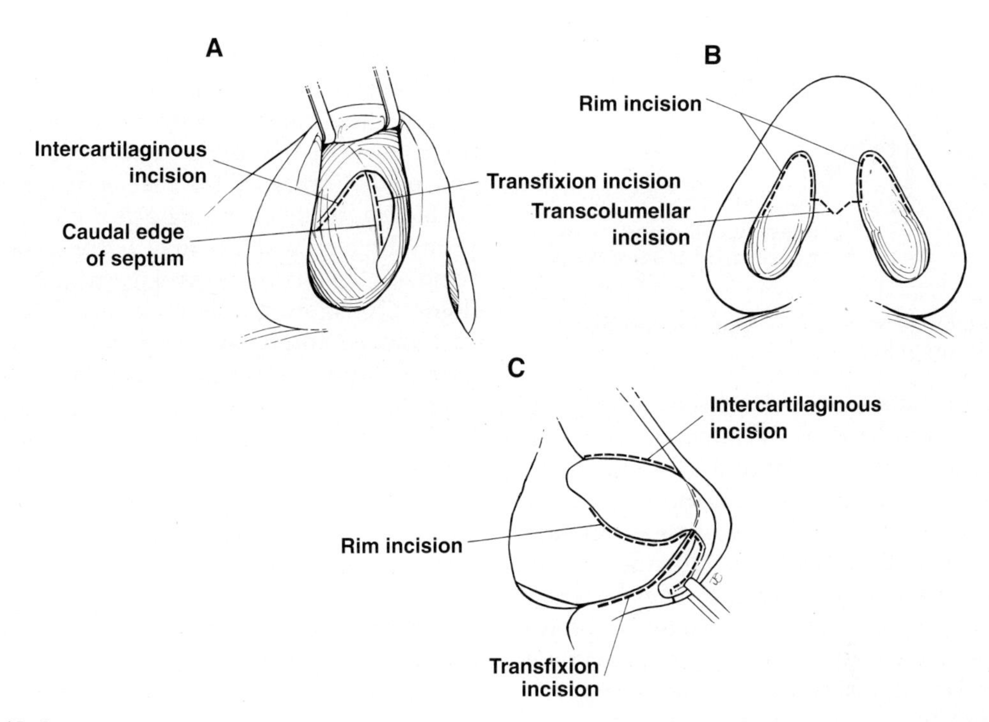

FIG 18–2.
A, the intercartilaginous and transfixion incisions. **B,** incision for open rhinoplasty. **C,** intercartilaginous and rim incisions to create a bipedicle flap.

the hump and make the nose smaller and/or narrower, the framework is reduced in its vertical and horizontal dimensions. If the patient's nasal skin is thick with prominent sebaceous glands, it may not adequately shrink postoperatively to fit the framework or permit visualization of the underlying changes, and the nasal tip may still be larger than the patient desires. The limitations placed on the postoperative appearance of the nose by thicker skin should be explained in advance to the patient. It is advisable to be conservative with resection of cartilage and soft tissue in the early stages of learning rhinoplasty, for it is easier to do a second procedure to take off more than to overresect and subsequently reconstruct. Care should be taken to remove as little nasal lining as possible since redundant nasal lining will shrink but resection of too much may cause increased scarring, nasal tip deformity, or nasal airway compromise.

Surgical Procedure

1. *Exposure of the structures.*—The vibrissae may be trimmed while waiting for the effects of the injectable anesthetic. The chosen incision is made and the skin and fat elevated from the upper lateral cartilages and nasal bones. Adequate freeing of the dorsal skin to allow hump removal is essential, but dissection should not be carried far down onto the nasal bones, or the bones will become unstable when fractured. The nasal mucosa at the junction of the upper lateral cartilages and the septum is dissected downward on either side of the septum (Fig 18–3). This allows the bone and cartilage cuts to remain isolated from the nasal cavity.

2. *Sculpting the dorsum.*—The cartilaginous and bony hump can be removed with a saw, guarded chisel, or rasp. Initial hump removal with a saw or chisel should be conservative because more can be removed than with a bone rasp. The bone edges are smoothed, and the dorsum of the cartilaginous septum is trimmed straight with a scalpel or scissors.

After the hump is removed, there is a space between the nasal bones/upper lateral cartilages and the septum. Separation of the nasal bones from the septum bilaterally may be completed by using a straight osteotome

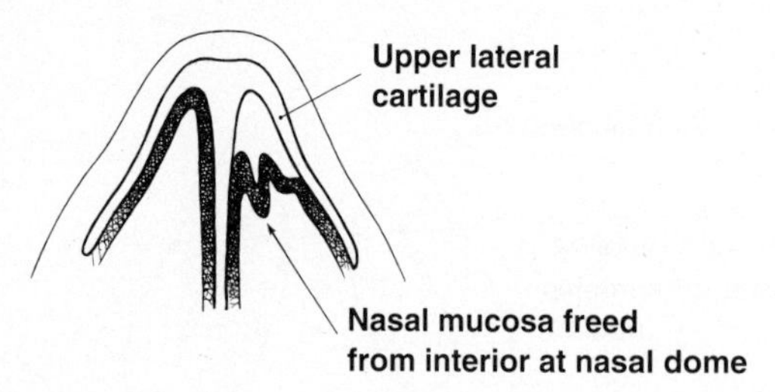

FIG 18–3.
The nasal mucosa removed from the internal dome of the nose.

(Fig 18–4). Subsequently it will be necessary to cut the nasal bone at the junction with the maxilla and then infracture to close the open dorsum (see "Infracture," below). The anterior borders of the upper lateral cartilages can then be trimmed flush with the dorsum of the septum. If the upper lateral cartilages overlap the septum, they can cause residual supratip fullness. If the midportion of the nose over the upper lateral cartilages is wide, soft tissue attached to the outer surface of the upper lateral cartilages should be removed to thin the nose. If following hump removal the dorsum cannot be made smooth, a temporalis fascia or dermal graft may be necessary to cover the irregular edges.

3. ***Reshaping the tip.***—Attention is then directed to the alar cartilages. If the tip is to be made smaller, the cephalad borders of the alar cartilages are removed bilaterally, with 5 mm of caudal cartilage left for tip support. If the tip is wide, fat can be removed from between the alar cartilage domes and/or sutures may be used to approximate the domes. Weakening of the dome with small alternating cuts in the superior and inferior borders will narrow the tip by making the angle between the lateral and medial crura of the alar cartilage more acute (Fig 18–5). If the nasal tip is long and protruding or wide, it may be necessary to remove a rectangle of cartilage from the alar dome. To shorten the nose, cartilage may be removed from the upper medial crus; to narrow the nose, cartilage may be removed from the medial portion of the lateral crus; and to shorten and narrow the nose, cartilage is removed from both areas (Fig 18–5). Complete transection of the cartilage is usually not done but may be necessary in an individual with thick nasal skin or a very large nose.

Care should be taken in a patient with thin nasal skin, for the cut edges of the alar cartilages may be visible through the skin, or "pinching" of the tip may occur. Unless an open rhinoplasty is performed with the cartilages in the normal position, the cut edges of the dome cartilages should not be sutured together, for if they are sutured incorrectly, irregularity of the tip may occur.

4. ***Revising the septum.***—To elevate the tip and shorten the nose it is necessary to remove a few millimeters or more of the caudal border of the septal cartilage after separating the mucoperichondrium (see Fig 18–2). In a patient with a deviated nose secondary to trauma, the cartilage has "memory," and it is difficult to get the septal

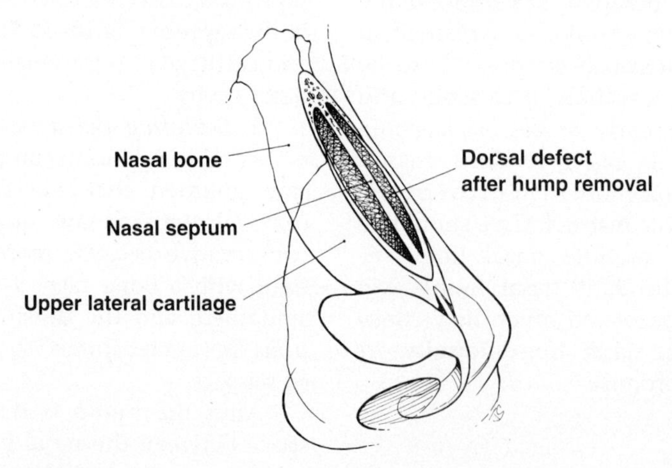

FIG 18–4.
The open roof of the nose following hump removal.

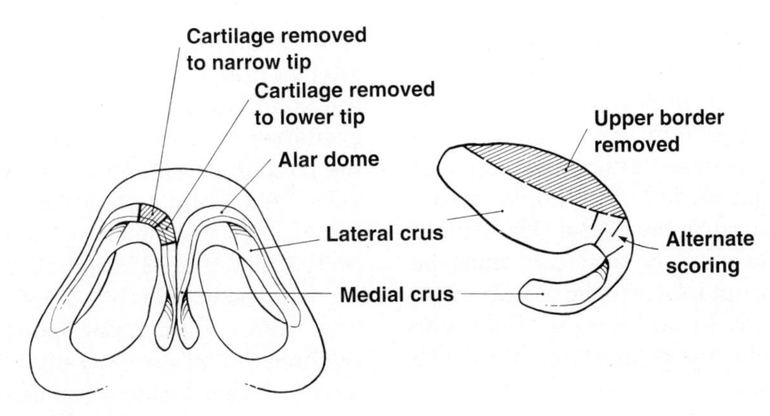

FIG 18–5.
Methods of weakening the alar cartilage and narrowing the nasal tip.

cartilage to remain straight. Therefore, after straightening the septum, it is frequently useful to place a fragment of removed alar or septal cartilage on the concave side of the nose to fill the concavity that will recur.

5. ***Infracture.***—The nasal bones are cut from the maxillary bone near the end of the operation since chisel or saw use will result in bleeding; the swelling and ecchymosis produced by the osteotomy can interfere with other operative steps. Combined infracture and outfracture of the nasal bones with instability of the nasal bones should be avoided. In most cases, infracture with finger pressure only at the desired level of fracture from the frontal bone is necessary. A 2-mm chisel can be used to score the nasal bone where fracture is desired.

Some surgeons prefer to close the various incisions at this point. A transcolumellar incision should be closed with fine nylon and a rim incision with either fine nylon or rapidly absorbing gut suture. The transfixation incision is closed with chromic catgut, and the intercartilaginous incision can be closed with similar suture or left open for drainage.

6. ***Alar wedges.***—After infracture, blood and fluid are evacuated from the nose by pressure, and the result is observed. At this point the final decision is made as to whether wedges of tissue should be removed from the nasal floor to narrow the base of the nose. In general, the nasal tip, when viewed from below, should be an equilateral triangle. If during the course of the other steps the distal tip has been lowered, the base of the triangle may appear wider. Therefore, small wedges of skin and subcutaneous tissue removed from just medial to the alar base will narrow the base of the triangle and restore an appropriate shape.

Once the surgical steps have been completed, tape or Steri-Strips are applied over the dorsum of the nose and around the tip. It is important to avoid strangulation and to allow swelling to separate the tape rather than strangulate the tip skin. Many different splint materials are available for placement over the nose to maintain the bony infracture.

Small nasal packs coated with ointment are used to approximate the intracartilaginous incisions for 24 to 48 hours. Care should be taken to not displace the infracture or open the intercartilaginous incisions with the packs. The nasal splint is left in place for 5 to 7 days. Some surgeons use a small padded metal splint over the nasal bones for 3 more weeks when the patient is sleeping or wearing glasses to prevent displacement of the fractured nasal bones. Preoperatively the patient should be told that the nose will be swollen for 4 to 6 months, thus delaying final evaluation of the result. Approximately 10% of rhinoplasties will require a secondary procedure to remove irregularities or further revise the result. Patients should be informed of this fact preoperatively.

Secondary Rhinoplasty

Secondary rhinoplasties require a careful preoperative analysis and a cautious surgical approach. If another surgeon performed the primary procedure, review of the operative notes becomes an important part of the preoperative evaluation. Secondary rhinoplasty varies from small "touch-ups" to major revision. As a rule, secondary rhinoplasties are more difficult because the dorsal skin is more adherent to the cartilage and care must be taken to not disrupt the cartilage or skin when gaining exposure. In addition, patients who are unhappy with the primary result may be difficult to satisfy.

Techniques in Secondary Rhinoplasty

The open rhinoplasty approach is more commonly used for complicated secondary procedures. Open rhinoplasty allows all structures to be visualized and corrected *in their natural position.* Cartilage grafts to provide tip projection and definition are sometimes necessary for a primary rhinoplasty, but they are more commonly used in secondary rhinoplasty. These grafts are usually taken from nasal septum or ear cartilage. One approach utilizes a shield-shaped cartilage graft to give projection to the nasal tip; this graft can be held in place with sutures to the medial crus of the alar cartilage and by transcutaneous sutures through the skin of the nose. Another method employs a rectangular cartilage graft on top of the alar cartilages for the same purpose. Dorsal cartilage grafts may be necessary when too much dorsum has previously been removed; cartilage "spreader" grafts may be necessary between the upper lateral cartilages and the septum if the nasal valve has been compromised. A variety of other steps may be employed to achieve secondary correction.

Complications

The most common complication of a rhinoplasty is supratip fullness ("polly tip"). This deformity may result from a variety of causes, including inadequate elevation of the nasal tip, hematoma with scar formation above the nasal tip, or improper resection of the dorsum.

Infection is a rare complication, but if the patient complains of discomfort beneath the splint or inordinate swelling around the splint after 24 hours, it may be necessary to remove the splint in order to perform an adequate examination. If there is evidence of infection, the patient is treated with appropriate antibiotics. Frequently a secondary revision is necessary after the infection has resolved, especially if the bones become displaced.

Nasal skin slough is a potential complication from a tight nasal splint or inordinate swelling. Metal postoperative splints seem to have a higher incidence of skin slough. Postoperative bleeding may occur, especially with pack removal, and the nose may need to be carefully repacked to avoid displacing the fractured nasal bones. Ecchymosis and swelling of the eyes are common following fracture of the nasal bones and may be minimized by use of head elevation and ice. If a plaster splint is used, it should not become wet and weakened from moist cold packs.

The dorsum of the nose will be numb for several months following rhinoplasty, and the patient must be warned to avoid excess sun exposure.

CLEFT LIP NASAL DEFORMITY

Techniques for repair of a cleft lip have advanced to the point where primary repair commonly produces a result that is aesthetically quite good. Advances in the primary surgical correction of a cleft lip *nasal* deformity have also been made, but residual deformity is very common.

Anatomy

The severity of the cleft lip nasal deformity may vary significantly, but the underlying structural abnormalities are similar (Fig 18–6). Deformities include general defects of the cleft-side lower lateral cartilage, the nasal septum, the columella, and the nasal tip; malpositioning of the maxillary segments; and deformity of the orbicularis muscle and the entire nasal pyramid. Different authors have attributed greater or lesser significance to the different aspects of the cleft lip nasal deformity; as a consequence, a great variety of

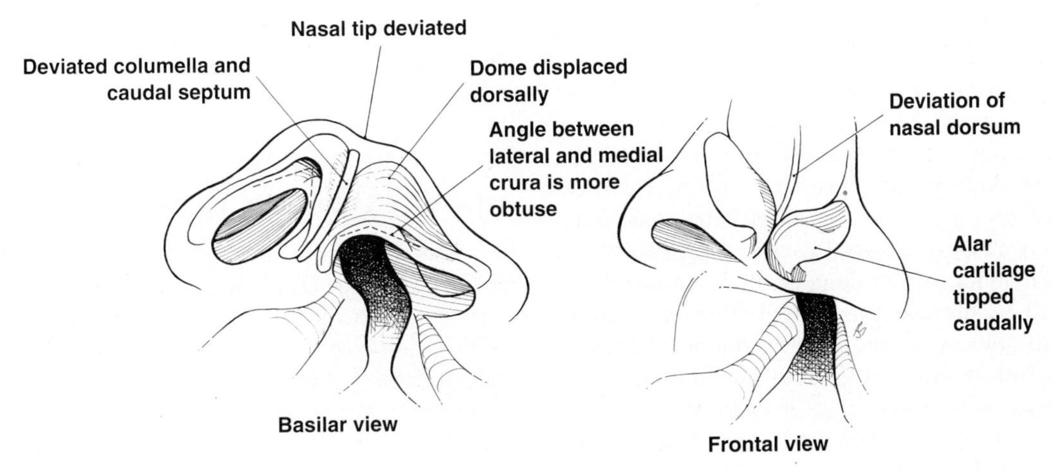

FIG 18–6.
Typical deformities of the cleft lip and nose.

repair techniques, each emphasizing correction of one or another of the structural abnormalities, now exists.

Surgical Principles

Asymmetry of the nasal tip, deficiency of projection, and deviation of the dorsum are the major aesthetic abnormalities of the cleft lip-nose; airway obstruction, speech abnormalities, and dental occlusal problems may be functional components. Both aesthetic and functional problems should be treated. The deformity may be addressed at the time of the primary cleft lip repair, prior to the start of school, during puberty, or in adulthood. Historically it was feared that early nasal surgery would interfere with growth, but this concern has lessened. Each surgeon must determine whether surgical repair of the small and delicate nasal cartilages of a child is superior to correction of the more developed structures of adulthood, even though uncorrected development may lead to more obvious deformity. To date, there is no good evidence that early surgical correction gives a better final result. Surgery prior to school is primarily done to avoid social problems.

Generally, osteotomy is not done during preschool correction. After the age of 16 years a formal rhinoplasty may be safely done, with steps that may include septal resection, osteotomy, cartilage or bone grafting, and extensive revisions of the alar and upper lateral cartilages to achieve symmetry. As a rule, the more severe the deformity, the earlier its correction should begin.

Surgical Technique

To restore nasal symmetry the alar cartilages should be equalized in size, repositioned, suspended, or augmented with cartilage grafts. Changes in the "normal" side of the nasal tip may be necessary to obtain symmetry. External incisions may allow better visualization of the nasal cartilages and improve the final result. To modify the alar cartilages it may be helpful to free them from both the vestibular mucous membrane and the external skin of the nose. Once the cartilaginous framework has been returned to as "normal" a position as possible, the skin is redraped over the framework. If the skin is not dissected free from the framework, it will interfere with repositioning. Maintaining the alar cartilages in the desired position usually requires suturing of the cartilages together, suturing of the cartilage to the opposite side, or cartilage suspension sutures brought out through the nasal skin. Alar columella webbing can frequently be corrected with excision of a portion of the web. Z-plasties may be necessary to correct the webbing in the lateral vestibule on the cleft side. It may also require repositioning of the lateral crus of the ala cartilage closer to the rim of the nostril. In all instances it is important to maintain the circumference of the cleft nasal orifice since it is extremely difficult to enlarge.

Cartilage augmentation of the cleft side of the nose may be necessary to adequately raise the dome. Cartilage for grafting may be obtained from the septum or the ear. A vertical cartilage graft in the columella has been advocated to elevate the tip when projection is inadequate. Cartilage grafts have also been used to elevate the nostril floor. Z-plasties, with one arm of the Z being the alar base and the other being tissue either lateral to or medial to the alar base, may be necessary to widen or narrow the nasal floor and alter the flare of the nostril.

Fracture of the nasal bones to obtain symmetry may involve both infracture and outfracture to allow enough mobility for the nasal bones to be brought into a symmetrical position. Dorsal grafts of cartilage or bone may be necessary to elevate the peak of the nasal triangle on the dorsum as well as on the tip. These may consist of cartilage obtained from the septum or ear or bone obtained from the calvarium or a rib.

AIRWAY OBSTRUCTION

Nasal airway obstruction may be the result of many causes, including septal deformities and turbinate abnormalities. In addition, a crooked septum may give rise to deviation of the external nasal structures. Therefore, submucous resection and septoplasty potentially improve both nasal appearance and function.

Surgical Principles

The septum is made up of thin segments of cartilage and bone, including a fixed (posterior) and a flexible (anterior) portion (Fig 18–7, A and B). Historically septal surgery

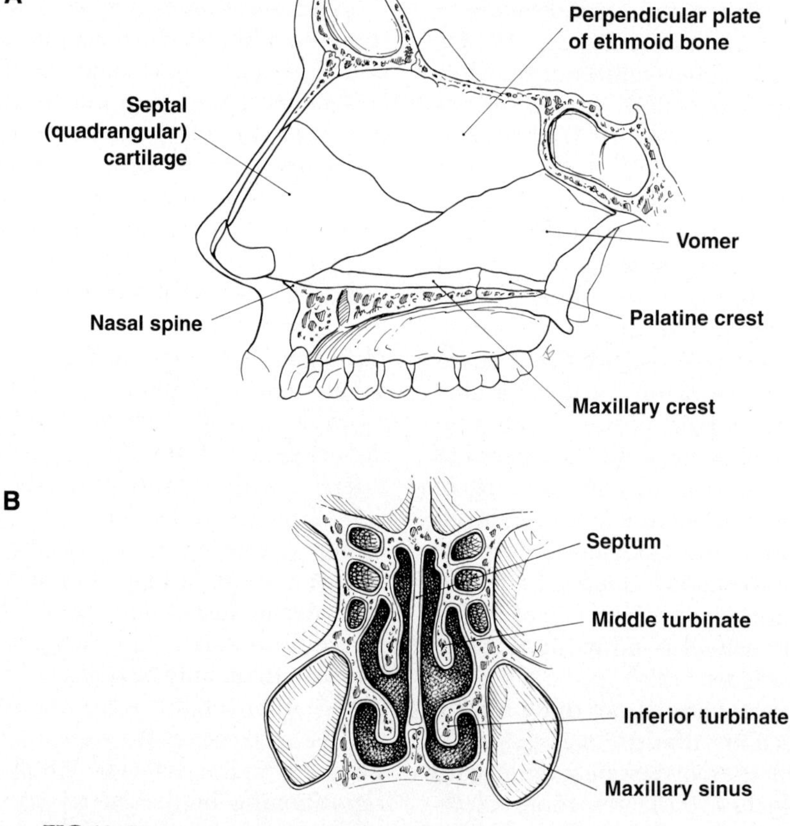

FIG 18–7.
A and **B,** internal nasal anatomy.

involved removal of large portions of cartilaginous and bony septum; in modern times, repositioning of cartilages and/or replacement of straightened cartilage and bone plus the use of various cartilage grafts has reduced the amount of tissue actually removed. With these newer approaches, the soft tissues of the nose and the respiratory epithelium are violated as little as possible in the correction of nasal airway obstruction, with a resultant reduction in complications.

Concern for interference with nasal growth has caused surgical procedures in children to be more conservative than in adults, but nasal obstruction has such a negative effect on the cardiopulmonary system that waiting for correction until after growth has ceased is not usually warranted. The aerodynamics of respiratory nasal airflow have an influence on the entire respiratory system and indirectly affect the metabolic function of body cells. Nasal obstruction diminishes lung compliance and alveolar oxygen concentration and can lead to chronic hypoxia.

Direct internal examination is essential to determine the causes of obstruction, although flow tests such as rhinomanometry may be helpful in the diagnosis and determination of the severity of airway obstruction. The most common cause of obstruction is a deviated or deflected nasal septum secondary to trauma or its sequelae. Congenital obstruction is possible. Injuries during growth may have more effect on the final structure of the nose than the same injury in adulthood. Allergies, neoplasm, and/or infection may also temporarily or permanently alter the nasal airway.

A variety of septal abnormalities exists: *deviation* most often involves the quadrangular cartilage and usually results in smooth, curving deformities; *deflection* is an angular deformity usually corresponding to an old fracture line; and *dislocation* represents partial or complete displacement from the V-shaped bony groove on the nasal floor.

Deviation of a portion of the septum to one side usually causes a compensatory deviation to the opposite side at another site and/or hypertrophy of the inferior and middle turbinate on the concave side. Prevention of septal deformities by acute reduction of septal fracture fragments gives a better result than secondary attempts at correction after healing has occurred.

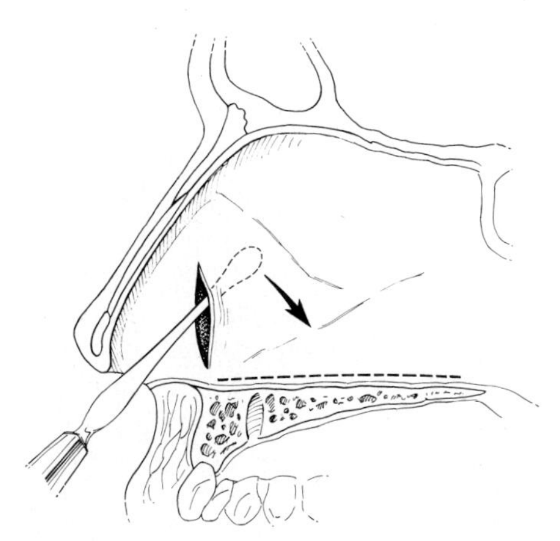

FIG 18–8.
An incision is made through the mucoperiochondrium and dissection carried posteriorly with an elevator. The *dashed line* along the floor of the nose indicates where an extension of the mucoperiochondrial incision may be made if necessary.

Surgical Procedure

An intranasal incision is made through the mucosa and perichondrium above the inferior margin of the quadrangular cartilage, usually on the right side (for a right-handed surgeon) or sometimes on the convex side. A plane is dissected between the perichondrium and cartilage over the area of deformity (Fig 18–8). An incision is made through the cartilage to reach the submucoperichondrial plane on the opposite side, and the mucoperichondrium is dissected from the deformed area of cartilage bilaterally (Fig 18–9). The mucoperiosteum is also freed from the bone over all areas of deformity. Care must be taken to avoid perforations on both sides of the mucoperichondrium or mucoperiosteum at the same level, or a permanent transseptal perforation may result. When two acute perforations occur at the same level, a piece of straightened cartilage can be placed between the perforations to obliterate the defect; healing without transseptal perforation will occur in most cases.

When the mucoperichondrium is free from the deformed cartilage bilaterally (Fig

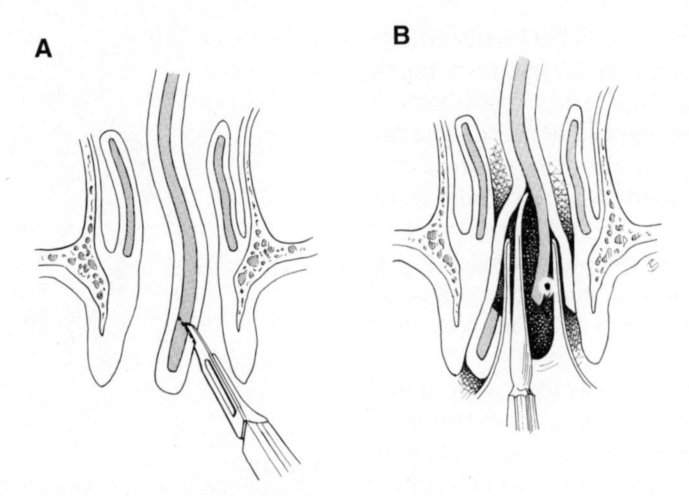

FIG 18–9.
A, a knife is used to perforate the cartilaginous septum. **B,** the mucoperiochondrium is dissected free from the cartilage on the opposite side with a Freer elevator.

18–10), a decision must be made whether to straighten the cartilage in place or remove it. Many times the dislocated footplate of the cartilage will be thick and hypertrophic; this must be removed to open the inferior portions of the airway. The superior cartilage can be removed, then scored or crushed until straight, and finally resituated between the mucoperichondrial walls to prevent septal flutter and stabilize the septum. Replacement of the straightened cartilage also helps to prevent scar contraction, which may cause external deformity or recurrent airway obstruction. If there is obstruction secondary to deviation or (more commonly) deflection of the vomer, the bone may be resected after the mucoperiosteum is freed bilaterally.

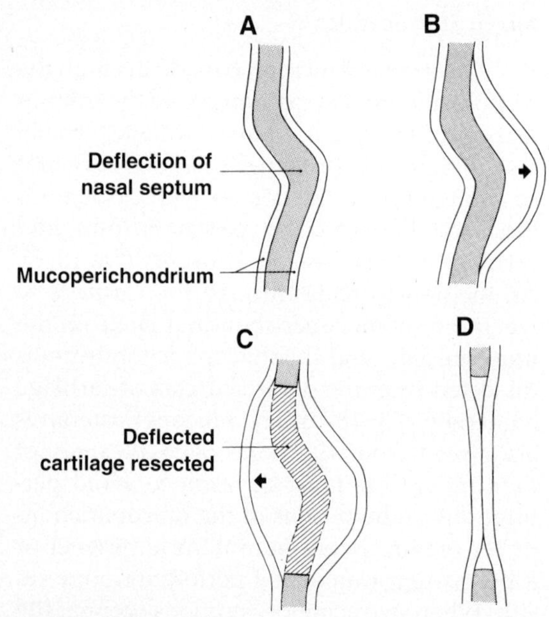

FIG 18–10.
Steps in submucus resection. **A,** deflection of the nasal septum is shown. **B,** the mucoperichondrium on one side is dissected free. **C,** both sides are dissected free from the cartilage. **D,** the deflected cartilage has been resected. (This cartilage can be straightened and replaced if desired.)

Nasal airway packs may be placed to hold the mucoperichondrium together, or absorbable mattress sutures can be placed through the walls of mucoperichondrium to obliterate the dead space. Usually nasal packs are coated with ointment to allow easier removal. The packs are left in place for up to 7 days and then gently removed. Occasionally bleeding will occur after pack removal, and repacking will be necessary for a few more days.

Turbinate Management

Protrusion of the turbinates from the lateral nasal wall increases the mucosal surface. Under normal circumstances, the turbinates control the heat and moisture exchange of the inspired air by their size change. Septal deviation frequently causes hypertrophy of the turbinate on the concave side of the deviation and makes it difficult to bring the septum to the midline without causing complete obstruction. In such cases, submucosal turbinectomy or crushing of the turbinate may be indicated. This is done by making an incision over the margin of the inferior turbinate and dissecting the mucosa free from the bone, followed by removal of the bone. Fracture of the turbinate bone downward out of the obstructing position may also be done. Cautery or injection of steroids into the turbinate to shrink the mucosa has also been advocated, but its benefit is usually only temporary.

Postoperative complications such as persistent nasal airway obstruction usually result from inadequate correction of the septal deformity, recurrent obstruction is usually due to scarring or reangulation of replaced cartilage, and nasal septal perforation often occurs after bilateral surgical perforation of the mucoperichondrium.

THE AGING FACE

The aging process of the face results from intrinsic changes in the skin combined with the effects of extrinsic factors. The intrinsic changes involve thinning of the skin, decreased elasticity, increased susceptibility to ultraviolet light, and increased occurrence of cutaneous malignancies. Extrinsic effects are primarily from sun damage, gravity, and factors such as smoking (which causes chronic vasoconstriction). Progressive loss of skin turgor coupled with the effects of gravity causes the skin to hang and permits bulging of subcutaneous tissues that have lost support. Upper eyelid skin redundancy and lateral "crow's-feet" usually appear in the fourth decade, while nasolabial folds, glabellar lines, and forehead wrinkles become more noticeable in the fifth decade. By the sixth decade the neck is often wrinkled and the jawline less distinct, and in the seventh decade wrinkling and ptosis occur in almost all Caucasians.

Several skin disorders may be manifested as or contribute to premature skin aging such as Ehlers-Danlos syndrome, cutis laxa, progeria, Werner syndrome, and pseudoxanthoma elasticum. (For additional discussion, see Chapter 13.)

In today's society we find that more and more individuals have the sense that they look older than they feel. When surgery is contemplated, realistic expectations are necessary to achieve a satisfied patient. Individuals who have difficulty describing their problem, who ascribe various personal inadequacies to the aging process, or who are desirous of surgery primarily for the benefit of another person are generally not good surgical candidates. (For further discussion of patient selection, see Chapter 6.)

Preoperative Evaluation

As with all preoperative evaluations, an appropriate history and a careful physical examination are important. A history of hypertension, aspirin use, or smoking are important because they are associated with a higher complication rate. Physical examination should proceed in an orderly and reproducible manner (e.g., beginning at the hairline and moving down the face to the neck). The level of the eyebrows and wrinkling of the forehead should be assessed. The nasolabial folds, the jawline and jowl areas, as well as the submental area and neck should all be evaluated. Voluntary contraction of the platysma to determine decussation across the midline should be examined. The nature and extent of skin wrinkles are noted. Preoperative photographs permit further study and are essential to document the patient's unoperated appearance, particularly if any medical/legal problems occur postoperatively.

Patient Counseling

It is essential to realistically communicate to the patient what can and cannot be expected from rhytidectomy. Forehead wrinkles, glabella wrinkles, crow's-feet, and malar pouches can be improved, but permanent wrinkles cannot be eliminated. The most difficult areas to improve by face-lifting are the nasolabial folds and the "marionette lines"; these can never be completely erased. An acute cervicomental angle may be aesthetically desirable, but a low anterior hyoid bone may prevent its creation. Fine wrinkles of the skin are not eliminated by a face-lift and may require a concurrent or subsequent chemical peel.

Anesthesia

Preoperative sedation should provide a relaxed, cooperative patient. If desired, a face-lift can be done under local anesthesia with preoperative and intraoperative sedation (frequently intravenous diazepam [Valium] and midozolam [Versed]). The presence of an anesthesiologist may allow for more profound sedation. Lidocaine (0.5%) or bupivacaine (0.25% or 0.5%) with epinephrine (1:200,000) is used for local infiltration. Epinephrine allows an increased total dosage of the local agent, prolongs the duration of anesthesia, and decreases the operative blood loss. The local anesthetic solution is injected in stages, with approximately 7 to 10 minutes between infiltration and incision.

"Classic" Rhytidectomy Surgical Procedure

The "classic" facial rhytidectomy consists of extensive subcutaneous undermining and is still used by many practitioners, especially in young patients with a thin neck and a good cervicomental angle. However, this does not routinely correct the effects of gravity on the tissues deep to the skin.

The hair in the temporal and postauricular area is combed away from the incision line, and 1 to 1 ½ cm of hair may be trimmed. The hair can be tied in bundles or ointment applied to keep it out of the incision. After the incision lines are drawn, the skin of the face is infiltrated with local anesthetic solution.

The incision starts in the temporal skin approximately 4 to 5 cm behind the hairline and 6 to 8 cm above the ear. Upon reaching the superior root of the helix it continues downward in the preauricular skin crease either anterior or posterior to the tragus, traverses the attachment of the ear lobule to the face, and then proceeds superiorly onto the ear 2 to 3 mm anterior to the posterior sulcus. At the level of the postauricular ligament the incision turns posteriorly into the hairline (Fig 18–11). The incision in the hairline is long enough to allow redraping of the neck skin and leave only a minimal "dog-ear" in the scalp.

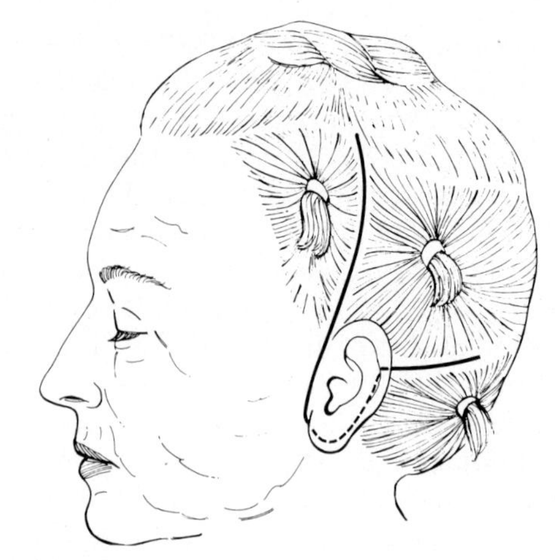

FIG 18–11.
The face-lift incision.

The incisions are made parallel to the hair follicles to prevent injury and hair loss. The incision in the temporal area extends to the temporalis fascia and then superficial to the fascia but deep to the hair follicles. Until experience is gained it is safer to use scissors to start the preauricular dissection by staying in the fat plane between the skin and the fascia of the face. Dissection is carried approximately to the midcheek. Skin and fat are dissected from the platysma and sternocleidomastoid muscle in the lateral portion of the neck. Care is taken to avoid injury to the great auricular nerve, which is just deep to the platysma and beneath the sternocleidomastoid fascia, 6.5 cm below the external auditory meatus. The skin of the neck is dissected free in the fatty plane while staying superficial to the platysma muscle (to avoid injury to the marginal mandibular nerve).

Following adequate dissection to allow smoothing of the wrinkles with traction, the flaps are advanced in a superior and posterior direction. With the amount of tension required to give the desired result, one suture is placed superior and one posterior to the ear to maintain the desired tension on the skin flaps. Care is taken to avoid rotation of the sideburns above the ear and leave a hairless area. It is sometimes necessary to excise a triangle of skin below the sideburns to prevent too much superior and posterior displacement. A suction drain can be placed if desired. Interrupted sutures are then placed beside the traction sutures to help distribute the skin tension and decrease the chance of skin slough. Redundant skin and scalp are excised prior to closing the wounds.

Superficial Musculoaponeurotic System/ Platysma Rhytidectomy

It has become apparent that many patients have a variety of problems besides the simple skin laxity that the "classic" lift corrects. These include deep tissue laxities, fat deposits in the submandibular and submental areas, microgenia, central platysma bands, and facial asymmetry. The superficial musculoaponeurotic system (SMAS) rhytidectomy is a technique that when combined with other ancillary procedures, is reported to give better, more long-lasting correction of facial laxity and associated deformities. Recently, facial rhytidectomy procedures at an even deeper plane, including subperiosteal face-lift, have been described. The superiority of such procedures over the SMAS-type lift has not been confirmed.

Anatomy

The SMAS is a deep tissue layer that lies in continuity with the frontal parietal fascia superiorly and the platysma muscle inferiorly. It is attached to overlying skin by numerous septa. The platysma muscle is a thin flat muscle lying beneath the skin and subcutaneous fat of the anterior and lateral portions of the neck. The main body of the platysma is innervated by the cervical branch, and the upper portion is innervated by branches of the marginal mandibular branch of the facial nerve. At its anterior border there are attachments to the depressor muscles of the lower lip that function synchronously. In most patients the platysma muscles decussate across the midline in the submental region and form a sling beneath the chin.

Surgical Technique

In contrast to the "classic" lift, this procedure requires relatively limited skin undermining. The SMAS and the platysma muscle are dissected free in continuity and advanced posteriorly as a single flap to tighten the deep structures of the face and neck. In some patients removal of submental fat, whether subcutaneous or between and beneath the medial borders of the platysma, is necessary to recreate the chin-neck angle. Liposuction may be used to remove excess submental fat for contouring prior to muscle plication or in place of plication when decussation of the muscles is present. The absence of decussation across the midline destroys the platysmal sling effect and allows a vertical fold of skin to appear over the anterior border of the platysma. To create a sling effect, the platysma muscles can be sutured together in the midline. As an alternate or adjunctive procedure, a portion of the anterior platysmal band can be incised or resected. The lateral border of the platysma muscle is then dissected free from the anterior border of the sternocleidomastoid, the external jugular vein, and the great auricular nerve and sutured posterior to the sternocleidomastoid fascia. Care must be taken to avoid injury to the great auricular nerve with dissection or sutures.

The SMAS is initially incised at the level of the inferior border of the zygomatic arch (Fig 18–12, A). This incision is 4 to 5 cm long and is carried to within 0.5 to 1 cm of the tragus. It is then carried downward toward the mandibular angle and connected with the lateral border of the previously elevated platysma. The SMAS and platysma are freed from the deep structures anteriorly. The SMAS is carefully elevated from the parotid gland to at least its anterior border. After the SMAS/ platysma flap is adequately freed, it is rotated and secured superiorly and posteriorly to lift the jawline and lower third of the face (Fig 18–12, B). Redundant SMAS and platysma are excised. Freeing the SMAS in the malar area is advocated by some to lift the upper anterior aspect of the cheek.

Postoperative Care

A bulky gauze dressing around the ear and over the cheek is held with an elastic dressing. This should not be a pressure dressing, which could increase the chance of skin

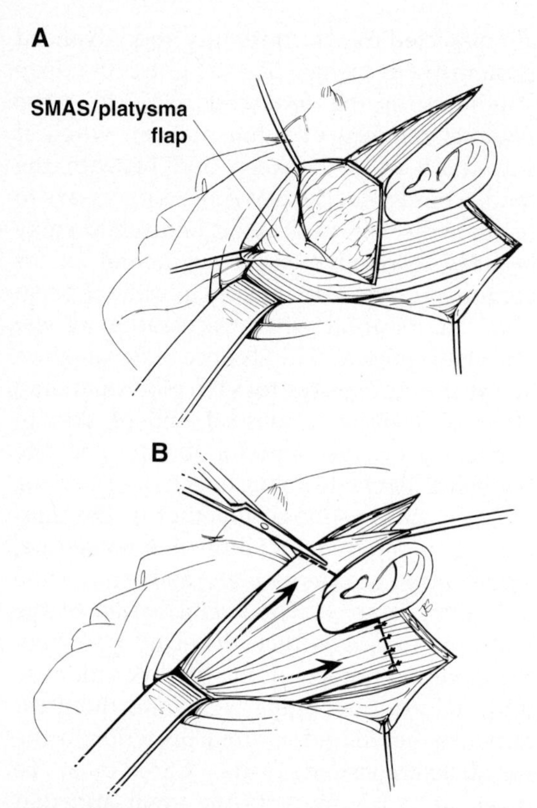

FIG 18–12.
A, the SMAS/platysma flap elevation. **B,** rotation and advancement of the SMAS/platysma flap posteriorly and superiorly.

loss; an elastic dressing helps the flaps conform in their new position. It is important to minimize retching, vomiting, and any masticatory movements postoperatively and to maintain at least 30 degrees of head elevation for 24 to 48 hours. In 2 or 3 days the patient is permitted to wash the hair and suture lines. The patient is instructed to use sun blocks on areas of skin that are anesthetic and may be easily sunburned.

Secondary Rhytidectomy

Secondary face-lifting as a rule removes less skin than the primary procedure and requires extra attention to tissue planes and facial nerve locations that may have been distorted by previous surgery. In addition, hair-bearing areas, particularly the sideburns, are at a higher risk of becoming malpositioned. Otherwise the procedure is similar to a primary face-lift.

Male Face-Lift

Male face-lifts have become increasingly popular; however, the scars are harder to hide and may be socially less acceptable. Therefore, it is more important in the male to not diminish or eliminate the sideburn and to hide the scars behind the ear and in the hair as much as possible. It is also important to emphasize that the patient may need to wear his hair longer than in the past to conceal the scars. Dissection of the flaps in the male is generally more difficult, and there is more intraoperative and postoperative bleeding because of the beard.

Complications

Hematoma is the most frequent significant complication of rhytidectomy and may vary from a small collection of blood found when the swelling goes down to a large expanding clot that can cause skin flap necrosis. The incidence of significant postoperative hematoma is approximately 2% to 5% and may be higher if perioperative hypertension occurs. The rate of hematoma formation is significantly higher in men than in women. An expanding hematoma must be recognized early and the sutures removed immediately to prevent vascular compromise of the skin. The hematoma must then be evacuated, the bleeding stopped, and the skin resutured.

Skin slough either behind the ear or extending onto the neck is usually superficial and generally heals with minimal or no residual scarring. Full-thickness loss usually occurs in the postauricular and mastoid areas where the advanced skin is the thinnest and the tension is the highest. The incidence of skin slough is related to thin skin flaps, excess tension on the wound closure, cigarette smoking, and hematoma formation. When skin slough occurs, careful observation rather than surgical debridement is advised. The slough area will contract dramatically as the eschar separates, although the scar may need later revision.

Sensory nerve injury most commonly produces numbness of the lower two thirds of the ear from compromise of the great auricular nerve. Numbness is almost universal a few centimeters anterior to the ear, secondary to skin undermining. Injury of the facial nerve is uncommon; when present, it is frequently due to local trauma to the nerve rather than division. If nerve transection is recognized intraoperatively, immediate microsurgical repair is indicated. Alopecia occasionally occurs after a face-lift either from tension on suture lines or injury to the base of hair follicles as a result of dissection or suturing. Hypertrophic scarring may occur and is most frequent in the postauricular incisions.

Other Associated Procedures

A recessed chin (microgenia) may be present, and a chin implant or mentoplasty can give marked enhancement of facial contour. Malar implants may also improve and accentuate the facial planes. Buccal fat pad excision through either the intraoral approach or the face-lift incision may help to eliminate fullness of the cheeks. Injections of fat and collagen give only temporary filling of wrinkles; long-term improvement (>1 year) is rare, which makes the use of these methods controversial.

A chemical peel may be indicated to treat fine wrinkles, superficial keratoses, or abnormal pigmentation. The best candidates for chemical peeling are patients with fair complexions since patients with darker skin have more problems with postoperative pigmentation. The most commonly used agent for chemical peeling has been phenol. However, there is an increasing interest in trichloracetic acid (TCA) peels. These are more superficial than phenol peels but have less morbidity and a shorter recovery time as well as a less dramatic result. Chemical peeling in the perioral area may be done in conjunction with a face-lift, but chemical peels over elevated face flaps should not be done since flap necrosis may be increased. Chemical peeling of the full face should be performed after the skin has recovered from the face-lift (i.e., 3 to 6 months later). The most common systemic complication of phenol peels is cardiac arrhythmia. To decrease cardiac problems, peeling should be done with a series of applications over the period of an hour in a well-ventilated room. Hypopigmentation and hyperpigmentation are the most common complications of chemical peels. Phenol peels are occasionally followed by hypertrophic scars, about which the patient should be counseled preoperatively. Dermabrasion has limited benefit in treating an aging face. (For additional discussion of chemical peels, see Chapters 5 and 13.)

Forehead- and brow-lifts are frequently done in conjunction with a face-lift to correct forehead wrinkling, brow ptosis, and lateral upper eyelid ptosis. Often ptosis of the forehead and eyebrows is the main cause for upper eyelid fullness and redundant skin. While a brow- and forehead-lift may restore the eyebrow to its proper position over the supraorbital rim, an upper lid blepharoplasty may still be needed. The frontalis muscle fibers are oriented vertically and cover most of the forehead. Contraction of the frontalis muscle elevates the eyebrows and over time gives rise to transverse forehead lines. The corrugator supercilii, procerus, and orbicularis oculi muscles counteract the pull of the frontalis muscle. The corrugator supercilii and procerus muscles are commonly resected with the brow-lift procedure.

The brow-lift is done through either a coronal incision or an incision in front of the hairline in a patient with a high hairline. The dissection is usually done superficial to the periosteum while avoiding injury to the supraorbital neurovascular bundles (which could produce anesthesia of the forehead). The fascial attachments to the supraorbital rim are frequently divided to allow elevation of the brow. A 1-cm-wide transverse portion of the frontalis muscle can be resected above the supraorbital nerves (carefully preserving the nerves), or the frontalis muscle can be crosshatched to decrease its functional pull. The forehead is then pulled upward and the tension adjusted so that the eyebrows are properly positioned. Complications, which are rare, include hematoma, alopecia, and decreased sensation of the forehead. Decreased sensation posterior to the incision occurs in all brow-lifts.

ALOPECIA/HAIR TRANSPLANTATION

The scalp consists of five layers; the most superficial is the skin, then the subcutaneous tissue, the epicranium (galea aponeurotica), the subepicranial space, and finally the pericranium (Fig 18–13). Its blood supply has six components: the supratrochlear and supraorbital arteries (arising from the internal carotid artery) and the temporal, occipital, intermaxillary, posterior auricular arteries (arising from the external carotid system). The veins, as a rule, accompany these arteries and drain the scalp. Preservation of this blood supply to ensure perfusion of the scalp in alopecia surgery is essential.

Sensation of the scalp is mediated by the supratrochlear and supraorbital nerves in the frontal area, the zygomatic nerve in the temporal area, the auriculotemporal nerve over the parietal area, the great auricular and lesser occipital nerve behind the ear, and the greater occipital nerve to the occiput and crown of the head.

A hair is a collection of dead cells composed of keratin that is formed in the hair follicle and pushed outward. The hair follicle extends into the skin at an angle, and in some cases, i.e., with curly hair, it may be curved or angulated. Each hair follicle has a single muscle called the *arrector pili.* This muscle elevates the hair and expresses secretions from the sebaceous gland associated with the hair follicle. The living cells in the base of the hair follicle grow by mitotic activity and form a hair column that is pushed out of the hair follicle. The cells become dehydrated and are converted into keratin after they die. An adult scalp contains approximately 100,000 hairs that grow at approximately 1 cm per month.

Hair growth consists of three phases. The *anagen* phase exists in approximately 90% of the hair at any one time, lasts about 3 years, and is the active growth period. The *catagen* phase, an involutional period, lasts between 1 and 2 weeks. The final *telogen* phase lasts from 3 to 4 months; during this period, no hair is produced by the inactive follicle.

Lanugo hair is found on the fetus and is usually shed approximately a month before birth. Vellus hair replaces lanugo hair in the postnatal period and is short, soft, and sometimes pigmented. It is spread over much of the body surface. Terminal hair replaces the vellus hair in specific sites on the body and is longer, coarser, and more pigmented. In the areas of scalp that will become bald the vellus hairs fall out and are progressively replaced by hairs of less vigorous growth; this process continues until baldness results. The hair follicles are still present in baldness but produce only a fine hair shaft.

Androgenic alopecia (male pattern baldness) is the most common type of hair loss and is controlled by a single dominant sex-linked autosomal gene. However, for baldness to occur, initiating agents such as androgen must be present. Bald areas are most often seen over the crown and in the frontal areas of the scalp.

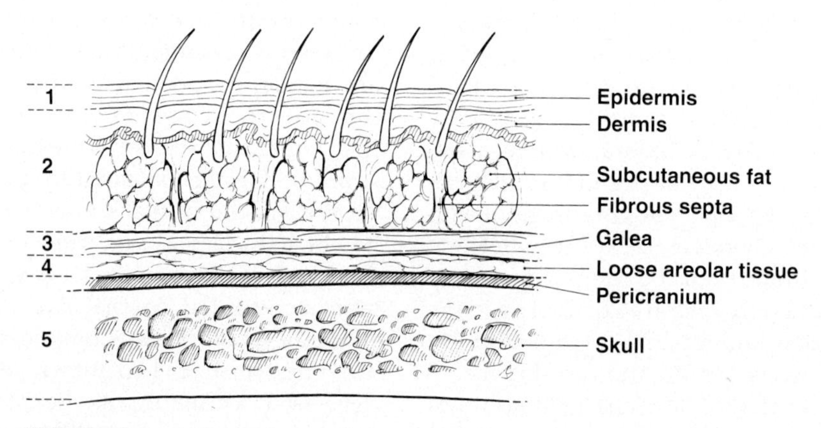

FIG 18–13.
The five layers of the scalp.

When a hair follicle is transplanted, it maintains the genetic capability to produce hair characteristic of the area of its original site rather than the area to which it has been moved. Therefore, hair taken from behind the ear and placed in the frontal area will produce hair until the other hair follicles behind the ear stop producing hair.

Medical treatment of male pattern baldness with minoxidil has been advocated, but controlled research studies indicate that only 10% of individuals treated with this agent show profuse enough growth of hair to continue its use. The drug is quite expensive, and when its use is discontinued, all previous benefits are lost.

Surgical Treatment

During surgical hair replacement, the anterior hairline is usually placed at an aesthetically acceptable level but not necessarily at the former hairline, thus requiring less hair transfer. Surgical treatment of male pattern baldness consists generally of three methods: hair-bearing free scalp *grafts,* scalp *flaps,* and scalp *reduction.*

Hair-Bearing Scalp Grafts

A patient with frontal hairline loss but good-quality hair is the best candidate for scalp grafts. In these patients, "plugs" of hair (actually, composite grafts) may be transplanted to deficient areas. Young individuals will have progressive loss, and the plugs that are placed may eventually become isolated. When a round punch is utilized, a slightly larger plug (e.g., 4 mm) is removed from the posterior inferior portion of the scalp and transplanted to a hole made by a slightly smaller (e.g., 3 mm) punch at the recipient site. It is important to leave enough length of hair in the graft to determine the direction of the hair growth. It is also important to hold the punch parallel to the hair shaft when taking the graft. Donor sites may be sutured or left open to heal by secondary intention. When creating the recipient sites it is critical to leave enough tissue between the holes to ensure adequate revascularization of the transplanted tissues. Enough space should be left so that a second group of plugs may be interspersed later.

Square or rectangular grafts may be used in place of round grafts. These are usually obtained by excision of a strip of scalp from the donor area and then cutting it into small squares or rectangles. The donor site can then be sutured. Square grafts include approximately 25% more hairs than circular grafts. Intact strips of scalp may be grafted to create a more uniform hairline, provided that the width is limited (usually 3 to 8 mm) to permit revascularization from the sides. Previous surgery in the area (e.g., scars or earlier grafting) makes a narrower strip (5 mm or less) advisable.

Scalp Flaps

The advantages of scalp flaps are that they bring a normal volume of hair into the area of loss and do not usually shed the hair following the procedure. (When hair plugs are used, the hair commonly falls out, and one must wait a period of time for hair regrowth.) For male pattern baldness the temporoparietal occipital flaps are most popular. These flaps are based on the temporal artery (which can be located by Doppler), measure 3 to 4 cm in width, and with delay, may reach 25 cm in length. Two shorter flaps from either side may be used to overlap in the midline, or two longer ones can be used to reach completely across the scalp from side to side. When the flaps are rotated, the hairs emerging from them grow posteriorly rather than anteriorly as in a normal frontal hairline, and the scars may be difficult to hide. Some surgeons have detached temporal flaps and transferred them to opposite sides of the scalp by microvascular anastomosis, thus creating hair that grows forward.

Scalp Reduction

Scalp reduction is most applicable to alopecia of the vertex of the scalp. In its simplest form this consists of serial excision of the hairless scalp. For larger defects, tissue expanders may be placed to stretch the surrounding hair-bearing scalp prior to excision and closure of the area of alopecia. A major disadvantage of tissue expanders is the temporary deformity of the scalp, which may be unacceptable for an individual who must go to work and appear in public.

It is important for patients to realize that all of these procedures for treating alopecia cause scarring of the scalp and, if the patient eventually becomes completely bald, all scars will likely be visible. In addition, if someone's hair is just thinning, the number of hairs removed in the donor site plug may be almost as many as those transplanted in the recipient site plug, and at least the initial result will show little improvement. Patients should be warned of such complications as infection, which can result in no hair growth at all, or ischemic loss of portions of the graft or flap, which may produce significant scarring and less hair growth.

EYELID SURGERY

The three most common plastic surgical problems of the eyelids are ptosis, the results of aging, and the desire to "westernize" an Asian eyelid.

Ptosis

Ptosis of the upper eyelid is usually due to decreased function and efficiency of the levator muscle. Ptosis may be present at birth; surgical correction is not needed in the first few weeks of life unless the child's vision is obstructed. Ptosis resulting from aging ("senile ptosis") is caused by stretching or avulsion of the levator muscle from the upper border of the tarsal plate with consequent decreased eyelid elevation. Three other common causes of eyelid ptosis are trauma resulting in compromised levator muscle function, injury to the levator nerve supply, or scarring in the upper eyelid that impairs lid mobility. As a rule ptosis is not the result of skin laxity and protrusion of periorbital fat, although these processes may occur simultaneously with senile ptosis.

Treatment of Ptosis

A history of the duration of ptosis and any initiating events is important. If myasthenia gravis is suspected, appropriate tests are essential, and consultation with a neurologist may be helpful. Correction of ptosis secondary to trauma is more difficult than treatment of either congenital or senile ptosis. Traumatic ptosis requires resection of scar with reapproximation of the muscle to obtain a more pliable and freely moving upper lid. Congenital and senile ptosis may be surgically treated through an external or an internal approach. In a patient who has only a few millimeters of ptosis, particularly of the senile type, a Fasanella-Servat procedure on the conjunctival surface may be adequate to achieve correction. In this procedure the upper border of the tarsal plate and the distal portion of the levator muscle are resected through a conjunctival incision. The disadvantage of this simple procedure is the lack of control of the amount of tissue resected and the amount of elevation obtained. Mild congenital ptosis may also be treated with this technique.

Surgical Technique

Frequently, senile ptosis can be corrected in conjunction with blepharoplasty. After redundant skin is removed from the upper eyelid for the blepharoplasty, dissection is carried through the orbicularis muscle to identify the tarsal plate. Superiorly the levator muscle attachment to the tarsal plate is encountered. If the fibers of attachment are stretched or thinned, dissection is carried higher freeing the muscle from the underlying conjunctiva. Then it is advanced, and reattached to the superior border of the tarsal plate. A few tacking stitches are placed between the muscle and the tarsal plate and then the patient placed in the sitting position to verify the accuracy of the eyelid elevation. It is useful to initially leave the extra muscle over the tarsal plate so that the attachment can be lengthened in the event that overcorrection is observed.

In congenital ptosis the external approach helps to create a scar that mimics the normal tarsal fold. In children with little function of the upper eyelid this fold is frequently nonexistent. The procedure may be done under local anesthesia but is commonly done under general anesthesia in children. First the level of the new lid crease is identified and marked, usually at the upper border of the tarsal plate or approximately 1 cm above the lashes. The skin is incised and dissection carried down to the tarsal plate. Immediately superior to the tarsal plate the levator muscle with its closely adherent Müller's muscle is identified. The levator muscle is freed from the conjunctiva; a ptosis clamp is placed between the levator muscle and the conjunctiva and clamped on the muscle. The dissection is carried superiorly on the anterior surface of the levator muscle and to the lateral borders of the muscle. The lateral attachments of the levator muscle to periocular soft tissue are freed to allow free downward movement of the levator muscle.

Although there is no general consensus, most authors feel that resection of 3 to 4 mm of muscle is necessary for each millimeter of elevation needed. The appropriate amount of muscle can be simply resected; alternatively, the muscle may be folded, with the free border of the muscle sutured to itself and the folded edge attached to the upper border of the tarsal plate. This leaves Müller's muscle intact and adds its sympathetic function to the lift of the eyelid. When local anesthesia is used, the patient may be asked to sit up and open the eye so that a comparison with the opposite side is possible. If the patient is under general anesthesia, slight overcorrection (compared with "normal") is usually required when the levator muscle is sutured to the upper border of the tarsal plate. Four to 5 mm of extra muscle should be overlapped over the tarsal plate so that the muscle can be lengthened by changing the suture position if overcorrection persists postoperatively. At the conclusion of the procedure a suture is placed through the lower eyelid and taped to the forehead for 3 days to prevent excess motion of the upper lid.

If there is no voluntary elevation of the upper eyelid, slings of temporal fascia or fascia lata can be extended from the frontalis muscle to the tarsal plate. This increases the patient's ability to elevate the eyelid by raising the brow, a compensatory mechanism most individuals with ptosis naturally use.

The Aging Eyelid

The aging eyelid results from excess skin with folding and wrinkling, redundancy of the orbicularis muscle, prolapse of orbital fat, and downward displacement of the eyebrow. Eye functions such as visual acuity and function of the intrinsic muscles should be evaluated in all patients preoperatively; in some patients, additional tests such as intraocular pressure measurement and tests for the adequacy of tear formation may be appropriate. The lower lid should be tested for excessive laxity since this may contribute to postoperative ectropion. When pulled outward, the lower lid should "snap back" quickly. A preoperative assessment should be made of the location of fat (i.e., which of the various pockets have extra fat) and a plan made for the amount of fat to be resected.

An important component in evaluating a patient for upper lid blepharoplasty includes an assessment of the contribution of the brow position to the eyelid deformity. If the eyebrows are no longer placed at or above the level of the supraorbital rim, then a brow-lift should be considered as an adjunct to (or in some cases in place of) blepharoplasty. When the brows are in a satisfactory position in relation to the orbital rim, then improvement in the appearance of the aging eyelid can be achieved by removal of excess upper eyelid skin.

In the lower eyelid, excess fat and skin similarly contribute to the aging appearance. At times, however, excess fat alone may be present, especially in younger people, and the patient will have more of a "tired" look than the appearance of aging. The treatment should be directed at the specific component causing the patient's problem, and fat removal without skin removal would be appropriate in such patients.

Surgical Technique

The incision (Fig 18–14, A) is marked in the main fold of the upper eyelid (approximately at the upper border of the tarsal plate) and extends medially to the area of the medial canthal ligament but not across the fold onto the nose. A line is drawn laterally along the crease and extended into one of the upper

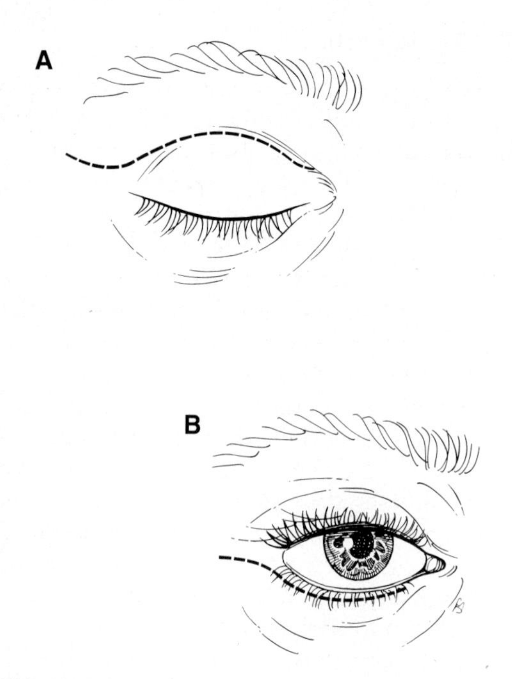

FIG 18–14.
A, the incision for upper eyelid blepharoplasty. **B,** the incision for lower eyelid blepharoplasty.

angled "crow's-feet." With the patient awake small forceps are used to pick up the skin above the line until the upper eyelid border is slightly elevated. An upper line of excision is then marked to permit removal of the amount of skin grasped in the forceps. At this point many surgeons would remove a strip of orbicularis muscle at the desired level for the lid fold postoperatively. Then the muscle is split in the direction of its fibers over the medial and middle fat compartments, and excess fat is removed. Fat protrudes from two pockets of the upper eyelid (medial and middle) and from three in the lower eyelid (medial, middle, and lateral). Weakening of the septum orbitale is primarily responsible for this fat protrusion. The amount of fat removed from each compartment should be compared with that removed from the corresponding compartment of the opposite lid to achieve a symmetrical result. The upper eyelid incisions are closed with interrupted or running sutures.

In the lower eyelid an incision is made approximately 2 mm below the lashes from just lateral to the lacrimal punctum to the lateral canthal area and then downward in one of the lateral "crow's-feet" (Fig 18–14, B). Either a skin or a skin-muscle flap is raised to the level of the infraorbital rim. If a skin flap alone is used, an incision is made parallel to the orbicularis muscle fibers to expose the three fat compartments. Now, with either technique and with gentle pressure on the globe, an incision or incisions are made in the septum orbitale to expose and remove the fat. Care should be taken to not place traction on the fat during resection since injury to the inferior oblique muscle may occur or too much fat may be removed. A strip of orbicularis muscle 2 to 3 mm in width may be removed to correct the hypertrophy of the muscle in the lower eyelid that causes thickening of the lid and wrinkling of the skin. The muscle edges are approximated without sutures and the skin of the eyelid draped upward and outward with gentle traction. With the eyes looking up and the mouth wide open, redundant skin is removed, the resultant lateral dog-ear is resected, and the incision is closed.

In patients with a lax lower lid with poor "snap-back," it may be necessary to resect a full-thickness wedge of the lower lid at the lateral canthal area to tighten the lid and prevent ectropion (a modification of the Kuhnt-Szymanowski procedure). Suspension of the lower eyelid to the lateral canthal area with a strip of orbicularis muscle may also be done.

Complications

Epiphora can result from pulling of the lower lacrimal duct out of the tear pool or from creating a space between the globe and eyelid that allows tears to pool and then pour over the lid margin. The "dry eye" syndrome (keratoconjunctivitis sicca) can also occur. This is usually present and at least minimally symptomatic by history prior to surgery; Schirmer's test can be used to make the diagnosis preoperatively. Following blepharoplasty more conjunctiva is exposed to the air, and more drying of the globe and conjunctiva occurs. Patients with preoperative dry eye symptoms should have very conservative resection and be warned that the use of artificial tears may be necessary after surgery. Some surgeons would not choose to perform cosmetic blepharoplasty on such patients. Blindness may occur as an extremely rare complication of blepharoplasty. If proptosis is noted intraoperatively or postoperatively, the surgeon must quickly open the incisions, administer diuretics (acetazolamide [Diamox] and mannitol), and obtain immediate ophthalmologic consultation.

Transconjunctival Blepharoplasty

Recently there has been growing interest in performing blepharoplasty without external scars. In a patient without lower lid skin redundancy but with bulging fat, incisions may be made on the conjunctival surface, thus eliminating visible scars. Particularly in a patient having a large amount of fat removed, the inferior oblique muscle should be identified to prevent inadvertent injury. Too much fat should not be resected, or a sunken eyelid appearance will result.

Postoperative Treatment

At the completion of the surgical procedure the eyelids are usually separated 2 to 3 mm, but full closure returns after local anesthetic distension and postoperative swelling abate. Postoperatively, cold compresses may be used to decrease swelling, but occlusive dressings should not be used.

The Asian Eyelid

In Asian eyelids, the fold at the superior border of the tarsal plate is absent as a result of a lack of attachment of the levator muscle to skin. "Westernization" of an Asian eyelid requires the creation of this fold. This is accomplished by intentionally creating a scar between the levator muscle and the skin at the upper border of the tarsal plate so that when the eye opens, a fold appears.

OTOPLASTY

Most of the common deformities of the ear are congenital in nature. Fairly sophisticated yet straightforward otoplasty techniques permit the correction of a wide variety of ear abnormalities, including the prominent ear (Figs 18–15 and 18–16) and the constricted ear. Partial (microtia) and complete (anotia) absence of the ear require much more complex reconstructive methods. The same principles are applicable to deformities of the ear acquired after trauma or ablative surgery. The benefits of these procedures are largely aesthetic in nature and contribute little to improvement of ear function. (For a detailed discussion of the principles and techniques of ear reconstruction and the

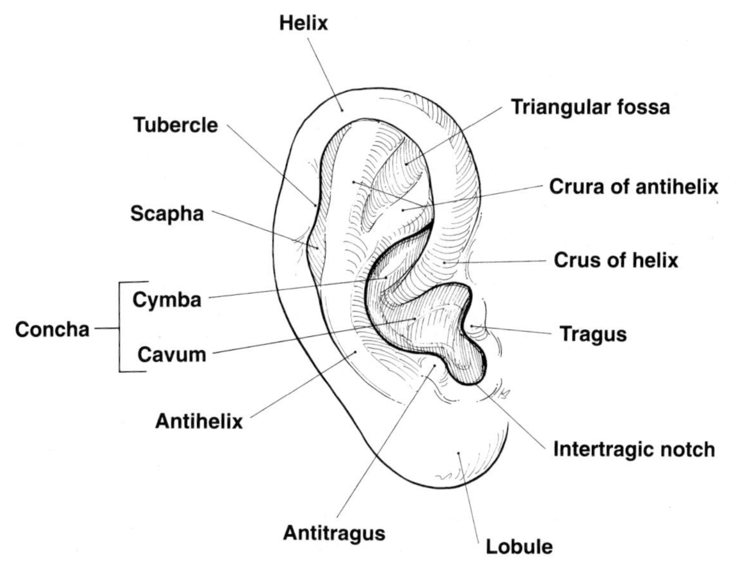

FIG 18–15.
The anatomy of the ear.

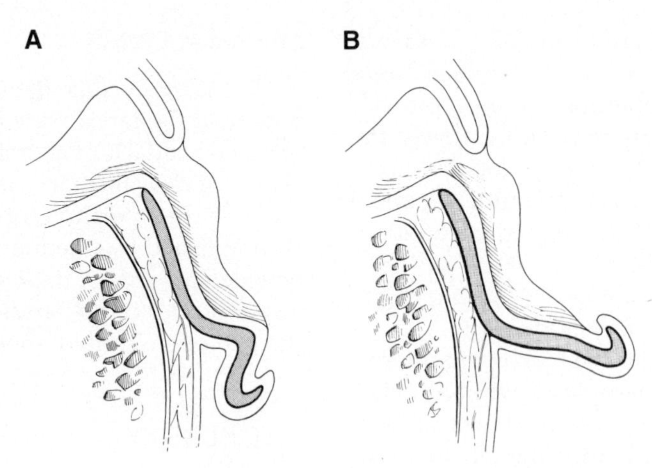

FIG 18–16.
Anatomy of the prominent ear. **A,** the antihelical fold in a normal-appearing ear (cross section). **B,** protrusion as a result of the absence of the antihelical fold.

correction of congenital abnormalities of the ear, see Chapter 15.)

The "Cauliflower" Ear

A "cauliflower" ear is the result of otohematoma from a blow or twisting of the ear. Bleeding occurs between the perichondrium and the cartilage and results in a scar that obliterates the visible convolutions of the ear. In the acute situation, the clots and serum should be drained with either needle aspiration or small incisions. The ear is then covered with moist cotton contouring dressings to obliterate dead space and allow readherence of the skin to the cartilage. Late correction of a "cauliflower" ear deformity is difficult; early treatment is the best approach.

TEMPOROMANDIBULAR JOINT

Women are more commonly affected by temporomandibular joint (TMJ) problems than men by a ratio of approximately 3:1. TMJ problems most commonly occur in young to middle-aged women. The common symptoms are limitation of mandibular motion, "popping" or "clicking" (Fig 18–17) in the joint, and pain in the preauricular area. A careful history and physical examination are essential to rule out other causes of symptoms in the TMJ area. An injection of lidocaine into the joint with relief of symptoms may further isolate the problem to the TMJ. Malocclusion and microtrauma over an extended period of time may be the cause or may at least contribute to the problem. The microtrauma may be the result of bruxism, masseter muscle spasm, or stress. If malocclusion is present, splints to change the condyle position in the fossa are indicated. This may relieve the pain/spasm cycle or prevent a subluxing disk.

Anatomy

The TMJ space consists of two compartments separated by a dense fibrous connective tissue structure (meniscus) (Fig 18–18). The lower space accommodates rotary movement, and the upper permits translatory motion (Fig 18–19). The disk is therefore a movable shim and shock pad.

Diagnostic Studies

Radiographs of the TMJ are valuable for diagnosis; these consist of transcranial tomography and arthrography. They are, however, at times difficult to evaluate. Transcranial views are limited since they visualize only the lateral pole of the mandibular condyle, but they have the advantage that they may be carried out with routine x-ray equipment. Tomography, with its series of cuts through

artificial or autogenous material. In less severe cases, sculpting of the condylar head may improve motion; more severe cases usually require some form of replacement for the condyle.

Other Problems of the Temporomandibular Joint

Other entities such as acute dislocation, recurrent dislocation, infectious arthritis, and avascular necrosis may occur in the TMJ. Anterior dislocation occurs when the condylar head subluxes into the infratemporal fossa. Dislocation usually corrects itself spontaneously; when this does not occur, sedation and manual reduction may be needed.

Recurrent dislocation may cause pain and degenerative joint changes. Intracapsular injection of sclerosing agents has been advocated but is rarely effective. Tightening of the capsule by excision or plication is the most effective treatment. Infectious arthritis of the TMJ may occur after violation of the joint with arthrography, aspiration, or injection. Incision and drainage are essential, but subsequent joint destruction is still common despite appropriate treatment.

Avascular necrosis of the TMJ is a rare problem that may appear several months after an untreated intracapsular fracture or devascularization of the head during surgical reduction of a fracture. Treatment is removal of the necrotic condylar head, usually followed by condylar replacement.

ORTHOGNATHIC SURGERY

Orthognathic surgery is used to treat a variety of problems, including congenital malformations (various syndromes); developmental malformations; posttraumatic deformities; the effects of abnormal neuromuscular patterns, infection, endocrine imbalance, and nutritional deficiencies; arthritis; and acquired postsurgical deformities. Dental malocclusion frequently accompanies the aforementioned entities, thus making close coordination between the orthodontist and the operating surgeon important.

Evaluation

Correct diagnosis and planning of the procedure are essential to obtain a good result.

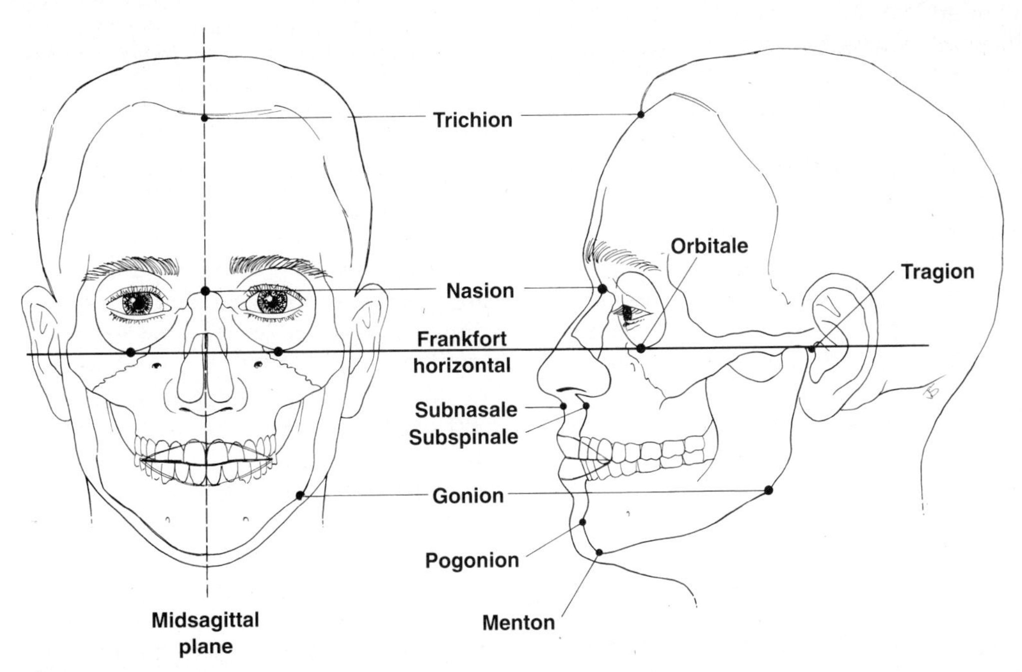

FIG 18–20.
Anthropometric landmarks are essential in measuring facial bony structures.

It is important not only to do an anatomic analysis but also to determine what deformity the patient actually sees and what the patient wants improved. Patient cooperation with the various preoperative and postoperative aspects of treatment over an extended period of time is essential. Examination of the patient's face from all angles with identification of the anthropometric landmarks is essential. Intraoral examination should determine the character of the occlusion and the state of oral hygiene. The common landmarks (Fig 18–20) are the trichion (midpoint at the hairline of the forehead); the glabella (the most prominent point in the midline between the brows); the nasion (the most anterior point of the midline of the frontal nasal suture); the subnasale (the point where the columella merges with the upper lip); the stomion (the interval between the lip); the menton (the lowest median point of the mandible); the pogonion (the most anterior point on the chin); the porion (the highest point on the external auditory meatus); the orbitale (the lowest point on the infraorbital margin); and the Frankfort horizontal, which passes through the porion and the orbitale. An "ideal" face is divided into thirds by horizontal lines through the nasion and the subnasale. Angle's classification of occlusion is widely accepted (Fig 18–21).

In most patients with occlusal problems, dental study models are essential to determine what abnormalities exist and how they can best be corrected. Cephalometric radiography provides a simultaneous record of dental, skeletal, and soft-tissue elements of the face. By tracing on acetate film one may determine the skeletal and soft-tissue relationships. There are many different methods of analysis that have been utilized to determine the appropriateness of these relationships of the various soft tissues and bony structures of the face.

Close coordination and planning between the surgeon and the orthodontist is necessary so that the teeth are moved to the position that is ideal for occlusion following the surgical procedure. This may involve temporarily making the occlusion worse preoperatively, particularly in people who have had previous orthodontic correction without appropriate surgical correction. Treatment goals of the presurgical orthodontic procedures may include adjustment of the mandibular and/or maxillary arch width to a normal position (Fig 18–22), adjustment of the occlusal plane, repositioning of the incisors to improve postsurgical lip position (Fig 18–23), and creation of interdental space for segmental osteotomies where indicated. Mock surgery on dental models and photographic records may be useful in preoperative planning.

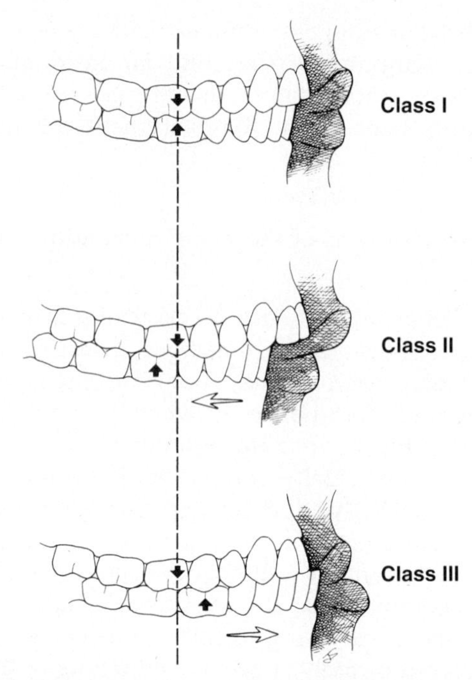

FIG 18–21.
Angle's classification of malocclusion. This classification is based on the anteroposterior (mesiodistal) relationships of the maxillary and mandibular first permanent molar teeth. In class I (neutroclusion), the facial profile is normal. The maxillary and mandibular first molar teeth are in an ideal anteroposterior relationship. The mesiobuccal cusp of the maxillary first molar is aligned correctly with the mesiobuccal groove of the mandibular first molar tooth. In class II (distoclusion), the mandible is retrognathic. The mandibular first molar occupies a more posterior position than normal. In class III (mesioclusion), the mesiobuccal groove of the mandibular first molar is anterior (mesial) to the mesiobuccal cusp of the maxillary first molar.

Among the common orthognathic procedures, genioplasty is perhaps the simplest. This procedure involves moving the chin forward for accentuation, height reduction, or

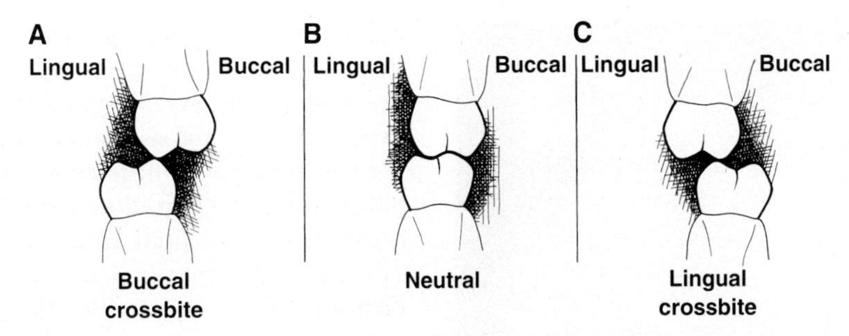

FIG 18–22.
The buccolingual relationships are shown. **A,** buccal version. Malocclusion is due to tilting of the maxillary tooth toward the cheek. **B,** neutroclusion—normal occlusion with the buccal cusp of the upper tooth overlapping that of the lower tooth. **C,** lingual crossbite—malocclusion caused by the lingual displacement of the upper teeth in relation to the lower teeth.

symmetry. Segmental alveolar osteotomies to reposition some of the teeth are also commonly done. For more significant problems, the entire mandible may need repositioning. Mandibular body osteotomies are rarely performed today because of the necessity of sacrificing a tooth and danger to the inferior alveolar nerve. Repositioning of the mandible is now usually done by sagittal splitting procedures of the ramus of the mandible. This may be done through either external or internal incisions. Intraoral vertical osteotomy is also commonly used for prognathism.

For maxillary malposition, the most commonly employed procedure is transverse osteotomy (Le Fort type I), which permits adjustment of occlusion in three planes. In this procedure, the incisions must be performed at least 4 to 5 mm above the maxillary teeth to prevent dental injury. Le Forte II and III osteotomies are most commonly used in the correction of congenital and posttraumatic abnormalities of the midface. It is common for multiple osteotomies to be carried out simultaneously to achieve the result desired.

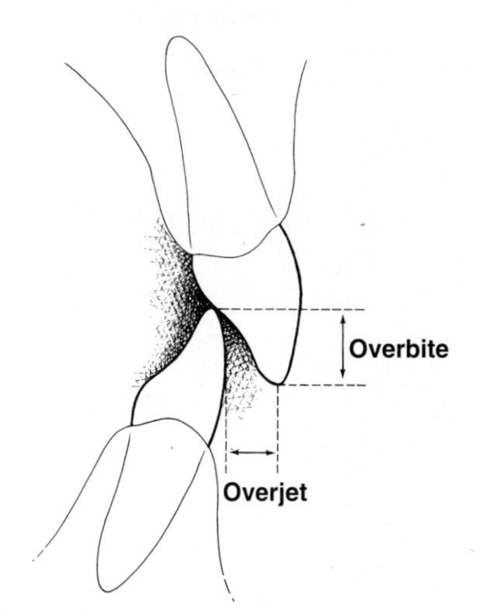

FIG 18–23.
Incisal edge relationship. Overbite refers to vertical overlap of the biting edges and overjet to the labiolingual relationship of the incisal edges.

MASSETERIC HYPERTROPHY

Masseteric hypertrophy is a functionally asymptomatic increase in the size of the masseter muscle; it is most commonly bilateral. While the etiology is unknown, it has been postulated that "jaw clenching" may cause muscle hypertrophy. This is primarily a cosmetic deformity that may have associated emotional problems.

Masseteric hypertrophy causes a square shape of the face by accentuating the lower lateral portion of the face in the area of the mandibular angles (Fig 18–24). The diagnosis may be made by asking the patient to bite down while palpating the masseter muscle. Other pathology in the area, such as parotid tumors, lymphangiomas, etc., should be ruled out. On x-ray studies there is commonly bone hypertrophy at the mandibular angle.

Treatment involves removal of the hyperostosis and reduction of the size of the muscle (Fig 18–25). Both the internal and external approaches have been advocated. The inter-

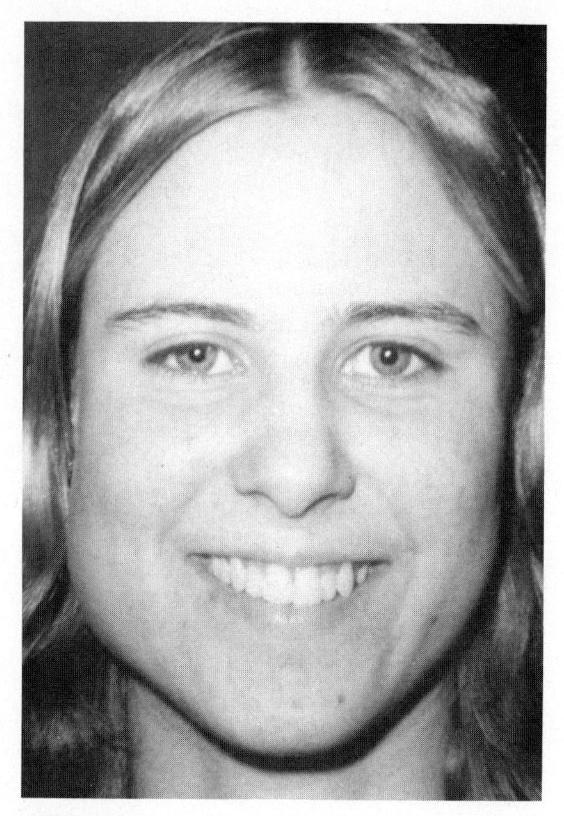

FIG 18–24.
The bulging of the masseter muscles can be seen bilaterally, but it is more marked on the right side.

nal approach avoids an external scar and decreases the incidence of facial nerve injury. Postoperatively, swelling and trismus may be expected. Early passive and active exercises of the jaw are important to prevent limitation of motion. It may be months before the swelling resolves and the final appearance is evident. The two sides may not be exactly the same postoperatively, a fact that the patient must fully understand preoperatively.

FACIAL PARALYSIS

Anatomy

The facial nerve leaves the skull via the facial canal of the temporal bone. In the facial canal it gives off three branches: the greater superficial petrosal nerve, the stapedial nerve, and the chorda tympani. The nerve then exits the stylomastoid foramen and enters the parotid gland. In the parotid gland the nerve usually has three major branches: the marginal mandibular, the maxillary, and the temporal. The marginal mandibular branch and the temporal branch have little or no interconnections with other branches, while the maxillary branch has

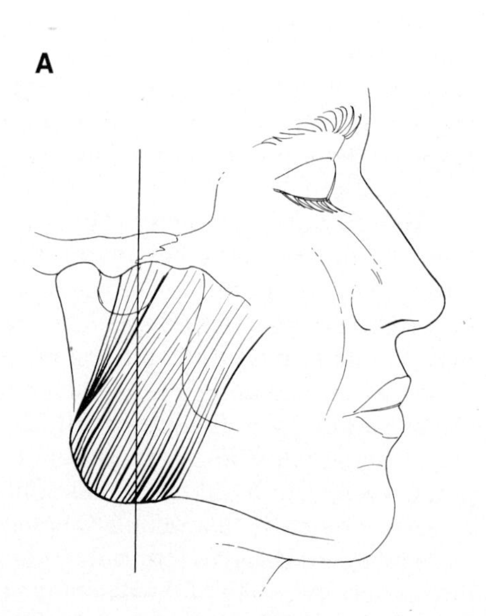

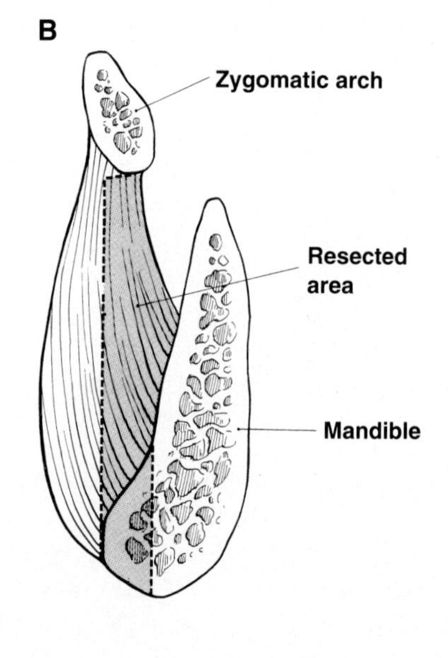

FIG 18–25.
Surgery for masseteric hypertrophy. The muscle and lateral edge of the mandible need to be resected.

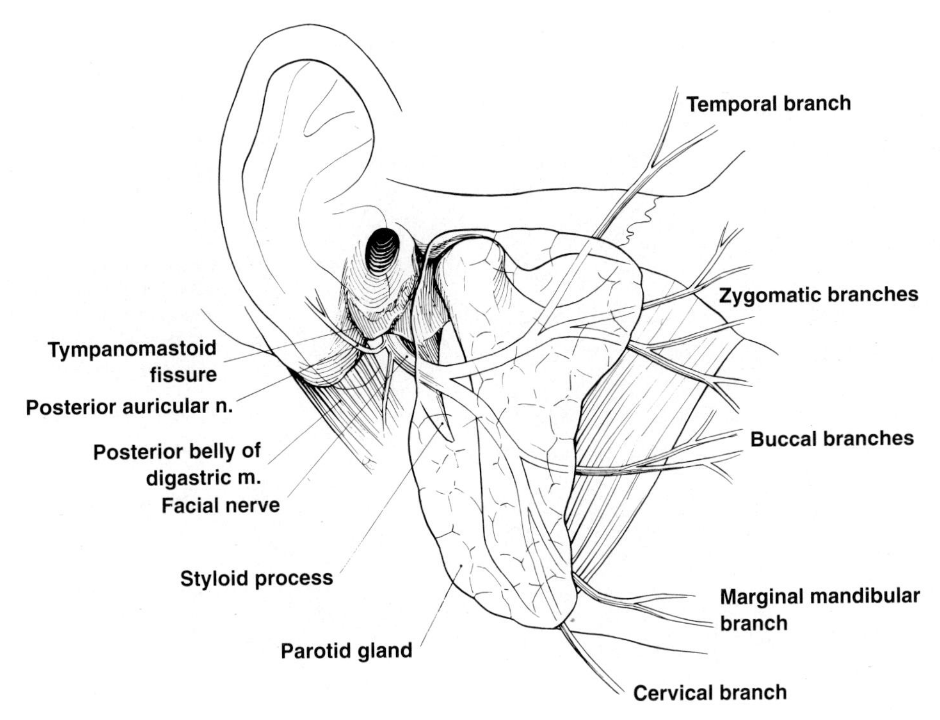

FIG 18–26.
The normal anatomy of the facial nerve.

frequent intermingling of fibers between its components (Fig 18–26).

There are 17 paired facial muscles that are innervated by the facial nerve (Fig 18–27). These muscles control the soft-tissue movements of the face. The nerves enter the muscles on their posterior surface.

Facial nerve paralysis usually occurs in one of three areas: the central or intracranial area, the area of the temporal bone, or the parotid gland area. Facial paralysis may be the result of neonatal developmental conditions, trauma, infection, metabolic causes, or neoplasm. Facial palsy also can be iatrogenic, toxic, or idiopathic.

Injury to the nerve may vary from neuropraxia to axonotmesis to neurotmesis. The muscles of facial expression maintain their motor end plates for 18 to 24 months following injury, which allows these muscles to avoid atrophy for longer periods of time than the usual denervated striated muscle. If, however, muscle does not eventually become reinnervated, it will ultimately atrophy.

Diagnosis

A history of the onset of paralysis including associated trauma, infection, or medications is important. The face should be examined at rest for asymmetries and motor tone. Motor function is tested by requesting the patient to show the teeth, pucker the lips as in a whistle, grimace, close the eyelids, and raise the eyebrows. There are two types of facial motor nerve weakness. A supranuclear paralysis involves the cortical bulbar pathways with sparing of the orbicularis oculi and frontalis muscles but paralysis of the lower portions of the face on the side opposite the lesion. A diagnosis of infratemporal causation requires testing the function of the branches given off in the temporal bone.

Various diagnostic tests may be used to locate the site of the injury, determine the type of injury, and show evidence of reinnervation. These tests consist of conduction test, strength duration curves, cronaxie, electromyography, and electroneurography. If an injury is peripheral in the maxillary branches, spontane-

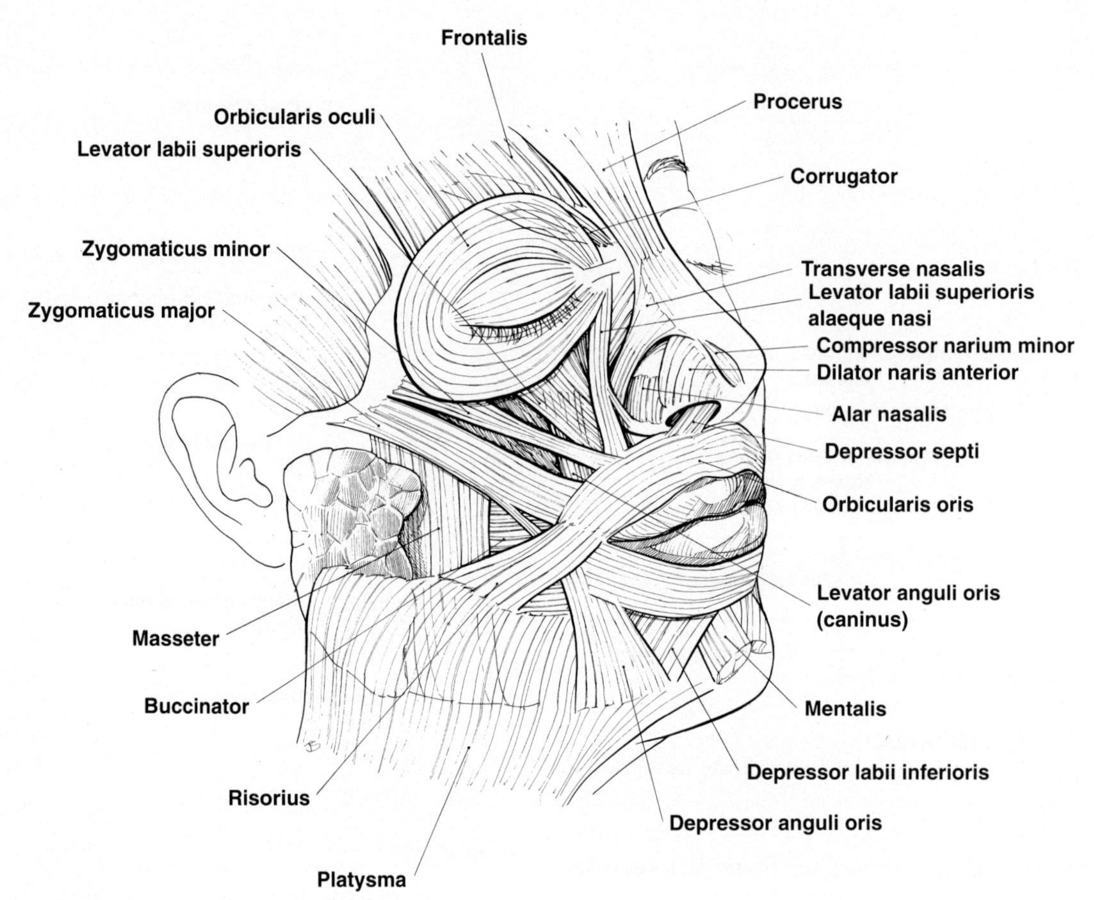

FIG 18–27.
The muscles of facial expression

ous return of function is common because of the multiple interconnections.

Treatment

Treatment may be divided into three stages: immediate repair (0 to 3 weeks postinjury), delayed (3 weeks to 2 years postinjury), and late (over 2 years postinjury). It is best to repair injuries to the facial nerve immediately or as soon in the intermediate phase as possible. (In most cases late functional correction requires transfer of muscle locally or as a free vascularized graft to restore function.) If the nerve ends cannot be approximated and nerve grafts are required, the most commonly used nerves are the great auricular, the sural, branches of the cervical plexus, or the lateral femoral cutaneous nerve. The great auricular nerve or cervical plexus is ideal, for it is found in the same field of dissection and has multiple branches that can be anastomosed distally.

If for some reason the proximal end of the nerve is not accessible, cross facial nerve grafts from the contralateral side may be necessary. Most commonly, a sural nerve graft is used for this purpose. Some advocate reversing the nerve graft, while others advocate secondary distal repair after the axoplasm has had the opportunity to reach the distal end of the nerve graft (this can be documented by Tinel's sign). The results of cross facial nerve grafting have been disappointing; the best use of this procedure is to innervate a free microvascular muscle transfer (see below).

In the past, the hypoglossal, spinal accessory, or phrenic nerve has been used to reinnervate the distal facial nerve. These procedures have been largely abandoned because of the functional loss in the muscles originally innervated and the achievement of only "mass action" of the reinnervated facial muscles (i.e., the entire face contracts at the same time).

Regional muscles have been transferred to animate the lateral commissure of the mouth and the eyelid. A fascial sling may be placed around the oral cavity either as a preliminary procedure or at the time of the muscle transfer. The most commonly used transfers are of the anterior portion of the masseter muscle, a turndown of the temporalis muscle, or detachment of the temporalis from the coronoid process and attachment to the circumoral sling with a tendon or fascial graft. The sternocleidomastoid and platysma muscles have also been used for transfers but rarely give results as satisfactory as the masseter or temporalis.

The temporalis muscle and its attached fascia can be used to close the eye. The fascia is dissected inferiorly from the temporalis muscle, left attached superiorly, and split into strips. One strip is placed in the upper and one in the lower lid, and both are attached to the medial canthal ligament. With temporalis muscle contraction the scissoring causes the lid to close. As an alternative form of treatment, the entire temporalis can be transferred to the lateral commissure to achieve reanimation of the mouth; at the same time, eyelid function can be enhanced by placement of a gold weight in the upper lid. Muscle transfer procedures require a great deal of time, effort, and dedication by the patient to learn to take advantage of the new muscle orientation.

As an ancillary procedure one may divide selected branches of the facial nerve to the normal side to decrease the strong pull and distortion and improve symmetry. This may be indicated as a primary procedure in older individuals or ones whose health does not allow more complicated and time-consuming operative procedures.

With the advent of microsurgery, several different muscles have been transferred via microvascular anastomosis to provide facial reanimation. Reinnervation is achieved through connection to the proximal facial nerve or to cross facial nerve grafts. Muscles that have been used to date are usually stronger in their pull than the original facial muscles; therefore, the search for the ideal muscle continues. The most common muscles presently used are the gracilis, the pectoralis minor, and the serratus anterior.

Several ancillary procedures such as brow-lift, face-lift, and excisions of redundancy at the nasolabial fold will sometimes aid in achieving symmetry after a facial reanimation procedure. Tarsorrhaphy, canthoplasty, lid magnets, springs, and upper lid weighting have all been used for closure and protection of the eye with varying success.

In many cases, significant improvement in facial animation is achieved by using the various procedures outlined above. However, perfect restoration of symmetrical function is rarely if ever achieved. Extensive preoperative discussion and counseling are essential when facial reanimation procedures are contemplated.

FACIAL ATROPHY (ROMBERG'S DISEASE)

Facial atrophy (Romberg's disease) is a poorly understood yet potentially devastating process. There is no evidence that this condition is inherited, and the incidence is unknown. Atrophy may occur at any age but most commonly begins before the age of 20 years with localized involvement of the skin and subcutaneous tissue (Fig 18–28). As it progresses, the underlying muscles, cartilage, and bone may become involved. The most severe deformity occurs in the child since normal tissue growth is adversely affected. This process is most commonly unilateral and may first appear as an isolated area of depression, thus warranting the name "coup de sabre." As a rule the atrophy progresses for a relatively short period of time (2 to 10 years), but in some cases the process may persist longer.

When the skin in the area of facial atrophy is examined histologically, one sees thinning of the stratum granulosum and rete papillae in association with atrophy of the adnexal elements. The subcutaneous tissue shows chronic inflammation and scarring. Muscle

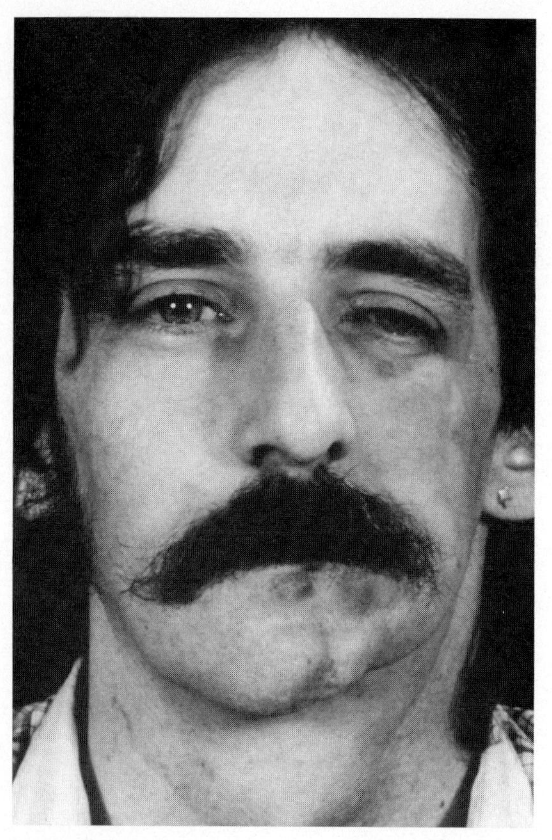

FIG 18–28.
Romberg's disease involving the left mandibular and maxillary portion of the face with a typical *coup de sabre* deformity of the chin.

atrophy is thought to be the result of overlying skin and subcutaneous tissue tightness. Romberg's original description in 1844 attributed atrophy to a "vasomotor trophoneuritis," and subsequent evidence supports this theory. Other causes that have been suggested are adjacent trauma, hemiplegic migraine, infection, and trigeminal neuralgia.

Treatment

Fat taken from the area of atrophy and placed elsewhere in the body hypertrophies, and fat brought from elsewhere and grafted into the area of atrophy tends to atrophy. Thus most surgeons postpone treatment until the disease has stabilized.

Commonly, patients require only soft-tissue augmentation. In the past, synthetic materials such as injectable silicone were used with encouraging results, although complications have now caused cessation of the use of silicone. Subcutaneous injection of fat with overcorrection has been advocated recently, but the results are too premature to judge its long-term efficacy.

The most commonly described treatment is free microvascular transfer of omentum, fascia, and fasciocutaneous tissue, particularly for irregular defects. There is some propensity for the omentum to sag, so multiple revisions may be necessary. Fascia and fasciocutaneous tissue are more stable and easier to design. It appears that bringing vascularized tissues into the area allows the filling of defects and brings enhanced blood supply to the atrophied area.

When bony involvement is significant, the atrophied and constricted bone should be reconstructed to build a framework on which to place the soft tissue. This may involve free bone grafts or vascularized free bone transfers.

SUGGESTED READING

Boies' L, Adams G, Paparella M: Diseases of the nose. In *Fundamentals of Otolaryngology: Textbook of Ear, Nose and Throat Diseases,* ed 5. Philadelphia, WB Saunders, 1978.

Denecke H, Meyer R: *Plastic Surgery of the Head and Neck.* New York, Springer-Verlag, 1967.

Furnas D: Facial aesthetic surgery: Art, anatomy, anthropometrics, and imaging. *Clin Plast Surg* 1987; 14.

Lewis J (ed): *The Art of Aesthetic Plastic Surgery.* Boston, Little, Brown, 1989.

McCarthy J: *Plastic Surgery.* Philadelphia, WB Saunders, 1990.

Menick F (ed): Aesthetic surgery of the face. *Clin Plast Surg* 1992; 19.

Smith B (ed): *Ophthalmic Plastic and Reconstructive Surgery.* St Louis, Mosby–Year Book, 1987.

Smith J, Aston S (eds): *Grabb and Smith's Plastic Surgery,* ed 4. Boston, Little, Brown, 1991.

Whitaker L (ed): Aesthetic surgery of the facial skeleton. *Clin Plast Surg* 1991; 18.

Chapter 19

Reconstruction

John J. Coleman, III, M.D.

CONTENTS

The scalp and calvarium
The midface
The oral cavity

CHAPTER OBJECTIVE

At the end of this chapter the resident understands the principles and is familiar with the techniques of reconstruction of the head and neck and applies this knowledge to a wide variety of deformities and disorders in this region.

LEARNER OBJECTIVES

On completion of this chapter the resident

1. **Understands the options for correcting a contour defect, including alloplastic material, autograft, and tissue transfers.**
2. **Understands the options for correcting a structural defect, including bone graft, vascularized bone graft, trays and bone graft, etc.**
3. **Understands the options for correcting functional defects including muscle transfers, nerve transfers and transections, slings, gold weights, etc.**
4. **Knows the techniques for bony fixation and the indications for and contraindications to each.**
5. **Is familiar with a wide variety of grafts and flaps for reconstruction of head and neck structures; understands the rationale for choices between different techniques.**
6. **Understands the principles and techniques available for appearance restoration.**
7. **Understands the specific reconstructive needs of special tissues such as oral mucosa, nasal lining, etc.**

CLINICAL PRACTICE ACTIVITIES

During the course of the training program, the resident

1. **Diagnoses and treats patients with functional and aesthetic defects of the head and neck.**
2. **Utilizes flaps, grafts, and/or alloplastic insertions for head and neck reconstruction.**
3. **Performs reconstruction of specific head and neck structures such as the eyelid, lips, nose, oropharynx, etc.**

The head and neck region is the anatomic area where structure, appearance, and function are more closely linked than any other site in the body. A significant defect, whether caused by infection, extirpation of neoplasm, trauma, or congenital error, is likely to impair the patient in numerous ways. The juxtaposition of the entrance of the digestive tract with that of the respiratory tract as well as the juxtaposition of the upper aerodigestive tract to the central nervous system (including the brain and cervical spinal cord) and the great vessels of the neck and mediastinum make each reconstructive effort one of considerable risk.

As with other therapeutic interventions, there is a hierarchy of priorities for reconstruction. Most important is *survival,* a consideration usually paramount only in resection of malignancy but also dependent on a reconstruction that will successfully separate the upper aerodigestive tract and central nervous system as well as allow alimentation and respiration. The second priority is preservation or restoration of *function* since the two main vegetative functions respiration and alimentation and their subsidiary functions, speech and swallowing, depend to a great degree on the synchronous action of various structures in this region. *Removal of painful stimuli* is an important corollary since resection of cancer or restoration of balance to the mobile structures is likely to alleviate pain. Preservation or restoration of normal or acceptable *appearance* is the next major priority. Because humans conduct most social interactions by speech and facial expression, this deformity is extremely disabling. Last in the hierarchy of priorities but most dependent on the skill, experience, and imagination of the surgeon is the parameter of *efficiency*. Efficiency is the ability to perform the reconstruction in a time period commensurate with the natural history of the disease. For example, hemifacial microsomia and carcinoma of the floor of the mouth both result in defects of the mandible. The necessity for single-stage reconstruction of this congenital disorder is not nearly as great as for the malignancy, where the 5-year survival rates are about 40% and 90% of recurrences are manifested within 2 years. In general, single-stage reconstructions, frequently with free tissue transfer, are more appropriate in disease processes with a high risk of failure. Staged reconstructive procedures are more appropriate in many cases for congenital disorders where remodeling and growth of tissue may change the needs of the wound.

Reconstruction of defects of the head and neck is frequently a complex undertaking. Many of the structures in the head and neck are mobile. They are three-dimensional and may be composed of skin and/or mucosa, bone, and muscle. The adjacent cavities are heavily colonized with bacteria that may become pathogenic. To overcome these problems, the surgeon should analyze the defect as a wound having certain characteristics to provide the single or multiple forms of reconstruction that will best reconstruct the wound. Wound characteristics include structural composition (skin, bone, cartilage, soft tissue, and mucosa); size or volume; dimensionality (uniplanar, biplanar, triplanar); sensory potential; propinquity to vital structures such as the great vessels, brain, and spinal cord; distensibility or volume of open space; presence of bacteria as a normal or abnormal situation; and mobility. The patient's past or future therapy and growth potential are also important. Nose, ear, and facial bone defects assessed before skeletal maturation may be underestimated. Previous radiotherapy or the likelihood of subsequent radiotherapy may also alter reconstructive options. After analysis of the wound, the surgeon should determine whether the defect is primarily one of *contour* or *three dimensions* and the impact of the reconstruction on *function.*

Crucial to the success of head and neck reconstruction is adequate blood supply to the defect. Whether grafts, flaps, or free tissue transfer is chosen, the ultimate success of the reconstruction depends on adequate blood supply (Fig 19–1). Ischemic tissue cannot withstand the indigenous bacterial colonization and will at best scar and result in a contracted dysfunctional area. When alloplastic materials such as stainless steel mandibular reconstruction plates or methyl methacrylate cranial reconstructions are used, they require ample, well-perfused soft tissue to prevent them from becoming exposed and contaminated.

The basic tools for reconstruction in the head and neck are grafts (skin, dermafat, fascia, cartilage, and bone), flaps (random cutaneous, axial cutaneous, fasciocutaneous, musculocutaneous, and axial fascia flaps with or without vascularized bone from local, cervical, or thoracic sites), and free tissue transfer. In addition, in selected cases alloplastic materials can be used. Just as defects or wounds have particular characteristics, so too do methods of reconstruction. Grafts are relatively homogeneous, but flaps, both local and distant, have various qualities rendering them more or less desirable. The potential size, volume, bulk, effect of gravity, arc of rotation, length of pedicle, homogeneity of perfusion or degree of perfusion gradient

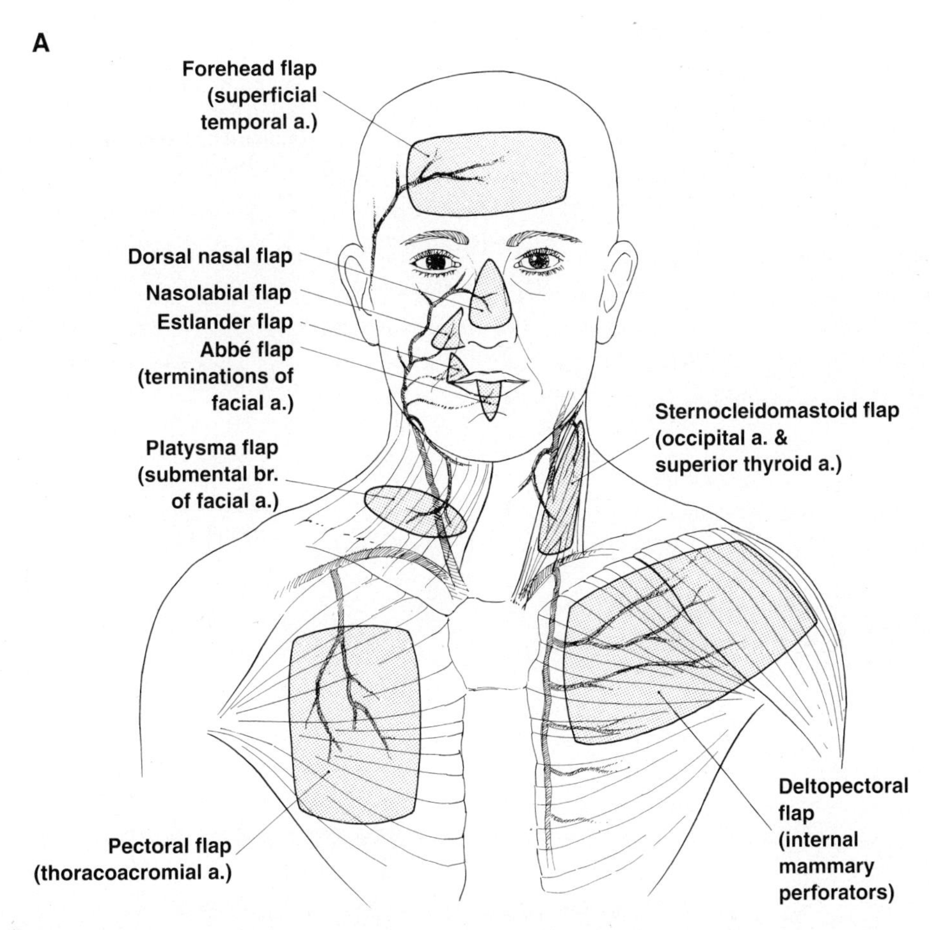

FIG 19–1.
Frontal **(A)** representation of axial cutaneous, fasciocutaneous, and musculocutaneous rotation flaps with their dominant blood supplies useful for head and neck reconstruction. *(Continued.)*

under normal conditions, presence of muscle, bone, or epithelial elements, durability and volume of bone, etc., may all be considered to make a reconstructive method more or less useful.

The following text addresses the various problems in head and neck reconstruction by anatomic site by considering wound characteristic and suggesting methods of reconstruction.

THE SCALP AND CALVARIUM

The scalp and calvarium can be considered a single unit for reconstruction in some cases. The main function is protection of the intracranial contents. Traumatic or malignant defects not involving the pericranium or periosteum of the skull can be resurfaced with split-thickness skin grafts. In fact, the dura mater of the brain itself can accept a skin graft if there is no central spinal fluid (CSF) leak. In adults with a distinct diploic layer, drill holes in the outer cortex may allow granulation tissue to cover bone denuded of periosteum and permit subsequent split-thickness skin grafting. Areas of alopecia or full-thickness skin loss may be closed by advancement of scalp flaps from the periphery of the defect. Transposition flaps as described by Orticochea, Juri, and others may be axial (based on temporal, frontal, or occipital arteries) or random. The surface area covered can be increased by scoring the galea to allow scalp expansion. This procedure may be repeated during staged advancements of the scalp as well. Mobilization of flaps into the temporo-

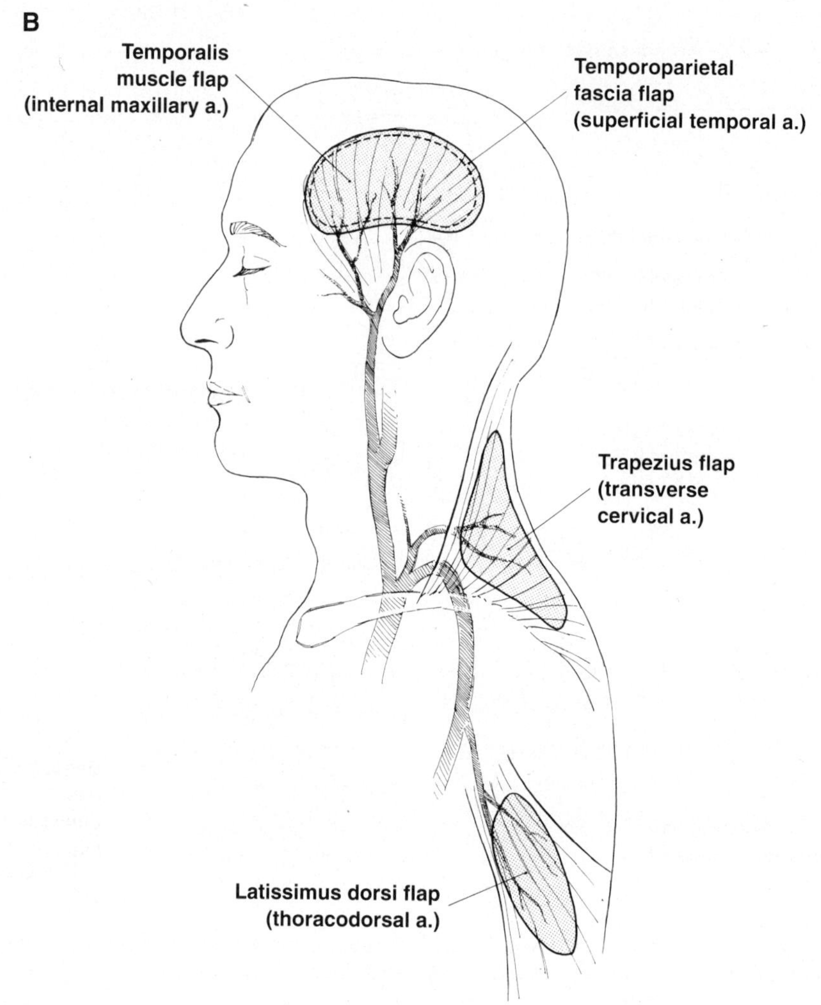

FIG 19–1 (cont.).
Lateral **(B)** representation of axial cutaneous, fasciocutaneous, and musculocutaneous rotation flaps with their dominant blood supplies useful for head and neck reconstruction.

parietal zone and beyond the occipital nuchae will allow optimal advancement.

The scalp is also amenable to tissue expansion, although too much pressure may cause necrosis of the hair follicles. The risk of partial alopecia and expander exposure, particularly in children, makes staged excision with scoring of the galea a reasonable alternative in selected cases. Damage to adjacent tissue, the vasculitic changes of radiotherapy, and other chronic changes in the scalp and neck may render the recipient bed unsuitable for grafting or make local or locoregional flaps unsafe. For lateral and posterior defects the trapezius musculocutaneous flap or muscle flap covered by a skin graft can provide well-vascularized tissue from outside the zone of injury. Latissimus and pectoralis musculocutaneous flaps have a limited ability to cover most calvarial defects but may be useful in the temporal or infratemporal areas. When limited areas of full-thickness scalp loss result in exposed bone, pericranial flaps based on the superficial temporal, frontal, or occipital vessels may provide an adequate recipient bed for skin grafting or other techniques.

Many free tissue transfers are suitable for soft-tissue coverage of the scalp. Moderate-sized areas are favorably covered with a scapular or radial forearm fasciocutaneous flap, which usually matches the thickness of the scalp. More extensive defects require larger flaps, and the latissimus dorsi muscle, serratus anterior muscle, rectus abdominis muscle, and omentum covered by a split-thickness skin graft are excellent alternatives. Musculocutaneous free flaps are usually too bulky for scalp reconstruction. The latissimus dorsi muscle is probably the most versatile because it has a large surface area and relatively long pedicle. The omentum has a very long pedicle but does not provide as durable coverage. Careful design of the serratus flap can provide the longest pedicle as well as a large segment of muscle. Despite the proximity of the superficial temporal vessels, microvascular anastomoses are most frequently performed in the neck. A preauricular or postauricular skin flap with extension into the neck gives access to the occipital or facial branches of the external carotid artery and to the posterior facial or external jugular vein. Venous outflow is better in these cervical vessels, and problems with the microvascular anastomosis are less frequent.

Bony defects of the calvarium may be dealt with in a number of ways depending on the condition of the surrounding soft tissue. (Replacement of the bony protection of the skull is not always necessary, particularly in the elderly or those with little likelihood of subsequent trauma to the area.) When full-thickness, well-vascularized soft tissue covers the defect, synthetic material such as methyl methacrylate or Vitallium mesh may be adequate. Obviously, synthetic substitutes are at a higher risk of infection when used in areas that may communicate with the paranasal sinuses or other parts of the upper aerodigestive tract. Restoration of the structural continuity of the skull when adequate, well-vascularized soft tissue is present or has been restored by free tissue transfer can be accomplished by split-rib grafts. The natural curvature and malleability of split-rib grafts allows them to be contoured to almost any defect. Interosseous wires in chain link fashion between the ribs and adjacent calvarium provide stability. Perhaps the best method of skull reconstruction is split calvarium. Improvement in craniofacial techniques and instrumentation has shown that harvesting of adjacent calvarium and splitting of the bone will provide cover for both the defect and the donor site. Miniplate fixation to surrounding bony structures provides stability, and the intervening areas show a high propensity for bony union, particularly in children.

Vascularized bone is not frequently required in skull reconstruction because of the lack of mobility and minimal bacterial exposure. Occasionally, however, a demand for this may be filled by free tissue transfers such as the scapula-latissimus osteocutaneous flap based on the circumflex scapulae or angular vessels and less frequently other methods. A more useful approach to vascularized bone in the skull as well as zygomatic malar or even mandibular reconstruction is to use pericranial or galeal pericranial flaps based on the superficial temporal or occipital vessels and carry the subjacent full- or partial-thickness bone with its periosteal blood supply (Fig 19–2).

THE MIDFACE

The midface is the anatomic area from the superior limits of the orbit to the plane of the palatal bone. It is the area of the face that gives the most clearly defined individual identity. The midface can be considered the watershed area between the orbital cavities and the oral cavity and is a complex three-dimensional truncated pyramid bordered by the anterior malar skin and bone, lateral nasal wall, choanae, soft tissues of the malar buccal area and lateral maxillary wall, floor of the orbit, and palate. This area, predominately composed of the maxillary and ethmoid sinuses and the nasal cavity, is the entrance to the respiratory tract and separates the orbits, eyes, and central nervous system from the alimentary canal.

Maxillofacial prosthetics have been extensively utilized in restoration of midface defects. The fundamental goal is usually to separate the oral cavity from the nasomaxillary complex. This allows speech without nasal escape and continence of the oral cavity distinct from the respiratory tract. This partitioning allows the tongue to push the food or liquid bolus on the palate down into the pharynx and facilitates the normal passage of

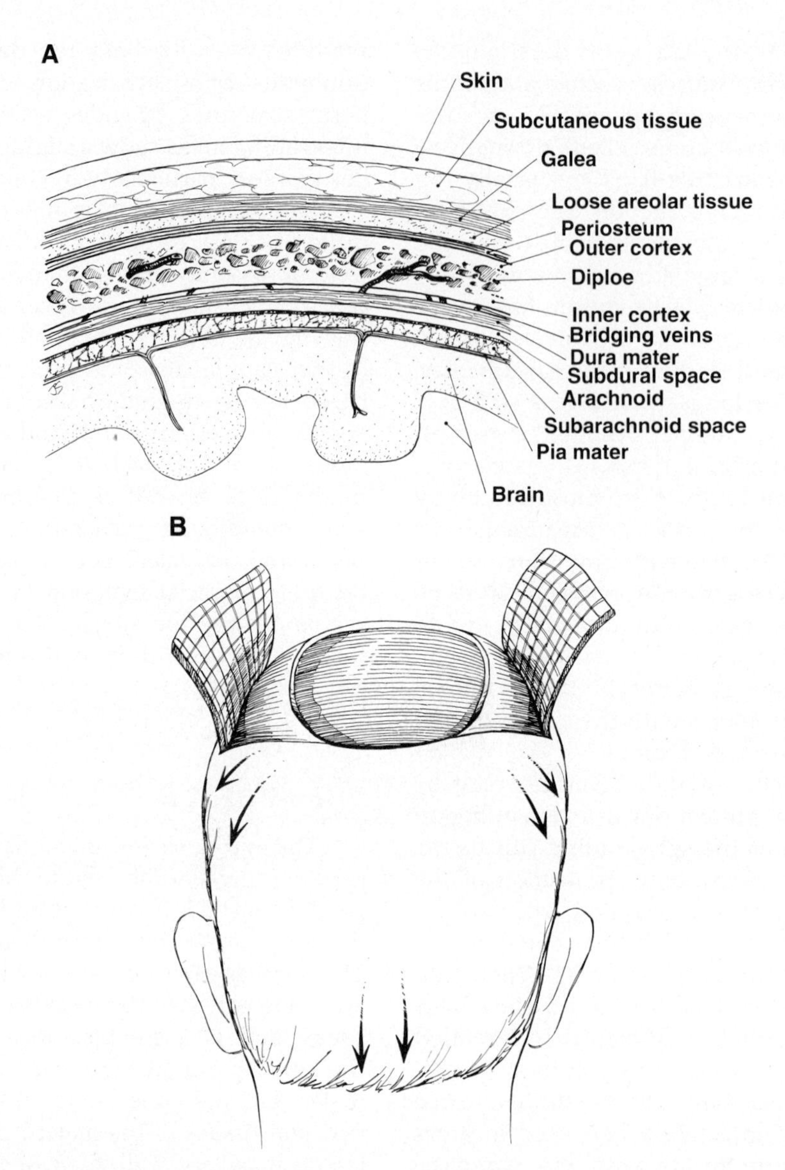

FIG 19–2.
A, Cross-sectional anatomy of the scalp and calvarium. Knowledge of this anatomy allows design of scalp flaps, harvest of calvarial bone grafts, and expansion of the scalp. **B,** Cross-hatching of the scalp allows expansion of the area of the scalp. Undermining below the junction of the temporoparietal fascia and temporalis muscle and into the neck beyond the occipital nucha allows the furthest advancement.

air through the nares into the nasopharynx and ultimately the larynx. When the defect is one consisting of the palate alone, an acrylic obturator attached to a denture can imitate the palate. For proper function of such a prosthesis two- to three-point support with surrounding tissue is necessary. The residual palate and teeth may provide one buttress, the buccal mucosa a second, and a superior nasal structure (such as the turbinates) a third pressure point. When the defect is so large that adequate support is not available, a prosthesis will not be effective. Sometimes the combination of several prostheses supported by different structures is effective—for example, an intraoral palatal prosthesis may separate the nose from the mouth, and an external prosthesis suspended on eyeglasses may cover the malar cutaneous deficiency in a radical maxillectomy defect where skin has been removed. In general, however, complex defects are rarely amenable to prosthetic rehabilitation because of expense, bulk, and difficulty with maintenance. If a patient is not a good candidate for total reconstruction, partial reconstruction to facilitate prosthetic rehabilitation may be appropriate.

There are numerous methods of midface reconstruction. Posttraumatic defects may be secondary to blunt or explosive forces and thus require different amounts of bone or soft tissue. Onlay rib grafts may be associated with considerable resorption. Cranial bone onlay grafts have less resorption if there is an adequate soft-tissue bed but are significantly less malleable. Complex three-dimensional defects such as those created by radical orbitomaxillectomy may be approached by meth-

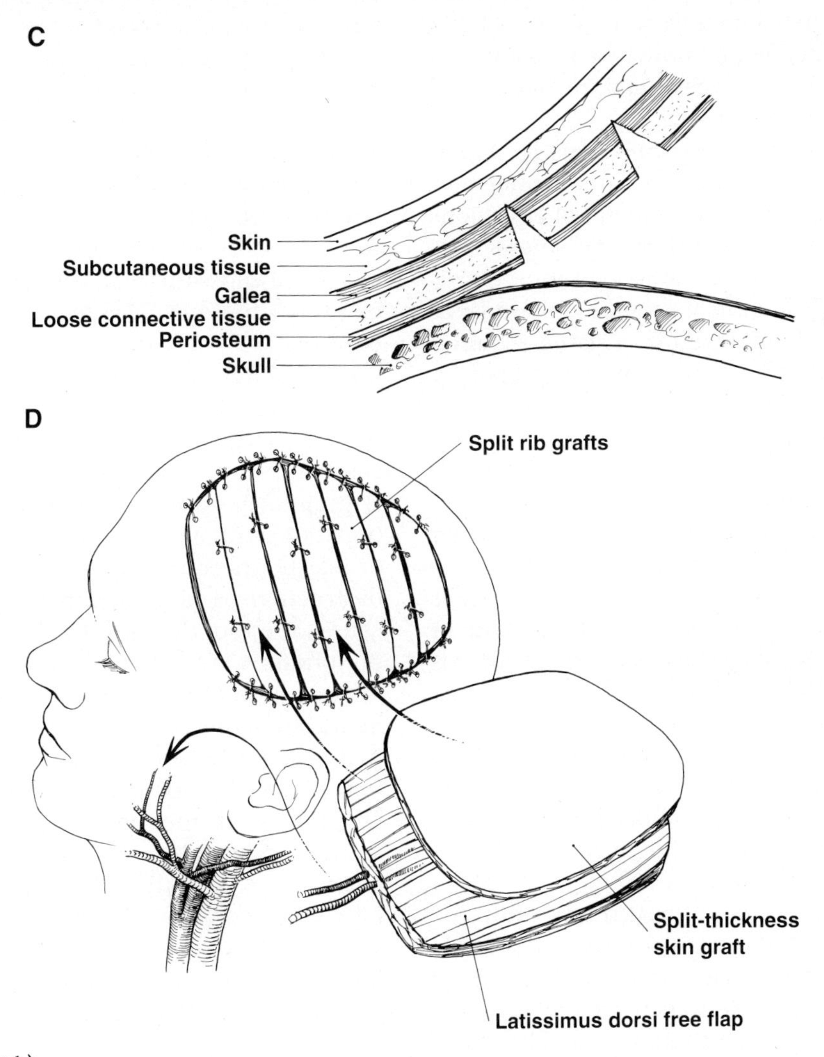

FIG 19–2 (cont.).
C, For best advancement of the scalp, the scoring and cross-hatching should extend into the subcutaneous tissue. Major blood vessels running in the subgaleal layers should not, however, be divided.
D, Reconstruction of massive resection of scalp and skull. Split rib grafts wired together with numerous interosseous wires reconstruct the vault of the skull. Alternatively, calvarial bone grafts split through the diploe can be used to cover both donor and recipient sites. The soft tissue coverage of the nonvascularized bone is provided by a latissimus dorsi free flap covered with a split-thickness skin graft. Microvascular anastomosis is performed in the neck, and the flap is sutured into the preauricular or postauricular skin depending on the site of the lesion, taking care not to compress the pedicle beneath the skin flaps.

ods involving restoration of not only bone but also epithelium and mucosa. One useful approach is to remove all remaining mucosal tissue and obliterate the three-dimensional defect with soft tissue forming the crucial epithelial-lined surfaces of the palate and the lateral nasal wall. The orbital floor may be reconstructed with bone or soft tissue. The alternative method of reconstructing the area in kind with multiple complex mucosa-lined flaps is somewhat unrealistic since exposure of unvascularized bone to the heavily colonized aerodigestive tract may lead to subclinical infection and resorption.

Although the temporalis muscle flap is useful for separating the base of the brain and the nasopharynx after craniofacial resections and may reach the palate and lateral oral cavity, local or thoracic muscle or musculocutaneous flaps are *rarely* useful for these large defects. The large amount of tissue required to resolve these defects is best supplied by free tissue transfer. There are two basic approaches: the first relies mainly on soft tissue to obliterate the three-dimensional defect alone or to provide a vascularized matrix for the placement of free bone grafts for malar bone or the orbit. The second method provides both vascularized bone and soft tissue as individual components of the defect. One of the major advantages of free tissue transfer is reversal of the usual reconstructive dilemma of inadequate tissue brought to the site by various methods to cover difficult, large, and complex defects. Now overcorrection of the defect with soft tissue allows for subsequent modification without the need for further importation of tissue.

The scapula flap (particularly with the bone based on the angular vessel), the fibula flap, the radial forearm flap, and the deep circumflex iliac artery flap can all provide vascularized bone and soft tissue to fill various three-dimensional defects, particularly those involving the palate. The latissimus dorsi, serratus, rectus abdominis, and omentum are excellent donor sites for soft tissue to support subsequent free bone grafts. Because of its amorphous nature, the omentum is best employed when it can be contained in a compartment (e.g., with the palate intact). Microvascular anastomosis should be performed in the neck through a cheek flap approach in the subcutaneous layer to avoid injury to the branches of the facial nerve. The facial vessels as they approach the mandibular notch are usually good recipient vessels.

The orbits, the periorbital tissues, and the eyelids may require reconstruction, particularly after craniofacial trauma or tumor resection or with congenital facial clefts and other birth defects. Of considerable concern after nasoethmoid trauma is the status of the nasolacrimal duct. Excessive tearing may signal transection of the duct. Direct repair is rarely feasible, so the usual approach is to allow secondary epithelialization of a connection between the punctum and the nasal cavity over a Silastic tube. Some claim improved results with small vein grafts to replace or restore the duct. The level of the globe in both the coronal and sagittal planes depends on the volume of the bony orbit, the volume of the periorbital soft tissue, its free mobility, and to some degree the correct position of the canthal tendons. The first of these parameters is preferably addressed by bony reconstruction, but synthetic materials such as Vitallium or Silastic sheeting may be used. Medial wall destruction is a sometimes unrecognized cause of enophthalmos. Loss of bulk in the periorbital area secondary to ischemia and fibrosis is another frequent cause of globe malposition that is more difficult to correct but may sometimes respond to bony augmentation of the floor or medial wall of the orbit. Disruption of the normal position of the medial or lateral canthal ligaments or misalignment secondary to fibrosis may result in telecanthus or other abnormalities. Bony reconstruction of the lateral and medial walls of the orbit must include proper positioning of the canthal tendons and fixation to stable adjacent bone.

The eyelids (upper and lower) provide reconstructive problems after resection for tumor (usually skin cancer), congenital colobomas, trauma including burns, and senile laxity. The lower eyelid is a more common problem, but in either case, analysis must consider whether the defect is partial or full thickness as well as the site, size, and condition of the surrounding tissue. The eyelid consists of skin with the lashes and meibomian glands covering the orbicularis oculi muscle. In the upper lid, the tarsus, the "skeletal" framework of the lids, is attached to the orbit by Müller's muscle and the levator palpebrae. The tarsus is connected to the orbital septum, which encloses the periorbital fat. Deep to this is the conjunctival layer. Defects superficial to the tarsus may be resurfaced with full-thickness skin grafts. The lax skin of the normal (opposite upper) lid may be a good donor site for such grafts, and overcorrection of the defect may be necessary to ensure healing without ectropion. Conjunctival synechiae may be released and contralateral conjunctival, buccal, or nasal mucosa grafts used for resurfacing.

Full-thickness defects are approached by primary closure, composite grafting with local flaps, or lid-sharing procedures, depending on the size of the defect. Up to one third of the normal lower lid and one fourth of the upper lid can be directly approximated, sometimes more on the lower lid if a lateral cantholysis is done. Closure must separately address the conjunctiva (which may be approximated with absorbable running suture), the tarsus (which may be closed with undyed nylon), and the skin (which may be approximated with silk). Larger full-thickness defects also require reconstruction of component layers. Composite reconstruction can be achieved by using a chondromucosal graft of nasal septum to replace tarsus and conjunctiva; the nasal septum is revascularized by a local skin flap such as the Mustardé cheek flap or by the Fricke flap from the forehead or upper lid. An alternative method of providing tarsoconjunctival or full-thickness tissue to the upper or lower lids is by lid-sharing procedures such as the Hughes method, where bipedicle flaps are inset into the defect and left attached to their native lid and the eye sutured closed for several weeks until the graft is revascularized from its edges, at which point the bipedicle attachment is divided and the donor site closed primarily. In relative importance of the eyelids, the upper lid is usually considered to be of greater importance (Fig 19–3).

The lips play an important role in facial expression, speech, maintenance of oral continence, and initiation of swallowing. Since all of these roles require both mobility and sensation, optimal reconstruction is from like tissue. Analogous in structure to the eyelids, the reconstructive principles are similar. Skin with hair to the vermilion border or a specialized mucosal margin covers the orbicularis oris muscle, which connects the subcutaneous layer to the muscles of facial expression, the depressor anguli oris, mentalis, levator anguli oris, quadratus labii superioris, buccinator, and zygomaticus at the modiolus. Deep to the muscle lie the minor salivary glands that drain into the oral cavity through the labial mucosa. Like the other muscles of facial expression, the orbicularis oris muscle, the sphincter of the oral cavity, receives its motor innervation from the facial nerve's marginal mandibular and buccal branches and its sensory innervation from the trigeminal nerve's termination of the mandibular nerve, the mental nerve, and the infraorbital nerve. The lower lip is usually more lax and protuberant than the upper lip, and therefore defects of larger size can be closed by primary approximation. Up to one third to one half of the lower lip and one fourth to one third of the upper lip can be directly approximated, depending to a great degree on the age of the patient. The relative symmetry of the upper and lower lips and the circular pathway of the labial artery, a branch of the facial artery lying just deep to the muscle, allow "lip switch" operations from either the upper or lower lip to fill defects of various sizes. The Abbe flap brings tissue from the lower lip to the upper and may consist of skin, muscle, and mucosa or muscle and mucosa alone. The Estlander flap transports similar tissue based on the labial artery from the upper lip to the lower. As a pedicle flap, these are inset and allowed to revascularize from the periphery; after 7 to 14 days the pedicle is divided. Each component layer should be approximated to its corresponding layer. The point of rotation of the flap is the most important site to be considered. There is some controversy over whether the muscle in the lip switch segment becomes innervated with motor or sensory supply, but independent of this, the segments usually provide adequate functional restoration.

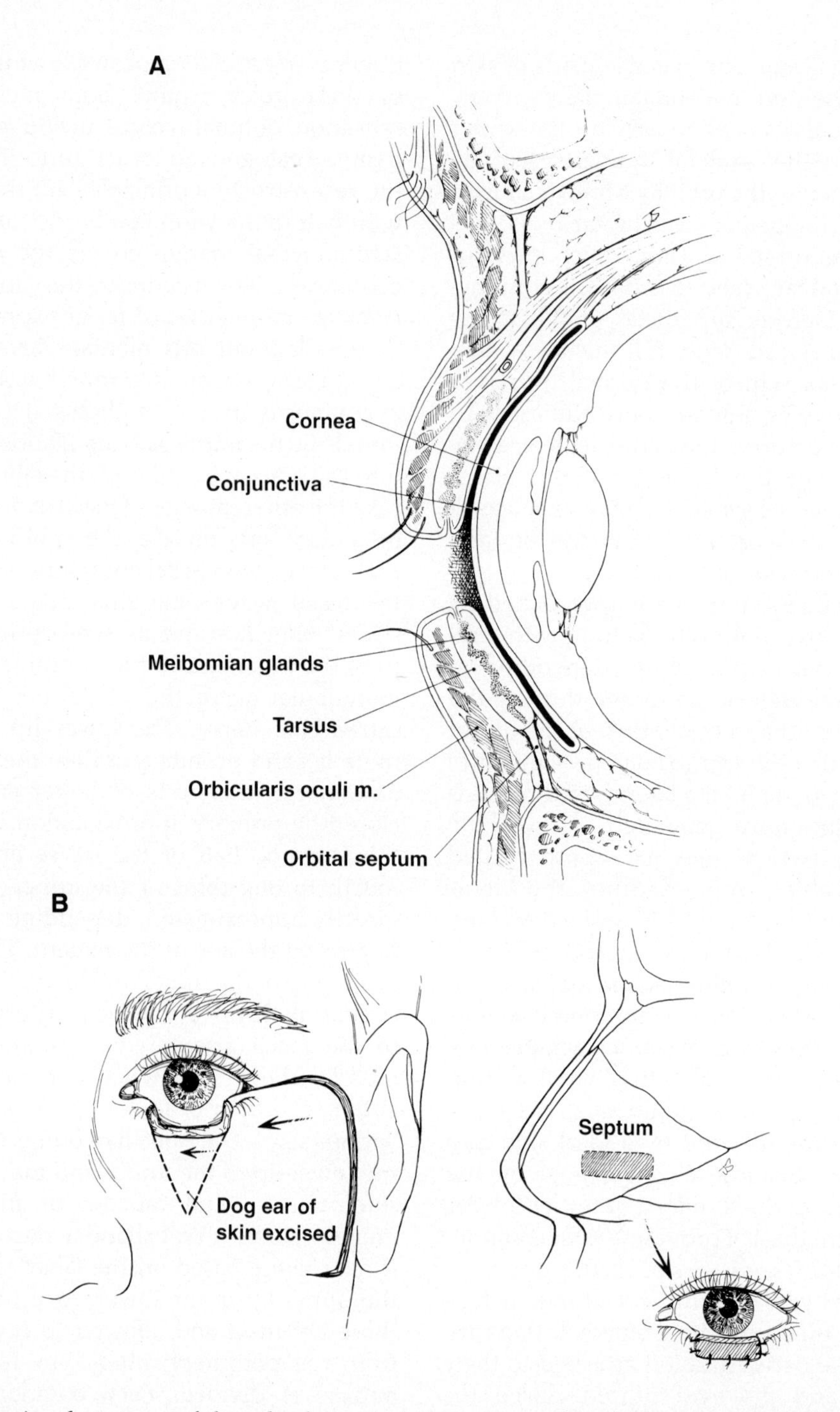

FIG 19–3.
A, Cross-sectional anatomy of the orbital area including the eyelids. **B,** The Mustardé flap method for closure of full-thickness defects of more than one third of the lower upper eyelid. The skin flap is mobilized superficial to the muscles of facial expression and extends lateral and upward over the malar and temporal areas. Superior extent must be sufficient to overcorrect the vertical defect to avoid ectropion. The excess skin resulting from medial rotation of the flap is excised as a dog-ear either at the time of the procedure or as a secondary revision. The donor area lateral and inferior can be closed by mobilizing temporal skin, neck skin, or by split-thickness skin grafts. The tarsus and conjunctiva are reconstructed with a free chondromucosal graft from the nasal septum, taking care to leave the contralateral mucosa intact.

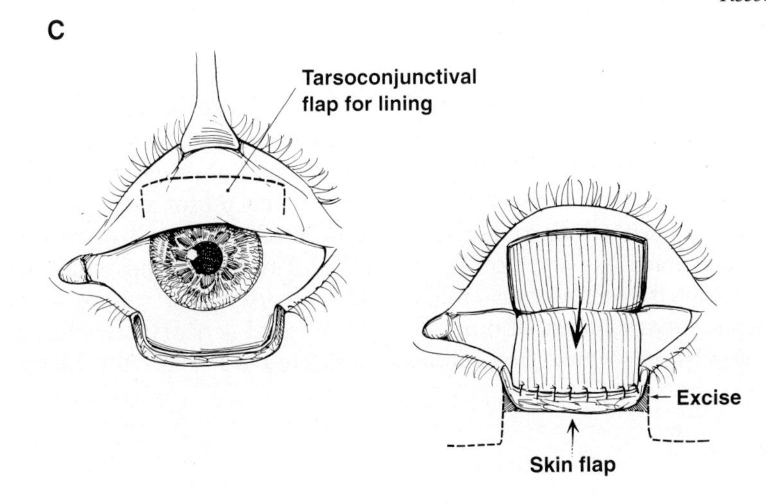

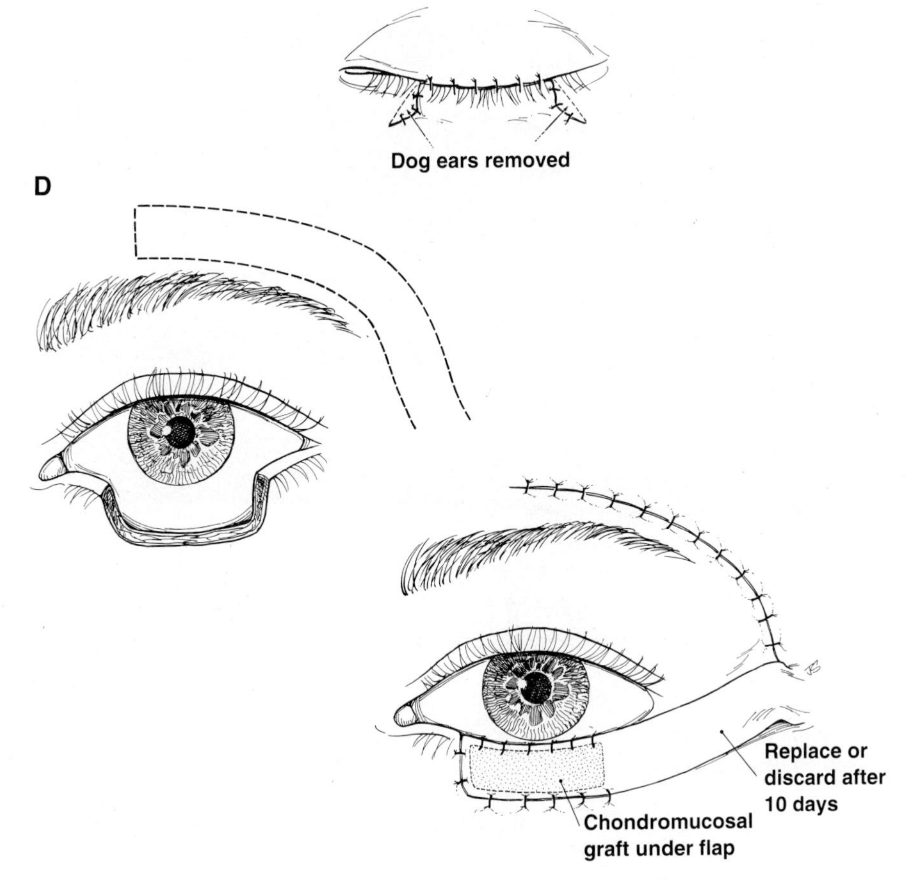

FIG 19–3 (cont.).
C, Reconstruction of a full-thickness defect of the lower lid by the Hughes technique. The upper lid is everted and a partial thickness quadrilateral superiorly based flap of conjunctiva and tarsus is separated from the overlying tissue. This is inset into the deep layer of the defect, securing conjunctiva to conjunctiva with absorbable suture and tarsus to tarsus with 4-0 or 5-0 nylon. The skin cover is obtained by an advancement flap of skin from below, and the dog-ears are excised laterally. The lids are sutured together to prevent an avulsion of the flap. After 2 to 3 weeks, the lid margins are divided and the tarso conjunctival flap separated and sutured to the skin margin. **D,** Closure of full-thickness defect with Frické flap. The tarsus and conjunctiva are reconstructed by a chondromucosal flap from the nasal septum. The skin is covered by a flap taken from the suprapalpebral skin of the forehead based laterally or medially. The donor site is closed primarily and the flap inset into the adjacent skin. The excess may be reinset into the donor defect or discarded.

Larger defects of the lip will not be satisfactorily reconstructed by primary closure or cross-lip flaps and may require mobilization of adjacent full-thickness flaps of cheek skin, muscle, and mucosa. Bernard flaps rely on advancement of buccal mucosa and skin with excision of the dog-ears in the nasolabial folds as Burow's triangles. Advancement of mucosa over the flaps results in a new vermilion margin. These advancement flaps serve only as dams; they are insensate because of division of the mental nerve and immobile because of loss of the motor nerve supply. Karapandzic described a method of reconstructing up to 80% of the lower lip while maintaining both the sensory and motor nerve supply. The motor and sensory branches of the nerve are dissected out with the blood supply to the

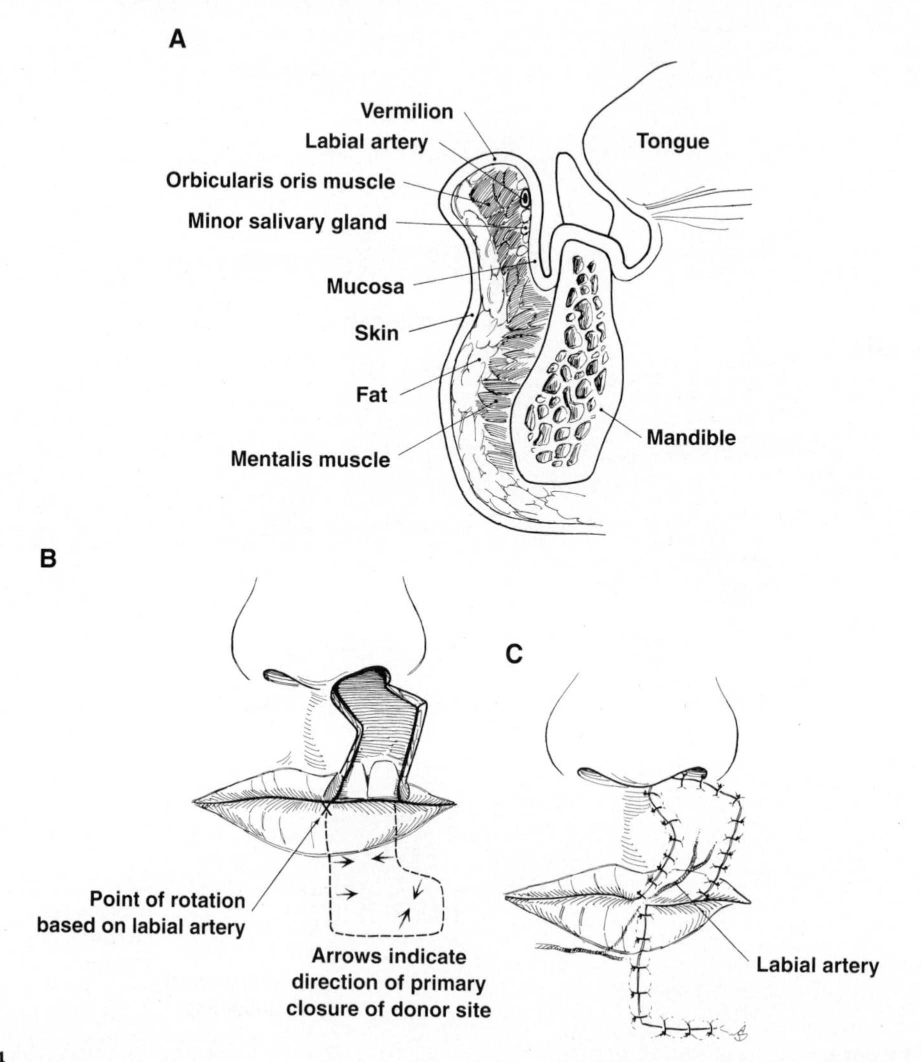

FIG 19–4.
A, Cross-sectional anatomy of the lip, floor of mouth, and mandible showing the relationship of the orbicularis oris to the other tissues including the labial artery. **B,** Large defect in the upper lip philtrum and columella and the nasal floor secondary to excision of malignancy. Reconstruction of more than one third of upper lip must address the vermilion mucosa and skin and soft tissue. The Abbé flap is designed to be rotated on the labial vessels, in this case based at the right edge of the lower lip and including enough tissue from the mental area to fill the floor of the nose and columella. **C,** The flap is rotated 180° with the labial artery left in continuity with the lower lip. The flap is inset to the upper lip approximating at least three layers, skin, orbicularis oris muscle and mucosa. The donor site is closed primarily. The vessels are left intact for 10 to 14 days and then divided, revising the upper and lower sites.

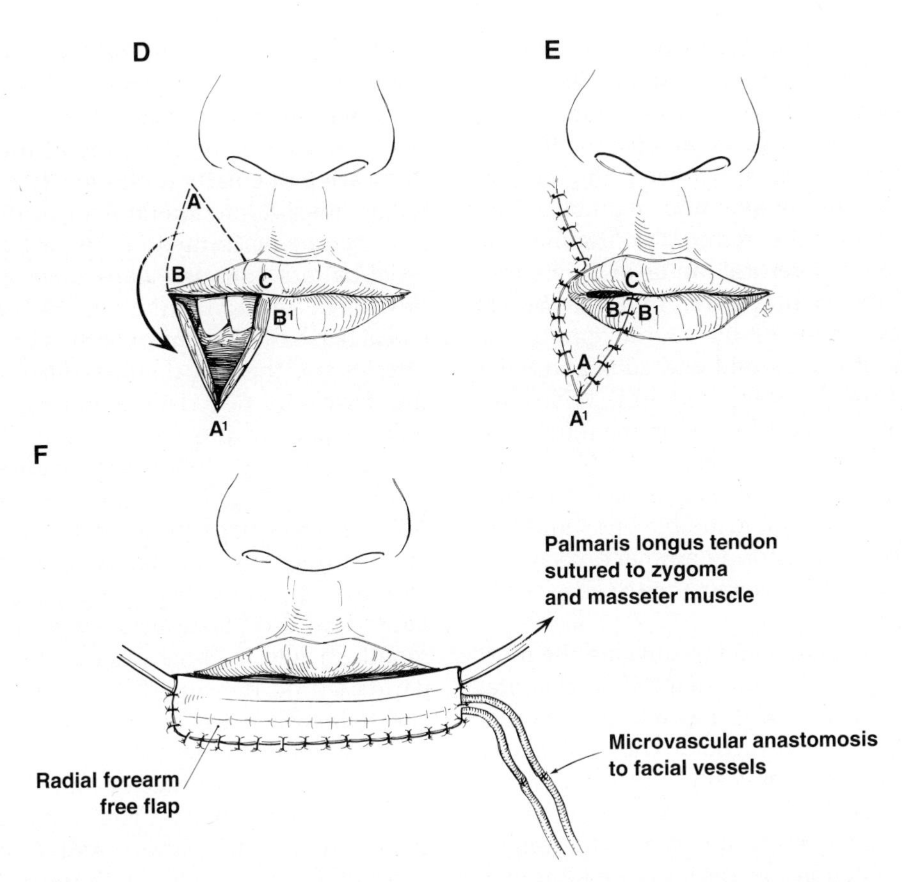

FIG 19–4 (cont.).
D, The Estlander flap based on the same principle as the Abbè flap is taken from the upper lip and based on the labial artery. **E,** It is rotated into the defect and sutured into place. At a later time the commissure can be lengthened by V-Y advancement of the mucosa onto the cheek skin. **F,** Reconstruction of total lower lip defects can be obtained by use of the radial forearm free flap draped over the palmaris longus tendon. The vascularized tendon graft is sutured into the zygoma, masseter, and muscles of facial expression. The flap is inset into skin and mucosa. Microvascular anastomosis is performed in the neck to the facial vessels. In young patients, anastomosis of the antebrachial cutaneous nerve and the mental nerve may provide some sensation.

orbicularis oris and the muscle detached from its insertion at the modiolus, lateral nares, and upper philtral area as necessary. The muscle is then bilaterally advanced to complete the circle of the mouth. Although relative microstomia is sometimes a problem, the preservation of oral continence is a major advantage.

Complete loss of the full thickness of the lower lip can be reconstructed by free tissue transfer. The radial forearm free flap with a segment of vascularized palmaris longus tendon inset into the modiolus and suspended from the zygoma or superficial musculoaponeurotic system (SMAS) fascia will provide a dam with some conducted motion from the adjacent muscles and may allow restoration of sensation by anastomosis of the mental nerve and anterior cutaneous nerve of the forearm. Loss of the vermilion and mucosa secondary to lip shaving for sun damage, hyperkeratosis, or noninvasive carcinoma can be restored by advancement of the adjacent mucosa over the orbicularis oris from the mandibulolabial sulcus. This procedure can also be used to thin lips for aesthetic improvement (Fig 19–4).

THE ORAL CAVITY

The oral cavity initiates digestion, serves as a reservoir and preparation site for food prior to swallowing, and refines exhaled air as the finished product of speech. It extends from the lips to the anterior tonsillar pillars and includes the labial and buccal mucosa, the mandibular and maxillary alveoli, the floor of the mouth, the area between the ventral surface of the tongue and mandible, the mobile tongue, the retromolar trigone, the mucosa-covered vertical ramus of the mandible, and the hard palate. Into the buccal mucosa and floor of the mouth empty the secretions of the parotid and submandibular glands through Stensen's and Wharton's ducts, respectively. The predominant function of the oral cavity is as a reservoir. Soft-tissue reconstruction is frequently linked to bony reconstruction of the mandible but should be oriented toward restoring normal capacitance and minimizing interference with the mobility of the tongue.

Tumor resection and trauma are the most common etiologies for defects of the oral cavity, and specific sites may require different methods of reconstruction. The oral cavity and tongue are basically mucosa-covered muscular structures, the mucosa being of the nonkeratinizing squamous type. The tongue is a combination of intrinsic longitudinal, transverse, and external muscles: the genioglossus, hyoglossus, palatoglossus, and styloglossus, all supplied by the hypoglossal nerve. The floor of the mouth is the mucosal covering of the mylohyoid muscles, and the cheeks have mucosa overlying the buccinator muscles and buccal fat pads. Conceptually the alimentary canal can be considered a long mucosa-lined muscular tube with a sphincter at both ends (the lips and anal muscles). The oral cavity is simply a modification of that tube to allow chewing and refined speech. The goal for partial-thickness defects of the oral cavity is to restore the epithelial lining. This can be done with split-thickness skin grafts in some cases. Grafts should be meshed and tightly fixed to the underlying bed with a tie over dressing to avoid shear from the constant motion of the tongue and jaws. The oral mucosa will reepithelialize relatively rapidly without grafting, but the concomitant contraction of the wound may interfere with function, particularly in the buccal area and along the floor of the mouth at its connection to the ventral surface of the tongue.

Because of the plentiful blood supply of the tongue, random myomucosal flaps can be designed to cover adjacent defects. These, however, may cause tethering of the tongue. They are particularly useful for defects of the palate, tonsils, and lateral floor of the mouth and may be performed in one or two stages. Axial-pattern intraoral flaps have also been described, including the palatal mucoperiosteal flap based on one or both of the palatine arteries and the buccal mucosal flap based on the facial arteries. The donor site for the palatal flap reepithelializes spontaneously. The buccal flap donor site requires either primary closure or a split-thickness skin graft. Adjacent skin flaps from the head and neck may also be useful. Before the advent of musculocutaneous flaps, bipedicle cervical flaps were used to resurface the floor of the mouth in two to three stages. The forehead flap based on the superficial temporal artery and vein will reach the floor of the mouth, palate, and buccal mucosa but is hampered by the necessity of two stages and the obvious donor site deformity. The nasolabial flap based on the facial artery and vein can be brought through a defect in the buccal mucosa to resurface small defects of the floor of the mouth or mandibular alveolus.

Unfortunately, most oral cavity defects, particularly those created by resection of malignancy, are such that local tissue is not adequate. Resection of oral cancer leaves a defect of muscle and mucosa or muscle, mucosa, and skin that requires closure with similar tissue with its own blood supply. Importation of tissue has been crucial to restoration of form and function of the oral cavity. Various "waltzed" thoracoepigastric flaps such as the dorsal scapula, Zovickian, or Mutter flaps preceded the deltopectoral flap, which was the mainstay of repair until musculocutaneous flaps were developed. The deltopectoral flap described by Bakamjian in 1965 is an axial cutaneous flap from the chest that is based on the perforating branches of the internal mammary vessels. It extends over the anterior deltoid area without delay and can be lengthened either to the posterior deltoid area or down the arm with one or more delay procedures. This flap provides relatively thin vascularized tissue, which is reasonably good lining for the buccal mucosa cheek skin or floor of the mouth. The disadvantages of this method are that it requires two stages and it is a thin axial skin flap that has a relatively high risk of ischemia at the distal margin, particularly in the presence of the highly contaminated oral cavity.

The elucidation of musculocutaneous flaps allowed for single-stage repair with a large volume of tissue. The pectoralis major musculocutaneous flap based on the thoracoacromial artery and vein can carry a large amount of anterior chest wall skin over the pectoralis muscle to the lower and mid oral cavity. Its arc of rotation easily reaches the floor of the mouth and tongue and possibly may reach the palate and zygomatic area. It can provide skin for epithelial lining, well-vascularized muscle, and bulk. The latissimus dorsi muscle or musculocutaneous flap based on the thoracodorsal vessels can also be transposed through the axilla to cover the buccal area or floor of the mouth. The trapezius musculocutaneous flap, particularly if vertically oriented, can achieve a wide arc of rotation based on the transverse cervical vessels. Although the pectoralis and trapezius have been touted as osseomusculocutaneous flaps carrying rib, sternum, or a spine of the scapula, neither bone segment is particularly reliable. The sternocleidomastoid flap based on the superior thyroid and occipital vessels has been used for reconstruction of the floor of the mouth but is not as reliable as other methods. Based on the submental branch of the facial artery as its superior pedicle, the platysma muscle can carry a skin paddle as a musculocutaneous flap and provide thin supple epithelial coverage for the buccal mucosa or the floor of the mouth.

Despite their numerous good qualities, the musculocutaneous flaps are not ideal for oral reconstruction because with their bulk, gravity tends to pull them toward the chest. Furthermore, the skin paddle of the pectoralis major flap, the most commonly used method, is relatively poorly perfused and carries a large amount of fat in most Caucasians. In the oral cavity this method is best suited for reconstruction of total glossectomy defects where its bulk does not interfere with the mobility of the tongue and for lateral defects where the mandible is no longer present. The bulk of these flaps makes them difficult to use when the mandible has not been removed.

Given the considerable motion and coordination required in the normal function of the oral cavity coupled with the need for supple tissue with a homogeneous blood supply to deal with the heavily contaminated environment, free tissue transfer may be ideal. The radial forearm free flap provides a large amount of pliable epithelial-covered tissue that can be shaped to the needs of the defect. The long pedicle may reach into the lower part of the neck if necessary, and sensory reinnervation is possible via the antebrachial cutaneous nerves. The lateral arm and medial arm flaps also provide thin pliable tissue; similar tissue can be supplied by a segment of jejunum opened as a patch. Defects with more bulk requirements are well dealt with by using a musculocutaneous free flap such as the rectus abdominis and the latissimus dorsi. Recent reports advocate free muscle flaps without skin coverage to be followed by atrophy and reepithelialization. In most cases, free tissue transfer can circumvent the problems inherent in the thoracic musculocutaneous flap—bulk, effect of gravity, and nonhomogeneous vascularization—and provide the watertight seal necessary to reconstruct the oral cavity.

When a defect of the oral cavity includes exposure of the great vessels in the neck, particularly if the patient has been previously irradiated, there may be an advantage to using a method that will cover the exposed carotid. This can be achieved with either a thoracic musculocutaneous flap or free tissue transfer and should be designed so that in the event of dehiscence of the repair, the flow of salivary contents is directed away from the vessels and they remain covered with well-vascularized tissue (Fig 19–5).

The pharynx consists of three relatively separate anatomic entities, each with a different function. The nasopharynx, the mucosa-lined vault above the soft palate and superior constrictor of the pharynx, is the receptacle of air from the nasal cavity prior to its entrance into the larynx. It also allows modulation of pressure between the pharynx and the middle ear via the eustachian orifices. The bony roof of the nasopharynx is the base of the brain. The oropharynx extends from the tonsils to the epiglottis and, along with the base of the tongue, soft palate, and lateral and posterior pharyngeal walls, is the beginning of the muscular tube that pushes the food bolus toward the stomach. As such it is intimately connected to and its actions synchronized with the larynx, oral tongue, and mandible. The hypopharynx, which includes the poste-

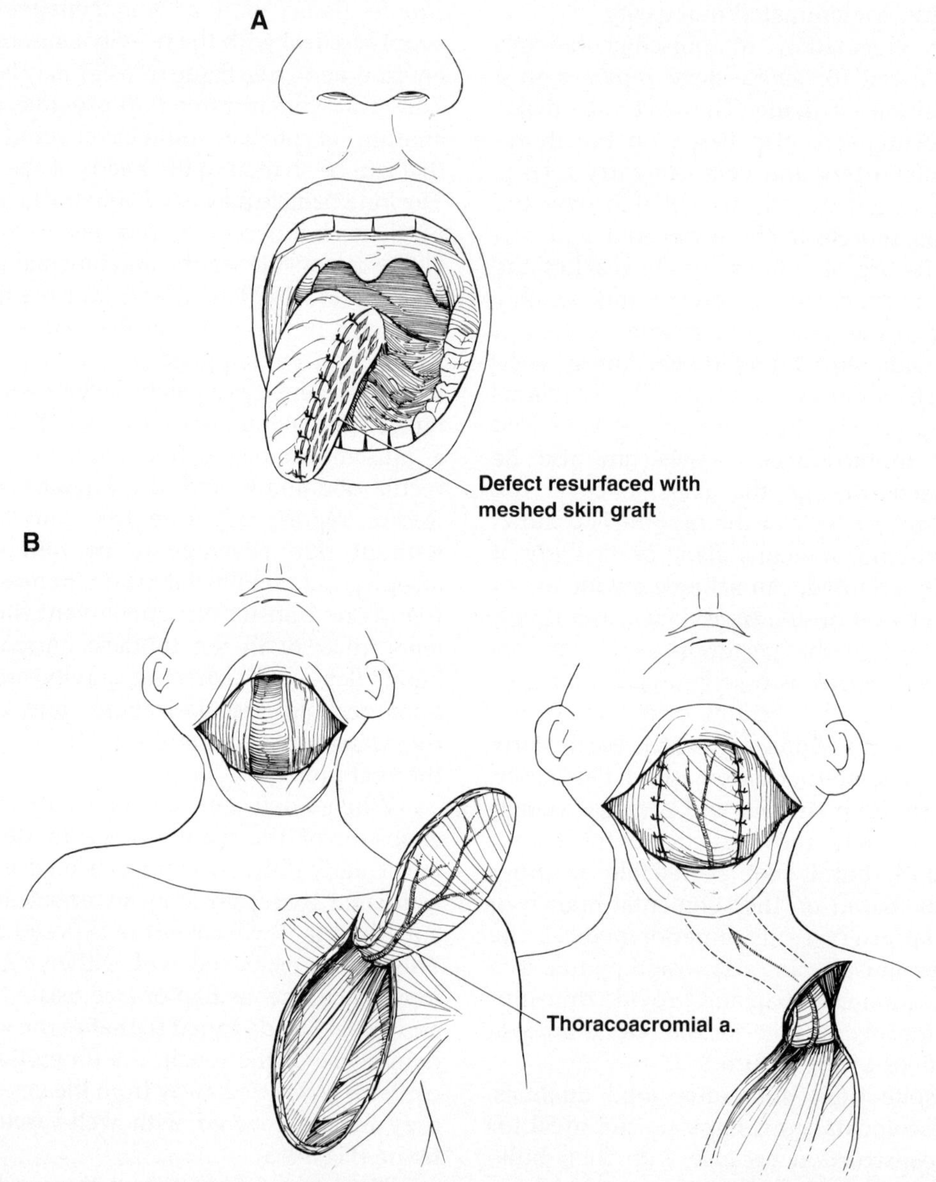

FIG 19–5.
A, Defects that are of small to moderate size and involve only soft tissue or occasionally bone with periosteum left intact can be covered with a meshed split-thickness skin graft sutured to the mucosa. In areas of concavity, the skin grafts should be immobilized with a tie-over bolster of some nonadherent material. **B,** Total glossectomy and laryngopharyngoectomy defect reconstructed with a pectoralis musculocutaneous flap. The flap raised from the chest is rotated 180° in the anteroposterior plane. The skin of the pectoralis major musculocutaneous flap is sutured to the posterior pharyngeal mucosa and prevertebral fascia, the mucosa of the retromolar trigone, and the remaining floor of the mouth mucosa. Excess muscle can be draped over the great vessels in the neck.

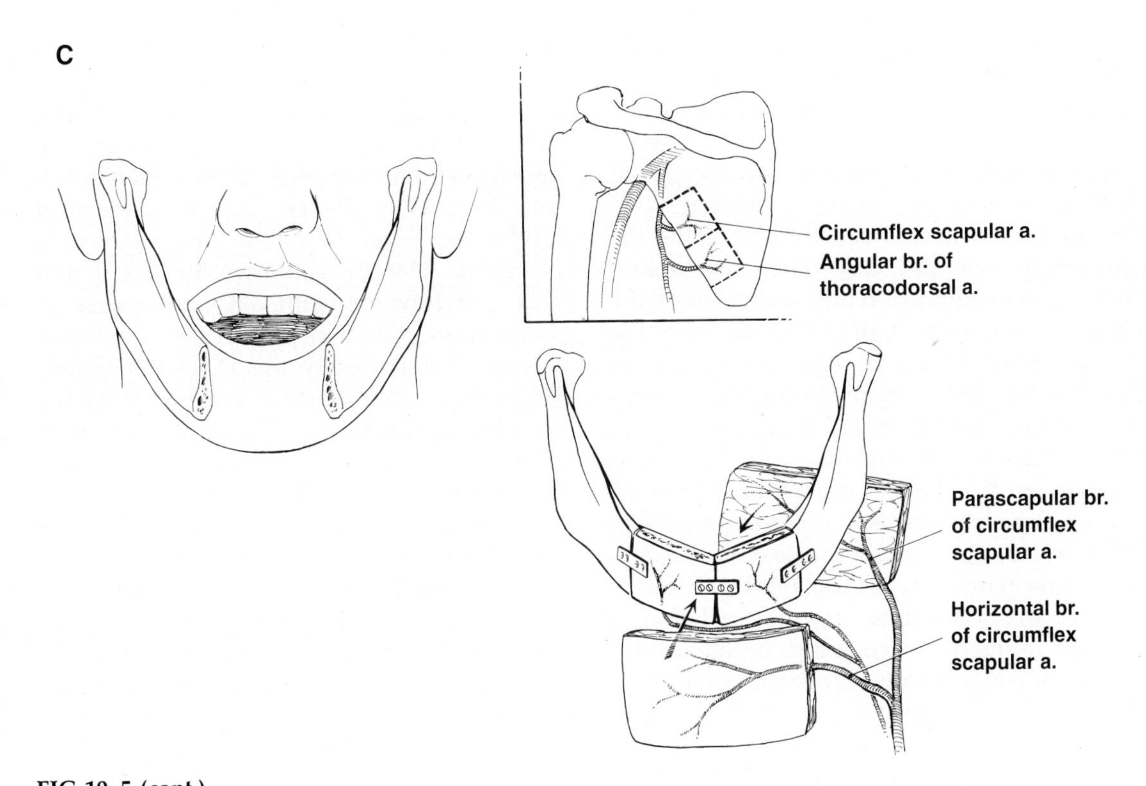

FIG 19–5 (cont.).
C, Resection of extensive carcinoma of the floor of the mouth involving skin, mandible, and mucosa of the floor of the mouth. The external coverage is provided by the circumflex scapula artery horizontal branch and the internal lining by the paddle of skin supplied by the parascapular branch. Bone is provided by two vascularized segments from the circumflex scapula and the angular branch of the thoracodorsal artery. Miniplate fixation of the segments is performed preserving as much of the periosteal blood supply to each segment as possible. The segments are similarly fixed to the remaining mandible replacing the symphysis. The skin paddles provide a watertight mucosal closure as well as external coverage and because of the freedom of each pedicle can be used in several arcs of rotation.

rior wall of the larynx, the postcricoid area, and the piriform sinuses, is the continuation of this passageway. Since these areas are so vitally related to respiration and swallowing, an understanding of the mechanisms of these actions is crucial to any reconstructive undertaking.

After the bolus of food is prepared in the oral cavity by mastication, crushing between the tongue and palate, and lubrication and partial digestion by the addition of saliva from the parotid, submandibular, and sublingual glands, it is moved to the back of the oral cavity by the tongue. As the tongue generates pressure, the superior pharyngeal constrictor closes, and the soft palate elevates to close the communication between the oropharynx and nasopharynx. Simultaneously the extrinsic muscles of the tongue and the mylohyoid elevate the larynx by pulling cephalad on the hyoid bone. This action allows the epiglottis to seal the opening to the larynx. While this is occurring, the cricopharyngeus and inferior constrictors relax and allow the bolus to be pushed behind and beside the closed larynx. The relaxation of the superior esophageal sphincter, the cricopharyngeus, initiates the peristaltic action of the esophagus, and the bolus continues on its path to the stomach. In addition, as the cricopharyngeus contracts to prevent regurgitation of the food bolus back up into the larynx, the relaxation of the suprahyoid muscles and the contraction of the infrahyoid strap muscles allow the larynx to descend. Naturally these actions must be coordinated with respiration, which is controlled primarily by the expansion and relaxation of the thorax and opening and closing of the glottis. Whatever the needs imposed by the defect, careful consideration must be given to preservation of these intricately connected functions. Bulk, interposition of insensate material, and other limitations may negate an otherwise seemingly adequate method.

Reconstructive considerations of the nasopharynx have two major elements: separation of the central nervous system from the pharynx and separation of the oral from the nasal cavity to allow normal speech and swallowing. The temporalis muscle or pericranial flaps based on the frontal portion of the anterior flap created by a coronal incision are excellent methods of separation of the base of the brain from the nasopharynx. A portion of a free tissue transfer can also be used to create a watertight seal. Problems that result in loss of the soft palate may be treated in a similar fashion to velopharyngeal insufficiency in patients with cleft palate: a flap, be it local, regional, or free tissue transfer, is inset between the palate and posterior of the pharynx and communication through the two cavities maintained by port holes created around rubber catheters. The radial forearm and lateral arm flaps are excellent methods of providing epithelial lining to both the oral and nasal portions of the pharynx.

Obviously no presently available method of reconstruction can replace the intricate synergy between sensate mucosa and muscle and cartilage in the oropharynx. The reconstructive consideration then becomes how to interfere least with the remaining function. Of particular importance is choosing a method that will minimize the risk of aspiration while allowing effective swallowing. If the risk of aspiration is high and there is reasonable concern that the patient will not tolerate some aspiration, then separation of the respiratory and alimentary tracts is indicated. In the case of extensive malignancy, this usually takes the form of laryngectomy. There are, however, reversible methods of closing the larynx that are occasionally appropriate for benign disease.

Defects of the oropharynx are usually the consequence of resection of malignancy or some complication of therapy for malignant disease. In analysis of such wounds, a history of radiotherapy or the need for prompt adjuvant postoperative radiotherapy is an important factor. The usual criteria of size, volume, proximity to the great vessels, etc., are also sometimes complicated by a mobile larynx. Whenever possible, primary closure of any defect adjacent to the intact larynx is advisable. This provides sensate tissue that may still function with adjacent muscle to allow coordination of respiration and swallowing. Unfortunately, this is rarely possible. Of paramount importance is maintaining the mobility of the larynx. If a large amount of oropharynx has been resected, lightweight tissue that will not tether the larynx is necessary for reconstruction. The radial forearm free flap or other fasciocutaneous flaps are excellent methods for reconstruction of the base of the tongue, lateral pharyngeal wall, soft palate, and occasionally the posterior pharyngeal wall. The pliability of these skin flaps allows them to be folded to recreate the complex anatomy of this compact area. Their homogeneous axial fascial blood supply allows them to be made large or small as needed and to be deepithelialized if necessary. Although free autografts of bowel share the pliability and excellent blood supply of fasciocutaneous flaps, their secretory epithelium increases the risk of aspiration, and they should not be used when the larynx is intact. In contrast to these methods, the pectoralis flap is usually much too bulky for partial defects of the pharynx because of the presence of the mandible and the larynx. When inset into the base of the tongue or adjacent to the larynx, it impedes motion and creates a higher risk of pharyngocutaneous fistulas as well as laryngeal dysfunction. Therefore, thoracic musculocutaneous flaps should rarely be used in partial pharyngeal reconstruction. There has been some interest in reinnervating free muscle flaps in an attempt to replace part or all of the mobile tongue. Anastomosis of the thoracodorsal to the hypoglossal nerve has been reported with inconclusive results.

A small but important subset of pharynx and oral cavity defects are those created by total glossectomy. Although previously condemned, it has recently been shown to be an effective method of both palliation and definitive therapy. When the oncologic dictates of the procedure do not require total laryngectomy, the larynx should be preserved. The defect created by removal of mucosa of the tongue and floor of mouth can be filled with either a pectoralis major musculocutaneous flap or free tissue transfer. Whatever method is chosen, care must be taken to suspend the larynx as far superior and anterior as possible by the pull of the flap from the mandible to the hyoid.

Another group of patients who may require partial pharyngeal reconstruction are those in whom orocutaneous or pharyngocutaneous fistulas develop. Small fistulas in areas where there are no bony structures frequently close without surgery. Larger defects, those in previously irradiated patients or those that occur at the base of the tongue or other extremely mobile areas, are less likely to resolve without surgery. The usual considerations for fistula evaluation and therapy apply. The presence of infection, a foreign body, residual tumor, or distal obstruction as well as a history of previous radiotherapy are all important. Effective reconstruction requires restoration of the site to a clean wound surrounded by viable tissue and introduction of well-vascularized epithelial tissue. For small pharyngocutaneous fistulas in the neck, the sternocleidomastoid musculocutaneous flap is useful. Rarely local cervical skin flaps or the deltopectoral flap is adequate. The weight and thickness of the skin on the pectoralis flap make it cumbersome. Free tissue transfer is excellent for large defects.

Since many surgical defects secondary to malignancy or resection of lye-damaged pharynx and esophagus result in total or subtotal pharyngectomy with associated loss of the larynx, an adequate method of restoring the conduit between the oral cavity and thoracic esophagus is necessary. The wound requirements range from a small circumferential defect to one extending from the nasopharynx to the inlet of the thoracic esophagus. The primary goal is restoration of a patent conduit that will allow the force of the tongue or whatever swallowing mechanisms remain to push the food into the peristaltic portion of the esophagus. Before the musculocutaneous concept, local cervical skin flaps such as the Wookey flap were utilized. These were, however, unreliable since the skin of the neck usually shared the same trauma from surgery and radiotherapy that affected the pharynx. The deltopectoral flap tubed on itself allowed a two-stage reconstruction but had a high risk of stenosis and fistula at both the proximal and distal suture lines.

Although numerous early small series reported successful use of the pectoralis major musculocutaneous flap tubed on itself for total pharyngeal reconstruction, recent experience has shown that whether used as a tube or a patch, the pectoralis major flap has a high fistula and stenosis rate. To decrease the likelihood of a fistula from the weight of the flap inset at the mobile base of the tongue, the usual recipient site for the anterior anastomosis, a 270-degree wrap of the musculocutaneous flap can be performed by insetting the edges to the prevertebral fascia and reconstructing the posterior of the pharynx with a split-thickness skin graft applied directly to the prevertebral fascia. The rigidity of the fixation of the flap to the prevertebral fascia maintains the patency of the conduit by preventing it from collapsing and also decreases the likelihood of a fistula at the base of the tongue. This same technique of 270-degree reconstruction can be effectively used with a free tissue transfer.

The jejunal free flap, either as a tube, a patch, or a fillet and tube, is an excellent method of total pharyngoesophageal reconstruction. It provides a number of the requisites for almost any wound: well-vascularized tissue with homogeneous perfusion, adequate length for virtually any neck defect, as well as secretion of mucus for lubrication. The random contractility can occasionally be a problem but almost always resolves with time. A mismatch in width at the proximal anastomosis can be avoided by end-to-side anastomosis. Adequate visualization of the proximal anastomosis is essential for avoidance of a fistula. This may require mandibulotomy to achieve and should always be performed if necessary. In addition to the bowel providing an excellent conduit, the mesentery can be used to cover the carotid vessels. By harvesting an excess of bowel, the site of microvascular anastomosis can be adjusted upward or downward by resecting the bowel at the mesenteric border, thereby changing the relative position of the main mesenteric vessels to the ends of the jejunum. In addition to the jejunum, segments of colon based on the ileocolic vessels and segments of stomach based on the gastroepiploic vessels may be useful for both partial and complete pharyngeal reconstruction.

When total esophagectomy is a necessary part of laryngopharyngectomy, the stomach based on the right gastric and gastroepiploic vessels can be transposed through the mediastinum to reach the pharynx or even occasionally the nasopharynx. This is a reliable method of reconstruction but has a higher mortality rate because of the concomitant violation of the abdominal and thoracic cavities. Furthermore, when a fistula does occur at the pharyngeal anastomosis, it is usually because of distal ischemia rather than a technical error as with free tissue transfer.

The mandible may require reconstruction for congenital abnormalities, trauma, osteomyelitis, osteoradionecrosis, or resection for tumor. In children, the presence of rapidly growing bone from the various growth centers must be weighted with the individual wound characteristics. Continuity of the mandible is required for strength in chewing and improves the likelihood of oral continence by creating a framework for the soft tissues of the lower portion of the face. The presence of teeth and the desirability of providing proper occlusion of the remaining mandibular and maxillary teeth are also important. There are a number of methods for mandibular reconstruction, each applicable under certain circumstances. Synthetic materials have long been used as mandibular replacements, usually as a secondary procedure by an external approach to avoid contamination by the oral cavity. Previously, single or double Kirschner wires, acrylic or silicone carved prostheses, and stainless steel bars were used. These all suffer from limitations imposed by the function of the muscles of mastication. The pressure generated by speech and chewing is great, and the lining between the mandible and oral cavity is thin. The constant motion of the jaw makes the risk of infection and extrusion high.

Recently, titanium or stainless steel reconstruction plates have increased the success of prosthetic reconstruction. These plates can be shaped to the size and contour of the missing mandible and fixed with intraosseous screws. Several series have reported high success rates for this method after tumor resection, but many areas, particularly the symphysis, remain problematic with high extrusion rates. In addition to short-term problems of infection and extrusion, long-term difficulties with stress fracture of the metal and loosening of the screws have been reported. Stainless steel, titanium, Dacron mesh, and other synthetic trays have also served as spacers to hold grafts of cancellous bone from the iliac crests or rib. These again require an excellent soft-tissue envelope surrounding them and are subject to the same problems as reconstructive plates. The basket serves as a stabilizer to allow "creeping substitution" from the remaining mandible. Free nonvascularized bone grafts from calvarium, iliac crest, or rib are also sometimes effective in a well-vascularized bed of tissue. Because all of these methods depend on either maintenance of a foreign body or creeping substitution from adjacent bone, rigid fixation is absolutely crucial. In addition to wire or screw fixation, intermaxillary fixation with arch bars is usually necessary.

Vascularized bone transfer has revolutionized mandibular reconstruction. Although there have been numerous reports of pedicled bone grafts, including pectoralis with rib, pectoralis with sternum, trapezius with scapular spine, sternocleidomastoid with clavicle, and temporalis muscle and fascia with calvarium, these methods are rarely satisfactory because of the quantity and quality of bone as well as the tenuous connection of the blood supply to the bone. Free tissue transfer provides numerous territories of vigorously perfused bone with different types of attached skin, fascia, or muscle that may be used to reconstruct adjacent soft-tissue deficits. Furthermore, healing of the grafted bone to the native mandible occurs as in a fracture rather than by creeping substitution, and the ultimate result is usually stronger.

Although serratus with rib and metatarsal with skin have been used in the past, the most frequently employed free tissue transfers for bony reconstruction of the mandible now are the fibula, scapula, deep circumflex iliac artery (DCIA) flap, and the radial forearm free flap. These vascularized bone grafts are useful in almost any situation, but particularly when the patient has been previously irradiated, there is inadequate soft-tissue lining or skin coverage, there is infection present, or other methods have failed. Properly cut and shaped, the fibula can provide enough bone to reconstruct the entire mandible. Supplied by the peroneal artery, it has both an endosteal and periosteal blood supply and is excellent when numerous osteotomies are required. The overlying skin is supplied by septocutaneous perforating vessels, and although not as reliable as some other skin paddles, it can be used for either intraoral or extraoral soft tissue. The DCIA flap can reconstruct a hemimandible and is particularly useful for ramus and angle reconstruction since the curvature of the iliac crest recreates that of the mandible. A skin island on the internal oblique muscle can be harvested with the bone but is frequently too bulky because of the high concentration of fat.

The scapula can provide 10 to 14 cm of vascularized bone based on either the circumflex scapular vessels or the angular branch from the thoracodorsal artery. Although this bone is not as thick as the fibula or iliac crest, it is satisfactory for mandibular reconstruction. The major advantage of the scapula is that two separate paddles of relatively pliable skin, one for intraoral lining and one for external coverage, can be obtained as well as bone on a single set of blood vessels. It is thus useful for complex defects including mucosa, bone, and skin as well as bone alone. If more soft tissue is necessary, the latissimus dorsi and serratus muscles can also be harvested by taking the vascular origin of the flap, including the subscapular vessels. The radial forearm flap can carry a segment of vascularized radius supplied by perforators through the flexor pollicis longus muscle. Although this bone is relatively thin, the excellent pliability of the overlying volar forearm skin makes this an excellent choice for symphyseal or short-segment body reconstruction. All of these free flaps have pedicles of reasonable to excellent length and vessel diameters of 2 to 3 mm.

The preservation or restoration of normal dentition is an important part of mandible reconstruction. Before the graft or implant is shaped and inset, the patient's maxillary and remaining mandibular arches are put into proper occlusion by intermaxillary fixation. With this spatial relationship fixed, the reconstruction is stabilized, preferably with intraosseous screws and plates but alternatively with wire suture or Kirschner wires. Miniplate fixation is usually adequate. Mandibular plates used on scapula or radial forearm osteocutaneous flaps may split the bone segments. When plate fixation has been used, the intermaxillary fixation can be released to allow mobility of the jaw immediately after surgery. When trays, nonvascularized bone grafts, or other methods have been used, intermaxillary fixation should be maintained for 6 to 8 weeks. In the elderly or in patients who have been previously irradiated or have major soft-tissue defects, immobilization of the jaw may result in trismus and fibrosis of the muscles of mastication and should be avoided if possible. The advent of osseointegrated implantation of artificial teeth has greatly improved the overall rehabilitation of the oral cavity. Almost any vascularized or nonvascularized bone graft will eventually remodel to adequate bone stock for implantation, but the fibula, the DCIA, and (with lesser certainty) the scapula flap provide adequate bone for early implantation.

The neck is the route of access for most resections of intraoral, pharyngeal, or other head and neck malignancies. When the neck has previously been irradiated, exposure of the carotid artery and jugular vein may result in catastrophic complications. Fibrosis and obliteration of the vasa vasorum of the carotid artery put the vessel at high risk for invasive infection if exposure and desiccation occur. Exposure of the irradiated carotid should be treated with urgency. Well-vascularized soft tissue such as the pectoralis major muscle must be used to cover the vessel and seal it off

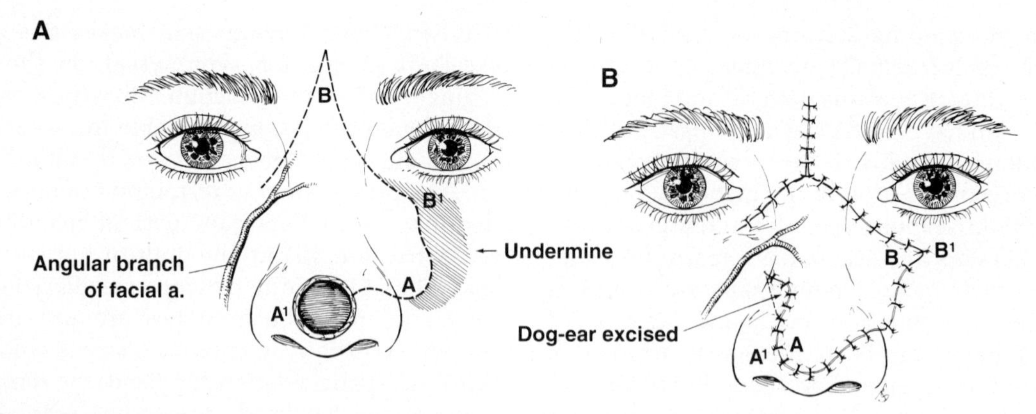

FIG 19–6.
A, Defects on the tip or alar rims of the nose may be resurfaced with similar skin by using the dorsal nasal flap based on the angular branch of the facial artery. This axial cutaneous rotation flap will reliably include the entire skin of the nose and glabella. Raised at the level of the periosteum and perichondrium, it may be mobilized from the nasomalar line on the side of the blood supply out into the malar area of the contralateral cheek depending on the tissue needs. **B,** The glabellar skin is closed primarily. The malar defect is closed by undermining or with the skin rotated from the glabellar area. The thin skin of the dorsum of the nose and malar area covers the tip. The dog-ear can be excised primarily if care is taken not to injure the angular vessels.

from the flow of salivary or cutaneous contaminants. This may be done by definitively closing the dehiscence or by creating a controlled fistula to divert flow away from the covered carotid. Intraoral or intrapharyngeal exposure of the carotid artery may occur as well and must be recognized and treated similarly. When an operation is planned in a heavily irradiated field, precautions should be taken to avoid exposing the carotid to the risk of invasive infection. If the carotid must be uncovered, it should be prophylactically ensheathed in well-vascularized tissue.

The nose, the center of the midface, is a complex aesthetic and functional structure with an external covering of thin, highly vascularized skin that reflects the definition of the underlying cartilaginous and bony skeleton. The integrity of this skeleton and its relationship to the turbinates and nasal septum determine the flow of air through the nose and the functioning of the internal nasal valve. Reconstruction of partial- or full-thickness defects is best done with like tissue because of the delicate synergy of the components and their high visibility. Superficial deficits in the skin such as those created by the excision of small malignancies can occasionally be closed primarily. This should, however, be done with extreme care to avoid deforming the nasal alae or the relationship of the cartilages at the dome of the nose. If there is adequate perichondrium, the defect may be skin-grafted from the postauricular or cervical area. Certain defects may also reepithelialize favorably without grafting, such as those in the canthal areas or at the nasomalar junction. Usually, however, achievement of optimal contour and color match requires a local flap. The best results are obtained when a skin cover of similar thickness to the adjacent part of the nose is used and junction lines such as the nasomalar, nasolabial, junction of the upper and lower lateral cartilages, and canthal areas are maintained. Bilobed rotation flaps are useful when they deliver skin of similar thickness and leave the line of closure along a normal anatomic crease. The nasolabial flap can provide a large amount of tissue based either superiorly or inferiorly, but this flap tends to be thick and fatty and must cross the nasomalar crease to reach the nose, thus violating one of the face's most obvious visual features. The dorsal nasal rotation flap based on either of the angular vessels at the medial canthal area can supply the entire thin skin of the dorsum of the nose all the way up into the glabellar area; it can also be carried laterally into the malar area to recruit even more thin skin. This can be rotated to cover defects on the tip and ala, and the resultant dog-ear can be excised primarily. The glabellar defect is closed primarily and the malar skin advanced to the nasomalar crease for primary closure. This is usually the first choice in flaps for the lower dorsal, tip, and alar areas of the nose (Fig 19–6).

Full-thickness defects of the nose require restoration of nasal lining in most cases plus a cartilaginous framework and external skin cover. Defects of the alar rim from 1 to 1½ cm (and occasionally larger in nonsmokers with reasonably healthy adjacent tissue) can be closed with composite grafts of skin and ear cartilage. Larger defects of the rim and tip require more extensive reconstruction. Lining for extensive defects is usually created by turn-in flaps from the adjacent skin, nasolabial flaps, or septal mucosal flaps. Cartilage framework may be obtained by trapdoor chondromucosal flaps of the nasal septum, free cartilage grafts from the septum, or conchal cartilage grafts (Fig 19–7).

The best source of skin coverage for large defects of the nose is one of the numerous variations on the median forehead flap based on the supraorbital or supratrochlear vessels. As a general rule, the total nasal unit should be reconstructed when subtotal resection or damage has occurred. When tissue in excess of that available from the forehead flap is necessary, tissue expansion of the forehead beneath the vascular supply may be carried out. This may also facilitate primary closure of the defect. Free tissue transfer is also a possible method of obtaining more skin, but the thin, pliable, highly vascularized (and like-colored) skin necessary is hard to match.

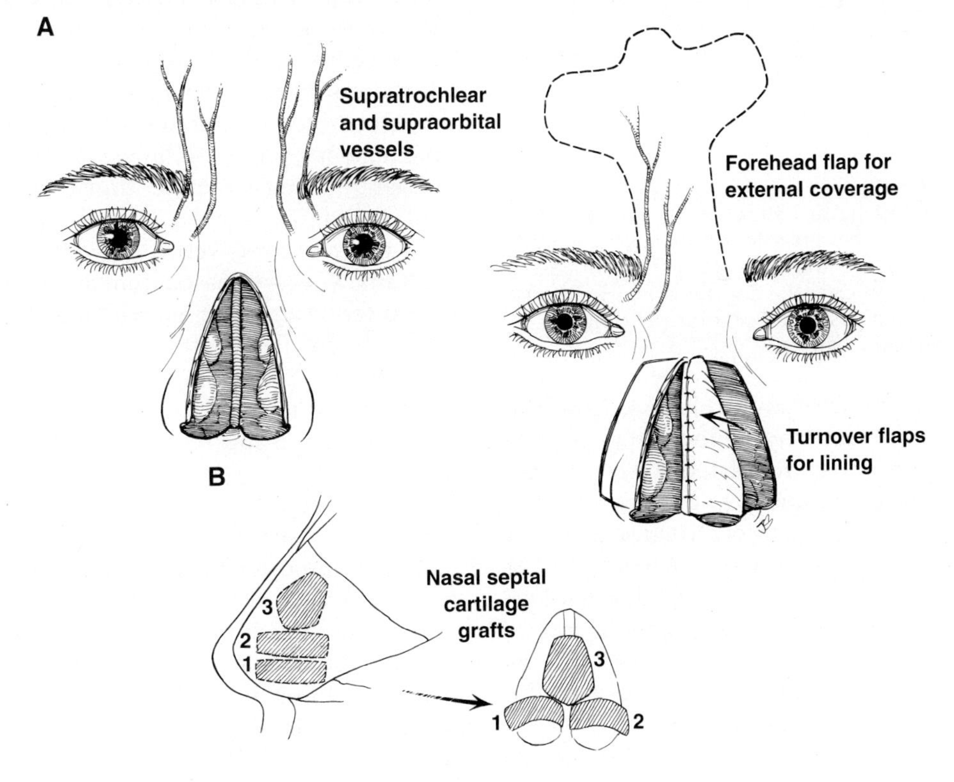

FIG 19–7.
A, Full-thickness defects of the nose require replacement of internal lining, skeletal framework, and skin coverage. The skin of the forehead is an excellent source of external coverage based on the supratrochlear and supraorbital vessels. **B,** Internal lining is provided by turnover flaps of adjacent skin or nasolabial flaps. Adequate lining is necessary to prevent internal exposure of the free cartilage grafts. Cartilage grafts of appropriate size and shape can usually be obtained from nasal septal or conchal cartilage. The median forehead flap usually provides adequate external coverage. It is inset based on the supraorbital or supratrochlear vessels and divided at a separate procedure. *(Continued.)*

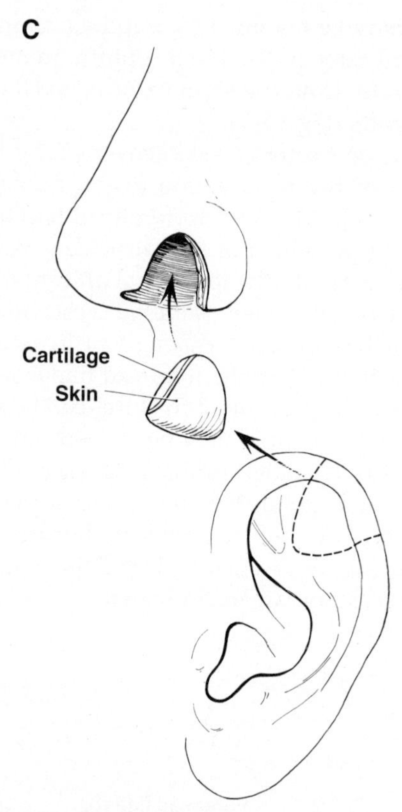

FIG 19–7 (cont.).
C, Small defects (1 to 1.5 cm) of the alar rim and columellar may be replaced with composite grafts of helical cartilage and skin, replacing skin and cartilage or skin cartilage and mucosa. The donor defect is closed primarily excising the dog-ear in the concha.

Ears asymmetrically projecting from the sides of the head may be indicators of congenital syndromes, an isolated congenital defect, the object of trauma, or the site of malignancy. The common reconstructive goal is a skeletal framework of a size matched to the opposite and covered with skin thin enough to show the detail of the cartilaginous framework. With abnormalities that consist of partial loss of the framework of the ear, the decision must be made whether total reconstruction is more advantageous than an attempt to use remnants of the ear. Usually the lack of cartilage is significant enough that total cartilaginous reconstruction is preferred. The lobule is usually in an abnormal position and requires repositioning at some later date.

Traumatic deformities must be evaluated similarly. Total avulsion may be treated by microvascular replantation, particularly if there is associated avulsion of the scalp. In some cases, removal of the skin of the ear or deepithelialization with implantation of the residual ear below the skin of the temporal scalp or temporalis fascia will allow subsequent coverage with a split-thickness skin graft. Traumatic avulsion may, however, require total ear reconstruction. Partial defects of the ear created by trauma such as human bites or resection of malignancy may be reconstructed by reducing the size of the ear somewhat, rotating the helical rim downward, and removing the cartilaginous dog-ear in the concha. Small composite grafts from the contralateral ear may also provide superior shape and symmetry. Total ear reconstruction requires the provision of an adequate skeletal framework (usually created by carving a helical and antihelical segment out of a block of cartilage obtained from the costal cartilage of the seventh, eighth, and ninth ribs) and adequate soft-tissue coverage. In most cases this is obtained by burying the cartilage in a subcutaneous pocket. If, however, the skin is deficient, it may require transportation of temporalis fascia or even a free tissue transfer. After the anterior coverage has been secured, the framework is released from the pocket and the posterior wall covered with a skin graft or advancement flap. Soft-tissue reconstruction of the lobule or helical rim may be performed with small rotation flaps. (For additional information regarding ear reconstruction, see Chapter 15.)

There have been many attempts in the past to reconstruct the ear with prostheses. Although the color match and shape may be replicated well, the lack of sensation in the area creates a major problem with adherence and pressure necrosis. Osseointegrated implants in the temporal bone may help to improve the quality of prosthetic rehabilitation of total-ear loss.

SUGGESTED READING

Beahrs OH: Surgical anatomy and technique of radical neck dissection. *Surg Clin North Am* 1977; 57:663.

Bunkis J, Milliken JB, Upton J, et al: The evolution of techniques for reconstruction of full-thickness cheek defects. *Plast Reconstr Surg* 1982; 70:319–327.

Coleman JJ: Reconstruction of the pharynx after resection for cancer. A comparison of methods. *Ann Surg* 1989; 209:554–561.

Coleman JJ: Reconstruction of the pharynx and cervical esophagus. *Surg Rounds* 1991: 855–864.

Hidalgo DA: Fibula free flap: A new method of mandible reconstruction. *Plast Reconstr Surg* 1988; 84:71–79.

Jabaley ME, Clement RL, Orcutt TW: Myocutaneous flaps in lip reconstruction. Application of the Karapandzic principle. *Plast Reconstr Surg* 1977; 59:680–688.

Matloub HS, Larson DL, Kuhn J, et al: Lateral arm free flap in oral cavity reconstruction: A functional evaluation. *Head Neck Surg* 1989: 11:205–211.

Sanger JR, Matloub HS, Yousif NJ: Sequential connection of flaps: A logical approach to customized mandibular reconstruction. *Am J Surg* 1990; 160:402–404.

Shah JP, Haribhakti V, Loree TR, et al: Complications of pectoralis major myocutaneous flap in head and neck reconstruction. *Am J Surg* 1990; 160:352–355.

Sultan MR, Coleman JJ III: Oncologic and functional considerations of total glossectomy. *Am J Surg* 1989; 158:297–302.

Surkin MI, Lawson W, Biller H: Analysis of the methods of pharyngo-esophageal reconstruction. *Head Neck Surg* 1984; 6:953.

PART V

Plastic Surgery of the Upper Extremity

Chapter 20

Anatomy/Physiology/Embryology

Susan Hobson, M.D.
Alan Seyfer, M.D.

CONTENTS

CHAPTER OBJECTIVE

At the end of this chapter the resident has a detailed knowledge of the anatomy, physiology, and embryology of the upper extremity and utilizes this knowledge in complete management of the hand, arm, and brachial plexus.

LEARNER OBJECTIVES

On completion of this chapter the resident

1. **Knows in detail the anatomy of the muscles, tendons, and ligaments of the hand and upper extremity.**
2. **Knows in detail the anatomy of the vascular tree of the upper extremity, including relationships to the surrounding structures.**
3. **Knows in detail the anatomy of the major nerves and their branchings in the upper extremity, including relationships to surrounding structures.**
4. **Understands the functional anatomy of the upper extremity, including the cutaneous cover.**
5. **Knows the clinical techniques for physical examination of the hand.**
6. Is familiar with the anatomy of the brachial plexus.
7. Knows the detailed radiographic anatomy of the bony structures of the upper extremity.
8. Understands the major aspects of embryologic development of the hand and upper extremity.
9. Understands the routine and special radiologic techniques (including CT and MRI) to discern the hard and soft tissues of the upper extremities.
10. Understands the principles of electrical evaluation and has knowledge

of the techniques of electrical examination of the upper extremities (including conduction studies and electromyographic evaluation).

CLINICAL PRACTICE

During the course of the training program, the resident

1. **Performs physical examination of the hand and upper extremity in normal and pathologic states.**
2. **Obtains and interprets radiographs and other diagnostic images for evaluation of traumatic, congenital, and degenerative problems of the hand and upper extremity.**
3. Performs dissections of upper extremity specimens.
4. Obtains and interprets electrodiagnostic studies of upper extremity problems.

EMBRYOLOGIC DEVELOPMENT OF THE UPPER EXTREMITY

In the fourth week of embryonic life, the lateral somatic mesoderm proliferates to form Wolff's crest (Fig 20–1). Shortly thereafter (around day 26), the proximal limb bud emerges from this crest as a projection of

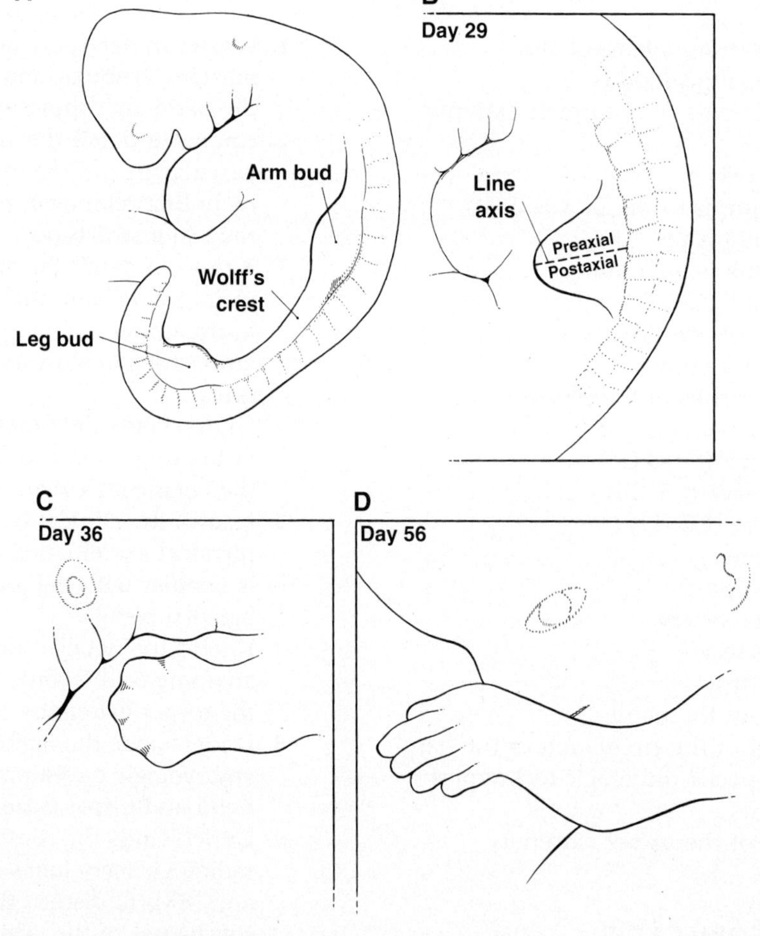

FIG 20–1.
A, 29-day-old embryo showing lateral wall somatic mesoderm proliferation (Wolff's crest) and developing limb buds. **B–D,** sequential development of upper limb bud.

unsegmented mesenchyme. The limb bud grows under the influence of the apical ectodermal ridge (AER), a critical condensation of layered cells on the distalmost aspect of the extremity. This transitory structure is essential to distal limb formation and exists only during days 26 to 38 of development. (The phocomelic effect of the teratogen thalidomide is thought to affect the AER and thereby disrupt distal growth of the limb) (see Fig 20–3).

On about day 32, the limb bud shows segmentation into the arm, forearm, and hand. The primordial hand is a paddle-shaped structure that develops radial ridges and grooves from the underlying mesenchyme. The normal segmentation of the AER overlying the radial grooves signals a resorptive process that forms digital interspaces while preserving the radial ridges and the five digital tubercles. Disruptions of this process may cause syndactyly or polydactyly.

The preliminary stages of innervation also begin around day 32 by the extension of C5–T1 nerve fibers toward the limb bud. At this stage the arm bud is flattened and possesses a cephalic preaxial margin and a caudal postaxial margin. The preaxial mesenchyme becomes associated with C5–8 and the postaxial mesenchyme with C8–T1. With further differentiation this segmental pattern is lost, and only the orderly dermatomal pattern remains.

By days 34 to 35 the anterior neural rami have united to form the brachial plexus, with its main axis extending into the root of the arm bud. The nerve fibers then branch and invade the limb bud. The resultant nerve pattern approximates adult innervation as early as day 40 and predates both muscular and bony development.

The muscles of the arm develop directly from the somatopleuric mesenchyme of the limb bud. Early in the seventh week a mesenchymal condensation appears at the root of the arm and migrates into the limb bud, later splitting to form flexor and extensor components. The muscles are initially segmental and then coalesce into distinct groups. By the end of the seventh week every muscle seen in the adult is identifiable. Muscular formation and differentiation occur in close association with innervation, each affecting the development of the other.

The development of the bony structures follows the invasion of the limb bud by the primordial nerves. These mesenchymal condensations appear in the fifth week and proceed in a proximal-to-distal direction. They are replaced by cartilage in all of the upper extremity skeleton except the clavicle. The clavicle forms by membranous ossification rather than endochondral ossification. By the seventh to eighth week primary ossification centers appear and transform the hyaline molds into bones. Secondary ossification centers are not present until after birth.

The vascular system begins with the formation of a large transitory marginal vessel containing blood-forming precursors. This vessel appears and regresses in concert with the AER. All further vascular development follows the adult pattern. At 5 weeks the axillary artery is present and extends into the arm bud as the brachial and median arteries. The radial and ulnar branches then develop as the dominant distal branches to the forearm with the median artery left to supply the median nerve.

FUNCTIONAL ANATOMY AND PHYSICAL EXAMINATION OF THE UPPER EXTREMITY

Skin

The skin of the hand may be divided into two types—the thin, mobile skin of the dorsum and the specialized thick skin of the palmar surface (glabrous skin). The thick palmar skin exhibits papillary ridges, seen best as the whorls and loops at the fingertips but present in linear arrangements throughout. The papillary ridges, designed for prehensile grip and moistened by eccrine sweat glands, overlie the fat pads of the fingertips, thenar and hypothenar eminences, and metacarpal heads. These pads and ridges are endowed with the highest density of sensory end organs in the body and supply texture and grip surface to the hand. The eccrine sweat glands add moisture to aid in adhesion. A peripherally denervated hand loses its sudomotor ability as well as its papillary ridges and eventually results in a dry, smooth hand devoid of fingerprints. This hand will have abnormal immersion test findings—no wrinkling of the denervated skin after immersion in water for 5 to 10 minutes.

The palmar skin is anchored by fibrous septa to the underlying palmar fascia. These septa traverse the fat pads to stabilize them. The coarse lines and creases of the fingers, palm, and wrist delineate skin that is adherent to the fascia without intervening fat. These creases do not move with flexion or extension and serve to stabilize the adjacent fat pads. The radial and ulnar skin of each digit is further anchored by filmy, yet strong retaining ligaments (Cleland's and Grayson's ligaments) that run directly to the underlying bone and prevent rotary displacement of the skin around the fingers in power grip.

The superficial (palmar) fascia is a fan-shaped aponeurotic structure that is continuous proximally with the palmaris longus and medially and laterally with the fascia of the thenar and hypothenar muscles and extends distally to the level of the metacarpal heads. In Dupuytren's disease, where the palmar fascia undergoes proliferation and contracture, the skin is secondarily tethered with resultant flexion deformity of the involved digit.

The deep fascia consists of the flexor sheaths of the fingers and thumb as well as the flexor and extensor retinacula of the wrist. These fibrous structures act as pulleys to prevent bowstringing of the extrinsic tendons (Fig 20–2).

General Aspects of Hand Anatomy

The most important functions of the hand are those of sensibility and grasp. Sensibility is so important that an insensate, yet mechanically intact hand will not be used.

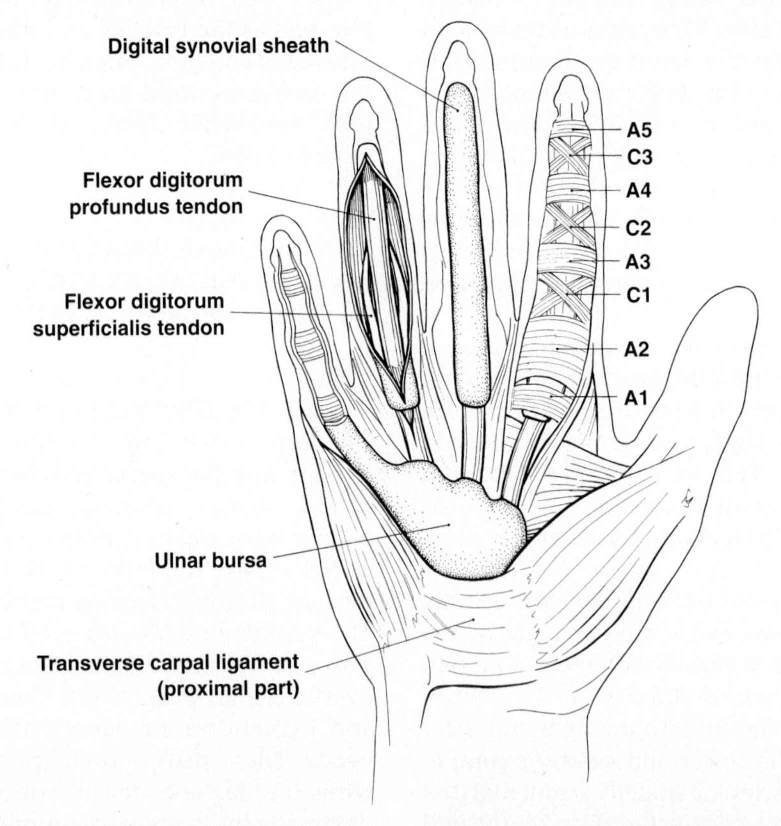

FIG 20–2.
Deep flexor structures of the hand. Pulley systems of the finger flexor sheath illustrating the "collapsible" cruciate pulleys overlying the joints, and the intervening thick annular pulleys.

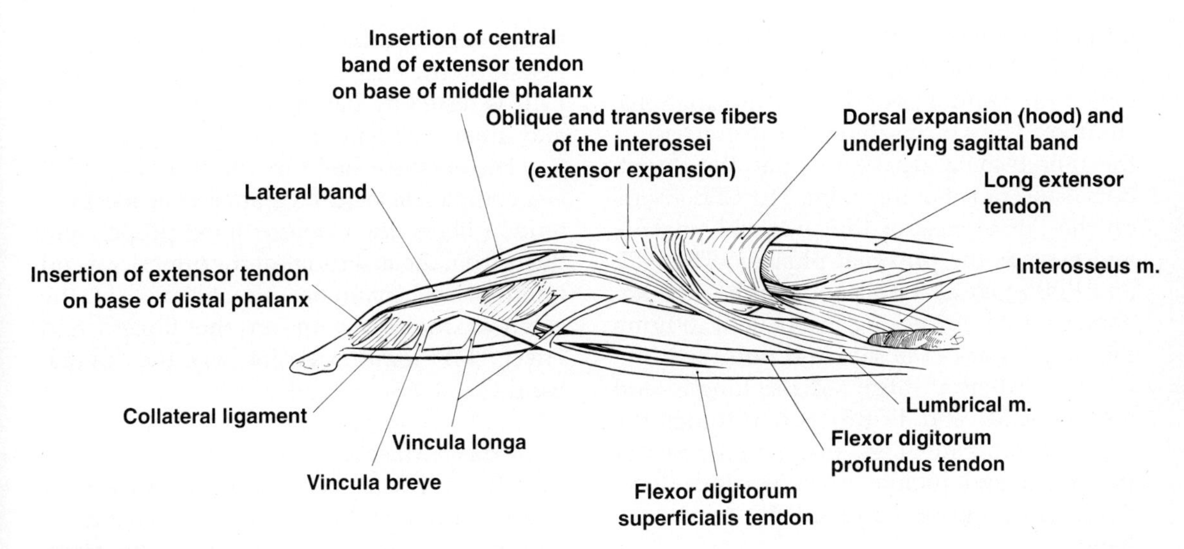

FIG 20–3.
Medial aspect of finger: flexor and extensor tendons, as well as dorsal expansion (hood) structures.

The extrinsic muscles of the hand and wrist originate in the forearm and elbow regions. The tendons of the wrist flexors lie superficial to the flexor retinaculum, while the digital flexor tendons pass deep to the retinaculum through the carpal tunnel.

The flexor carpi radialis (FCR) inserts on the palmar aspect of the index metacarpal, while the flexor carpi ulnaris (FCU) inserts on the pisiform and base of the fifth metacarpal. These motor units palmar-flex the hand as well as move it in radial and ulnar deviation. The FCR, FCU, and palmaris longus (PL) tendons can be palpated by asking the patient to flex the wrist against resistance.

The flexor pollicis longus (FPL) is the primary flexor of the interphalangeal (IP) joint of the thumb and inserts on the volar base of the distal phalanx. This muscle can be tested by asking the patient to flex the tip of the thumb while stabilizing the thumb metacarpophalangeal (MP) joint in extension.

There are two sets of long flexors to the fingers (see Fig 20–2). The flexor digitorum superficialis (FDS) is the primary flexor of the proximal interphalangeal (PIP) joint. These tendons pass through the carpal tunnel to insert on the base of the middle phalanx of each of the middle digits. Each FDS tendon bifurcates in the palm and allows the tendon of the flexor digitorum profundus (FDP) to pass distally. The FDP is the primary flexor of the distal interphalangeal (DIP) joint and inserts on the base of the distal phalanx. It also serves as an origin for a lumbrical muscle.

The FDP can be tested by stabilizing the PIP joint in extension and asking the patient to flex the distal joint. Because of a common FDP muscle mass for digits 3, 4, and 5, the FDS is tested by stabilizing all of those fingers in extension except the finger to be examined. The patient is then asked to flex the free finger at the PIP joint.

The FDS and FDP tendons pass through a specialized structure called the fibro-osseous tunnel. The tunnel is made up of the palmar surface of each phalanx and the volar plate of each joint. The sides and roof consist of five annular (A1 through A5) and three cruciate (C1 through C3) pulleys (see Figs 20–2 and 20–3). The most important are the A2 and A4 pulleys of the fingers and the A1 pulley of the thumb since these are critical to maximal flexion.

The Extrinsic Extensors

The muscle bellies of the long extensors lie in the dorsal part of the forearm, and their tendons pass through the compartments of the extensor retinaculum at the wrist before inserting in the hand. There are six retinacular compartments numbered 1 to 6 in a radial-to-ulnar direction.

The first compartment contains the abductor pollicis longus (APL) and extensor pollicis brevis (EPB) tendons. These two tendons define the ventral boundary of the anatomic snuffbox. The APL inserts on the dorsal base of the thumb metacarpal and pulls the thumb dorsal and radial to the palm. The EPB inserts on the dorsal base of the proximal phalanx and extends the proximal phalanx. The APL and EPB work as a unit and can be simultaneously tested by asking the patient to bring the thumb out to the side and dorsally.

The extensor carpi radialis longus and brevis (ECRL and ECRB) run through the second compartment and insert on the base of the index and middle metacarpals, respectively. These dorsiflex and radially deviate the hand.

The long extensor of the thumb is the extensor pollicis longus (EPL). It forms the dorsal boundary of the snuffbox after passing through the third compartment and then inserting on the base of the thumb's distal phalanx. It extends the thumb IP joint and is tested by asking the patient to lift the thumb with the hand palm down on a flat surface.

The fourth extensor compartment transmits the extensor indicis proprius (EIP) and the four extensor digitorum communis (EDC) tendons. The EDC tendons insert on the middle phalanges and become an integral component of the extensor hood mechanism of each finger. The EDC tendons work en mass primarily to extend the four fingers at their MP joints. This is tested by having the patient extend the MP joints while maintaining the IP joints in flexion.

The EIP passes just ulnar to the index EDC and inserts on the dorsal base of the middle phalanx to allow independent extension of the index MP joint.

The extensor digiti minimi (EDM) passes through the fifth compartment and, analogous to the EIP, passes ulnar to the fifth-finger EDC tendon and inserts on the dorsal base of the middle phalanx. The EDM allows for independent extension of the fifth-finger MP joint. The EIP and EDM can be tested simultaneously by having the patient extend the index and small fingers while flexing the middle and ring fingers.

The sixth compartment contains the extensor carpi ulnaris (ECU) tendon, which inserts on the base of the fifth metacarpal. The ECU is tested by having the patient dorsiflex and ulnarly deviate the hand.

The extensor hood mechanism (Fig 20–3) is a complex structure composed of the EDC tendon fibers, the extensor hood proper, and fibers from the insertions of the lumbricals and interossei. It maintains the balance of the extensor forces acting on the fingers and effects MP joint extension via the sagittal bands.

Intrinsic Muscles

The intrinsic muscles have both their origins and insertions within the hand. In addition to their individual actions, the intrinsic muscles as a group support the normal arches of the hand. The absence of this system is demonstrated by the flattened hand of an ulnar nerve palsy.

The adductor pollicis (AP) arises from two heads—the oblique, which originates from the volar ligaments over the trapezium, trapezoid, and capitate, and the transverse head, which arises from the shaft of the middle metacarpal. Both heads insert on the base of the thumb proximal phalanx. The AP adducts the thumb and stabilizes it in pinch. It can be tested by having the patient firmly hold a piece of paper between the thumb and radial aspect of the index finger while the examiner attempts to pull the paper away. Flexion of the thumb IP joint during this maneuver is called "Froment's sign" and indicates weakness of pinch (i.e., weakness of the AP and first dorsal interosseous muscles), sometimes indicative of an ulnar palsy.

The thenar muscles arise from the radial carpal bones and associated ligaments and include the abductor pollicis brevis (APB), opponens pollicis (OP), and flexor pollicis brevis (FPB). The OP inserts on the radial border of the thumb metacarpal, and the APB and FPB insert on the base of the proximal phalanx. The opponens can be used as a test for the motor branch of the median nerve since it is the most distal muscle innervated by this branch. It is tested by palpating the muscle while the patient touches the tip of the thumb to the base of the small finger. The thenar muscles can also be tested as a group by asking the patient to place the dorsum of the hand flat and raise the thumb to form a right angle with the palm.

The hypothenar muscles are the abductor digiti minimi (ADM), opponens digiti minimi (ODM), and flexor digiti minimi (FDM). They arise from the volar ulnar carpal bones and associated ligaments. The ODM inserts midshaft on the fifth metacarpal, which it adducts and rotates for opposition. The ADM and FDM insert on the base of the proximal phalanx and aid in abduction and MP joint flexion. The hypothenar muscles are tested as a group by having the patient abduct and flex the small finger at the MP joint.

The interossei and lumbrical intrinsic muscles serve the same function. There are seven interossei, four dorsal and three palmar, with variable anatomy. In general, they arise from the metacarpal shafts and insert distally into the extensor hood of the respective digit. The dorsal interossei abduct the index, long, and ring fingers. The palmar interossei are the primary adductors of the index, ring, and small fingers. The interossei also flex the MP joints and extend the IP joints.

The lumbricals serve the same function but are weaker than the interossei. They originate from the FDP tendons in the palm and insert on the radial aspect of the extensor hood mechanism.

The interossei can be used to test for the motor branch of the ulnar nerve. The examiner stabilizes all but the middle finger and asks the patient to "move the middle finger like a windshield wiper." Palsy of the ulnar motor nerve makes this impossible.

Intrinsic muscle tightness can occur following ischemia or with fibrosis or spasm. This results in the so-called intrinsic-plus position, which is flexion of the affected MP joint, hyperextension of the PIP joint, and flexion of the DIP joint. (In its severe form a swan-neck deformity results.)

To test for intrinsic tightness, the MP joint is stabilized in flexion, thus relaxing the intrinsics, and the PIP joint is passively flexed. The MP joint is then stabilized in extension, thereby stretching the intrinsics, and the PIP joint is again passively flexed. If PIP joint flexion is easier with MP joint flexion than extension, intrinsic tightness has been demonstrated. If PIP motion is greater with MP extension, extensor tightness is present. If PIP motion is equally restricted with MP joint extension and flexion, decreased joint motion is likely due to joint or periarticular tightness.

The Metacarpophalangeal and Interphalangeal Joints

Intrinsic tightness is one reason for loss of motion of the MP and PIP joints. Other causes are Dupuytren's contracture, palmar scarring, collateral ligament contracture and tendon adhesions, articular damage, or blockage by exostosis or a bone spur.

JOINTS AND LIGAMENTS OF THE UPPER EXTREMITY

The wrist joint is a highly complex joint characterized by a wide range of motion and substantial stability. There are actually multiple joints at the wrist, including the distal radioulnar joint, the radiocarpal joint, the intercarpal joints, the midcarpal joint, and the carpometacarpal joints. The radiocarpal joint is often thought of as "the" wrist joint.

The primary stabilizer of the distal radioulnar joint is the triangular fibrocartilage. A complex array of interosseous, volar, and dorsal ligaments interconnect the carpus and radius, the volar ligaments being the most substantial. Important ligamentous stabilizers of the radial aspect of the carpus are the scapholunate interosseous ligament, the radioscaphocapitate ligament, and the radioscapholunate ligament. The ulnar aspect of the carpus is stabilized at the distal end of the ulna by a ligamentous and cartilaginous complex termed the "triangular fibrocartilage complex" or the "ulnocarpal ligament complex." This complex is composed of the radioulnar ligaments, the ulnar collateral ligament, the meniscus homologue, the ulnolunate and ulnotriquetral ligaments, the articular disk, and the sheath of the ECU tendon.

The bones of the carpus are extensively interconnected by the interosseous, dorsal, and volar ligaments. The proximal carpal row articulates with the distal carpal row at the intercarpal joint, which is involved in wrist flexion and extension as well as radial and ulnar deviation. The distal row forms the proximal transverse arch. This arch is permanently fixed as a result of the tough intercarpal ligaments and the arch configuration of the carpal bones, with the capitate serving as the keystone. Further support is added by the volar carpal ligament.

The metacarpal bases articulate with the distal carpal row. The metacarpotrapezial joint of the thumb is a biconcave saddle joint allowing great mobility. Its stability is provided by the ulnar collateral and radial collateral ligaments as well as the tough joint capsule. Strongest of the ligaments is the ulnar collateral ligament, which attaches the volar lip of the first metacarpal base to the trapezium and resists hyperextension and radial subluxation of the thumb. The first metacarpal is attached to the second at their bases by the anterior and posterior intermetacarpal ligaments.

The second and third metacarpals are rigidly bound to the proximal arch at their carpometacarpal joints by the volar and dorsal carpometacarpal ligaments, with essentially no movement allowed at those articulations. In contrast, the fourth and fifth metacarpals have significant flexion-extension mobility at their carpometacarpal joints. All four finger metacarpals are bound together at their proximal and distal ends by the volar and dorsal intermetacarpal ligaments.

The bicondylar MP joints of the fingers allow radial and ulnar deviation as well as circumduction while in extension. This is a result of the configuration of the metacarpal heads, which causes their collateral ligaments to be loose in extension. However, in flexion the collateral ligaments become taut to stabilize the joint and prohibit side-to-side deviation. Additional stability is afforded by the volar plate, which resists hyperextension. The collateral ligaments of the condyloid thumb MP joint are taut in both flexion and extension; therefore this joint functions more like the IP hinge joints.

The bicondylar IP joints of the thumb and fingers are hinge joints that permit only flexion and extension. They are stabilized by the collateral ligaments as well as the volar plate.

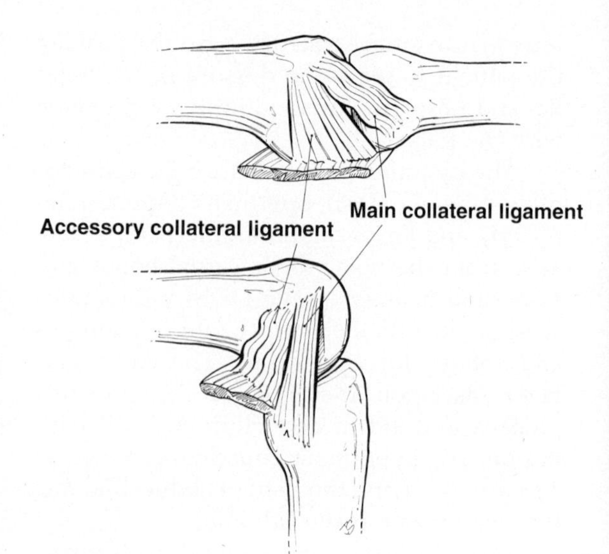

FIG 20–4.
Illustration demonstrating slackness in extension and stretch in flexion of the collateral ligaments of the MP joint.

The "protected" or "safe" position of mobilization of the hand is one in which the MP joints are flexed 45 to 60 degrees, the IP joints flexed 0 to 10 degrees, and the wrist extended 20 to 30 degrees. Because of the cam-like structure of the MP joints the collateral ligaments are slack in extensionand taut (favorable) in flexion (Fig 20–4). If the MP joint is immobilized in extension, the main collateral ligaments can shorten, thereby preventing flexion on remobilization.

INNERVATION

Brachial Plexus

The brachial plexus is formed from the anterior rami of nerves C5–T1. It is divided into roots, trunks, divisions, and cords (Fig 20–5). At the base of the neck, the roots emerge between the scalenus anterior and medius muscles and continue as trunks and divisions in the posterior triangle. Within the axilla (in the axillary sheath), the plexus is arranged in medial, lateral, and posterior cords as determined by relationship to the axillary artery. The cords then divide into terminal branches (Table 20–1).

Common Injuries to the Plexus or Its Proximal Branches

Upper Trunk (C5–7) Injury

Violent displacement of the head and neck to the contralateral side with simultaneous depression of the shoulder on the ipsilateral side (as seen in motorcycle injuries in which the helmet and shoulder strike the ground simultaneously) can avulse the upper trunks of the plexus. Upper trunk injuries result in an Erb-Duchenne–pattern palsy or "waiter's tip" hand where the upper extremity hangs limply by the side in medial rotation with the forearm pronated.

Lower Trunk (C8–T1) Injury

Both excessive abduction of the arm and cervical rib syndrome can result in traction injury to the lower trunk, most often affecting T1. The result is a Klumpke-pattern palsy or "clawed hand" as a result of loss of the ulnar nerve.

Long Thoracic Nerve Injury

This can be caused by blunt trauma or stab wounds in the axilla. The serratus anterior is paralyzed, and protrusion of the inferior angle of the scapula ("winged scapula") results.

Axillary Nerve Injury

Caudal dislocation of the humerus into the quadrilateral space or fracture of the surgical neck of the humerus can cause axillary nerve injury. This results in paralysis and atrophy of the deltoid with weakness in lateral rotation and abduction of the arm. There is also a loss of sensation over the lower half of the deltoid muscle.

Terminal Branches of the Plexus—The Radial, Median, and Ulnar Nerves

Radial Nerve (C5–T1)

After sending off the axillary nerve, the posterior cord becomes the radial nerve (Fig

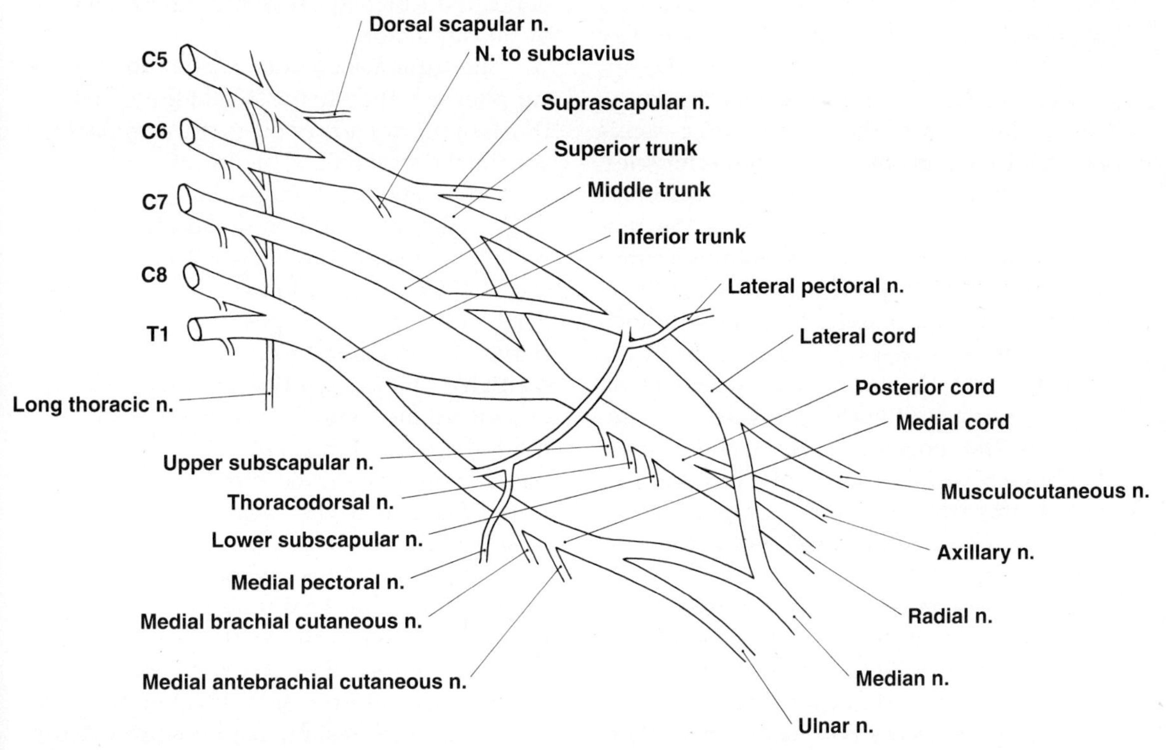

FIG 20–5.
Schematic of the brachial plexus.

TABLE 20–1.
Branches of the Brachial Plexus

Level	Nerves	Muscles Innervated
Roots C5–7	Long thoracic n. (C5–7)	Serratus anterior
	Dorsal scapular n. (C5)	Rhomboids
Upper trunk	N. to subclavius (C5–6)	Subclavius
	Suprascapular n. (C5–6)	Supraspinatus Infraspinatus
Lateral cord	Lateral pectoral (C5–6)	Pectoralis major Pectoralis minor
	Musculocutaneous n. (C5–C7)	Coracobrachialis Brachialis Biceps
Medial cord	Medial pectoral n. (C8–T1)	Pectoralis major
	(Medial antebrachial and medial brachial cutaneous nn.)	
	Ulnar n.	(see Figure 20–5.)
Medial and lateral cords	Median n.	(see Figure 20–5.)
Posterior cord	Upper subscapular n. (C5–6)	Subscapularis
	Thoracodorsal n. (C7–8)	Latissimus dorsi
	Lower subscapular n. (C5–C6)	Subscapularis Teres major
	Axillary n. (C5–C6)	Deltoid
	Radial n.	Teres minor (see Fig. 20–5.)

20–6, A). It descends into the arm, passes into the posterior compartment, and winds its way to the forearm in the spiral groove of the humerus along with the profunda brachii artery. Within the groove the radial nerve sends branches to the triceps and anconeus muscles. Piercing the lateral intermuscular septum, it becomes anterior again, innervates the brachioradialis and ECRL, and then divides into superficial and deep branches at the level of the lateral epicondyle. The deep branch then descends between the two heads of the supinator into the forearm to reside along the posterior aspect of the interosseous membrane as the posterior interosseous nerve. This branch supplies the remaining muscles of the forearm posterior compartment—ECRB, supinator, APL, and all of the extensors to the digits.

The most common site of compression of the radial nerve in the forearm is where the deep branch dives beneath the proximal edge of the superficial head of the supinator to lie between the muscle's two heads. Here there often exists a fibrous band known as the arcade of Frohse that may compress the nerve beneath the medial half of the superficial head of the supinator.

The superficial branch of the radial nerve supplies sensation to the skin of the radial two thirds of the dorsum of the hand, as well as the proximal dorsal half of the thumb, index, and middle fingers and radial half of the ring finger. Also, it should be noted that in about half of the people studied, the motor branch to the ECRB was found to arise from the superficial rather than the posterior interosseous nerve. Its branches to the digits, like the median and ulnar sensory nerves, are roughly in concordance with the arterial supply to the digits. Because of this, a bleeding vessel in the hand should never be blindly clamped because damage to the accompanying nerve may result.

Sensory testing of the radial nerve is done on the dorsum of the thumb-index web space because this area possesses the least amount of crossover innervation. A sharp object lightly applied (such as a pin or broken tongue blade) can be used for testing. A two-point discrimination test carries little meaning here. Motor integrity can be demonstrated by function of the long digital extensors or the EPL specifically.

The posterior interosseous syndrome, a consequence of injury to or compression of the posterior interosseous branch of the radial nerve, results in the inability to open the palm effectively because of loss of the finger and thumb extensors.

Complete radial nerve lesions can be caused by an epicondylar fracture of the humerus and should be distinguished from a posterior interosseous palsy. A complete radial nerve lesion results in loss of the sensory branch to the dorsum of the hand and loss of wrist extension, whereas the posterior interosseous syndrome involves the digital extensors only. If triceps muscle function is impaired, the injury is high, and this usually implies a complete division of the radial nerve.

Median Nerve (C5–T1)

The median nerve is formed by the terminal branches of the medial and lateral cords of the brachial plexus (Fig 20–6, B). It descends medially in the anterior compartment of the arm, lateral to the axillary and brachial arter-

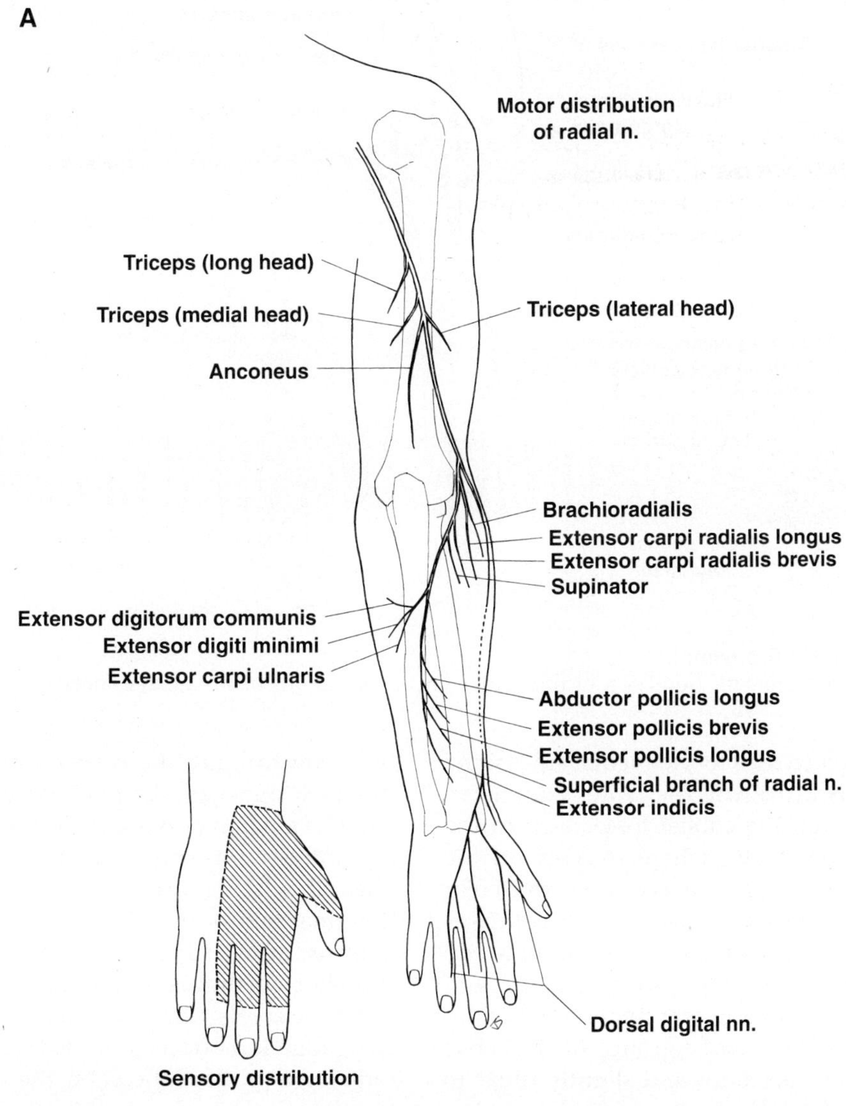

FIG 20–6.
A, Schematic depiction of the course and innervations of the radial nerve.
(Continued.)

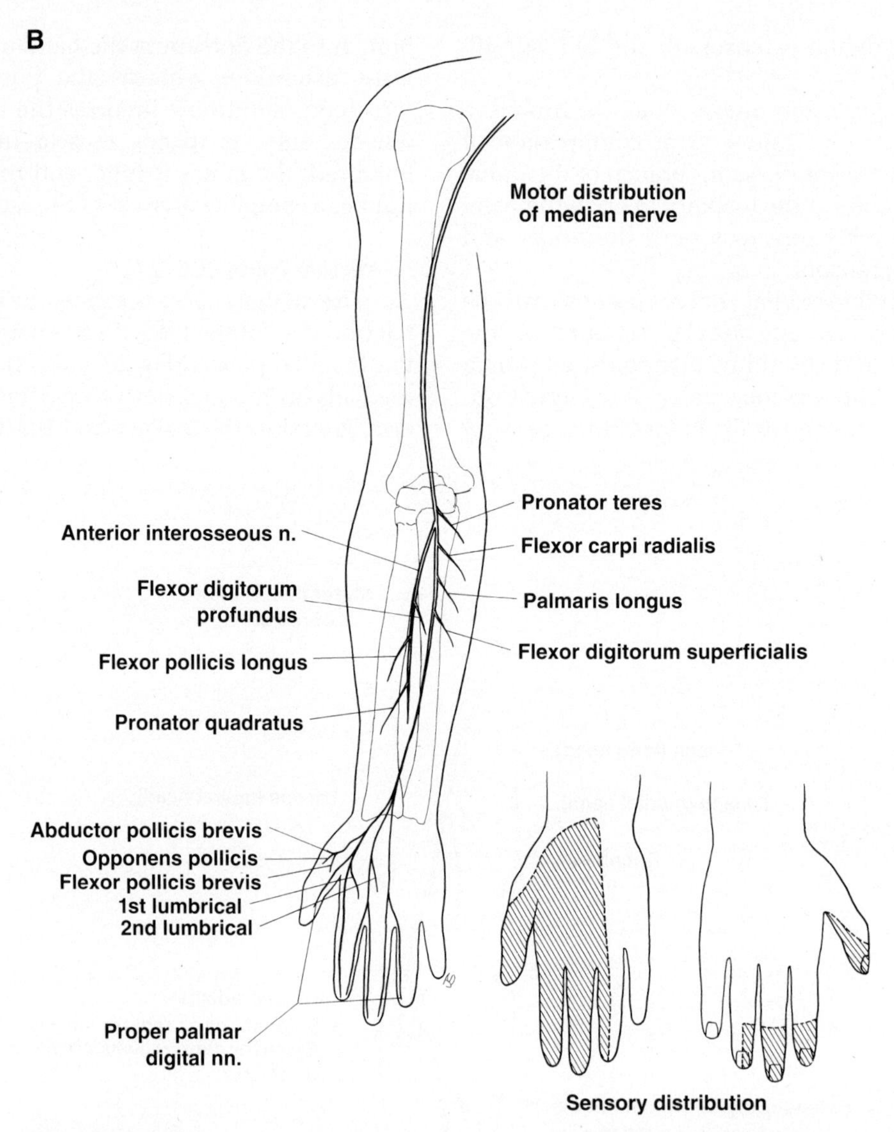

FIG 20–6 (cont.).
B, Schematic depiction of the course and innervations of the median nerve.

ies, and then crosses to the medial side of the artery midway down the arm. The nerve passes through the cubital fossa deep to the bicipital aponeurosis, where it gives off the anterior interosseous nerve and muscular branches to the superficial anterior compartment muscles. It enters the forearm between the two heads of the pronator teres and continues in the forearm where it resides beneath the FDS muscle group. At the wrist, the nerve lies posterior and slightly ulnar to the palmaris longus tendon and then enters the hand through the carpal tunnel beneath the thick transverse carpal ligament.

The median nerve is the primary nerve to the anterior forearm compartment and supplies all muscular groups except the FCU and the ulnar half of the FDP. The anterior interosseous nerve supplies the FPL, FDP, and pronator quadratus. In the hand, the median nerve innervates three thenar muscles and the two radial lumbricals. It is also sensory to the radial two thirds of the palm, the volar skin of the thumb, the index, middle, and radial half of the ring fingers, as well as the distal and dorsal half of those fingers.

The motor branch of the median nerve can be tested by palpating the action of the OP (described earlier). Sensory function is tested by two-point discrimination at the distal half of the pulp of the finger. The ends of a bent paper clip can be touched to the skin in a longitudinal direction with just enough pressure to blanch the skin. The patient, with eyes averted, reports whether one or two points are felt. The distance between the points is then varied until the critical distance is found, that is, the minimal distance at which the patient can distinguish two separate points. The normal value is 4 to 6 mm on the distal half of the pulp skin. It is important to orient the points longitudinally so that each of the two digital nerve areas can be tested independently.

Injury to the median nerve may be caused by a supracondylar humeral fracture. Also, because of its superficial position, it is subject to injury from lacerations at the wrist. Such injury may result in loss of abduction and opposition of the thumb, as well as loss of sensation to the skin of the radial half of the palm and 3½ digits. Injuries at the humeral

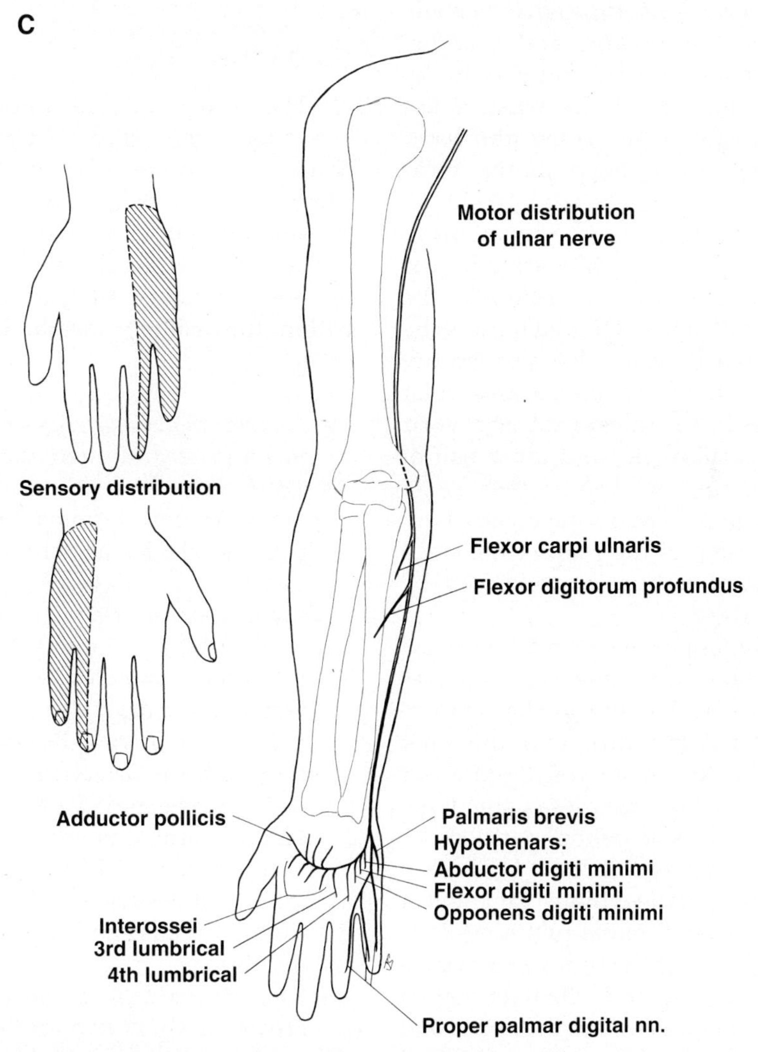

FIG 20–6 (cont.).
C, Schematic depiction of the course and innervations of the ulnar nerve.

level may additionally cause loss of flexor function of the index and middle IP joints. Atrophy of the thenar eminence and external rotation of the thumb are evident with long-standing paralysis and result in a flattened "ape hand."

Ulnar Nerve (C8–T1)

The ulnar nerve is the last branch from the lateral cord and enters the anterior compartment of the arm medial to the axillary and brachial arteries (Fig 20–6, C). Midway down the arm, the nerve dives posteriorly beneath the triceps and becomes superficial behind the medial epicondyle of the humerus. It courses anteriorly again, through the cubital tunnel and into the forearm, and runs between and supplies the FCU and FDP to the ring and small fingers. At the wrist, it lies radial to the pisiform and enters the hand through Guyon's canal deep to the volar carpal ligament.

Like the median nerve, the ulnar nerve gives off no branches in the arm. In the anterior portion of the forearm it supplies the FCU, the ulnar half of the FDP, and most of the intrinsic muscles of the hand. It is also sensory to the ulnar third of the dorsal and volar surfaces of the hand, the dorsal and volar aspects of the small finger, and ulnar half of the ring finger.

Sensory testing is performed with two-point discrimination of the pulp of the small finger, and motor testing is performed by testing the interossei.

Ulnar nerve lesions are primarily caused by injuries at sites where the nerve courses superficially, i.e., behind the medial epicondyle or at the wrist. Interruption of the ulnar nerve proximal to the wrist paralyzes the vast majority of the intrinsic muscles of the hand. With time, an intrinsic-minus position, or "claw hand" deformity, will result because of the loss of these muscles. Intact function of the median innervated radial two lumbricals will maintain flexion of the index and middle fingers. Sensory loss involves the ulnar half of the palm and dorsum as well as the dorsal and volar aspects of the small finger and ulnar half of the ring finger.

At the wrist the ulnar nerve divides into its deep and superficial (sensory) branches. Lacerations of the ulnar nerve at the wrist therefore may involve only the superficial sensory branch and affect cutaneous sensation to the ulnar half of the palm with no motor deficits.

VASCULAR ANATOMY

The blood supply to the upper extremity is served by three arteries (axillary/brachial, radial, and ulnar) but is rich in collateral anastomoses (Fig 20–7).

The Axillary Artery

The primary arterial supply to the upper extremity is the axillary artery—a continuation of the subclavian artery. It begins at the lateral border of the first rib and continues to the inferior border of the teres major. The axillary artery is closely related to the cords of the brachial plexus, all of which are enclosed within the axillary sheath. It gives off six branches:

- *Supreme thoracic artery.*—Supplies the first and second intercostal spaces.
- *Thoracoacromial artery.*—Immediately divides into four terminal branches: pectoral, clavicular, acromial, and deltoid.
- *Lateral thoracic artery.*—Supplies the pectoralis major and minor and the serratus anterior muscles as well as the female mammary gland.
- *Subscapular artery.*—Divides into (1) the thoracodorsal artery to the latissimus dorsi muscle and (2) the circumflex scapular artery, which winds around to the infraspinous fossa where it divides and anastomoses with branches of the dorsal scapular and suprascapular arteries.
- *Anterior and posterior humeral circumflex arteries.*—These two arteries encircle the surgical head of the humerus and anastomose.

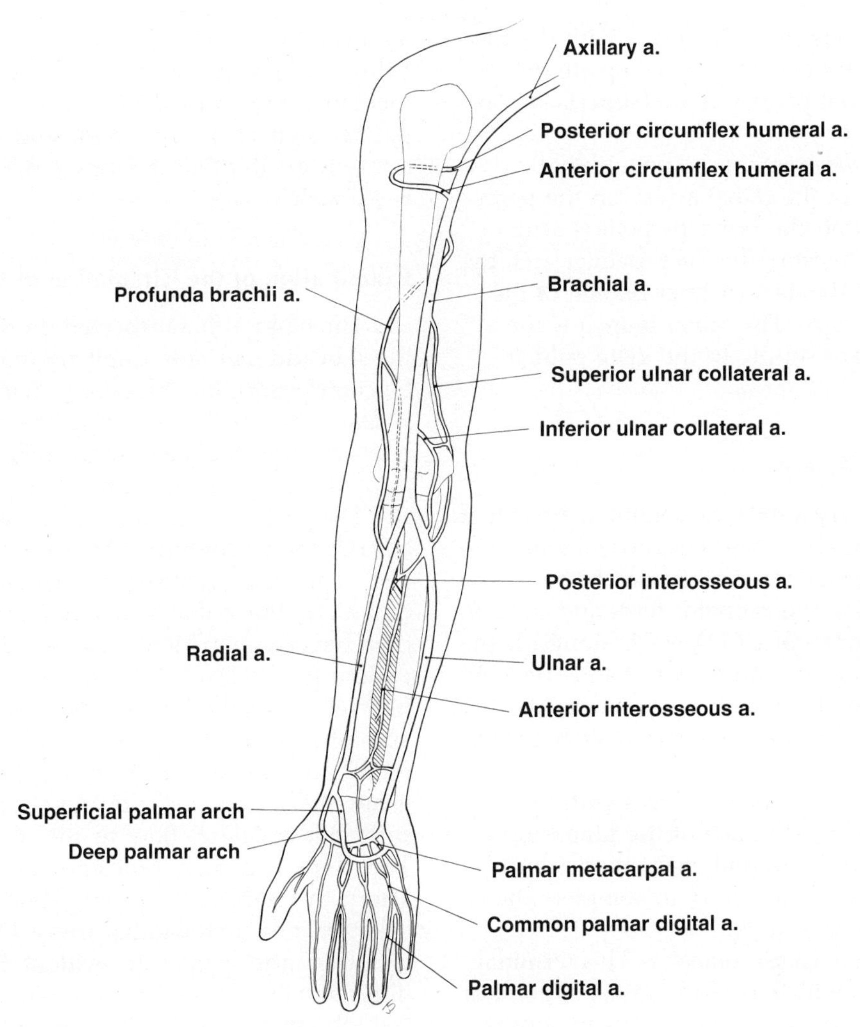

FIG 20–7.
Major arterial blood supply of the upper extremity.

The Brachial Artery

The axillary artery becomes the brachial artery at the inferior border of the teres major. It descends medially in the anterior compartment of the arm, enters the cubital fossa deep to the bicipital aponeurosis, and splits into its two terminal branches, the radial and ulnar arteries.

The Radial Artery

Originating as the lateral bifurcation of the brachial artery in the antecubital fossa, the radial artery passes through the forearm to lie posterior to the brachioradialis muscle and becomes superficial at the wrist. Curving over the radial aspect of the carpal bones, it passes under the APL and EPB tendons to lie within the anatomic snuffbox. It then dives ventrally between the heads of the first dorsal interossei to enter the palm between the heads of the adductor pollicis. It has three main branches:

- *Palmar carpal branch.*—Originates proximal to the flexor retinaculum and anastomoses with the palmar carpal branch of the ulnar artery to form the palmar (deep) carpal arch ("deep" to the flexor tendons).
- *Superficial palmar branch.*—Descends through the carpal tunnel and the the-

nar muscles to anastomose with the ulnar artery and thereby complete the superficial palmar arch ("superficial" to the flexor tendons).

- *Deep palmar branch.*—The terminal branch of the radial artery. In the palm it gives off the princeps pollicis artery before forming the deep palmar arch by joining the deep palmar branch of the ulnar artery. The radial branch is the dominant supply to the deep palmar arch.

The Ulnar Artery

This artery is the larger terminal branch of the brachial artery and lies more medially in the antecubital fossa. It passes beneath the ulnar head of the pronator teres and runs on the posterior surface of the FCU alongside the ulnar nerve. It enters the hand through Guyon's canal between the pisiform and the hook of the hamate. It has two main branches:

- *Deep palmar branch.*—Dives with the deep palmar branch of the ulnar nerve through the hypothenar muscles and joins the radial artery to complete the deep palmar arch.
- *Superficial palmar branch.*—This terminal branch, which joins the radial superficial palmar branch, is the dominant supply to the superficial palmar arch.

The Arteries of the Hand

The blood supply to the hand is rich in anastomoses between the radial and ulnar arteries. The superficial and deep palmar arches in turn anastomose with each other to form the common palmar digital arteries. These bifurcate to form the proper palmar digital arteries that supply the adjacent fingers and then again anastomose at the distal ends of the fingertips. In addition, the radial and ulnar arteries join on the dorsum of the hand to form the dorsal carpal arch, which sends dorsal digital arteries to each of the fingers. These anastomose with the palmar digital arteries.

The "classic" complete superficial palmar arch is only found in 34% of cases, with 37% being entirely ulnar in supply. A persistent median artery contributes to the superficial palmar arch in 20% of cases, and in 3% the artery is greater than 1.5 mm in diameter and is palpable.

Examination of the Circulation of the Hand

The hand is first inspected for the color of the skin and nail beds. Capillary refill is tested by compressing the fingertip or nail bed until it blanches and then noting the time after release until the color and turgor return, normal being less than 2 seconds.

The patency of the radial and ulnar arteries can be confirmed by using the Allen's test. This is performed by simultaneously occluding the radial and ulnar arteries and then having the patient make a tight fist. The patient then relaxes the hand, and the examiner releases only the radial artery. The hand and all five digits should fill with blood and return to color within 5 seconds. This establishes the patency of the radial artery with sufficient collateral flow to the ulnar artery. The steps are then repeated for the ulnar artery to establish its patency and adequate collateral flow to the radial artery. Dominance of either artery may be evident by grossly different filling times. The results of the Allen's test should be described as "normal" or "abnormal" for each artery tested.

The Allen's test may be performed on the digits as well.

ROUTINE AND SPECIAL RADIOLOGIC TECHNIQUES

Conventional radiography remains the cornerstone for defining bone structure and diagnosing trauma in the upper extremity. Although newer techniques provide superior contrast resolution, plain x-ray studies offer excellent spatial resolution and provide information about alignment and arrangement, fractures, joint space widths, and bone density changes resulting from metabolic or neoplastic processes.

Standard studies exist for the examination

of the upper extremity. For example, the initial hand study is generally the three-view series—frontal (posteroanterior), oblique, and true lateral. If the thumb is of special interest, it may be necessary to order an isolated frontal view because the thumb is seen in oblique projections in all three standard hand views. The wrist has a standard four-view series that includes the same three views as the hand with an additional specialized view to visualize the scaphoid.

Arthrography, utilizing injectable contrast material, further defines the joint spaces and demonstrates the articular surfaces, extensions, and capsular recesses. Tears or defects in joint connective structures are visualized by abnormal communications between compartments.

Angiography demonstrates vessel patency or possible vascular anomalies. It can also be used to demonstrate dominance of flow into collateral systems such as the arches of the hand.

Computer-assisted tomography (CT) consists of a series of sections through the extremity. Although this results in a loss of spatial resolution, it overcomes the problem of superimposition encountered with plain radiography, thereby showing the exact location of foreign bodies, etc., with respect to the neighboring bone. Furthermore, CT offers increased contrast resolution for better visualization of soft-tissue structures.

Magnetic resonance imaging (MRI) offers the best contrast resolution of all of the techniques. MRI imaging can delineate individual muscles, tendons, fat, bone, marrow, fluid, and blood as well as abnormal soft-tissue masses.

Radionuclide bone imaging is a specialized technique with applications that include the imaging of vasculature; early recognition of bone changes such as occult fractures, inflammatory disease, and osteonecrosis; and further evaluation of lucent or cystic lesions as seen on routine radiographs.

ELECTRODIAGNOSIS

Standard electrodiagnostic techniques are electromyography (EMG) and nerve conduction velocity studies. EMG records action potentials within a muscle by means of needle electrodes. The pattern of these potentials reveals denervation as well as specific stages of nerve regeneration.

Nerve conduction velocity studies measure the velocity of signal transmission through a specific portion of a nerve. The nerve is stimulated by a surface cathode generating a depolarization, which is then recorded at a given distance from the site of stimulation.

EMG can be used to distinguish between single-nerve entrapment, peripheral neuropathy, or radiculopathy. With peripheral nerve injury, the EMG can assist in the initial documentation of the localization, character, and completeness of the lesion and can supplement the assessment of recovery. Nerve conduction studies can differentiate between and localize conduction block (neurapraxia), axon death (axonotmesis), demyelination, remyelination, and axon regeneration. The combined use of EMG and nerve conduction velocity studies can distinguish among true motor neuron disease, peripheral nerve disease, and myopathy.

BIOMECHANICS OF THE UPPER EXTREMITY

Reconstructive surgery of the upper extremity must be based on a firm understanding of the basic mechanics of each of its functional subunits. Smooth, integrated function of these subunits is dependent on their precise architecture and a balanced distribution of the forces that act upon them. These forces are dependent not only upon muscle power but also upon the vectors and the lever arms associated with a given joint. Any upset in this delicate balance will compromise the function of the whole extremity. Proceeding distally from the shoulder, each subunit is involved with progressively finer adjustments of the hand in space. Movement at the shoulder and elbow is responsible for movement of the hand into proximity with its task. The forearm adjusts the rotary position of the hand through pronation and supination. The final adjustments of hand position are made at the wrist, which then serves as a stable base from which the hand functions. It is important to appreciate that maximal performance of the hand is highly dependent on the proper functioning of the upper extremity's constituent parts.

The hand is under the dynamic forces of its associated musculotendinous units and ligaments. At rest, the hand adopts the so-called functional position, the position from which prehension is most easily assumed. The fingers lie in a cascade, thumb slightly opposed, fingers progressively more flexed radially to ulnarly. This characteristic resting posture results from the muscle tone and viscoelastic forces of the attached musculotendinous units.

The wrist is essential in properly positioning the hand for maximal function, and any anatomic deformity will compromise digital function. The ranges of motion of the digits and wrist are interdependent because of the effective length of the extrinsic finger muscles, which are not long enough to allow both the fingers and wrist to be simultaneously maximally flexed or extended. The functional implication of this system is that maximal finger flexion power requires that the wrist be neutral or slightly extended and maximal extension requires that the wrist be neutral or slightly flexed. Likewise, strong wrist action requires fingers that are neither fully flexed nor fully extended.

The hand can be structurally divided into transverse and longitudinal arches. The two transverse arches are the fixed proximal transverse arch formed by the distal carpal row and the adaptable distal transverse arch at the level of the metacarpal heads. The longitudinal arches are formed by the five digital rays. With their concavities toward the palm, these arches allow the hand to be formed into a cup.

Functionally, the hand consists of fixed and mobile units. The fixed unit of the hand is composed of the proximal transverse arch and the rigidly attached second and third metacarpals. The proximal transverse arch is permanently fixed by the arch configuration of the distal carpal bones, with the capitate serving as the keystone, and by the tough intercarpal ligaments. Further support is added by the volar carpal ligament, which spans the extreme ends of the arch, the hamate, and trapezium. The second and third digital rays are rigidly attached to the arch as well as firmly bound to each other at their intermetacarpal joints. The fixed unit is controlled by the wrist extensors ECRL and ECRB and by the wrist flexor FCR.

Suspended from the central fixed unit are the mobile units of the hand, which are the thumb ray, the index finger, and the ring and small digital rays along with the middle finger.

The basal joint of the thumb, the metacarpotrapezial joint, allows the thumb its wide range of motion. This articulation is the primary site for rotation of the thumb about its longitudinal axis and, along with the secondary rotational contribution of the MP joint, allows opposition of the thumb to each of the other digits.

The index finger projects from the central fixed unit of the hand and articulates with the fixed second metacarpal. The MP joint acts as a hinge joint in flexion but allows a substantial amount of mediolateral mobility in extension. Three intrinsic and four extrinsic muscles supply the index finger with a relative independence of function.

The middle finger along with the ring and small digital rays function together to grasp and stabilize objects. This is important during power grasp and when stabilization of an object for precision handling by the thumb and index finger is desired. The fourth and fifth metacarpals are tethered to the central fixed unit of the hand with significant mobility at the carpometacarpal and intermetacarpal articulations. This mobility, along with the wide range of motion of the first metacarpal, provides the adaptability of the distal transverse arch through the metacarpal heads. Thus, the arch can be pulled into a semicircle by the thenar and hypothenar muscles or flattened by the extensors.

SUGGESTED READING

American Society for Surgery of the Hand: *The Hand: Examination and Diagnosis,* ed 3. New York, Churchill Livingstone, 1990.

Aulicino PL, Dupuy TE: Clinical examination of the hand, in *Rehabilitation of the Hand.* St Louis, Mosby–Year Book, 1984.

Gilula LA (ed): *The Traumatized Hand and Wrist: Radiographic and Anatomic Correlation.* Philadelphia, WB Saunders, 1992.

Green DP (ed): *Operative Hand Surgery.* New York, Churchill Livingstone, 1982.

Hoppenfeld S: *Physical Examination and Diagnosis of the Spine and Extremities.* New York, Appleton-Century-Crofts, 1976.

Jupiter JB (ed): *Flynn's Hand Surgery,* ed 3. Baltimore, Williams & Wilkins, 1991.

Netscher DT, Peterson R: Normal and abnormal development of the extremities and trunk. *Clin Plast Surg* 1990; 17:13–21.

Sadler TW: *Langman's Medical Embryology,* ed 6. Baltimore, Williams & Wilkins, 1990.

Chapter 21

Congenital Disorders

Vincent R. Hentz, M.D.

CONTENTS

CHAPTER OBJECTIVE

At the end of this chapter the resident is familiar with the spectrum of congenital abnormalities of the upper extremity and performs comprehensive diagnostic and surgical management of such problems.

LEARNER OBJECTIVES

On completion of this chapter the resident

1. Understands a classification system for congenital hand anomalies including
   a. Failure of part formation
   b. Failure of differentiation
   c. Duplication
   d. Overgrowth
   e. Undergrowth
   f. Congenital bands
   g. Generalized musculoskeletal anomalies
2. Understands physiologic theories that explain the etiology of anomalies in each category.
3. Knows the incidence and inheritance pattern of the more frequent of the anomalies.
4. Knows the anomalies of other body parts that may be associated with the particular hand anomaly.
5. Understands the range of deformity that can exist within a category and the specific anatomic changes that define that anomaly.
6. Knows indications for surgery for each category, including timing of the operation.
7. Knows specific operations used in the surgical management of conditions within each category.
8. Understands the normal embryologic developmental sequence of the hand and the postnatal ossification pattern (bone age).
9. Understands the indications for and the application of nonoperative casting and splinting for conditions within each category.

CLINICAL PRACTICE ACTIVITIES

During the course of the training program, the resident

1. Performs preoperative evaluation of patients with congenital and developmental anomalies of the upper extremity; applies proper nomenclature in the diagnosis of these patients.
2. Performs surgical procedures for the treatment of congenital and develop-

mental anomalies of the upper extremity.
3. Performs postoperative care of patients with congenital and developmental anomalies of the upper extremity.
4. Applies casts and splints for the preoperative and postoperative care of these patients.
5. Provides pre- and postoperative teaching to parents of children with congenital anomalies of the upper extremity.

Congenital disorders of the hand occur in only a small fraction of patients with hand disorders seen by the plastic surgeon. However, the plastic surgeon is often asked to see a newborn with a congenital hand disorder and is therefore in a position to relieve ever-present parental anxiety if he is sufficiently well informed to educate the parents about the current state of knowledge of the incidence, genetic peculiarities, timing, treatment, and anticipated outcome of their child's deformity. It is important not to be pinned down to exact dates or procedures at this initial consultation. On the other hand, it is a great disservice to merely tell the parents that the child will be able to "do almost everything" or that "it's too early" to do anything except see the child in the future.

INCIDENCE, GENETICS, AND EMBRYOLOGY

Previous studies have provided varying data regarding the incidence of hand anomalies. A large study of skeletal deficiencies gave an incidence of 1/4,000 live births. Other studies indicate an incidence for all upper limb anomalies of approximately 1/626 live births. Clearly some deformities have a strong familial predilection, including such common conditions as syndactyly and polydactyly. Others, such as phocomelia associated with maternal ingestion of the drug thalidomide, are clearly environmental in origin. However, the majority of anomalies cannot be definitively traced to defective genetic material or to some external or environmental event. Many series show only a 5% to 7% incidence of inheritance patterns in congenital hand defects. Most anomalies are probably the result of some interaction between genetic and environmental influences.

Knowing the orderly sequence of developmental events allows one to understand the pathophysiology involved in many congenital hand anomalies. The human limb develops during the fourth week of gestation in the form of lateral swellings called limb buds (really ectodermal sacs filled with mesoderm). Nerves and blood vessels sprout into the limb buds from central or trunk nerves and vessels. There soon develops a thickening of the ectoderm, termed the apical ectodermal ridge (AER), that acts as a pacemaker for the developing limb and influences subsequent development in a proximodistal direction through a process termed induction.

The limb appears on about the 26th day. By the 37th day, the primary divisions of the limbs have been established, including a hand plate, a proximal arm and shoulder region, and primordia of most of the osseous elements. The hand plate is marked by digital ridges with evidence of deepening of interdigital clefts. By 42 days, muscles are recognizable, and all skeletal elements except the distal phalanges exist as cartilage, the limb resembling that of the adult. By 90 days the limbs have rotated into their typical position, where they undergo only enlargement during the remaining 6 months of gestation.

Distortion of the inductive pattern, loss of inductive capacity, or failure of proper ectoderm-mesoderm contact may cause anomalies. Genetic or environmental defects that interfere with the normal proximal-to-distal development will have more or less severe sequelae of skeletal deficiency depending on the time of presentation. Prolonged survival of cells normally programmed to degenerate in order to sculpt digits from the digital plate will result in syndactyly. An extra fold of AER may result in duplication of a part. In summary, abnormal morphogenesis may involve anomalies resulting from aberrations of progressive events of primary limb establishment or limb pattern or anomalies resulting from regressive phenomena such as degeneration of well-formed structures, extensions of regions of normal degeneration, or failure of occurrence of normal degeneration.

CLASSIFICATION OF LIMB ANOMALIES

The most useful classification system is one adopted by the International Federation for Societies of Surgery of the Hand. Eight categories are described (Table 21–1).

GENERAL CONSIDERATIONS

Several factors common to most congenital hand disorders require consideration, including cognizance of the high incidence of associated anomalies and decisions regarding the timing of treatment. It is relatively standard today to provide genetic counseling to parents either personally or via consultation with a pediatric geneticist. Close coordination with the child's pediatrician is very important, particularly with some defects known to be associated with anomalies of other organs such as complex polydactyly or thumb agenesis. Such problems influence the timing and priorities of care.

The optimal age for surgery of various deformities remains controversial, although the current trend is toward surgery at younger ages. Those surgeons who favor early surgery emphasize the relief of parental anxiety as well as the possibility of allowing the child to use the part in a more normal manner early in his functional development, thus avoiding the need to overcome bad habits. In addition, earlier use of the part may promote growth. In contrast, those surgeons who favor surgery at a later age are influenced by certain physical factors such as the difficulty in performing precise surgery on the infant's small parts, the difficulty with postoperative immobilization of the infant's hand, somewhat greater scarring of the very young child, and the inability to determine the ability and useful functions of the deformed parts at a very young age.

In general, all agree that procedures that endanger growth potential (such as fusion of joints) should be postponed as long as possible, while parts that have no value (such as a poorly attached floating thumb) should be removed very early. As much restoration as possible should be accomplished prior to school age, but when a distal defect may have a great effect on the growth of more proximal

TABLE 21–1.
Classification of Congenital Hand Deformities*

- I. Failure of formation of parts (arrest of development)
  - A. Transverse deficiencies
    - 1. Amputations: arm, forearm, wrist, hand, digits
  - B. Longitudinal deficiencies
    - 1. Phocomelia: complete, proximal, distal
    - 2. Radial deficiencies (radial clubhand)
    - 3. Central deficiencies (cleft hand)
    - 4. Ulnar deficiencies (ulnar clubhand)
    - 5. Hypoplastic digits
- II. Failure of differentiation (separation) of parts
  - A. Synostosis: elbow, forearm, wrist, metacarpals, phalanges
  - B. Radial head dislocation
  - C. Symphalangia
  - D. Syndactyly
    - 1. Simple
    - 2. Complex
    - 3. Associated syndrome
  - E. Contracture
    - 1. Soft tissue
      - a. Arthrogryposis
      - b. Pterygium cubitale
      - c. Trigger digit
      - d. Absent extensor tendons
      - e. Hypoplastic thumb
      - f. Thumb-clutched hand
      - g. Camptodactyly
      - h. Windblown hand
    - 2. Skeletal
      - a. Clinodactyly
      - b. Kirner's deformity
      - c. Delta bone
- III. Duplication
  - A. Thumb (preaxial) polydactyly
  - B. Triphalangism/hyperphalangia
  - C. Finger polydactyly
    - 1. Central polydactyly (polysyndactyly)
    - 2. Postaxial polydactyly
  - D. Mirror hand
    - 1. (Ulnar dimelia)
- IV. Overgrowth—all or portions of the upper limb
  - A. Macrodactyly
- V. Undergrowth
- VI. Congenital constriction band syndrome
- VII. Generalized skeletal abnormalities
  - A. Madelung's deformity

* Adapted from Swanson AB: *J Hand Surg* 1976; 1:8–22.

structures (for example, radial clubhand), early correction is indicated.

MANAGEMENT OF SPECIFIC DEFORMITIES OR FAILURE OF FORMATION

Radial Aplasia

Failure of proper longitudinal development of preaxial elements is termed radial deficiency, and the most common disorder is termed radial clubhand, with deficiencies ranging from total absence of the radius to absence or hypoplasia of the most distal preaxial element, the thumb. Radial deficiency occurs in 1 per 100,000 births and is equally common bilaterally and unilaterally. This condition is frequently associated with other anomalies, especially septal defects of the heart.

Treatment of significant deformities begins at birth with serial casting or splinting and stretching exercises to correct the radial deviation. Some patients lack adequate elbow flexion and may be unable to place the straightened hand to the mouth, and these extremities perhaps should not be treated. For the others, very early surgical centralization (at 6 months of age) of the carpus on the ulna is indicated, especially where splinting has not corrected the deviation. The carpus is approached via an ulnarly located incision plus a radially located Z-plasty incision with three essential goals in mind: adequate soft-tissue release to allow placement of the hand over the ulna, adequate balance by tendon transfer or shortening, and capsular stabilization. If severe ulnar bowing is present, it may be corrected simultaneously by ulnar osteotomy. A K-wire maintains the hand centralized on top of the ulna, and prolonged postoperative splinting, initially full-time and then nightly, usually throughout childhood, seems mandatory. Unfortunately, recurrence of the wrist deformity is frequent, and the ulnar osteotomy may need to be repeated. Even with successful treatment, wrist motion will be very limited but functionally helpful.

Other Longitudinal Deficiencies—Aplasia or Hypoplasia of the First Ray

The functional and cosmetic stigma of aplasia or severe hypoplasia of the first ray is great. The thumb is the pillar of manual dexterity; therefore, considerations for providing an opposable thumb assume supreme importance. A wide spectrum of thumb deformities exists. The thumb may be totally absent as part of severe aplasia of all the preaxial elements (radial clubhand), diminutive and attached by a thin soft-tissue thread (pouce floutant), or skeletally better formed but malpositioned and imbalanced because of abnormal development or placement of supporting structures.

The history of reconstruction of the absent thumb has somewhat paralleled the evolution of plastic surgery principles and techniques, and many clever operations have been proposed, including microvascular toe transfer. For total or near-total absence of the thumb, however, the benchmark remains pollicization of the index finger by the neurovascular pedicle technique, usually carried out between 1½ and 3 years of age. The goal is the creation of a radially positioned, opposable digit of proper length and the establishment of stability, a feature more important than mobility. This requires carefully placed incisions to allow adequate exposure, skeletal shortening by subtotal metacarpal resection, repositioning and Kirschner wire fixation of the digit to its own metacarpal base in a thumb-like projection by radial and palmar angulation and rotation of the digit, and finally, extrinsic-intrinsic muscle rebalancing (Fig 21–1). Factors found important for success, aside from superb surgical technique and a detailed knowledge of the anatomy, include ablating the metacarpal epiphysis to prevent overgrowth, striving for a thumb slightly shorter rather than longer than normal, and using the metacarpophalangeal joint as the new carpometacarpal joint and fixing this to the metacarpal base with the joint in a fully flexed position to obviate the tendency of this joint to become unstable in hyperextension. The result is a three-fingered hand with a well-positioned opposable thumb. Occasionally,

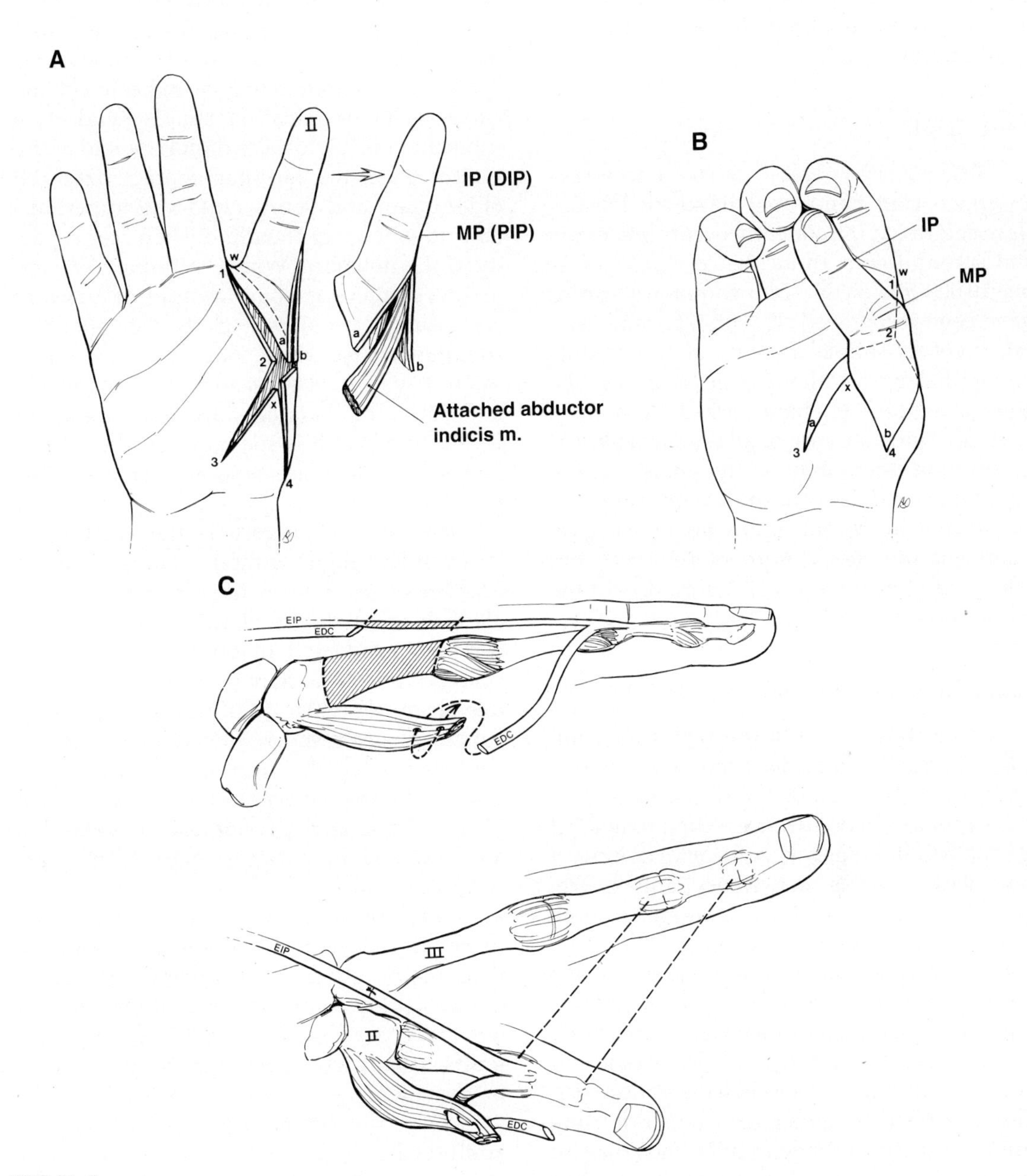

FIG 21–1.
A, skin incisions must allow sufficient exposure for reconstruction and permit the reconstruction of an adequate first web space. Scars should fall along the borders of the normal tetrahedral space to avoid later compromise. The small palmar flap helps to cover the extra bulk of the relocated abductor indicis, now the abductor pollicis brevis. **B,** the metacarpal is shortened appropriately and its epiphysis ablated. The metacarpal head is fixed to its own metacarpal base in the normal mean thumb projection of 20 degrees of radial abduction and 35 degrees of palmar abduction. **C,** Proper opposition requires that the index metacarpal be rotated (pronated) almost 100 degrees. Note how the extrinsic and intrinsic muscle-tendon units are rebalanced by shortening the extrinsic tendons and using part of the extrinsic tendon mechanism to provide an attachment for the relocated abductor indicis to create an abductor pollicis brevis.

insufficient strength or stability can be corrected by subsequent transfer of the abductor digiti minimi muscle.

Cleft Hand

Absence or hypoplasia of the central rays is termed cleft hand, split hand, or lobster-claw deformity. It frequently occurs bilaterally and is found with an incidence of 0.4 to 0.14 per 10,000 live births. Two common patterns have been recognized. The first, termed typical, involves simple absence of the middle finger phalanges with intact metacarpals. The atypical pattern is characterized by a deep cleft indicating absence of all the metacarpals. In addition, there may be hypoplasia of the remaining middle rays and syndactyly between the thumb and index finger. Surgical treatment involves closure of the cleft and release or correction of any deformities of the border digits.

Failure of Differentiation—Syndactyly

Syndactyly is one of the two most common congenital limb disorders. It occurs in approximately 1 of 2,000 births, with 80% of cases sporadic in occurrence. When familial, it is usually inherited as an autosomal dominant trait with variable penetrance and is frequently associated with other anomalies such as Poland's or Apert's syndrome.

Syndactyly may be *simple* and involve only soft-tissue attachments between two adjacent digits or *complex* with associated bony union, absence of extensor or flexor tendons, and overlapping patterns of innervation. It is also described as either *complete,* indicating union over the entire lengths of the adjacent digits, or *incomplete,* indicating union over less than the full length. The third web is the most frequently involved, followed by the fourth and then the second. Regardless of the type of syndactyly, there is almost always an absolute deficiency of skin that must be replaced at the time of separation, usually in the form of full-thickness skin grafts. Timing of surgery is controversial; however, most children undergo surgery between 8 months and 3 years of age for the most common types of simple syndactyly. If terminal phalangeal fusion exists between border digits, the shorter digit may deform the longer. In such cases, very early bony separation may be indicated. Some surgeons favor releasing simple syndactyly soon after birth while the digit is devoid of the typical excessive fat that characterizes the older infant and young child and to perhaps take advantage of the diminished scar capacity of the newborn. Where multiple clefts are involved, there is some danger of vascular compromise if adjacent clefts are separated simultaneously. Here, separation is more safely staged. If all clefts are involved, the first and third are separated at the first procedure. If the thumb web is spared, then the second and fourth clefts are separated at the initial procedure.

The goal of surgery is the creation of independent digits without deformity, and a number of procedures have been described, all sharing certain similarities. For a simple, complete syndactyly involving only one web space, typically a flap of proximally based dorsal and/or volar full-thickness skin and subcutaneous tissue is elevated to form the commissure at the appropriate level with respect to the adjacent normal digits (Fig 21–2). Additional flaps of dorsal and volar skin are designed in a zigzag pattern to create reciprocal volar and dorsal flaps that after separation of the digits, can be interdigitated to cover the majority of the raw surfaces, particularly about the proximal interphalangeal (PIP) joint. The remainder of the defect is covered with full-thickness skin grafts, usually harvested from the groin crease or abdomen.

When the syndactyly is more complex, additional operative steps are required. The conjoined nail must be separated and a new eponychial fold created either from adjacent tissue or from a composite graft harvested from the toe. Bony phalangeal unions must be separated by saw or osteotome. Frequently a decision must be made regarding the neurovascular structures within the cleft. The nerve is rarely a problem. Even when the nerve branches very far distally, it can be split as far proximally as desired. Often, however, a single digital artery exists, or the artery

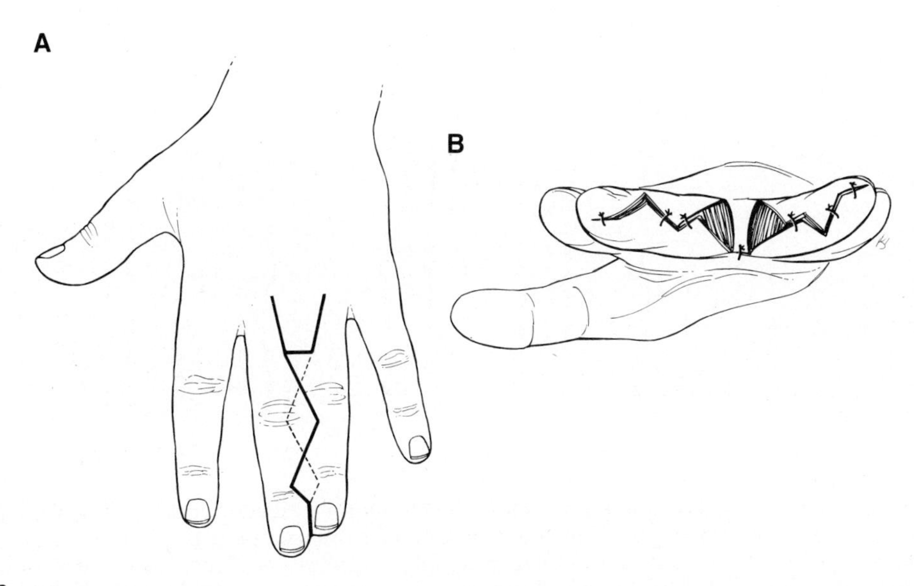

FIG 21–2.
A, dorsal view of the incisions for separating syndactylized digits. The dorsally based truncated rectangular flap ensures a well-formed commissure. The dorsal incisions are designed to fall along areas that undergo very little change in dimension with motion. Note the relationships of the incisions to the level of the axis of rotation of the various joints identified by the dorsal skin wrinkles. **B,** the largest skin deficits are located proximally, areas where accurate sensation is unnecessary. Full-thickness skin grafts are accurately cut from the hairless areas of the groin.

branches too far distally to be retained with both digits. In such cases the arterial contribution to one of the two digits must be divided. This is rarely a problem in simple cases with only one cleft involved. However, when adjacent clefts are affected, this step must be carefully recorded so that at subsequent separation of the adjacent cleft, the digit whose artery has been sacrificed at the previous procedure can be preferentially awarded the artery if necessary. Postoperatively, the limb is immobilized for 2 to 4 weeks.

Duplication (Polydactyly)

Polydactyly may involve any of the digits. It is frequently described as either preaxial, postaxial, or central in presentation. Postaxial polydactyly may be the most common congenital limb disorder (occurring eight times as frequently as preaxial polydactyly), but its incidence is surely underreported because small supernumerary fifth digits are routinely removed in newborns by obstetricians or pediatricians. Postaxial polydactyly is very common in blacks, where it is usually inherited as an autosomal dominant trait. In the Caucasians its presence is frequently associated with other serious abnormalities. However, the treatment of most cases of postaxial polydactyly is relatively straightforward and involves excision of the ulnar element. In contrast, the incidence of preaxial polydactyly among the black and white races is about 0.08 per 1,000 live births, and a variety of types have been described. The classification system of Wassel based on the degree of skeletal duplication is most commonly used (see Fig 21–3). Thumb polydactyly is seldom syndrome associated.

A wide range of pathologic findings may exist, depending on the type of polydactyly. Various skeletal parts may be duplicated, hypoplastic, or abnormally shaped. Frequently, duplicated tendons have abnormal insertions resulting in abnormal inclinations of the skeletal elements. Intrinsic muscles may be absent, hypoplastic, or anomalous in insertion.

Treating the common preaxial duplication requires surgical restoration of a more functional and aesthetic unit, which involves either amputation of the supernumerary digit or reducing and combining two digits into one. Generally, some components of a seg-

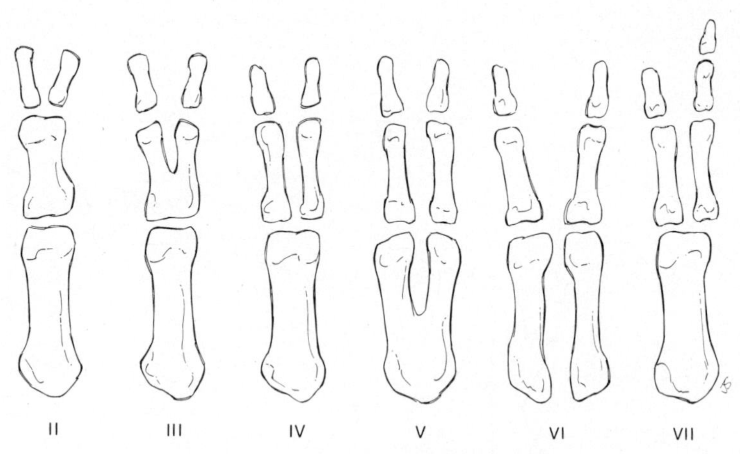

FIG 21–3.
Wassel's classification of thumb duplication is most commonly used. Seven types are described. It is a simple and easily remembered system. The odd numbers refer to incomplete duplication of the three skeletal elements, while the even numbers refer to complete duplication. Type 7 refers to the many different presentations of so-called triphalangeal thumbs. (From Wood VE: *J Hand Surg* 1978; 3:436–444. Used by permission.)

ment to be ablated are preserved to augment the remaining part. This concept of salvage typically includes skin and subcutaneous tissue but may also include parts of the skeleton, collateral ligaments, and tendons. When a definite separation exists, usually one segment will have a greater flexion-extension arc and more power. Its twin should be amputated, and collateral ligaments at the amputation site must be reconstituted. Typically, the ulnar twin of the duplicated elements is the more dominant, and its radial twin is excised. Careful consideration is given to the final placement of incisions so that a straight midaxial closure is avoided. There is always extra skin, and a loose Z-shaped closure with skin flaps can be accomplished. A careful search for duplicated extensor and flexor tendons is carried out. The duplicated portion is excised close to its point of duplication from the main elements to avoid tethering of the tendon by attachment of the amputated remnant to surrounding scar. In contrast, the detached tendon can be reinserted at a point adjacent to the insertion of its twin to help achieve balance at the joint if this has been pulled into radial deviation by a malattached tendon. Occasionally, a midphalangeal osteotomy is required to correct a deviated distal segment.

Less commonly performed is a procedure that combines major and symmetrical components from each half of a duplicated pair. It is generally restricted to type I or II duplications, i.e., either complete or incomplete separation of the distal phalanges. If more than distal segment combinations are attempted, the procedure becomes more technically complex, thus making it more difficult to achieve a satisfactory aesthetic and functional result. Typically, some combination of ablation and sharing is performed.

Overgrowth

Terms such as macrodactyly, gigantism, localized hypertrophy, or macrodactylia fibrolipomatosis are used to describe a disproportionately large digit. True macrodactyly involves overgrowth of all elements as opposed to the enlarged digit seen with an arteriovenous fistula or hemangioma or with congenital lymphedema. It is a rare congenital limb anomaly and appears to be noninherited and therefore unassociated with other anomalies. It may be *static,* with the initially enlarged digit growing proportionally to the other fingers, or *progressive,* with disproportionate growth.

Management must be individualized but includes such procedures as total ablation for the unsightly huge digit, epiphyseal arrest, angulation osteotomies, and bulk reduction procedures, usually performed in two or more stages. If amputation is chosen, the most appropriate level is ray resection of border digits and ray resection combined with digital transposition for the central digits. Admirable results are rare.

Undergrowth

Most congenital hand deformities have some element of hypoplasia. The group of deformities categorized as "undergrowth" are those with relatively symmetrical shortening and are termed brachydactyly or ectrodactyly. The digits may be represented by only a small, poorly attached bubble of skin or by a sizable part lacking only some length in the middle phalanx. Treatment, especially for the more severely hypoplastic digit, remains controversial. Many surgeons feel that no treatment is indicated, particularly if the opposite hand is normal. Others feel that any additional length will be useful to the child, especially if the hypoplastic digits are at least a third the normal length.

Many different operative procedures have been proposed, depending upon the extent of the deficiency. If a sufficient skin tube is present but is skeletally underserved, then bone grafts from common sites have been promoted, as has the transfer of complete nonvascularized toe phalanges. Commonly, the second toe becomes the donor site. There is controversy regarding whether epiphyseal growth persists after transfer and whether the phalanx should be harvested subperiosteally or extraperiosteally. Receiving mixed reviews also is skeletal lengthening with distraction. This technique, developed for traumatic loss, has been applied to congenital defects and involves the application of a device fixed by wires to both sides of an osteotomy site in the phalanx or metacarpal. Usually at least 3 cm of bone length is required before this technique can be employed. The device allows the divided bones to be gradually stretched apart slowly enough to permit the elongation of surrounding soft tissues. Several centimeters of additional length can be obtained with this method. Usually the distraction site requires subsequent bone grafts. Although controversial, transfer of entire toes by microvascular technique has also been performed for the amelioration of these defects.

Constriction Bands

This deformity is also termed congenital ring constriction, and a variety of manifestations exist, including a simple encircling band about a digit plus or minus distal swelling, acral absence of one or many digits with simple or complex fusion of the remaining digital elements, or so-called intrauterine amputations (amniotic band syndrome.) The incidence is reported to be about 1/15,000 births. There is controversy regarding the etiology of this deformity, with two prominent theories emerging. The first attributes the deformity to defective germ plasm, while the second believes that the deformity is secondary to amniotic band strangulation of the developing or developed part.

Shallow bands may require no treatment. Deep bands associated with massive distal edema may require surgery during the newborn period. However, even deep grooves are completely compatible with adequate arterial and venous circulation, and mild enlargement distal to the groove is not in itself an indication for neonatal surgery. Surgery between 1½ and 2 years of age seems more acceptable. When the ring encircles the entire digit, typically half of the ring is released at a time by excision of tissues constituting the ring, and Z-plasty of adjacent skin is performed to redirect the scars. While there are advocates for total correction at one operation, it seems safer to stage this procedure. When acrosyndactyly exists, the operative procedure must be individualized, and the goal of surgery varies according to how far proximal the deformity exists. Imperfect digits may be separated from the fusion mass, but numbers are less important than proper spacing, length, and stability. The same types of procedures utilized for the management of complex syndactyly (which exists with acrosyndactyly) are employed, including flaps from the sides of digits and full-thickness skin grafts.

Generalized Musculoskeletal Defects

There are a number of deformities that defy easy categorization, such as arthrogryposis and Madelung's deformity. Arthrogryposis is a syndrome of persistent joint contracture. Clinical findings include multiple, usually symmetrical contractures present at birth, dimpling on the involved joints, a waxy skin appearance with little subcutaneous tissue, and association with other congenital anomalies. Madelung's deformity is classically a shortening of the radius at the wrist with the ulnar half of the radius much more affected, although the entire forearm may be slightly short. It usually does not become obvious until late childhood or adolescence. Many of these problems are truly orthopedic in nature and are rarely treated by the nonhand specialist.

SUGGESTED READING

Dobyns JH, Wood VE, Bayne LG: Congenital hand deformities, in Green DP (ed): *Operative Hand Surgery,* ed 2, New York, Churchill Livingstone, 1988.

Flatt AE: *The Care of Congenital Hand Anomalies.* St Louis, Mosby–Year Book, 1977.

Hentz VR: Congenital anomalies of the thumb, in McCarthy JG (ed): *Plastic Surgery,* vol 8. Philadelphia, WB Saunders, 1990, pp 5106–5134.

Kelikian H: *Congenital Deformities of the Hand and Forearm.* Philadelphia, WB Saunders, 1974.

Upton J: Congenital anomalies of the hand and forearm, in McCarthy JG (ed): *Plastic Surgery,* vol 8. Philadelphia, WB Saunders, 1990.

Chapter 22

Benign and Malignant Tumors

Earl J. Fleegler, M.D.
Brentley A. Buchele, M.D.

CONTENTS

CHAPTER OBJECTIVE

At the end of this chapter the resident understands the principles of diagnosis and treatment of upper extremity tumors and undertakes comprehensive management of a wide variety of such lesions.

LEARNER OBJECTIVES

On completion of this chapter the resident

1. Knows the pathology of soft- and hard-tissue upper extremity tumors.
2. Is familiar with the epidemiology, modalities of treatment, and results of such treatment in upper extremity tumors.
3. Knows diagnostic techniques for upper extremity tumors.
4. Understands the principles and techniques of management of other soft-tissue upper extremity tumors.
5. Understands the principles and techniques of management of bony upper extremity tumors.
6. Knows the reconstructive principles and techniques for restoration of anatomy and function after surgical resections.
7. Knows the indications and use of adjunctive therapy in the management of these tumors.

CLINICAL PRACTICE ACTIVITIES

During the course of the training program, the resident

1. **Evaluates and performs extirpative surgery for patients with upper extremity tumors.**
2. **Reconstructs soft- and hard-tissue defects after the removal of upper extremity tumors.**
3. **Performs evaluation of short- and long-term results after the treatment of upper extremity tumors.**
4. *Utilizes radiotherapy, medical oncology, hand therapy, occupational therapy, and prosthetics where appropriate for patients with upper extremity tumors.*

For the sake of brevity, discussion in this chapter will be limited to the diagnostic and therapeutic activities appropriate to the care of benign and malignant lesions when they occur in the upper extremity. More fundamental biology or particular features of these tumors when they occur elsewhere are covered in other chapters.

INCIDENCE

Data pooled from three series of upper extremity tumors show that ganglion cysts and giant-cell tumors of the tendon sheath account for greater than 60% of all benign tumors (Table 22–1). When the additional common conditions of epidermal inclusion cyst, mucous cyst, hemangioma, benign skin lesion, and lipoma are added, they total 80% of the masses.

TABLE 22–1.

Incidence of Tumors in the Upper Extremity—Pooled Data from Three Series*

Tumor	No.	Benign (%)	Malignant (%)	Percentage of Total Tumors
Benign				
Ganglion cyst	1,428	56.22		52.60
Giant-cell tumor, tendon sheath	291	11.46		10.72
Epidermal inclusion cyst	149	5.87		5.49
Mucous cyst	123	4.84		4.53
Hemangioma	122	4.80		4.49
Lipoma	78	3.07		2.87
Neurilemoma, etc.	53	2.09		1.95
Glomus tumor	43	1.69		1.58
Fibroma	49	1.93		1.80
Enchondroma	35	1.38		1.29
Osteochondroma	15	0.59		0.55
Aneurysm, arteriovenous malformation	12	0.47		0.44
Osteoid osteoma	7	0.28		0.26
Gout	4	0.16		0.15
Synovioma	5	0.20		0.18
Lymphangioma	3	0.12		0.11
Myxoma	4	0.16		0.15
Nodular fasciitis	2	0.08		0.07
Leiomyoma	4	0.16		0.15
Myositis ossificans	2	0.08		0.07
Myxolipoma	1	0.04		0.04
Boeck's sarcoid	1	0.04		0.04
Benign skin lesions	108	4.25		3.98
Parosteal chondroma	1	0.04		0.04
Total benign	2,540	100.00		93.55
Malignant				
Fibrosarcoma	6		3.43	0.22
Squamous cell cacinoma	120		68.57	4.42
†Keratoacanthoma	15		8.57	0.55
Malignant melanoma	8		4.57	0.29
Kaposi's sarcoma	1		0.57	0.04
Malignant giant-cell tumor	4		2.29	0.15
Malignant schwannoma	2		1.14	0.07
Synovial sarcoma	3		1.71	0.11
Liposarcoma	3		1.71	0.11
Hemangioendothelioma	1		0.57	0.04
Basal cell carcinoma	6		3.43	0.22
Granular cell myoblastoma	2		1.14	0.07
Malignant fibrous histiocytoma	1		0.57	0.04
Epithelioid sarcoma	1		0.57	0.04
Osteosarcoma, chondrosarcoma, clear-cell sarcoma	0		0.00	0.00
Metastatic tumor	1		0.57	0.04
Ewing's sarcoma	1		0.57	0.04
Total malignant	175		100.00	6.45
Total tumors	2,715			

* Data from Bogumill GP, Sullivan DJ, Baker GI: *Clin Orthop* 1975; 108:214; Butler ED, Hammill JP, Seipel RS, et al: *Am J Surg* 1960; 100:293–300; and Posch, JL: In Flynn JE (ed): *Hand Surgery*, ed. 2. 1975.
† There is still question as to the behavior of this tumor.

The most common malignancy is squamous cell carcinoma. If this primary skin tumor is excluded, other malignancies total less than 2% of all hand tumors.

The high incidence of benign lesions emphasizes the importance of not sacrificing hand function during the treatment of a mass of unknown etiology. The small yet significant number of malignancies that occur in the hand emphasizes the importance of an accurate diagnosis.

TABLE 22–2.
Clinical Staging of Hand Tumors*

Stage	Grade	Tumor	Metastasis
Benign	0		
IA	1	1	0
IB	1	2	0
IIA	2	1	0
IIB	2	2	0
III	Any	Any	1

* See the text for specific definitions. (From Enneking WF, Spanier SS, Goodman MA: The surgical staging of musculoskeletal sarcoma. *Clin Orthop* 1982; 153:106. Used by permission.)

PREOPERATIVE EVALUATION

The high incidence of benign conditions and the relative ease of diagnosing these conditions preoperatively minimizes the need for extensive preoperative evaluation in most cases. A thorough history and physical examination may reveal systemic conditions (e.g., neurofibromatosis) or preexisting diseases (e.g., lung carcinoma) that explain the presence of a mass. Plain radiographs may reveal a bony lesion or a mass effect from a soft-tissue lesion that was not palpable.

The ease of diagnosis of the common benign masses and the diagnostic appearance of certain benign bone lesions imply that a lesion that is not easily diagnosed should be considered suspicious. Bone scans, computed tomography (CT), and magnetic resonance imaging (MRI) are helpful in diagnosing these tumors and determining the local extent of the tumor. Even so, tissue diagnosis is usually the method of definitive diagnosis. Small lesions that are within one anatomic compartment and can be completely removed with no functional loss can be definitively treated by excisional biopsy. Other lesions should have incisional biopsies through incisions that would not interfere with future resection or reconstruction.

While the specific natural history of a particular malignancy must dictate its treatment, some general staging principles for sarcomas exist. Three elements contribute to clinical staging: histologic grade, tumor extent, and metastases.

Sarcomas are graded G0, benign; G1, low grade (mature cells with low cell density relative to stroma; less than five mitoses per high-powered field); and G2, high grade (immature cells with less stroma; greater than ten mitoses per high-powered field). A T1 sarcoma exists in one anatomic compartment (intraosseous, intrafascial, intraarticular, etc.), while a T2 sarcoma extends beyond one compartment. M0 represents no detectable metastatic disease, and M1 has detectable metastases. Table 22–2 shows a clinical staging scheme based on these parameters.

Soft-tissue and bony malignancies have a tendency to involve local nodes (demonstrated clinically) and the lungs (examined by chest radiography and/or chest CT). If a malignant bone tumor is suspected or diagnosed, laboratory work should include a complete blood count, alkaline phosphatase determination, a myeloma profile, and a sedimentation rate (elevated in Ewing's sarcoma).

ABLATIVE TREATMENTS AND RECONSTRUCTION

Bony and soft-tissue sarcomas may require amputation or function-impairing resections. Functional considerations must not interfere with lifesaving ablations, yet as adjunctive therapies improve, less radical resections are possible. Resections need adequate pathologic examination and frequently require decalcification to ensure satisfactory margins. Reconstruction should be delayed until this pathologic information is confirmed, which may be as long as 4 to 8 weeks after therapy. Reconstructive priorities are based on function, not appearance. For example, a sensate pinch is a high priority and may be established by pollicization or toe-to-hand transfer.

GANGLIA

Extrasynovial accumulations of synovial-type fluid surrounded by a pseudocapsule are termed "ganglia." These can be classified according to location and presumed etiology (Table 22–3).

In general, ganglia occur in patients 20 to 40 years old but are not uncommon in the teenage years. They are more frequent in women. Only 10% have specific antecedent trauma; most have symptoms varying from weakness or pain to the simple presence of a bulge. The valve-like stalk allows for changes in size. This valvular mechanism has been confirmed by continuity of the cyst with the joint on arthrography but not cystography. Malignancy has not been reported.

Dorsal wrist ganglia contribute 60% to 70% of hand and wrist ganglia. The majority originate from the scapholunate ligament. The cyst may have a long neck or may put pressure on the posterior interosseous nerve and result in pain. Adequate excision, usually through a transverse incision, results in a 13%–40% recurrence rate.

Volar wrist ganglia account for 18% to 20% of hand and wrist ganglia. Most are present at the flexor crease, just radial to the flexor carpi radialis. The cyst is frequently intimately associated with the radial artery. A preoperative Allen's test is helpful. Usually a longitudinal incision turning transversely at the wrist crease provides best exposure. Freeing the radial artery from the cyst prior to formal dissection of the cyst decreases the chance of arterial injury. The cyst origin is frequently the scaphotrapezial or radiocarpal ligament.

Mucous cysts are ganglia of the distal interphalangeal joint. Grooving of the nail may precede the presence of a mass. Radiographs usually reveal osteoarthritic osteophytes, which should be removed at the time of cyst excision. The skin over the cyst is frequently thin, and the incision must be carefully designed. The entire width of the extensor tendon should be visualized to avoid missing an occult cyst on the margin opposite the cyst in question. The patient should be cautioned about possible postoperative nail abnormalities.

Proximal interphalangeal joint cysts are dorsal masses whose neck is usually between the central slip and the lateral band of the extensor apparatus. The joint capsule at the base of the neck should be excised.

Cysts that originate in the flexor apparatus are referred to as *volar retinacular cysts.* They usually originate at the distal edge of the A1 pulley. Their stationary position with finger motion distinguishes them from trigger finger nodules.

Cysts can occur in other synovial surfaces. Ganglion cysts may be associated with de Quervain's disease. Nerve compressions from cysts in the carpal tunnel and Guyon's canal have been reported.

While the osteoarthritic spur of a *carpometacarpal boss* is not a true ganglion, a ganglion is associated with the bossing in 30% of cases. This mass of bone at the base of the index or long metacarpal may be confused with a routine dorsal ganglion. Correct treatment is excision of any associated ganglion, the affected joint capsule, and the spur down to normal cartilage.

In patients with unexplained wrist pain, the rare finding of an *interosseous ganglion* may occur on radiographs. If no other source of the patient's pain can be found, curettage and bone grafting are indicated.

TABLE 22–3.
Ganglia by Site of Origin

Joint etiology
Dorsal surface of the wrist
Volar surface of the wrist
Mucous cyst
DIP* joint
PIP* joint
Tendon sheath
Volar retinacular
Flexor tendon sheath
Extensor tendon
First dorsal compartment
Carpel tunnel
Ulnar (Guyon's) canal
Bone
Carpometacarpal boss
Interosseous ganglion

* DIP = distal interphalangeal; PIP = proximal interphalangeal.

GIANT-CELL TUMOR OF THE TENDON SHEATH

A *giant-cell tumor of the tendon sheath* is also called xanthoma of the tendon sheath. A more accurate but rarely used term is "localized pigmented vilonodular tenovagosynovitis." The lesion is manifested as a slowly growing mass with minimal pain, although nerve compression is possible. Grossly there is a yellow-gray mass attached to the tendon sheath that is rarely fixed to the skin. Histologically the number of giant cells may vary. Excision should be complete to avoid recurrence.

A patient with multiple nodules, which if single might represent giant-cell tumor, would suggest *xanthoma tuberosum.* This condition has lipid deposits that infiltrate fibrous tissues as a manifestation of familial hyperlipidemia.

OTHER BENIGN CONDITIONS

Cutaneous horns, keratoacanthomas, actinic keratoses, warts, and nevi (dysplastic, congenital, and acquired) occur in the upper extremity. Their treatment is the same as in other locations (see Chapter 11).

Lipomas of the upper extremity are histologically similar to lipomas elsewhere. Their excision should be prompted primarily by symptoms. Avoidance of injury to cutaneous nerves during excision is important.

Epidermal inclusion cysts are common in the hand and may be related to frequent local trauma. Their management is the same as when located elsewhere.

Tumors of the peripheral nerve including *neurilemoma* and *schwannoma* are uncommon. They are usually excised only when symptomatic. A 15% to 30% potential for malignant degeneration has been described in lesions associated with von Recklinghausen's disease.

Glomus tumors are benign neoplasms of the thermoregulatory neuromyoarterial apparatus. There are five specific parts to the glomus: afferent artery, the arteriovenous canal, neuroreticular elements, lamella of collagen, and collecting veins. Large numbers of these structures are in the pads and under the nails of the fingertips. Glomus tumors are manifested by pain (often severe) and pinpoint tenderness. Cold sensitivity is common, and distortion of the nail bed is possible. Excision is appropriate and may require elevation of the nail and incision through the nail bed.

Hemangiomas and vascular malformations, when isolated to the skin, should be treated no differently from other skin hemangiomas. When in the bone, pathologic fractures may result. Phantom disease of bone, a condition where bone resorption occurs, is histologically a hemangioma. *Maffucci's syndrome* is the association of soft-tissue hemangioma and skeletal chondromas. Large hemangiomas of the upper extremity, as in other locations, may result in thrombocytopenic purpura, also known as the Kasabach-Merritt syndrome.

Dupuytren's disease may start as a palmar nodule, possibly attached to the skin. In the absence of contracture, asymptomatic, small nodules need not be excised. When excision is indicated, adequate exposure, preservation of the neurovascular bundles, and meticulous hemostasis are critical.

BENIGN BONE TUMORS

Enchondroma is the most common primary tumor of the bones of the hand. The lesion may be solitary or multiple, with the proximal phalanx a common site. Radiographs show a lucent lesion with calcium flecks and a thin cortex. Histologic examination shows lobules of hyaline cartilage with areas of calcification. Pathologic fracture is common and often the initial manifestation. If fracture is present, it can be allowed to heal prior to definitive curettage and bone grafting. Recurrence is less than 1%. The risk of malignancy is very low in solitary lesions but must be considered when multiple lesions exist.

Osteochondroma represents an aberrant focus of cartilage on the surface of a bone that ossifies enchondrally. These are most frequent in the metaphyses. They are usually multiple when seen in children. If no fracture develops, delay of excision is warranted. A decrease in range of motion would, however, prompt excision.

Unicameral or solitary bone cysts may occur in the hand but are more common in the radius. On x-ray studies there is a hint of chambers or cells within the overall lucent lesion. Traditional therapy has been curettage and bone grafting. However, intralesional methylprednisolone has been reported to be successful.

Osteoid osteoma is a sclerotic lesion with a small lucent center. It produces pain that is very responsive to aspirin. Treatment is by curettage and bone grafting.

Osteoblastoma has mature bone cells in an osteoid matrix. On radiography it is usually an expanding lucent lesion with scattered calcifications.

Giant-cell tumor of bone may be manifested as a growing lesion or a pathologic fracture of the tubular bones of the hand, but most commonly the metacarpals and radius. Histologically it is indistinguishable from a giant-cell tumor of the tendon sheath. Malignancy is rare. Therefore, curettage and bone grafting of small lesions and resection of larger, more locally destructive lesions are appropriate. This lesion has a high recurrence rate with curettage.

MALIGNANT TUMORS OF SKIN AND SOFT TISSUE

Basal cell and squamous cell carcinomas occur in the hand. Prior solar or x-ray therapy exposure increases the incidence of squamous cell tumors. Melanomas also occur, and the acral lentiginous form may occur as a subungual melanoma. Benign pigmentation can occur under the nail. Longitudinal streaks of pigment, *melanonychia striata longitudinalis,* is such a condition. It is more common in the Afro-American population. A melanoma remains stationary with nail growth, while a small hematoma moves distally with time. Eccrine sweat gland tumors, while rare, may be manifested as a mass in the palm. Patients with these sweat gland tumors are usually in the sixth to eighth decades of life.

Kaposi's sarcoma, a form of angiosarcoma, occurs in chronically immunosuppressed patients, including patients with acquired immunodeficiency syndrome (AIDS). Initially, these lesions are usually purple discolorations in the skin. They are more common in the lower extremity but may be found in the upper extremity.

Malignant fibrous histiocytoma, the most common adult soft-tissue sarcoma, can occur in the upper extremity. Preoperative oncology and radiation therapy consultation should be obtained.

Epithelioid sarcoma is an unusual tumor seen in younger patients. It has slow persistent growth. In addition to lymph node and lung metastases, fascial and perineural spread occurs. Recurrence as late as 10 years postoperatively has been reported.

Synovial sarcoma is rare and frequently detected late. Calcification may exist in the tumor. Histologically it has epithelial and spindle cells. Wide excision or amputation is frequently required, yet the prognosis remains poor.

Lymphangiosarcoma may develop in patients with long-standing lymphedema.

Rhabdomyosarcomas occur in four types: embryonal, pleomorphic, alveolar, and botryoid. This tumor is more common in the pediatric than the adult population. Chemotherapy, when combined with major resection, has improved the prognosis.

MALIGNANT TUMORS OF BONE

Malignant bone tumors are uncommon. The bone changes seen on radiography are not pathognomonic. Only after tissue diagnosis and staging can the appropriate resection and adjunctive therapy be planned.

Lung, breast, and kidney tumors may metastasize to bone, including the hand. These foci of tumor rarely involve the carpus and are most commonly seen in the distal phalanx. They are radiolucent. Metastatic disease to the hand is a poor prognostic sign, with most patients dying within 6 months.

Chondrosarcoma may be more common than previously thought. Clinically, the tumor may be present in the medullary cavity (central) or on the bony surface (peripheral), or it may exist separate from bone. If the malignancy develops in a lesion (e.g., enchondroma), it is classified as a secondary chondrosarcoma.

Ewing's sarcoma occurs in younger patients as a lytic lesion.

Osteogenic sarcoma is a sclerotic expansile lesion. Chemotherapy should supplement operative therapy.

CONCLUSION

Mass lesions of the hand are common. Fortunately, most are benign, and in the majority of cases excision is satisfactory treatment, provided that the underlying etiology is treated simultaneously.

There are classic radiographic presentations of certain benign bone conditions, but only histologic examination of the removed tissue can confirm the diagnosis. A variety of malignant tumors of bone can exist in the hand, but the frequency of any specific lesion is small.

SUGGESTED READING

Bogumill GP, Fleegler EJ: *Tumors of the Hand and Upper Limb.* New York, Churchill Livingstone, 1993.

Bogumill GP, Sullivan DJ, Baker GI: Tumors of the hand. *Clin Orthop* 1975; 108:214–222.

Butler ED, Hammill JP, Seipel RS, et al: Tumors of the hand. A ten-year survey and report of 437 cases. *Am J Surg* 1960; 100:293–300.

Enneking WF, Spanier SS, Goodman MA: The surgical staging of musculoskeletal sarcoma. *Clin Orthop* 1982; 153:106.

Fleegler E: Tumors involving the skin of the upper extremity. *Hand Clin* 1987; 3:187–212.

Fleegler EJ: Skin tumors, in Green DP (ed): *Operative Hand Surgery,* ed 2. New York, Churchill Livingstone, 1988.

Fleegler EJ: Tumors of the upper extremity, in Smith JW, Aston SJ (eds): *Grabb and Smith's Plastic Surgery,* ed 4. Boston, Little, Brown, 1991.

Huvos AG: *Bone Tumors—Diagnosis, Treatment and Prognosis,* ed 2. Philadelphia, WB Saunders, 1991.

Mankin HJ: Principles of diagnosis and management of tumors of the hand. *Hand Clin* 1987; 3:2.

McFarland GB Jr: Soft tissue tumors, in Green DP (ed): *Operative Hand Surgery,* ed 2. New York, Churchill Livingstone, 1988.

Chapter 23

Trauma

Leland Chick, M.D.
Graham Lister, M.D.

■ CONTENTS

Digital pulp
Tendon sheaths
Web space
Deep palmar space
Specific types of infection

CHAPTER OBJECTIVE

At the end of this chapter the resident understands the principles of diagnosis and treatment of upper extremity trauma and performs comprehensive management of acute injuries and other trauma-related problems of the hand and arm.

LEARNER OBJECTIVES

On completion of this chapter the resident

1. **Is thoroughly familiar with the anatomy and pathophysiology of injuries to the hand and upper extremity.**
2. **Understands the principles and applications of diagnostic techniques for the evaluation of hand and upper extremity trauma.**
3. **Knows the techniques for operative management of traumatic injuries of the upper extremity, their indications and contraindications, and their potential complications and the treatment thereof.**
4. **Understands the indications for, contraindications to, and techniques for nonoperative management of traumatic injuries of the hand and upper extremity.**

CLINICAL PRACTICE ACTIVITIES

During the course of the training program, the resident

1. **Evaluates the traumatized upper extremity and performs initial emergency treatment.**
2. **Debrides and closes simple wounds.**
3. **Evaluates and manages nerve injuries.**
4. **Evaluates and manages tendon injuries of the hand.**
5. **Diagnoses, evaluates, and treats upper extremity infections.**
6. **Manages nail bed and fingertip injuries.**
7. **Performs skin grafting and flap closure of soft-tissue defects of the upper extremity.**
8. **Directs rehabilitation of upper extremity trauma following surgical treatment.**
9. **Manages fractures of the hand, including reduction and immobilization.**
10. Evaluates and manages joint, muscle, and tendon injuries of the arm.
11. Recognizes, evaluates, and manages Volkmann's and other ischemic contractures.
12. Manages upper extremity fractures (exclusive of the hand), including reduction and immobilization.
13. Performs disability evaluations following upper extremity trauma.

One third of all injuries involve the upper extremity. Each year in the United States there are 16 million upper extremity injuries severe enough to restrict activity. Hand injuries alone result in more days lost from work annually (some 16 million) than any other form of occupational accident. In the United States, the total cost of upper extremity trauma was $42.4 billion in 1987.

TENDON INJURIES

Hand Posture

If a completely relaxed or anesthetized normal hand is raised with the forearm supinated, the weight of the hand causes the wrist to fall into about 30 degrees of dorsiflexion. The metacarpophalangeal (MP) joints lie in increasing flexion from 40 degrees in the index finger to 50 degrees in the middle, 60 degrees in the ring, and 70 degrees in the small finger; the proximal interphalangeal (PIP) and distal interphalangeal (DIP) joints adopt a similar posture. Thus, the distance from the digital pulp to the palmar crease decreases in smooth progression from the index to the small finger—the so-called cascade. The MP and interphalangeal (IP) joints of the thumb both lie in 30 degrees of flexion, the thumb abducted to the extent that the pulp lies closely adjacent to the pulp of the index finger.

When an unsupported, relaxed arm is then turned into pronation, the wrist falls into 40 to 70 degrees of palmar flexion, depending on whether the elbow is extended or flexed, and the fingers and thumb all extend, the thumb fully and the finger joints to within 20 degrees of the neutral position.

Flexor Tendon Injuries

Complete division of all flexor tendons at the wrist results in full extension of all fingers in the supinated limb.

Complete division of both flexor tendons to one finger results in that finger lying in full extension, in marked contrast with the normal posture of those adjacent. Division of the flexor digitorum profundus alone results in loss of flexion at the DIP joint. This causes the fingertip to fall out of alignment with the others. Hyperextension of the DIP joint suggests that the profundus tendon has been avulsed. On the other hand, *division of the superficialis tendon without injury to the profundus* will result in *no* detectable change in posture. Division of the flexor pollicis longus results in full extension of the IP joint of the thumb which, depending upon the normal range of the joint, may appear to be hyperextended.

It is not possible to flex the ulnar three DIP joints independently of one another because of the common origin of the profundus tendons. If two of the three are fixed in extension by the examiner and the patient asked to flex the third, this movement will be produced by the flexor digitorum superficialis and will occur at the PIP joint. That the flexor digitorum profundus is not responsible for any flexion during this test can be confirmed by passively moving the relaxed DIP joint. The integrity of the flexor digitorum superficialis to the ulnar three fingers can thus be demonstrated. It should be noted that in one third of normal patients the superficialis cannot achieve flexion of the small finger—in approximately half of those it will do so if the ring finger is permitted to flex simultaneously.

This test *cannot* be applied reliably to the index finger, its flexor digitorum profundus muscle being independent. To test the index flexor digitorum superficialis the patient is asked to perform a pulp-to-pulp pinch with the thumb and index finger as, for example, by gripping a piece of paper taken from the dressing pack. The more strongly this is performed by the hand, the more it becomes an action of the flexor digitorum superficialis to the index finger with the flexor digitorum profundus relaxed, as is shown by the hyperextension of the DIP joint. In contrast, if this test is performed in the presence of flexor digitorum superficialis division, the DIP joint becomes progressively more flexed as the flexor digitorum profundus substitutes for the flexor digitorum superficialis.

Anatomy and Repair

Fibrous Flexor Sheath

The fibrous flexor sheath commences over the palmar plate of the MP joint to which the most proximal pulley (A1) attaches. The arrangement of pulleys and sheath in the fingers is logical. Where the tendon lies over a joint, the sheath must be sufficiently thin and resilient to allow free flexion. This structural limitation does not apply over the phalanges, where the sheath can be much more rigid and therefore stronger. Thus there are strong annular pulleys attached to the major portion of the proximal and middle phalanges of the fingers, which are referred to as A2 and A4, respectively. Over the three palmar plates, those of the MP, the PIP, and the DIP joints, there are much narrower annular pulleys, called A1, A3, and A5, respectively.

On either side of these annular pulleys over the joints the sheath has a more cruciate structure that gives a loose retinacular and often transparent appearance. The pulley system in the thumb is similar in function but differs somewhat in design. The proximal pulley is similar in all respects to the A1 pulley in the finger. It arises from the palmar plate of the MP joint of the thumb and is annular in structure and therefore strong. The other major pulley of the thumb passes diagonally across the proximal phalanx from a proximal ulnar to distal radial direction. Like the A2 and the A4 pulleys in the finger it is very strong and equally indispensable for efficient flexion.

The A2 and A4 pulleys in the fingers are necessary to prevent bowstringing of the flexor tendons. Division of these pulleys during tendon repair is to be avoided because closure is extremely difficult. As a corollary, these two pulleys should be reconstructed if divided by injury. While dissimilar tissue such as tendon has been recommended for pulley reconstruction, identical tissue is preferable. Sources include adjacent fingers, either uninjured or so badly damaged as to warrant amputation, the extensor retinaculum and adjacent synovial sheath, both at the wrist and the ankle, and the digital sheaths of the toes.

The flexor zones of the fingers are determined by the pulley system. Zone I contains the area distal to the insertion of the flexor digitorum superficialis tendon and contains the distal tendon sheath and insertion of the flexor digitorum profundus tendon. Zone II, or "no man's land," contains both flexor tendons within the rigid flexor tendon sheath. It begins at the distal palmar crease (which is also the proximal end of the tendon sheath) and ends at the middle phalanx with the insertion of the flexor digitorum superficialis tendon. Zone II is notable for its tendency to form scar adhesions between tendons that have been repaired within the sheath. Zone III includes the midpalm to the distal extent of the transverse carpal ligament. The unique feature in this zone is the origin of the lumbrical muscles from the flexor digitorum profundus tendons. Zone IV covers the territory of the carpal tunnel. Zone V is proximal to the carpal tunnel.

Tendon Repair

When a tendon is injured, the initial surgery has the greatest influence on the ultimate outcome. Digital flexor tendon injuries should be managed in the operating room. If hand surgery expertise is not available, the wound should be closed and the patient referred to a surgeon having the proper training and experience. A delayed primary repair should be optimally performed within 6 days. Emergency room care of tendon injuries should be reserved for isolated extensor tendons that lie within the initial wound and are clean and tidy.

In injuries involving loss of overlying soft tissue, wound conditions may require debridement and wound coverage followed later by tendon repair.

Optimal repair of flexor or extensor tendons requires the use of atraumatic technique involving gentle handling of tissues, judicious debridement, and the use of fine sutures and instruments, as proposed by Bunnell. The tendons must be kept moist with frequent irrigation, and their handling should be limited to cut surfaces only.

Nutrition

The vinculum emerges from the recess between the two checkrein ligaments to gain the dorsal, deep, or periosteal surface of the flexor tendon. This intratendinous blood supply is confined to the dorsal surface of the tendon. Intratendinous, or "core," sutures should therefore be restricted to the palmar half of the tendon. Those areas of tendon that appear to be avascular, including the entire palmar surface, receive their nutrition from the synovial fluid.

Healing

Healing of tendons is initiated by proliferation of the epitendinous cells that grow along the tendon and into the laceration, thereby forming a "callus" in a manner very similar to healing skin or bone. Somewhat later the fibroblasts within the tendon, or tenocytes, invade the callus and produce collagen, which subsequently realigns to produce a strong tendon. The nutrition provided by the synovial fluid is sufficient to support this process. The adhesions that so frequently form are not essential for either healing or nutrition.

Skin Incisions

Considerations for making incisions on the hand include the position of old scars; the location of underlying structures such as

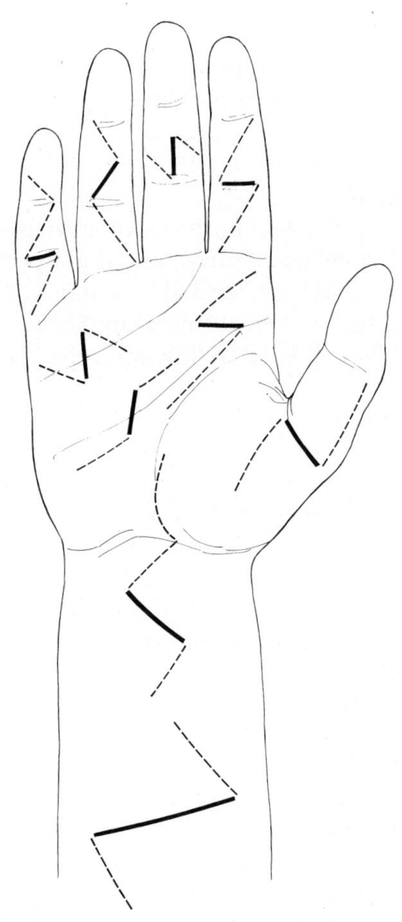

FIG 23–1.
Exposures for primary suturing of tendons. *Solid lines* highlight skin lacerations; *broken lines* indicate options for enlargement to obtain additional exposure. (Adapted from Milford L: *The Hand.* St Louis, Mosby–Year Book, 1988.)

tendon sheaths, joints, nerves, and blood vessels; and the vascularity of the surrounding skin. The incisions begin at the extremes of the wound and usually parallel the skin creases or follow the midaxial lines of the digits. They should not cross skin creases at right angles, or contracture will result in restricted motion (Fig 23–1).

Flexor Exposure

The midlateral incision provides good exposure of the flexor apparatus of the finger. The incision should be placed at the extremes of the digital flexion creases to avoid crossing the creases. This midlateral incision may pass anterior or posterior to the ipsilateral neurovascular bundle. The latter necessitates division of the fine vascular branches to the flexor sheath and indirectly to the vincula, which can impair tendon healing and nutrition.

A zigzag incision of the palmar digital skin provides excellent exposure of the flexor sheath. The incision is made obliquely across each palmar segment of the digit, with opposite ends of adjacent creases joined alternately. Dorsal digit incisions are best directed longitudinally to avoid injury to the veins. Oblique or longitudinal incisions are preferred in the palm and give excellent exposure to the longitudinal tendon. Incisions should not cross the palmar creases at right angles. The flexion and extension surfaces of the wrist should be exposed through incisions that course obliquely in a curvilinear or zigzag configuration. Care should be taken to avoid the radial or ulnar cutaneous sensory nerves dorsally and the palmar cutaneous branch of the median nerve on the flexor surface of the wrist.

Tendon Repair Techniques

The basic requisites of tendon coaptation are that (1) the ends should be precisely aligned, (2) the repair technique should be sufficiently strong, and (3) the suture configuration and placement should cause minimal trauma to and devascularization of the tendon.

The Kessler suture technique or one of its modifications is used most frequently (Fig 23–2). Suture loops should exit the tendon at least 1 cm from the ends for better holding capacity, whereas the longitudinally aligned limbs of the suture should exit the cut ends in the palmar half of the tendon to prevent ischemia. Placement of the transverse suture superficial to the longitudinal suture to form a "locking loop" suture tightens its hold on the

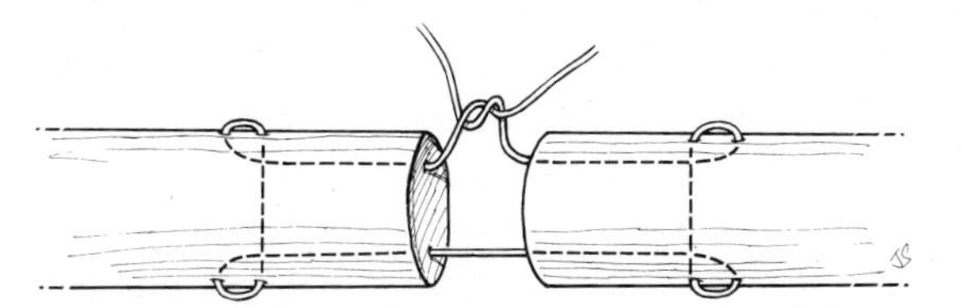

FIG 23–2.
Modified Kessler technique of flexor tendon suturing. A transverse suture is passed palmar to the longitudinal sutures.

tendon bundles as the tension is increased. A fine running inverting 6-0 or 7-0 suture is placed around the tendon juncture to approximate the epitenon.

Specific Flexor Tendon Injuries

Zone I

Closed rupture of the profundus tendon is a relatively common injury that most frequently occurs at the bony insertion of the tendon. This injury can occur at any age and involve any digit, but most commonly it involves the ring finger. Many of these injuries occur in football players when the fingers grasp the jersey of the opposing player; as the player pulls away, the fingers are extended forcibly while the profundus muscle mass is maximally contracting. Delays in diagnosis are common. The main factors having an influence on prognosis are the level to which the tendon retracts and whether the remaining blood supply to the stump of the avulsed tendon is preserved. The time between injury and treatment does not affect the prognosis.

Type 1. The tendon retracts into the palm when the vinculum is ruptured, and this results in a substantial loss of the distal tendon blood supply. These injuries should be repaired to bone within 7 to 10 days of injury.

Type 2. This is the most common type of zone I injury. The tendon retracts to the level of the PIP joint and is tethered by the vinculum. The tendon is reattached to bone with suture or wires passed through the distal phalanx and tied over a button for 6 weeks (Fig 23–3).

Type 3. These injuries are characterized by a large bony fragment of the base of the distal phalanx, which usually catches on the A4 pulley and prevents proximal retraction. These injuries are characterized by swelling, ecchymosis, and tenderness over the middle phalanx and the inability to flex the distal joint. Diagnosis is confirmed on radiographs that reveal the large bony fragment. Treatment is early reduction and internal fixation of the bony fragment.

Injuries of the flexor digitorum profundus tendon distal to the superficialis insertion are repaired by the techniques described above.

Zone II

The portion of flexor mechanism between the proximal flexor pulley and the superficialis insertion has been termed "no man's land" to reflect the rather dismal functional results formerly achieved following repair in this region.

Division of both flexor tendons in zone II results in the inability to flex the PIP and DIP joints. Because most zone II flexor tendon injuries occur with the finger in flexion, the site of tendon division is distal to the skin wound. For this reason the digital wound is usually extended distally to expose the sheath injury and to determine the position of the digital tendon ends.

Clinical results following superficialis excision are poorer than with primary repair of both tendons. For this reason, most surgeons repair both tendons whenever possible. The superficialis repair provides a gliding bed for the profundus and also functions as a checkrein ligament of the PIP joint, as well as allows greater individual finger motion. Repair is performed either proximal or much more commonly distal to the A2 pulley.

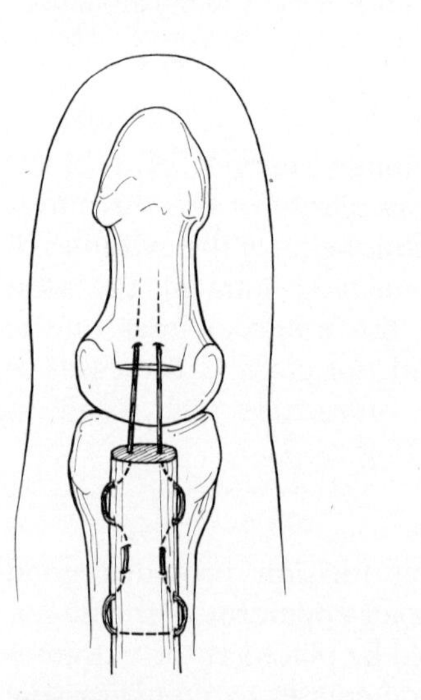

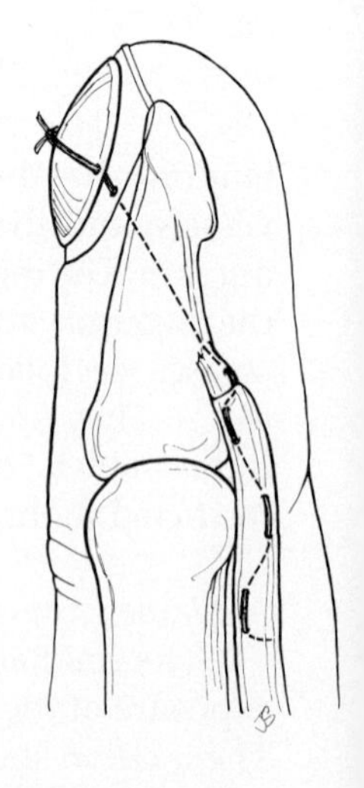

FIG 23–3.
Reattachment of the profundus tendon to its bony insertion.

Proximal Flexor Tendon Injuries

In zone III, or the midpalmar area, the tendons lie outside the fibro-osseous sheath, and pulley mechanisms are absent. The tendons are loosely bound to folds of paratenon and are separated from the adjacent neurovascular structures by vertical septa from the palmar fascia. Injuries in zone III are usually accompanied by injuries to neurovascular structures.

Flexor tendon injuries within the carpal canal (zone IV) are similar to those in zone II in that the tendons are in an unyielding fibrous canal. As in zone II injuries, adhesion formation is not well tolerated. The median nerve is the most superficial structure of the carpal canal and is frequently injured. Division of the transverse carpal ligament may be necessary to gain adequate exposure but should be avoided if possible.

Injuries to tendons in zone V are frequently associated with injury to the adjacent median and ulnar nerves and arteries. In more proximal lesions, it may be difficult or impossible to effect a primary tenorrhaphy because no tendon substance is available proximally. In these cases, repair to an adjacent tendon or muscle group may be indicated.

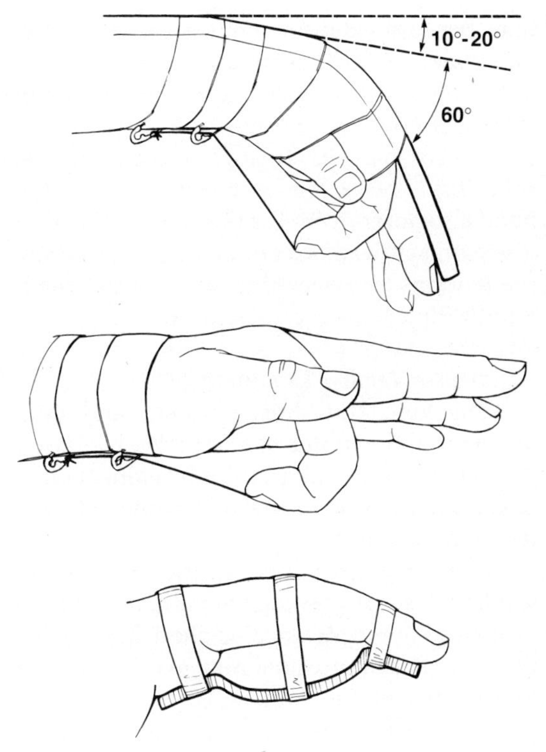

FIG 23–4.
Immediate controlled motion of flexor tendon repairs controls the amount of extension while allowing passive flexion. (Adapted from Hunter JM, Schneider LH, Macklin EJ: *Tendon Surgery in the Hand.* St Louis, Mosby–Year Book, 1987.)

Postoperative Management of Flexor Tendon Injury

Postoperative management of injuries to flexor tendons in zone II requires special consideration because of the propensity of these flexor tendon repairs to develop scar adherence to the fibro-osseous canal. The controlled passive motion advocated by Duran and Houser is a technique designed to prevent this adherence. They found that 3 to 5 mm of active extensor motion in the tendon repairs combined with a passive exercise program helped to prevent adherence of the repaired tendon to the surrounding fibro-osseous canal. In the immediate postoperative period dynamic splinting may also be used for zone II injuries to prevent adhesion formation (Fig 23–4). Tension on a rubber band attached to the fingernail and proximally at the wrist should permit the patient to extend the finger fully with the normal extensor mechanism. A dorsal splint flexes the wrist to 45 degrees and allows extension of the IP and PIP joints but maintains the MP joint in approximately 20 degrees of flexion.

Extensor Tendon Injuries

The extensor mechanism consists of extrinsic and intrinsic components interwoven in a complicated system that balances the flexor tendon system and makes possible hand motion that is precise and delicate.

Extensor tendon injuries are common because of their exposed position in the dorsum of the hand. Because they are thinner and more delicate than their flexor counterparts, they are more subject to rupture with even moderate forces. Extensor tendon injuries differ from those of the flexor tendon in that the loss of continuity is not usually associated with immediate proximal retraction. Because extensor tendons do not separate widely when lacerated or avulsed, many of these tendon injuries, particularly those in the digits alone, may be overlooked and, when diagnosed, may be treated successfully by splinting. The extensor mechanism of the hand also differs from the flexor system in that it is extrasynovial, except at the wrist where the tendons are covered by a synovial sheath within the extensor retinaculum.

Extensor Tendon Examination

The long and short extensor and long abductor of the thumb can be tested by asking the patient to extend his thumb against gentle resistance applied to the nail while the tendons are palpated.

The long extensors of the fingers are similarly tested by asking the patient to extend against gentle resistance applied first to the dorsum of each proximal phalanx and second to the tips of the fingers with the middle phalanges supported on their palmar aspect. The second maneuver detects the presence of a *mallet finger.* With the use of gentle resistance to extension, division will be revealed by some lag in extension when compared with adjacent fingers and by pain over the site of division.

Traumatic dislocation of a digital extensor, usually the long extensor, results from a tear of the radial transverse fibers of the extensor hood over the MP joint, which permits ulnar dislocation of the long extensor tendon. The occurrence is acute and associated with pain and a snapping sensation. The result is chronic dislocation with pain but normal extension.

The extensor tendons are divided into five zones.

Zone I and II Injuries

Laceration or avulsion of the terminal extensor tendon results in a mallet finger deformity. The cause is often a blow to the extended distal phalanx that pushes it into forced flexion. On examination, the patient cannot actively extend the distal joint, but passive extension is possible. Later, hyperextension of the PIP joint may result in a swan-neck or recurvatum deformity. Whether from open or closed injury, it can often be managed nonoperatively.

When nonoperative treatment is preferred, a splint should be taped in place with the joint in extension and used continually for 6 weeks or longer if an extensor lag persists. Splints are not successful in noncompliant patients or in patients who must repeatedly get their hands wet, such as health professionals. In these patients, an internal K-wire splint with the wire cut off beneath the skin is preferable. This should also be protected by external splintage whenever possible.

Fresh lacerations of the extensor mechanism of the distal joint after irrigation and debridement can be repaired by simple figure-of-8 reapproximation of the tendon or with through-and-through sutures approximating the tendon and the skin simultaneously. When forced flexion of the extended distal phalanx results in a distal phalanx fracture involving one third or more of its articular surface, treatment requires open reduction and internal fixation of the fracture.

Zone III and IV Injuries

Zones III and IV include the area of the middle phalanx, the central slip of the long extensor tendon, and the lateral bands. These injuries commonly result from direct trauma, deep burns affecting the extensor mechanism, or fracture-dislocation at the PIP joint. Loss of the extensor mechanism over the middle joint results in unopposed action of the flexor digitorum superficialis characterized by flexion at the PIP joint. As contracture occurs, the characteristic boutonniere position results, with the middle joint in flexion, the terminal joint in hyperextension, and the MP joint in slight hyperextension. In closed injuries the characteristic boutonniere deformity may not be present at the time of injury and may develop 1 to 2 weeks after injury.

Injuries resulting from disruption of the central slip of the extensor expansion require splinting of the PIP joint to maintain full extension for 6 weeks while leaving the DIP joint completely free for active flexion exercises.

Indications for operative treatment of disruption of the central slip are a long delay between injury and initial presentation, avulsion of a bone fragment from the base of the middle phalanx, dislocation of the PIP joints, or complicating factors including soft-tissue loss or a phalangeal fracture. Where tissue has been lost, the central slip may be reconstructed with a free graft or transposition of one or both lateral bands, with soft-tissue closure effected by local rotation or cross-finger flaps. When the joint is so severely injured that recovery of reasonable function is unlikely, arthrodesis may be the only feasible method available for reconstruction.

Zone V Injuries

Zone V injuries are usually easily repaired because the intertendinous connections prevent proximal retraction. The laceration generally involves three layers—the capsule, tendon, and joint capsule—but may be repaired as a single layer with horizontal mattress sutures. After repair, the wrist should be immobilized at 45 degrees of dorsiflexion, with the MP joint at 45 degrees of flexion to minimize contractures. A removable palmar extension splint may be desired to hold the IP joints at 0 degrees between exercise periods.

Injuries to Proximal Zones

Extensor tendon injuries proximal to the fingers can be troublesome. First, clinical recognition may be difficult because of intertendinous connections. Careful exploration of the wound is necessary. Second, if the laceration is proximal to the junctura, retraction of the tendon may occur and require separate incisions to locate the tendon end. Third, the extensor retinaculum may present problems similar to those encountered with the flexor tendons and lead to limitations of excursion by adhesion. Primary suturing is the best procedure at these levels. With tissue loss, tendon grafts may be necessary, or transfer of the index or little finger extensors may be used.

Postoperative Management of Extensor Tendon Injuries

Positioning of the digits and wrist after extensor tendon repair is determined by the level of injury along the course of the tendon. Repairs at the level of the DIP joint are splinted in neutral or mild hyperextension while the PIP joint is allowed to flex without restriction. Injuries at the level of the PIP joint are maintained with the PIP joint in full extension while allowing for flexion of the DIP joint. For injuries to the extensor tendons at the level of the MP joint and proximal to that level, the wrist is immobilized in approximately 45 degrees of extension, the MP joint in 45 degrees of flexion, and the PIP joints flexed to only 10 degrees.

INJURIES TO THE NERVES OF THE UPPER EXTREMITY

The anatomy of the nervous system of the extremity is described in Chapter 20, but a review of the physical examination following specific injury is presented here.

Sensory Loss

Sweating is lost in the distribution of a divided peripheral nerve. An initial determination that a nerve injury is present or not can be made simply by lightly stroking a digit on the uninjured hand with the barrel of a plastic pen and then a digit in the dermatome in question on the injured side. Frequently a distinct difference will be detected, the digit in the denervated region being smooth and dry by comparison with the slightly adherent and moist finger in the uninjured side. While doing this, the examiner can ask an alert patient whether the touch is perceived and whether it differs between the two sites. When doubt still exists, a simple alternative remains. Each side of each digital pulp and the dorsum of the metacarpal region of the thumb should be tested for *moving two-point discrimination* by using a paper clip or a caliper. The nerves divided can then be deduced by knowing the site of the wound and the sensory distribution of the extremity nerves.

Motor Examination

Testing of muscle action evaluates the integrity of the muscles, their tendons, and their innervation. The examiner should carefully distinguish the cause of abnormal findings.

Key to motor examination is knowledge of anatomy and muscle actions. Palpation of muscle activity is more important than mere observation. Muscle evaluation is done against resistance and designed to isolate the muscle action.

Testing should proceed in an organized fashion from a proximal-to-distal direction. Motor examination of the extremities has been described above under tendon injury. All extensors are innervated by the radial nerve and flexors by the median nerve (apart from the flexor carpi ulnaris and flexor digitorum profundus to the ring and small fingers, which are supplied by the ulnar nerve).

Intrinsics

The median innervated thenar intrinsics are tested by thumb-to-little finger opposition. The thenar musculature is palpated during this action.

The hypothenar intrinsics are innervated by the ulnar nerve and are tested by abduction of the fifth finger against resistance.

Interosseus function is tested by placing the palm on a flat surface with the fingers abducted. With intact function, each finger should be able to deviate from side to side when extended off the surface. The first dorsal interosseous is tested by palpation during abduction of the index finger.

Types of Nerve Injury

Nerve injuries have been classified by both Sunderland and Seddon (see Table 23–1).

Injuries in Continuity

When characteristic sensory and motor loss have been identified but despite exhaustive exploration the nerve in question is found to be intact, axonotmesis or neurapraxia is present. In order to facilitate possible secondary neurolysis the exact site and extent of any bruising or swelling of the nerve should be recorded at exploration. If such swelling is significant, primary epineurotomy may reduce nerve damage and speed recovery.

Traction Injury

A long section of the nerve may be damaged in traction injuries; it is swollen throughout to a varying degree and may be visible through the epineurium. If this is creating tension evidenced by induration of the nerve on palpation, then it should be released by incising the epineurium.

Compression

Prolonged compression sufficient to produce lasting nerve disturbance is an unusual primary injury but occurs in acute carpal tunnel syndrome and is usually associated with significant wrist fractures or dislocations.

Nerve Repair

Nerve repair is accomplished by primary suturing or by interpositional grafting. Neurorrhaphy is preferred over grafting when there is a clean laceration with easily identifiable fascicles and if the repair is possible in the total absence of tension. Nerve grafting results are actually better than nerve suturing done under tension. Grafting should be done for nerve gaps of greater than 2.0 cm or in cases where the nerve must be dissected

TABLE 23–1.
Classifications of Nerve Injuries

Sunderland	Seddon	Injury	Recovery Potential
I	Neurapraxia	Ionic block; possible segmental injury	Full
II	Axonotmesis	Axon severed; endoneurial tube intact	Full
III	Neurotmesis	Endoneurial tube torn	Slow, incomplete
IV	Neurotmesis	Only epineurium intact	Neuroma in continuity
V	Neurotmesis	Loss of continuity	None
VI	Neurotmesis	Combination of the above	

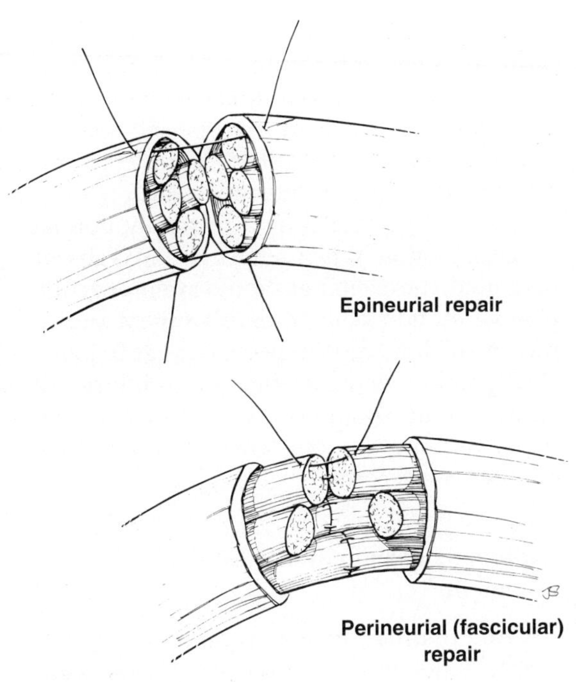

FIG 23–5.
Representations of fascicular and epineural repairs.

proximally or distally more than 6 cm in order to release tension.

Suturing of nerves may be done either as an epineural repair or as a fascicular (perineural) repair. The latter repair attempts to match identifiable bundles of nerve fascicles proximally and distally and repair each bundle separately with one of two sutures (Fig 23–5). The fascicular repair has the theoretical advantage of better fascicular alignment with more axons entering appropriate distal endoneural tissues. It is possible, although difficult, to histochemically identify motor and sensory nerve endings and suture these fascicles appropriately with fascicular techniques. Disadvantages include more internal scarring and foreign-body reaction and the requirement of microsurgical skills by the surgeon.

The epineural repair, suturing the connective tissue of the epineurium, is the more common repair done in clinical practice. Its advantages include relative ease of repair, minimal magnification requirements, and less internal scarring of the nerve.

To date, there have been no controlled randomized studies comparing epineural vs. fascicular repair. Moreover, other experimental and clinical studies do not prove the superiority of fascicular repairs over the simpler epineural repair. Some authors suggest the use of epineural repairs in most clinical situations, especially in more proximal extremity lesions. Here the nerves are generally monofascicular and lend themselves easily to the technique. Clean, sharp lacerations of more distal nerves leaving easily identifiable bundles can best be managed by rotating the nerves to obtain bundle apposition and epineural repair. Other more distal polyfascicular nerve lacerations or nerve grafts are perhaps better served by the use of microsurgical fascicular repairs.

For nerve grafting, common donor nerves include the sural nerve (most used), the anterior branch of the medial antebrachial cutaneous nerve, and the lateral antebrachial cutaneous nerve. The latter two nerves are located in the forearm adjacent to the basilic and the cephalic veins, respectively.

Microsurgical transfer of "vascularized" nerve grafts has been suggested for use in heavily scarred beds. The saphenous neurovascular bundle is more commonly used, or the sural nerve. Clinical results, however, do not conclusively show better results than standard nerve grafting.

Allografts currently in experimental and clinical study include Silastic tubes, polyglycolic acid (Dexon) tubes, and the use of cadaver nerve grafts protected with a short course of cyclosporine. The use of autogenous vein has also been described. No evidence has yet been shown to justify the widespread use of any of these techniques.

Timing of nerve repairs may significantly improve clinical results. Primary suturing of open nerve injuries is indicated at initial presentation if the wound is clean and tidy and repair can be done without tension. Nerve ends should have been sharply transected with identifiable fascicles. If the nerve has been injured over a long segment or in the case of actual loss of nerve tissue, it is better to repair the nerve at a later date. Nerve grafting done in the initial procedure is rarely indicated. It is better to wait several weeks for the actual nerve loss/degeneration to become apparent. Clean wounds expected to heal without significant scarring are best reexplored with nerve repair at 6 to 8 weeks after the edema is gone. Untidy or extensive wounds (such as from a chain saw) are best reexplored earlier, 3 to 4 weeks before massive scarring has occurred. This 3-week interval will allow the extent of nerve injury to become apparent.

BONE AND JOINT INJURY

The skeleton is injured by force, either direct or indirect. *Direct* blunt force to metacarpal and phalangeal bones produces transverse or comminuted fractures. However, the majority of the injuries sustained by the skeleton of the hand result from *indirect* force transmitted (1) *axially,* often causing articular fractures; (2) by *leverage,* producing a ligament injury, a condylar fracture, or an oblique diaphyseal fracture; or (3) by *torsion,* resulting in a ligament injury or a spiral diaphyseal fracture.

Major open injuries result from great force, which commonly also produces significant indirect but closed injuries more proximally in the limb. The patient, because of considerable pain from the open injury, rarely complains about the proximal injury. Radiologic assessment in such cases should include the humerus, the shoulder girdle, and the cervical spine. Occasionally minimal trauma causes a fracture, and radiologic evaluation may reveal an unsuspected disease or tumor (pathologic fracture).

Examination—General Comments

Certain symptoms and signs are common to all fractures and dislocations—*swelling, deformity, loss of motion,* and the presence of *abnormal motion* and *tenderness.* Significant swelling around a bone or joint should arouse suspicion of underlying skeletal injury. Any *bruising* beneath the skin, in the absence of any other cause, is pathognomonic of a fracture or ligament tear. Absence of skeletal injury is most expeditiously checked by asking the patient to put each joint through a normal range of motion. Apart from direct injury to the joint or the bones that form the joint, limitation or a lack of active motion may result from nerve or tendon injury or lack of patient cooperation. When *pain* limits active motion, note should be made of that specific point in the joint range. The *stability* of fractures already suspected or later revealed on x-ray studies will be shown by a relatively normal range of motion. When active motion is absent or limited, the examiner should attempt gentle passive motion both to detect injury and to record any limitation of normal range in joints clearly not involved in the current injury. All neutral joint positions, i.e., when the two bones forming the joint are in line with one another, are recorded as 0 degrees.

Radiologic Examination—General Comments

All injured hands should be radiographed, not only for medicolegal reasons but also because previous injury should be recorded and because the most confident clinical exclusion of fractures can be wrong. Even a small flake of bone at a point known to have a ligament or tendon attached is important; in such instances an unstable joint or tendon imbalance may result. The mallet finger and posttraumatic boutonniere deformity may both result from such situations.

If intra-articular fragments are displaced even minimally, accurate reduction is imperative; otherwise early osteoarthritis is likely. Many intra-articular fractures have ligaments or tendons attached to one or more fragments. This makes any closed reduction inherently unstable and internal fixation necessary.

On posteroanterior views of any phalanx the articular surfaces at either end should parallel one another. Fractures confined entirely to cartilage occur but are not revealed by radiography. If the injury is closed, such patients are usually seen later with persistent swelling and pain.

Epiphyseal Fractures

Fractures that encroach on the epiphyseal plate have been classified by Salter and Harris into five categories (Fig 23–6):

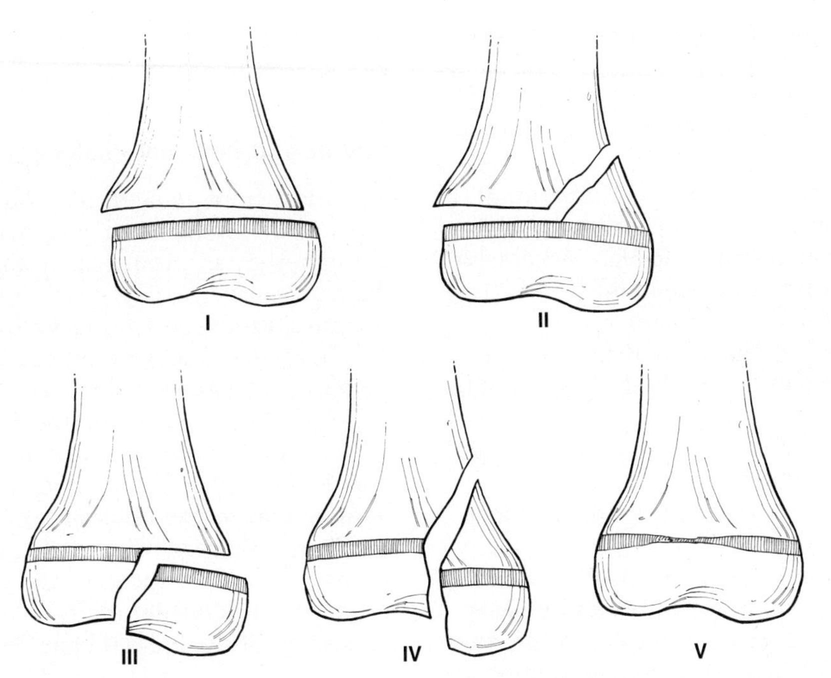

FIG 23–6.
Epiphyseal fractures as categorized by Salter-Harris.

- *Type I.*—Separation of the epiphysis from the metaphysis through the plate in a shearing manner.
- *Type II.*—Separation of the epiphysis, a small angle of the metaphysis being broken off with it.
- *Type III.*—An intraarticular fracture of part of the epiphysis without interference with the epiphyseal plate.
- *Type IV.*—A vertical, displaced fracture passing from the articular surface through epiphysis, plate, and metaphysis.
- *Type V.*—A compression fracture of the cartilaginous plate with no evident injury to the epiphysis or metaphysis.

Type I injuries of the distal phalanx commonly produce a mallet finger deformity in children, the extensor tendon being attached to the epiphysis and the flexor profundus to the metaphysis.

Types I and II remodel well, but reduction should be attempted. With accurate reduction, type III injuries carry a good prognosis because they do not interfere directly with the epiphyseal plate. However, type IV and V injuries may arrest the growth of all or part of the bone with consequent shortening or angulation because of epiphyseal plate injury. Overall, fractures are often underestimated. Remodeling only occurs in those fractures angulated in the line of pull of the extrinsic tendons (anteroposterior) and is best at the metaphysis. Lateral angulation and rotational malalignment require accurate reduction.

Management of Fractures—General Comments

Ideal fracture management should adhere to the aims proposed by the Arbeitsgemeinschaft für Osteosynthesfragen (AO) group:

1. Accurate anatomic reduction
2. Rigid internal fixation
3. Early, active motion of adjacent joints

In the fingers, the most significant of these is early institution of joint motion. With this in mind, fracture management should answer the following sequential questions: If the fracture cannot be reduced or made stable without surgery, what will be necessary to make it so? Is that surgery justifiable? Is the fracture reduced? If displaced, is the displacement acceptable? If not, can it be reduced in a closed manner? If it is reduced, can be reduced, or is acceptable, is it then stable? If it is not stable, can it be made so in a closed fashion?

"Acceptable" fractures are important to recognize since they require no treatment provided that they are stable. "Acceptable" fractures include the following:

- *Tuft* of the distal phalanx
- *Chips* only if minimally displaced, for they are usually attached to ligament or tendon
- *Anteroposterior angulation* of metaphyseal fractures in *children*
- *Nonarticular comminution* with minimal angulation
- *Metacarpal neck* fractures with 15 degrees of angulation in the index and middle fingers and 20 to 70 degrees in the ring and small fingers (the variation depends on the author)
- *Nonarticular metacarpal base* with 20 degrees of angulation in adults and 40 degrees in children

PHALANGEAL INJURIES

Distal Phalanx

The most common fractures of the distal phalanx are as follows:

1. *Comminuted.*—Resulting from a direct crushing force, these are almost invariably associated with injuries of the nail bed and are often confined to the *"tuft,"* or distal margin of the phalanx.

2. *Intraarticular.*—These are mainly avulsive injuries and include mallet fractures resulting from traction by the extensor tendon, fractures of profundus avulsion, and condylar fractures in which the fragment remains attached to the collateral ligament (less common here than in the PIP joint).

3. *Transverse.*—Transverse fractures are through the waist of the distal phalanx and invariably adopt an apicodorsal configuration. The entire nail bed rides with the distal fragment, and the proximal edge of the germinal matrix often dislocates onto the superficial surface of the eponychial fold—it must be replaced to achieve fracture reduction.

Middle and Proximal Phalanges

Aside from *intraarticular* fractures, fractures of the middle and proximal phalanges are either *spiral,* produced by torsion of the digit, or transverse diaphyseal or comminuted fractures, produced by direct blows.

Transverse fractures of the middle and proximal phalanges adopt an apicopalmar angulation as a result of the forces of the superficialis and intraosseous insertions. This angulation will not only threaten the flexor tendon, which may be impaled, but will also result in a "zigzag" deformity whereby the change in pull on the extrinsic tendons will produce a flexion deformity of the joints at either end of the broken bone.

Interphalangeal Joints (and the Metacarpophalangeal Joint of the Thumb)

The most commonly injured joints in the hand are the ginglymus, or hinge, joints, probably because they are constrained to only one plane of movement. These include all the IP joints and the MP joint of the thumb. The latter is considered here rather than with the other MP joints because it differs markedly in anatomy and mechanisms of injury. Ginglymus joints have a similar structure. The true and *accessory* collateral ligaments together form a fan of fibers that radiate out from a recess on the lateral aspect of the head of the proximal bone. The true collateral ligament inserts into the base of the distal bone, whereas the accessory ligament inserts into the lateral aspect of the palmar plate. In children the ligament attaches to both the epiphysis and the metaphysis in the phalanges. The fibers are tight in all positions of the joint, with no freedom for lateral motion. The palmar plate has two distinct portions. The fibrous part attaches to the palmar aspect of the base of the distal bone and by proximal lateral extensions to the margins of the anterior surface of the proximal bone.

These extensions—the checkrein ligaments—when viewed anteriorly give the appearance of a swallowtail. The fibrous palmar plate serves both to restrict hyperextension of the joint and as an extension of the articular surface of the base of the distal bone. It is through the fibrous part that tears of the palmar plate occur. Such tears extend to a varying degree into the collateral ligament and split the fibers of the true and accessory elements. The membranous part of the palmar plate lies between the checkrein ligaments and serves to transmit blood vessels to the vincular system of the flexor tendons. The extensor tendon closes the circle of attachments to the base of the distal bone. The head of the proximal bone is enveloped by these structures, through which it tears in dislocation.

True lateral dislocations of the hinge joints of necessity tear the true collateral ligament. Hyperextension injuries and dorsal dislocations tear the palmar plate but need not tear all of either of the collateral ligament even when completely dislocated dorsally. Such hyperextension injuries commonly occur in sports when the tip of the finger is struck by the ball. The axial load tears the palmar plate or avulses its bony attachment. If this injury is at the PIP joint, as is most frequent, the middle phalanx is often subluxed by the pull of the extensor. This injury is often disregarded at the urging of athletic staff and has been referred to as "*coach's finger.*" With use the joint rapidly deteriorates. Oblique dislocations cause tears *between* the fibers of the collateral ligament and through the palmar plate, but often only partially.

Anterior dislocations tear the palmar *and* one or both collateral ligaments. In the ginglymus joints of the hand, the ligaments and tendons tear most frequently from their distal attachment, often with an accompanying bone fragment. The larger the bone fragment, the more likely the phalanx from which it is torn will sublux from its proper articulation with the head of the proximal bone.

The palmar plates are tested by hyperextension. All collateral ligaments should be stressed by lateral angulation of the joint. Angulation of more than 20 degrees indicates a complete tear. Those especially prone to injury are the collateral ligaments of the PIP joints and the ulnar collateral ligament of the MP joint of the thumb, injured in forced abduction (gamekeeper's thumb). *Gamekeeper's thumb* (or ski pole thumb) is a tear of the ulnar collateral ligament of the MP joint of the thumb. The injury most commonly results from falling on an outstretched hand. The injury involves avulsion of the collateral ligament from the base of the proximal phalanx, with or without a fragment of bone, together with tearing of the palmar plate and accessory collateral ligament. The torn ligament in the thumb may lie superficial to the adductor expansion, which normally overlies it, and eliminate any chance of healing and result in the Stener lesion.

Management of Closed Phalangeal Injuries

Certain closed fractures can only be reduced and stabilized by surgery. In others, however, nonoperative management consisting of initial *rest and elevation* for 5 days followed by *early active motion* allied with the use of a *splint for rest and protection* may effect an equally good result.

Angulated, rotated, or shortened nonarticular phalangeal fractures, whether spiral, oblique, or transverse, should be reduced and fixed. The single exception may be modest anteroposterior angulation in the child—one in which the child can obtain full IP extension. This will remodel.

Closed reduction with percutaneous fixation can often be achieved, especially with spiral fractures. The transverse, sometimes comminuted fracture of the diaphysis of the proximal phalanx is often associated with severe soft-tissue trauma. If the circulation is intact, there is merit in avoiding further injury from incision and dissection for open reduction. Closed reduction can be obtained by firmly flexing the MP joint by pressure on the head of the proximal phalanx and placing a pin through the metacarpal head and the MP joint and down the medulla of the phalanx.

Many nonarticular fractures require *open reduction and internal fixation.* Various fixation techniques are available: *screw fixation* of spiral fractures, *type A intraosseous wiring, intramedullary Steinmann pin fixation,* and microplate and screw fixation (Fig 23–7).

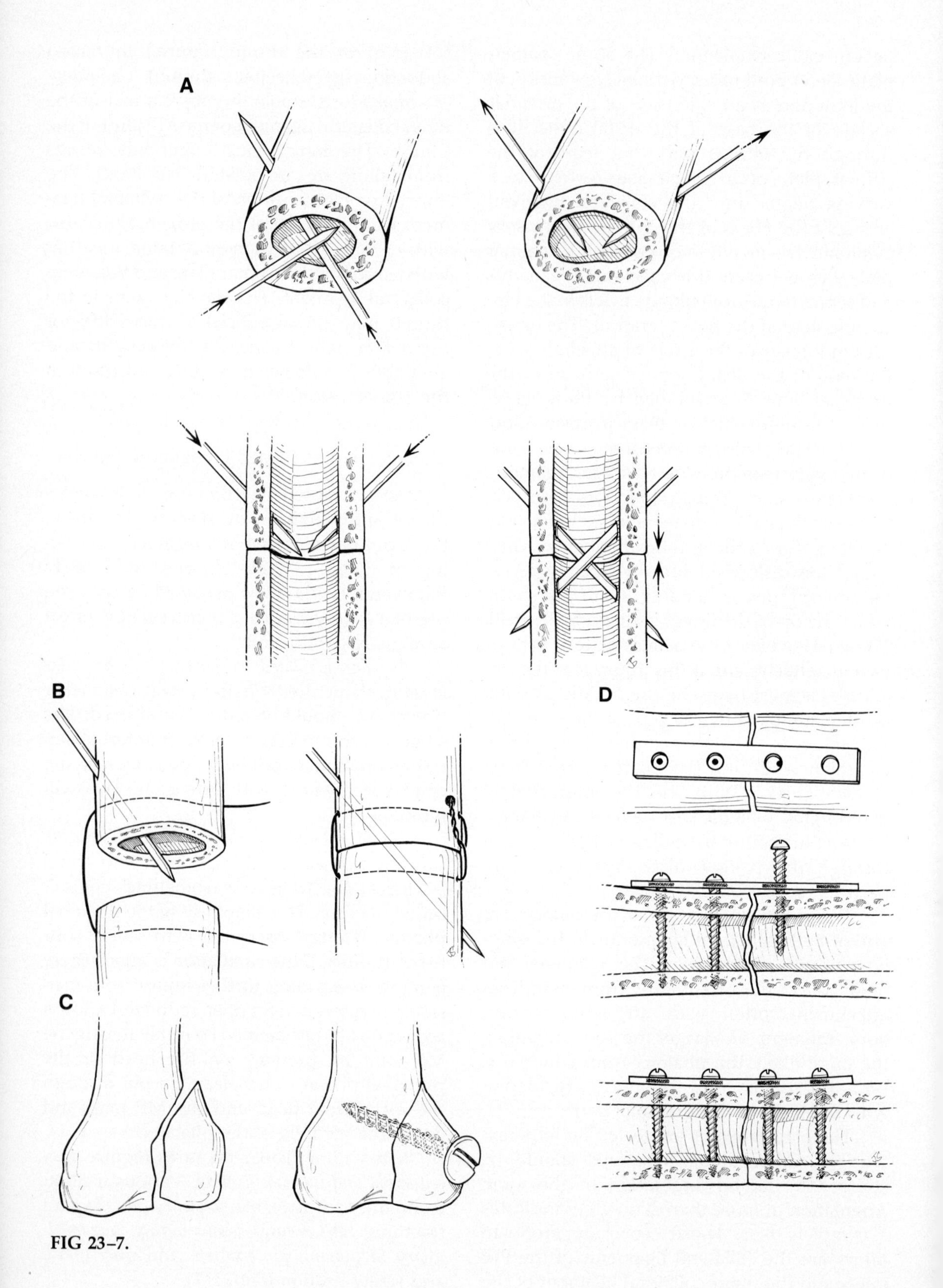

FIG 23–7.

Intra-articular fractures should be reduced and fixed with absolute precision. While this may be achieved in closed fashion, the authors prefer direct visualization of the articular surface, with fixation by a *screw,* two *Kirschner wires,* or *type B intraosseous wiring.*

Ligamentous tears following dislocation may be managed by *protective splinting* or *open repair. Extension block* splinting will protect the palmar plate. *Buddy* splinting will protect the collateral ligament of the PIP joint in cooperative patients but should not be applied until 5 days after injury to permit swelling to resolve, during which time the hand and wrist should be supported in a volar splint. Open repair is indicated in either situation when patient compliance is in doubt.

Although methods have been reported to confirm the presence of a Stener lesion in *ulnar collateral ligament* injuries of the MP joint of the thumb, they have not gained widespread acceptance. The authors open all ligament injuries with a suggestive history and bruising over the appropriate region.

METACARPOPHALANGEAL JOINT INJURIES (OF THE FINGERS)

The MP joint of the fingers is classified as ellipsoid. The head of the metacarpal is narrower on its dorsal than its palmar surface.

As a result of two facts—the wider palmar aspect of the head and the differing tension in the true collateral ligament, which has an eccentric proximal attachment—the collateral ligament is tight and unyielding when the MP joint is flexed. When the joint is extended, it is loose, and the proximal phalanges have considerable lateral play into abduction and adduction. In injury, edema fluid in the joint and the periarticular soft tissues tends to force the MP joint into extension. If left in that position, the collateral ligament shortens to produce an extension contracture. The palmar plate is similar in construction to that of the PIP joint. It is connected to adjacent plates by the deep transverse metacarpal ligament. Sesamoid bones are always present in the palmar plate of the thumb (where their fracture may be an obscure source of pain) and are often in the index and less commonly in the other fingers.

The laxity of the collateral ligament of the MP joint (as compared with the PIP joint) allows the ligament to avoid frequent injury. The collateral ligaments of the MP joints of the fingers can only be tested for integrity or injury by lateral stress on the proximal phalanx with the MP joint in maximum *flexion.*

A recognized *dislocation* of the MP joint of the fingers is relatively uncommon and takes two distinct forms:

- *Simple.*—A posterior dislocation that can be readily and effectively reduced in closed fashion.
- *Complex.*—A posterior dislocation in which the metacarpal head becomes trapped between the palmar fascia on its palmar aspect and the displaced and ruptured palmar plate on its dorsal aspect and between the flexor tendons on its ulnar side and the lumbrical muscle on its radial side.

The posture of the dislocated finger is distinct for each of these dislocations. In simple dislocations the proximal phalanx tends to lie in almost 90 degrees of hyperextension, while in complex dislocations, the angle of hyperextension is appreciably less. In complex dislocations, the displaced metacarpal head forms a marked prominence in the palm, which also shows deep puckering of the proximal palmar crease because of traction on the skin attachments of the palmar fascia.

Simple dislocations can be readily reduced, usually in the emergency room and often without anesthesia. The hand should then be placed in an anterior *rest and protection* splint, with the commencement of early motion sessions protected by a buddy splint between the injured and an adjacent finger. Reduction of complex dislocations, by contrast, requires anesthesia.

The finger may then be reduced in closed manner by wrist flexion and traction on the digit, but often the joint must be opened dorsally, which permits easy reduction of the palmar plate. Ligament tears are treated by protected mobilization after an initial brief period of rest. Chip fractures attached to the ligament can be ignored.

METACARPAL AND CARPOMETACARPAL INJURIES

Metacarpal head fractures are primarily intraarticular and include (1) human bite injuries and chondral fractures; (2) ligament avulsions; (3) epiphyseal injuries, which may go unrecognized and result in brachymetacarpia; (4) single fractures in any plane; and (5) comminution (most frequently).

Neck fractures are common and result from the fist striking a relatively immovable object—*boxer's fracture.* The anterior cortex proximal to the articular surface is comminuted, with resultant apicodorsal angulation that is recognized clinically by the loss of the prominence of the metacarpal head dorsally and its appearance in the palm of the hand. *Shaft* fractures may be transverse, comminuted, or frequently, spiral, for the diaphysis of the metacarpal is the frequent target of torsional forces on the finger. Deformities of *angulation, shortening,* and *rotation* are common.

Fractures of the *base* are intra-articular and are an integral part of a complex that includes *dislocations* and *fracture-dislocations* of the carpometacarpal joints most frequently found in but not limited to the thumb:

1. *Bennett's fracture* of the first metacarpal is the most common; as a result of traction of the abductor pollicis longus, which attaches to the base, the main portion of the metacarpal subluxes, with the anterior beak of the base (which is attached to the ulnar or palmar collateral ligament) left in its correct anatomic position.
2. A similar fracture-dislocation of the *fifth metacarpal* is sometimes called a *reversed Bennett's* fracture because the displacement is similar and has similar cause (the extensor carpi ulnaris subluxing the main portion of the fifth metacarpal as well as the abductor pollicis longus subluxing the first).
3. The *Rolando fracture* resembles a Bennett's fracture but differs from it only in the addition of a fracture of the dorsal portion of the base to which the abductor pollicis longus attaches, thus creating a so-called T-condylar fracture.
4. *Carpometacarpal dislocations* have been reported on all the rays in varying patterns, usually with the base dorsal.

Management of Metacarpal and Carpometacarpal Injuries

Since fractures of the *metacarpal head* are intra-articular, they demand precise open reduction and internal fixation with the institution of an early motion program.

In fractures of the *metacarpal neck,* since the second and the third metacarpals have virtually no motion at their carpometacarpal joint, no angulation can be accepted; otherwise the anterior displacement of the metacarpal head may produce a painful grasp. By contrast, since there is motion in the basal joint of the fourth and fifth metacarpals, some angulation can be accepted. In the common *boxer's fracture* of the fifth metacarpal neck, 40 degrees of angulation is widely recommended as acceptable, and some advocate as much as 70 degrees. However, hand function should dictate management. If the patient can fully flex and fully extend his small finger *without any tendency to claw,* then the angulation should be corrected in closed fashion as best as possible and the finger immobilized in a splint. If motion is abnormal, open reduction and fixation will be necessary.

Shaft fractures can be treated by closed means, simply with a protecting splint, provided that (1) there is *no rotation,* for as little as 5 degrees of rotation produces 1.5-cm overlap in the fingertips on flexion, and (2) the shortening and angulation are deemed acceptable (what is acceptable varies widely between authors). However, mobilization early enough to maintain full MP joint function is likely to lead to delayed union or nonunion. The authors' preference is for open reduction and internal fixation, followed by early protected motion. *Screw* fixation for spiral fractures and *plate and screw* fixation for transverse fractures are preferred. If comminution exists, the fracture should be treated by closed means, but if open management is necessary, *external fixation* or an *intramedullary Steinmann pin* with a *tension band wire* is the primary alternative.

Carpometacarpal fractures and dislocations

should be reduced. In many instances reduction is done in closed fashion, but this often proves unstable, in which case percutaneous Kirschner wires are used to fix the reduced metacarpal to the carpus. This is a method commonly used in the management of Bennett's fracture.

CARPAL INJURIES

Mechanisms of Injury

Direct blows to carpal bones, especially their prominences, may result in isolated fractures such as those of the trapezoid ridge, the hamulus, or the pisiform. These do not interfere with the dynamics of the carpus.

The vast majority of injuries to the carpus occur when the patient falls on an outstretched hand. With impact the carpus extends, deviates ulnarly, and supinates relative to the forearm. Because the radial end of the carpus is relatively less mobile than the ulnar, it is more prone to injury in heavy falls. The force inflicted in such falls, which is dissipated at the ulnar end in many instances by midcarpal hyperextension, meets resistance in the radial column, which is levered at the waist of the scaphoid around the fulcrum of the dorsal lip of the radius. Three structures may be involved: (1) the distal end of the radius as in a Colles' fracture, (2) the ligamentous tethers of the proximal pole of the scaphoid; and (3) the scaphoid itself.

Pure ligamentous injuries pass around the lunate from a radial to distal to ulnar direction and produce four stages of instability according to their extent (Fig 23–8):

I. *Scapholunate instability*
II. *Dorsal subluxation of the capitate*
III. *Fractures of the triquetrum*
IV. *Lunate dislocation* (the lunate so displaced may produce acute carpal tunnel syndrome)

Injuries that follow this perilunar pattern are said to occur in the *"lesser arc"* of the vulnerable zone for carpal fractures and dislocations. The *"greater arc"* passes through the waist of the scaphoid and the bodies of the capitate,

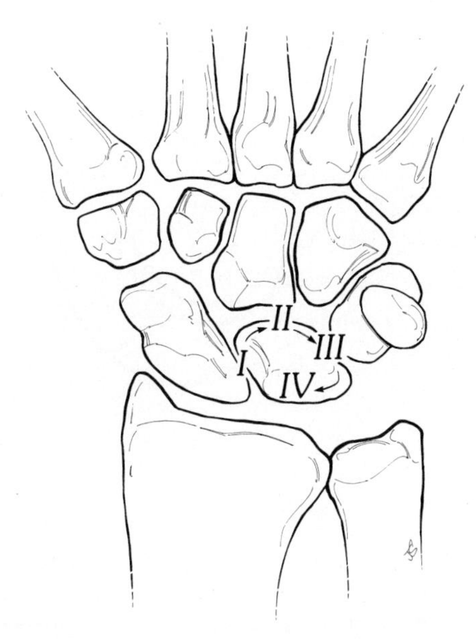

FIG 23–8.
Progressive perilunar instability. (See the text for a description.) (Adapted from Mayfield JK: *Clin Orthop* 1980; 149:50. Used by permission.)

hamate, and triquetrum in turn. Extensions of the arc may occur and cause fractures of the radial and ulnar styloids. Combinations of lesser and greater arc injuries produce the apparently diverse and confusing variety of carpal fracture-dislocations, which are simply combinations and extensions of the two arcs: transscaphoid perilunate fracture-dislocation, scaphocapitate syndrome, and others.

Radiologic Examination

In *posteroanterior* views of the wrist, apart from examining each carpal bone in turn for evidence of a fracture, four features, three of which are likely to reveal ligamentous disruption, should be studied:

1. The *carpal arcs* (these are not to be confused with the arcs of injury mentioned above) (Fig 23–9): arc 1 is the proximal convex outline of the scaphoid, lunate, and triquetrum; arc 2 is the distal curve of the same bones; and arc 3 is the convex surfaces of the capitate and hamate. A break in any arc indicates disruption of ligamentous integrity.

2. The *width of the intercarpal joint spaces*—all should be equal.

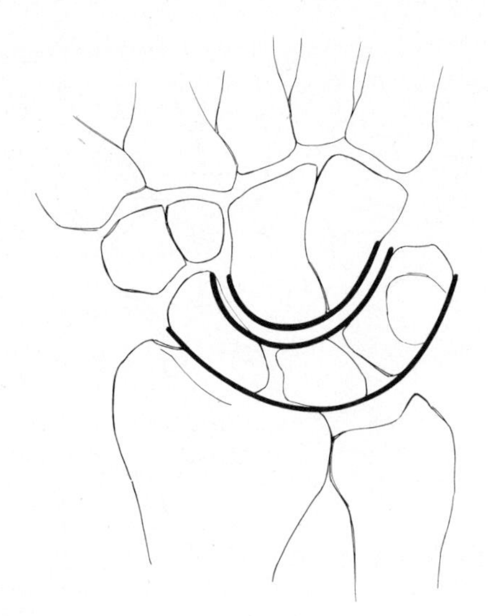

FIG 23–9.
Gilula's carpal arcs denoting normal radiographic carpal relationships. (See the text.)

3. The *shape* of the various *carpal bones.*
4. *Ulnar variance,* which is the relationship of the distal outline of the ulnar head to that of the articular surface of the radius. The variance is *negative* if the ulnar head fails to reach that line, *positive* if it projects beyond it, and *neutral* if it lies in the exact line.

The *lateral* view should be taken with the radius in the same line as the third metacarpal and radial or ulnar deviation avoided. Again, as in the anteroposterior view, four features should be observed:

1. The *angle of the distal radius.* The normal palmar tilt of 10 to 15 degrees may be reversed, usually after a Colles' fracture.
2. The *colinearity* of the radius, lunate, and capitate.
3. The *angle of the lunate* relative to the axis of the radius. Its axis may point dorsally, in which case it is dorsiflexed, and vice versa.
4. The *scapholunate angle* should be measured. The angle measured is that created by the *two axes extended distally.* The normal angle averages 47 degrees, with a normal range of 30 to 60 degrees.

Special additional views may be required to investigate incongruencies established clinically or by study of the standard radiographs.

Management of Closed Carpal Injuries

As a general rule, fractures or dislocations of the carpus that are *undisplaced and stable* are treated by immobilization in an anterior splint until swelling has subsided, at which time a cast is substituted. Qualifying comments to this generality are appropriate for certain fractures.

Scaphoid fractures, as is evident from the above discussion of mechanisms of injury, can occur in two quite distinct ways:

1. An *isolated* scaphoid fracture that results from a pure extension vector will commonly be undisplaced and stable. While controversy exists on every aspect of immobilization, suffice it to say that a long-arm thumb spica circular cast with the wrist in radial deviation, slight palmar flexion, and pronation for 6 weeks, followed by a similar short-arm cast for a further 6 weeks, offers a high chance of union.
2. An apparently isolated, undisplaced fracture may be the only evidence of a *reduced transactinide perilunate fracture-dislocation.* This circumstance can be recognized by the presence of an offset of more than 1 mm between the fragments or by evidence of proximal row instability as seen by changes in the alignment of the lunate on the true lateral view. Such fractures should be opened, reduced, and internally fixed with Kirschner wires or with screws, including that designed by Herbert.

Fractures of the hook of the hamate should be excised despite isolated recommendations to fix the fracture. Fractures or dislocations of the carpus that are *displaced* should be reduced. Reduction can be attempted by closed means but should be done in sterile conditions with finger trap traction and fluoroscopic control. Repeat radiographs should be taken with *release of traction after* successful reduction, for frequently such views will demonstrate that the reduction has been lost or that a collapse pattern has ensued. In such circumstances, the surgeon should proceed with open reduction, internal fixation, and ligamentous repair.

VASCULAR INJURY/AVULSIONS/ AMPUTATIONS

Viability

In clean lacerations viability is less likely in doubt than in injuries resulting from crushing or avulsion. Depending upon the quality and integrity of the collateral circulation, division of the brachial artery or the radial and ulnar arteries may or may not result in insufficient perfusion of the distal portion of the limb. When either the radial or the ulnar artery but not both have been divided at the wrist, the viability of the hand is usually not compromised. The lack of frank vascular inadequacy should not imply that the vessels should not be repaired, for otherwise late problems with hand function may arise.

The nonviable digit is characteristically very white with areas of pale violet. The pulp is collapsed and the temperature of the digit palpably lower than adjacent ones. With fingertip pressure, there is no blanching or refill. Rotating the digit that is hanging loosely will not aid in determining whether or not vascular torsion or frank division is the cause of the pallor. Only exploration and fracture fixation can do so. If both arteries to a finger are cut or occluded, vascular repair is necessary for survival of the digit.

In untidy injuries the paramount and often the most difficult question is "what is viable?" No final decision regarding viability should be made until fractures are reduced and immobilized. Torsion and compression of otherwise uninjured vessels may well arise through the instability of fractures, and apparently nonviable parts may be amputated needlessly if this is not appreciated.

Replantation

Replantation of totally severed parts and revascularization of incomplete amputations are routinely possible. In macroreplantation the amputated part contains significant muscle bulk; speed is important, and a high level of microsurgical skill is not necessary. In microreplantation the amputated parts are usually digits—speed is of secondary significance, and a high level of microsurgical skill is essential. Certain factors have come to be recognized as contraindications to replantation.

Strong Contraindications

1. Significant associated injuries of the torso and head, common in macroreplantation candidates
2. Extensive injury to the affected limb or to the amputated part, i.e., multiple-level degloving or widespread crushing
3. Severe chronic illness such as to preclude transportation or prolonged surgery

Relative Contraindications

These are often present in combination and therefore more discouraging.

1. Single-digit amputation, especially proximal to the insertion of the flexor digitorum superficialis
2. Avulsion injuries as evidenced by
   a. Mechanism
   b. Structures dangling from the part, usually nerves and tendons (this often indicates vessel avulsion from the part)
   c. "Red streak"—bruising over the neurovascular pedicle indicating vessel disruption
3. Previous injury or surgery to the part
4. Extreme contamination
5. Lengthy warm ischemia—in practice only applicable to macroreplantation
6. Age—increased chance of vessel disease and systemic illness

Salvage Replantation

Despite much of the above, replantation should be attempted in children or following amputation of the thumb or more than two fingers.

Replantation combines repair of all digital/extremity structures as previously out-

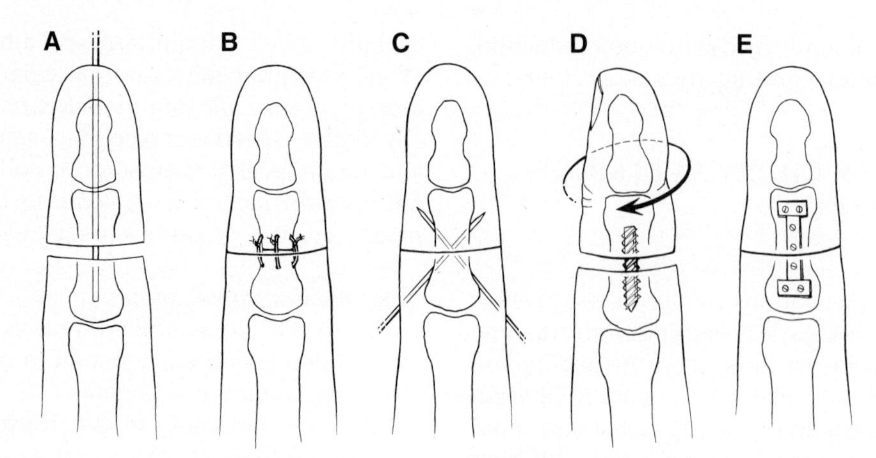

FIG 23–10.
Methods of bone fixation. **A,** one or two intramedullary K-wires. **B,** intraosseous wiring. **C,** a chevron-type fusion. **D,** a bone screw inserted into the amputation stump, the screw head cut off, and the digit literally *"screwed on."* **E,** miniplate and screws.

lined. A generally accepted order of repair is (1) bony fixation (Fig 23–10), (2) extensor tendon repair, (3) flexor tendon(s) repair, (4) digital nerve repair, (5) venous repair, and (6) arterial repair. The last three repairs almost always require use of the operating microscope. If one is judicious in choosing digits to replant, a 90% success rate can be accomplished.

Open Vascular Injuries

Complete arterial lacerations may be distinguished by a history of dramatic blood loss at the time of injury, sometimes described as pulsatile, that has ceased by the time of examination because of longitudinal and circumferential retraction of the arterial wall. The wound is filled with a thick, shiny, gelatinous, dark red clot that may continue oozing. Examination of peripheral pulses is of little value since retrograde flow may fill a lacerated vessel. If the suspected laceration is in the radial or ulnar artery, obliteration of the other may eliminate the pulse. In theory, the Allen's test could reveal an injury of either forearm vessel. In practice, this maneuver is often too painful and may also provoke renewed bleeding.

Partial lacerations of a major vessel may be associated with continued hemorrhage since the absence of normally hemostatic retraction serves to increase blood loss. Such lacerations are the *only cause of death in the upper extremity.* They may be characterized by no active bleeding, a large wound clot, and distal pulses present because of occlusion of the defect in the wall by the clot, thereby reestablishing the vascular conduit.

Lacerations in the correct site and of sufficient depth to have produced an arterial injury require prompt exploration.

Closed Injuries (Including Penetrating Wounds)

In open injuries, the surgeon need only speculate on what the necessary exploration will reveal.

By contrast, potential injury in relatively closed spaces presents a much greater diagnostic challenge, for the surgeon must decide whether or not exploration is necessary.

Arterial compromise may result from several mechanisms:

1. Gunshot wounds
2. Fractures of the humerus and clavicle
3. Dislocations of the elbow and shoulder producing either partial division (false aneurysm) or extensive intimal disruption (thrombosis)

The findings in the acute situation in the upper extremity may be remarkably few. This is especially so and particularly hazardous in injuries to the subclavian and axillary arteries, where a neglected false aneurysm may result in later brachial palsy with less than a 50% chance of recovery. In order of appearance, the following are signs of major arterial trauma in the arm:

1. Diminution or absence of distal pulses. In a swollen limb or in an ischemic digit the use of the Doppler flowmeter to check pulses is valuable.
2. Pallor, especially evident in the nail beds, which show very poor refill after blanching.
3. Pain, most evident on handling the limb.
4. Paresthesia, hypoesthesia.
5. Paralysis. When this degree of muscle ischemia is present, compartment syndromes are inevitable; correction of the vascular interruption may increase the problem by inducing postischemic edema—it should be accompanied by fasciotomy.

It should be reemphasized that many peripheral signs may be absent. Delay may be disastrous, so if suspicions are still present, further steps must be taken, either by arteriography or exploration.

Arteriography is not indicated in open injuries since exploration gives direct answers, thus saving time. The value of arteriography in closed injuries has been questioned for similar reasons. However, exploration simply because major vessels are possibly injured may be unnecessary, especially if other injuries or illnesses are present. Physical findings are unreliable since they gave false negative indications in 20% and false positive indications in 42% of 86 patients subsequently evaluated by angiography.

Arteriography is commonly employed in evaluating all patients who *may* have sustained an arterial injury from blunt trauma or a proximate penetrating injury, even if they have no peripheral evidence of arterial occlusion. Such studies may reveal intimal fractures, pseudoaneurysms, or mural stenoses that do not impede flow—a positive finding in an asymptomatic patient.

The simple *Doppler pencil probe* is valuable since it permits detection of flow in vessels that cannot readily be palpated because of pain, swelling, or their relatively small caliber. Closed injuries of digits may produce sufficient swelling to reduce arterial flow so that survival is in doubt. Such injuries may also eliminate blood flow by damage to the vessel over such an extent as to render doubtful one's ability to restore flow. Both circumstances have the same presentation. If the vessel can be followed into the digit with the Doppler probe, the problem can be deemed to be one of compression. If there is clear loss of the signal proximally in both digital vessels, then occlusion or disruption exists. When available, color duplex ultrasonography can give more detailed information regarding flow and vessel caliber.

Management of Closed Vascular Injuries

Closed injuries with vascular tree occlusions causing peripheral symptoms require *exploration.* At exploration, *embolectomy* or localized arterial resection with direct repair may suffice, but more commonly, resection and interpositional *vein grafting* are required. In digits with Doppler verification of occlusion, midlateral *fasciotomy* may be done and peripheral flow reexamined. When surgery is unlikely to relieve a very distal occlusion or angiography shows no distal refill of vessels for grafting or when surgery has failed, thrombolytic therapy should be attempted.

Fasciotomy should be considered in *all* major closed vessel injuries and should certainly be done if the standard indications are present or if ischemia has exceeded 6 hours—less if the patient has been hypotensive for much of that time. It may be done as a preliminary step if delay is anticipated.

Compartment Syndromes

The investing fascia of extremity muscles is firmly attached to bone by a relatively inelastic intermuscular septum. Any fluid accumulation within the fascial compartment may cause a rise in pressure and increase tension in the compartment. The critical closing pressure of the vessels serving the muscles appears to be 40 mm Hg. Should intercompartmental pressure exceed that level, muscle ischemia may result with an initial onset of *pain,* followed within 2 hours by irreversible muscle necrosis—*Volkmann's ischemia.* Pain may well subside with muscle necrosis.

Nerves passing through the compartment are affected most, with *paresthesia and hypoesthesia* occurring. By contrast, major vessels contain a pressure equal to systolic pressure. Flow through these vessels will continue unimpaired, with palpable distal pulses long after muscle necrosis has become irreversible. As the fascial compartment attempts to accommodate the increased fluid volume, it approximates the configuration that contains the largest volume in the smallest area—a sphere. This "balling up" of the muscles accentuates the initial pain. Thus, in the most common anterior forearm compartment syndrome, this results in flexion of the digits with resistance to passive extension (the *passive stretch test*), which will be positive whether or not the patient is conscious. The physician may compound the problem by the application of external splints or casts, by elevation of a limb at risk, or by failing to correct hypovolemia.

Upper extremity compartment syndromes most frequently afflict the forearm flexor compartment and the interosseus spaces but can also occur in the dorsal muscle compartment.

The symptoms and signs, in sequence, are as follows:

1. Pain out of proportion to the injury
2. Weakness of the compartment muscles
3. Increased tenseness of the compartment envelope
4. Hypoesthesia in the sensory distribution of nerves that pass through the compartment

Pain on passive stretching of the muscles of the compartment will be present in increasing degrees from the outset of injury.

Interosseous Compartment

Interosseous compartment syndromes are more difficult to detect than forearm compartment syndromes since several of the criteria are more subtle. Inappropriate pain may pass unheeded in the injured hand; hypoesthesia does not occur, and weakness of the muscles and raised compartment pressure are difficult to detect. The diagnosis therefore rests heavily on suspicion. Physical examination may be particularly helpful in the passive stretch test for the interosseous compartment. The MP joint is held in hyperextension, the IP joints flexed, and the finger then deviated both radially and ulnarward. If pain is elicited, decompression may be required. It should be emphasized that initially the pulse is not lost in either the forearm or the interosseous compartment syndrome since main arterial pressure is well above the critical closing pressure of vessels supplying the compartment tissues. An absent pulse is probably evidence of major vascular impairment, which will coincidentally worsen the compartment syndrome by lowering the perfusion pressure. Both problems require urgent attention.

FINGERTIP INJURIES

The fingertip is an area in which the configuration of skin loss and the nature of the exposed tissue are particularly important in selecting the method of reconstruction and thereby influencing the outcome.

Pulp

Sensation, adequate padding, and freedom from discomfort are essential. Treatment principles depend on the following:

1. Is the bone exposed? If not and the defect is smaller than 1 cm^2, good results have been reported merely by dressing the wound. If the defect is larger than 1 cm^2 in an adult, a skin graft is indicated. Split-thickness skin is used for small defects, particularly on the ulnar side of the digit where contraction will draw in normal sensitive skin. Full-thickness grafts are employed for larger areas of well-vascularized soft tissue, especially on the radial, or contact, aspect of the finger. If bone is exposed, a flap is required to maintain length.

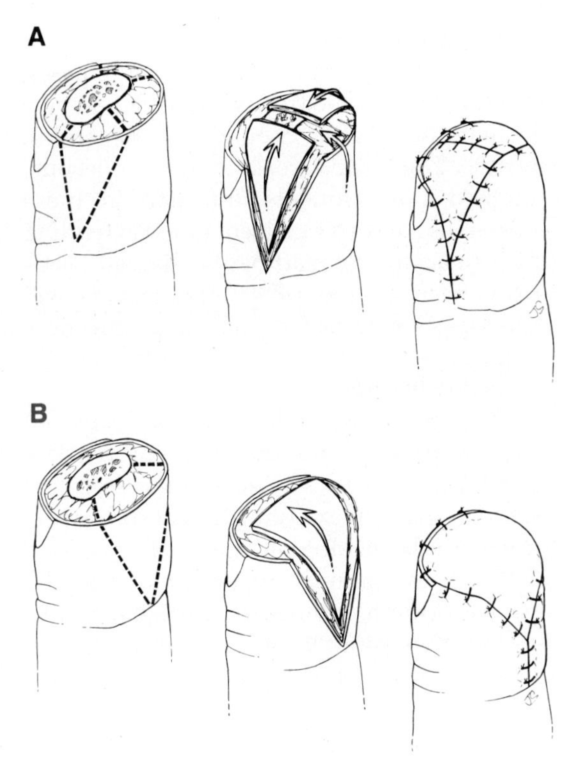

FIG 23–11.
Two methods of V-Y advancement of tissue onto the distal part of the fingertip. **A,** the Kutler lateral V-Y flap works well for nearly transverse amputations. **B,** the Atasoy-Kleinert volar V-Y flap works well for more dorsal losses of tissue, with sparing of volar tissue.

2. Where is the tissue loss? If more tissue has been lost from the dorsal than the palmar aspect, a local V-Y advancement flap may be an excellent choice (Fig 23–11). If the angulation is reversed (i.e., more lost from the palmar than from the dorsal aspect), any local flap would fail because of tension. In the thumb distal to the IP joint, a palmar angled defect may be closed by a Moberg advancement flap or by a dorsal neurovascular island flap from the thumb itself.

When bone is exposed and the angulation of the wound is unsuitable for local flap repair, the choices include the following:

1. Cross-finger flap—the most common solution. The main excluding factor is injury to the dorsum of the adjacent donor finger. The cross-finger flap to the thumb can be taken from the proximal phalanx of the index finger or from the middle phalanx of either the middle or ring fingers.

2. Thenar flap. This pedicled flap from the MP crease of the thumb may be restricted to patients under 40 years of age because unacceptable PIP joint contracture may result in older patients. It is the flap of choice in younger women since it avoids an unsightly donor scar on the dorsum of the finger.

3. Immediate neurovascular island—only applicable for thumb pulp loss, experienced surgeons, and a clean wound. Amputation revision—sacrifice of length is unfortunate, but may be needed to provide a sensitive, well-healed stump. It is appropriate in isolated loss of a fingertip in older patients where a cross-finger flap is contraindicated.

Nail Bed

Adequate nail support without nail distortion is necessary to prevent the nail from becoming a nuisance functionally or an embarrassment cosmetically. The injured nail bed should be inspected under magnification. Treatment principles include the following:

1. If the distal half of the terminal phalanx is present and fractured, it should be stably reduced with a fine Kirschner wire. The more phalanx missing, the greater the likelihood of a curved nail, which can only be avoided if the nail bed is supported by bone throughout its length.

2. Accurate localization and matching of both the germinal and sterile nail bed should be accomplished prior to careful repair; otherwise, deformity will result.

3. The eponychium should be carefully inspected. Any adhesion between the eponychium and nail bed will result in a grooved or split nail. This can be prevented by careful repair of all layers of the new fold and insertion of a splint to keep the cul-de-sac open during healing.

4. If any nail bed is missing, it is best replaced with a split-thickness nail bed graft taken either from the injured finger or from a toe. These have been shown to be most effective on the sterile matrix.

5. When the nail bed is completely destroyed but distal phalanx remains, length can be preserved by covering the soft-tissue defect with a reversed deepithelialized cross-finger flap.

HAND INFECTIONS

Classification

Hand infections may be bacterial, viral, fungal, protozoal, chlamydial, or metazoal. While most infections are polymicrobial, the most commonly isolated organisms are *Staphylococcus* (60%), *Streptococcus* (16%), *Enterobacter* (16%), and *Pseudomonas* (2%).

Infections are generally categorized by their anatomic distribution in the hand. Localization to one area is a function of both the type of infecting organism and the fact that the hand has distinct anatomic compartments.

Deeper abscesses may communicate with more superficial layers. With subfascial abscesses, three pockets may develop—one beneath the fascia, one subcutaneous, and one subcuticular. The surgical implications are clear—the superficial abscesses may be drained and the deeper abscesses left undrained.

Anatomic Compartments

The palmar surface of the hand and the tissue around the distal phalanx are divided into compartments that limit the spread of infection.

Nail Fold

The nail fold is especially susceptible to injury. Infections are common, probably because they are initially neglected and the area is subjected to repeated trauma. Infection of the nail fold is called paronychia.

Apical Spaces

The skin of the fingertip is firmly attached to the distal phalanx by numerous fibrous septa that divide the soft tissue immediately beneath the nail into a large number of relatively closed compartments.

Digital Pulp

The middle and distal digital creases, which overlie the joints, are attached respectively to the A3 and A5 pulleys of the tendon sheath. The pulp areas therefore become confined compartments. Infection in these pulp areas remains localized, rarely extending into adjacent compartments. Indeed, soft-tissue necrosis and phalangeal osteitis will develop sooner than extension of infection.

Tendon Sheaths

The attachment of overlying skin to the A3 and A5 pulleys and the adjacent cruciate sheath means that there is no intervening fat between the skin and sheath to absorb puncture wounds. In addition, the cruciate portion of the sheath is much more flimsy than the annular portion. Injuries to the digital creases are therefore more likely to result in tendon sheath infections (Fig 23–12).

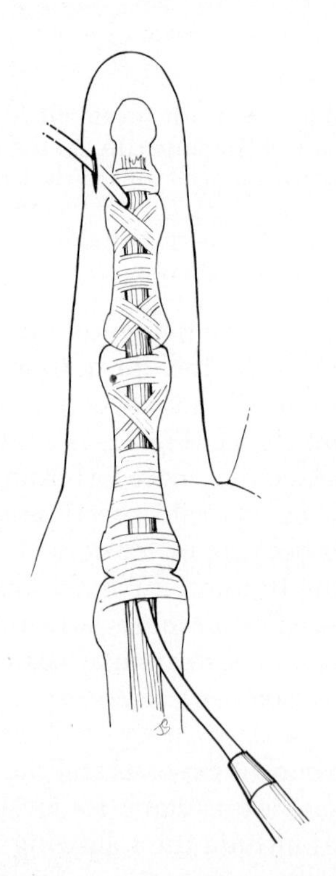

FIG 23–12.
Drainage of suppurative tenosynovitis. A small irrigation catheter is placed just proximal to the A pulley, and a second drainage catheter exits distally. Continuous irrigation aided by dependent drainage is maintained for 24 to 48 hours.

In over 80% of hands the tendon sheath of the small finger communicates with the ulnar bursa. That of the thumb almost invariably communicates with the radial bursa. Infection involving the sheaths of these digits may easily communicate with the wrist and lower part of the forearm. These sheaths may also connect with one another and create a "horseshoe" abscess involving the tendon sheaths of both the thumb and small finger. The tendon sheaths of the other fingers rarely communicate with the ulnar bursa; more commonly they end proximally at the MP joint beneath the palmar crease.

Web Space

Less well defined anatomically than the other compartments, the web space is nonetheless clearly circumscribed when infected. It is bounded by the margin of the web containing the natatory or superficial transverse palmar ligament distally, by the deep attachments of the palmar fascia proximally, and by its attachment to the tendon sheaths laterally. The deep transverse metacarpal ligament forms the floor of the space that extends dorsally between the fingers around the distal edge of that ligament.

Deep Palmar Space

This space lies deep to the palmar fascia. The fascia resists infectious penetration but results in considerable tension, and consequent pain, in the relatively rare case of infection.

Specific Types of Infection

Septic arthritis should be suspected in the presence of a wound overlying the finger joints dorsally. If such a wound continues to discharge small quantities of seropurulent fluid for more than a week after injury, septic arthritis should be suspected. By far the most common cause of septic arthritis is a human "bite." On the other hand, septic arthritis can develop without such a wound or indeed any recent injury. In such a situation, gonorrhea, or noninfective causes of acute arthritis such as gout and rheumatoid disease should be considered. The clinical features of septic arthritis include swelling out of proportion to the inflammation present in the skin around the wound and, at later stages, restricted joint motion. This is often surprisingly slow to develop, but eventually both flexion and extension produce pain.

Instability may be evidenced by increased laxity in the collateral ligaments, a motion that may be accompanied by crepitus. Discharging sinuses may develop if drainage is unduly delayed. Radiologic changes, only the first of which are apparent in the initial two weeks, include the following:

- Dorsal soft-tissue swelling evident on lateral views
- Decalcification of the juxta-articular bone
- Narrowing of the joint space
- Progressive fragmentation of the bone ends

It should be emphasized that joint instability, sinus formation, radiographic changes, and even severe pain on motion may not be present when the patient can best be helped. The diagnosis must be considered when disproportionate swelling accompanies a wound that is in the appropriate site and that continues to discharge long after injury. Cultures from both effusion from the wound as well as the synovial fluid are important.

Cellulitis is dramatic in onset. The patient may have a history of acute onset of swelling (12 to 24 hours from injury), redness, and pain often following a minor injury. Examination may show an ill, pale, and sweating patient, often with a marked elevation in temperature. The most striking feature in the hand is the extensive puffy redness with streaks of lymphangitis often obvious in the forearm. Axillary nodes are occasionally enlarged but more often are simply tender in the early stages. There may be a hemorrhagic blister present that can be removed without pain. If a wound is present, it is usually unremarkable and exuding only a few drops of serous fluid. Culture of the serous fluid from either the blister or the wound usually yields hemolytic

Streptococcus. Incision and drainage are not indicated in cellulitis.

Herpetic whitlow occurs mainly on the digital pulp of medical and dental workers. Commencing with pain, redness, and swelling, it is often confused with a distal pulp infection. However, after 24 to 36 hours, the characteristic vesicles appear and are clear at first but quickly become opaque and apparently purulent. Culture is sterile, but the causative virus can be demonstrated within 6 hours. An accurate diagnosis is important since incision and drainage are contraindicated. With observation, the lesion will regress spontaneously.

Human bites are serious injuries because of the plethora of organisms encountered in the oral cavity; the wounds require vigorous treatment. The majority of human "bites" are not in fact bites but are rather tooth wounds sustained in a fight. For this reason patients may delay treatment and lie about the cause of injury. It should be assumed that a wound over the metacarpal is from a tooth and communicates with the joint space. These should be explored. The wound should be excised at each level while remembering that the posture at exploration is entirely different from that at the time of the blow. For this reason successive wounds in the skin, extensor apparatus, joint capsule, and metacarpal head do not correspond and indeed are far removed from each other. The injury to the metacarpal head will not be seen on radiography since it is a chondral "divot" fracture, but it is frequently found on exploration. *Eikenella corrodens* is commonly cultured from human bite wounds and is sensitive to crystalline penicillin.

Staphylococcal as well as gram-negative infections are also common. Aerobic and anaerobic cultures should be routinely taken.

Drug addiction has contributed significantly to the incidence of hand infection. Often the patient will be seen at a late stage and give an inaccurate history. Dorsal abscesses are most common, but septic arthritis may be the initial disorder, with *Serratia* and *Pseudomonas* being frequent causative organisms. It is unlikely that the infection will follow the first patient use of drugs, and often extensive soft-tissue changes will be present. The hand of an established addict may show extensive indurated puffy edema, chronic tenosynovitis, and/or inflexible ankylosis of the small joints.

Previously uncommon organisms are now being isolated more commonly, especially among immunocompromised patients such as patients with acquired immunodeficiency syndrome (AIDS) or transplant patients. *Mycobacterium fortuitum, kansasii, marinum, tuberculosis, chelonei,* and *avium* have all been reported in recent years to involve tendon sheaths, bursae, joints, fascia, and bone in that order of frequency. The more chronic forms may be mistaken for gout or rheumatoid disease.

SUGGESTED READING

Lister, Graham: *The hand: diagnosis and indications,* ed 3, New York, Churchill Livingstone, 1993.

Mackinnon SE, Dellon AL: *Surgery of the peripheral nerve,* New York, Thieme Medical Publishers, 1988.

Schneider, Lawrence H: *Flexor tendon injuries,* Boston, Little, Brown & Co, 1985.

Chapter 24

Aesthetic and Functional Problems

Charles L. Puckett, M.D.
Matthew J. Concannon, M.D.
Gregory H. Croll, M.D.

CONTENTS

CHAPTER OBJECTIVE

At the end of this chapter the resident is familiar with aesthetic and functional problems of the hand and arm, understands the principles of rehabilitation of the upper extremity, and performs total management, including comprehensive rehabilitation of the upper extremity dysfunction.

LEARNER OBJECTIVES

On completion of this chapter the resident

1. **Demonstrates knowledge of the common nerve compression and entrapment syndromes of the upper extremity.**
2. **Understands the basic principles of medical and surgical treatment of nerve compression and entrapment syndromes of the upper extremity.**
3. **Is familiar with the pathologic anatomy and physiology of upper extremity joint contractures and Dupuytren's disease.**
4. Knows the basic pathophysiology of rheumatoid arthritis of the upper extremity.
5. Is familiar with the pharmacologic treatment of rheumatoid arthritis and the details of its prescription, use, and side effects.
6. Is familiar with surgical treatment of rheumatoid arthritis: timing of therapy, types of treatment, and interactions with medical therapy.
7. Demonstrates knowledge of the common circulatory disorders of the upper extremity, including but not limited to arterial thromboses, aneurysms, embolic disease, arteriovenous fistulas, and vasospastic disease.
8. Is familiar with the basic principles of medical treatment of circulatory disorders of the upper extremity such as anticoagulants and vasodilators.
9. Has detailed knowledge of the surgical aspects of treatment of patients with circulatory disease of the upper extremity.
10. Understands the manifestations and surgical treatment of aesthetic upper extremity deformities.
11. Understands the diagnosis and treatment of common pain syndromes.
12. Understands the physiology of management of patients with upper extremity lymphedema.
13. Demonstrates detailed knowledge of the surgical treatment options for upper extremity contractures.
14. Is familiar with all aspects of hand and upper extremity rehabilitation, including but not limited to splints,

prostheses, physical therapy, and sensory reeducation.

■ CLINICAL PRACTICE ACTIVITIES

During the course of the training program, the resident

1. **Evaluates and performs surgery on patients with nerve compression and entrapment neuropathies of the hand.**
2. Evaluates and performs surgery on patients with nerve compression and entrapment neuropathies of the upper extremity.
3. Performs surgery on patients with problems related to rheumatoid arthritis in the upper extremity.
4. Evaluates and treats with medical and surgical modalities patients with upper extremity circulatory disorders.
5. Evaluates and performs surgery on patients with aesthetic deformities of the upper extremity.
6. Completes reconstructive surgical procedures on patients with contractures and Dupuytren's disease of the upper extremity.
7. Prescribes splints, prostheses, physical therapy, etc., for patients requiring upper extremity rehabilitation and follows these patients through their rehabilitation by coordinating all aspects of care.
8. *Utilizes pharmacologic agents for the treatment of rheumatoid and related arthritides of the upper extremity.*

NERVE COMPRESSION AND ENTRAPMENT SYNDROMES

The symptoms of entrapment neuropathy arise from segmental vascular compromise. Venous congestion in the epineural and intrafascicular tissues produces axonal anoxia, which interferes with the integrity of the cell membrane and ultimately leads to a loss of conduction along the nerve. The relative ischemia also produces capillary dilatation, which contributes to endoneural edema, further compounding the original compression. With prolonged ischemia, eventual fibroblast proliferation within the nerve may result in intraneural scarring.

Carpal tunnel syndrome (the most frequently occurring nerve entrapment syndrome of the upper extremity) is produced by compression of the median nerve at the carpal tunnel. The most common reason for this compression appears to be either specific (rheumatoid) or nonspecific tenosynovitis, which by increasing carpal tunnel volume, results in nerve compression. Symptoms include weakness or awkwardness of the hand, complaints of altered sensation in the median nerve distribution, frequent worsening of the symptoms with use of the hand, awakening from sleep with pain or numbness, and pain proximally in the forearm and even the arm. Advanced signs of this syndrome are thenar atrophy and dense anesthesia in the distribution of the median nerve. Phalen's test (reproduction of symptoms with wrist flexion) is a key diagnostic maneuver, as is testing for Tinnel's sign at the wrist. Electrodiagnostic studies are important in confirming the diagnosis and are commonly demanded as corroborative evidence by third-party payers (see Fig 24–1).

Conservative management includes

1. Paresthesia or numbness in median nerve distribution
2. Awakening at night with pain or numbness
3. Positive Phalen's test
4. Positive Tinnel's test at the wrist

= Carpal tunnel syndrome

+/− confirming electrodiagnostic studies

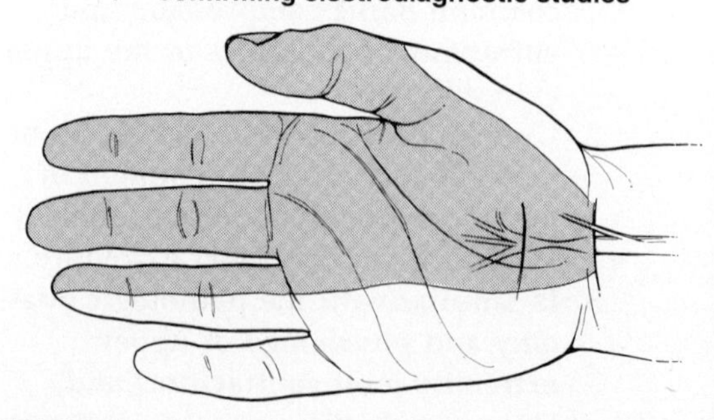

FIG 24–1.
Diagnostic criteria for carpal tunnel syndrome.

splinting of the wrist in slight extension, a trial of an oral nonsteroidal anti-inflammatory drug (NSAID), and corticosteroid injection into the carpal tunnel. The indication for operative intervention (release of the transverse carpal ligament) is failure of conservative management. While open release of the ligament is the gold standard of treatment, endoscopic release is apparently associated with less morbidity and an earlier return to work.

Entrapment of the median nerve more proximally can produce the pronator syndrome. This syndrome, which is also exacerbated with activity, mimics carpal tunnel syndrome in a sensory pattern but is less likely to awaken the patient at night; pain in the proximal portion of the forearm should suggest this syndrome. The possible sites of entrapment are at the ligament of Struthers, at the lacertus fibrosus, within the pronator teres muscle bellies, and at the arch of the origin of the flexor digitorum superficialis. The diagnosis is difficult but may be confirmed by electrodiagnostic studies. If pronator muscle–relaxing splints are unsuccessful as conservative management, operative treatment involves exploration and decompression of the median nerve along its course in the proximal part of the forearm.

The anterior interosseous syndrome (much less common than those conditions noted previously) is caused by entrapment of the median nerve in the proximal part of the forearm. This syndrome generally has no sensory symptoms. Individuals usually have dysfunction from weakness or paralysis of the flexor digitorum profundus of the index finger, the flexor pollicis longus, and the pronator quadratus. There is no role for conservative management; surgical release is indicated promptly because recovery of muscle function is diminished after prolonged compression.

Ulnar nerve entrapment at the elbow (cubital tunnel syndrome) is the second most common nerve compression syndrome of the upper extremity and is characterized by pain in the proximal medial portion of the forearm, accompanied by paresthesia or anesthesia of the palmar aspect of the ulnar 1½ fingers. Wasting of the ulnar innervated muscles is a late finding. The diagnosis is suggested by a positive Tinnel test over the ulnar nerve at the elbow (although this can be elicited in many normal individuals) and by increased numbness with elbow flexion. Electrical studies are very valuable in this syndrome. The surgical treatment involves decompression alone (division of the fibrous arcade of the flexor carpi ulnaris) or its combination with transposition of the nerve and/or medial epicondylectomy. With severe symptoms, the best long-term results seem to be associated with anterior transposition of the nerve, but this maneuver results in increased operative morbidity.

Ulnar nerve entrapment at Guyon's canal, although commonly discussed, is much less frequent. A variety of signs and symptoms are possible, depending on whether the entrapment is distal or proximal to the bifurcation of the ulnar nerve into its deep motor and superficial branches. If both motor and sensory symptoms are present, the entrapment is at Guyon's canal or more proximally. Motor signs include ulnar nerve–innervated intrinsic muscle weakness or paralysis; sensory symptoms are localized to the palmar surface of the little finger and the ulnar half of the ring finger. This entity may be associated with an occupational cause (hypothenar hammer syndrome) or some local condition such as a ganglion or lipoma. In examining the patient, it is important to perform an Allen's test to confirm ulnar collateral circulation, which may suggest a vascular etiology. The surgical treatment includes release of Guyon's canal and complete nerve decompression.

Radial tunnel syndrome is the most common entrapment syndrome of the radial nerve and may involve compression from the radial head to the supinator muscle. Symptoms are primarily complaints of pain in the extensor musculature of the proximal part of the forearm that are exacerbated by activity. This compression is often confused with tennis elbow, but the point of maximal tenderness is more anterior. The middle finger test (pain upon extension of the middle finger against resistance with the wrist in neutral position and the elbow extended) is frequently used but is not diagnostic. Maximal tenderness is over the extensor digitorum communis muscle, 5 to 6 cm distal and anterior to the lateral epicondyle. Initial management involves immobilization of the extremity. If the pain persists or recurs, exploration of the radial nerve in the radial tunnel may be indicated, through either an anterolateral or posterior approach. The muscle-splitting incision of Lister is expedient. Four distinct compression points have been identified and include recurrent vessels overlying the nerve, fibrous bands, the arcade of Frohse, and the tendinous margin of the extensor carpi radialis brevis.

Thoracic outlet syndrome can have equivocal and puzzling symptoms, including shoulder pain that radiates down the extremity in a radicular pattern and typically involves the medial aspect of the forearm. It is usually precipitated by specific extremity positions. The syndrome is caused by compression of the lower trunk of the brachial plexus (the C8, T1, and occasionally C7 nerve roots) as it passes superiorly and laterally across the first rib between the medial and anterior scalene muscles. The diagnosis is suggested by reproduction of symptoms (numbness and paresthesia) when the upper extremity is abducted to 90 degrees and externally rotated. Simply altering sleep posture or muscle strengthening exercises may provide relief. Resection of the first rib has replaced anterior scalenectomy as the operation of choice for intractable symptoms; the transaxillary approach is preferred.

Brachial plexus neuritis is most often associated with scarring related to previous surgery, irradiation, or tumor. This devastating syndrome is frequently associated with intractable pain, and while surgical decompression and scar excision may provide some relief, most patients are relegated to chronic pain endurance.

RHEUMATOID AND NONSPECIFIC ARTHRITIS

The various arthritides affect the joints, supporting ligamentous structures, or the musculotendinous units that move them. Arthritis of any etiology generally results in joint pain and ultimately in dysfunction from either instability or contracture. Two major patterns are prevalent (see Fig 24–2): rheumatoid and rheumatoid-like arthritis (RA) and osteoarthritis, or degenerative joint disease (DJD). RA is a systemic autoimmune disease whose major target organ seems to be synovium. Any area in which synovial cells reside can be affected by RA. In joints, the synovium becomes hypertrophic and may invade ligaments or even subchondral bone and destroy articular cartilage. Ligaments are stretched by expansion of the hypertrophic synovium, and invasion further weakens them to render joints unstable. Subsequent subluxation may result in destruction of the architecture and balance of the hand. The hypertrophic synovium of tendon sheaths may affect tendons in a similar way. Synovial invasion and swelling of the tendon can result in triggering with further progression possibly leading to rupture. Cartilage degeneration and loss of synovial-lined gliding surfaces may leave rough bony protuberances that can erode, weaken, and cause tendon rupture. Precisely how RA affects muscles, particularly the intrinsic muscles of the hand, is less well understood. Intrinsic muscle contractures add additional distracting forces to the digits that compound flexion contracture and dislocation of the metacarpophalangeal (MP) joints and result in swan-neck deformities distally.

A diagnosis of RA can frequently be made clinically once the deforming stage has been reached. However, sophisticated testing and comprehensive medical management require the services of a rheumatologist to specifically categorize and separate RA from the many rheumatoid-like arthritides. Nonsurgical treatment includes splinting, various forms of physical therapy, and early NSAID treatment, but gold and ultimately steroids will be necessary in advanced cases.

Surgery is directed at both prevention of progressive deformity and correction or compensation for existing dysfunction. Prophylactic surgery consists mainly of synovectomy; while not halting the disease, this can delay progression of deformities and tendon disruptions. Dorsal wrist synovectomy may be indicated in medically controlled patients with

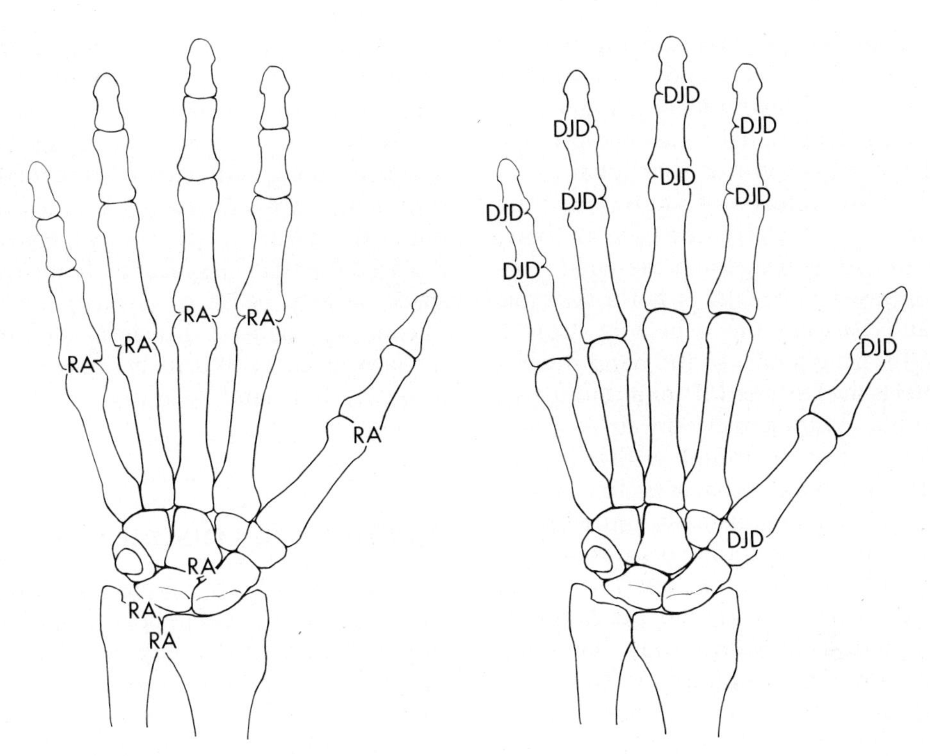

FIG 24–2.
Most common patterns of joint involvement of rheumatoid arthritis *(RA)* and degenerative joint disease *(DJD)* (osteoarthritis).

pain or swelling at the extensor retinaculum to prevent tendon ruptures. There is a similar but less well defined role for MP and even proximal interphalangeal (PIP) joint synovectomy prior to overt joint instability and dislocation. Unfortunately, many patients who could benefit by synovectomy progress to tendon rupture, joint subluxation, and contractures prior to referral. Once disruption and deformity occur, recapturing hand function is more difficult.

Tendon ruptures frequently occur as attrition ruptures of the extensor tendons at the wrist. Here denuded and abrasive bony edges literally shred the tendon over time. Flexor tendon ruptures seem to be more commonly related to direct invasion and weakening by the tenosynovium. When extensor tendon rupture has occurred, it is rarely possible to do end-to-end repair. Tendon transfer to adjacent intact tissues will usually recapture adequate function. Tendon grafts fare poorly in patients with RA. Correction of the offending bony edges is indicated, and interposition of the extensor retinaculum between the newly repaired tendons and the bone should restore a satisfactory gliding surface. Flexor tendon ruptures may be more of a problem since tendon grafts are not desired and shortening of the tendon may result in flexion contracture. When necessary, profundus superficialis transfers may provide the needed length. Alternatively, distal interphalangeal (DIP) joint fusion may be considered.

RA of the wrist with involvement of the radioulnar, distal ulnar, and other joints may require a Darrach procedure (resection of the distal ulnar head with/without extensor and/or flexor tendon rebalancing). Limited fusions have some application, but total wrist joint replacement or fusion may ultimately be necessary. Once subluxation of the MP joints has occurred, soft-tissue rebalancing alone is rarely possible because of intrinsic muscle contractures. Joint replacement with Silastic and/or metallic artificial joints and centralization of the extensor can restore valuable functional ability. Repair of joint capsules and intrinsic muscle division or transfers may aid in correcting ulnar drift.

Tendon transfers and rebalancing may aid in correcting swan-neck and boutonniere-type deformities of the thumb and fingers, but often interphalangeal (IP) fusions provide more reliable and pain-free functional restoration. However, osteoporosis and poor bone quality result in a decreased rate of bone fusion here, just as they do in the wrist.

In contrast to RA, DJD is not a systemic disease and typically affects heavily stressed or weight-bearing joints. In the hand it commonly affects the DIP and PIP joints but spares the MP joints. Quite characteristically it affects the basilar joint of the thumb at the trapeziometacarpal interface and may occur in accelerated fashion in any previously injured joint, particularly if cartilaginous disruption has occurred. The etiology is unknown, but chronic stress or wear as the cartilaginous surface is gradually worn away has been implicated. Primary symptoms are pain with some limitation of motion. Women are affected approximately twice as often as men. At the DIP joints, Heberden's nodes and loss of cartilage thickness often result in visible deformity with angulation. These patients usually remain remarkably functional. For pain, the drug of choice is aspirin followed by other NSAIDs. Surgical debridement of osteophytes and reefing of the joint will provide both aesthetic and some functional improvement. Fusion is the only acceptable treatment for a clearly unstable and painful DIP joint. Indeed, the debridement procedure may result in fusion itself. Fusions are relatively simply accomplished by rigid fixation with microplates.

PIP joint involvement is more of a problem and may be associated with more disabling pain. Fusion is the ultimate solution, and many surgeons have abandoned intermediate steps. Joints that do not move do not hurt! The problems with trapeziometacarpal arthritis at the base of the thumb are even more complex. Because of the progressive subluxation of the metacarpal and its contracture into the palm, compensatory hyperextension at the MP joint occurs. Correction at the base of the thumb without attention to the MP joint may result in a flail thumb despite the improvement in the base joint. Considerations for surgery depend upon the degree of arthritis (pantrapezial vs. that confined to the carpometacarpal surface, etc.). Typically, resection of the trapezium and ligamentous balancing along with release of the metacarpal contracture are necessary. A rolled tendon graft (the anchovy procedure) has usually replaced the silicone spacer to fill the trapezial space, largely because of the possibility of silicone synovitis. Correction of MP joint hyperextension will usually allow restoration of nearly full hand span and grasp of large objects.

CIRCULATORY DISORDERS

Excluding direct trauma and tumors or malformations, circulatory disorders are largely disturbances in flow resulting in inadequate tissue perfusion (ischemia). Disorders include arterial thrombosis, embolic problems, aneurysms and arteriovenous fistulas, various vasospastic disorders, and other diseases resulting in arterial or arteriolar compromise (collagen disorders, Buerger's disease).

Arterial thrombosis may result from external trauma (hypothenar hammer syndrome), be associated with intimal disruption, or result from emboli of central origin. Arterial occlusion or significant diminution in arterial flow will eventually result in distal tissue ischemia and, ultimately, tissue death. Treatment of these disorders of flow often requires surgical intervention, although in some (atherosclerosis, Buerger's disease, collagen diseases) the potential for improvement is very limited.

The most common manifestation of arterial thrombosis in the upper limb is ulnar artery thrombosis as seen in the "hypothenar hammer syndrome." This is typically produced by recurrent trauma to the hypothenar area with resultant contusion of either the ulnar artery or a portion of the superficial volar arch against the hook of the hamate. It may be seen in laborers when the fist is used as a hammer. Patients commonly note ischemic symptoms (cold or pain in the fingers), and occasionally ulnar nerve symptoms of either numbness or paresthesia are apparent in the fifth digit and the ulnar portion of the fourth. The differential diagnosis includes a ganglion in Guyon's canal, ulnar artery aneurysm, embolic phenomena, and disease-related ulnar artery occlusion (e.g., atherosclerosis or Buerger's disease). While thrombectomy may be successful in a small percentage of patients, most occlusions are too long-standing, and resection of the involved segment and direct vascular reconstruction with a vein graft are probably indicated. Recent reports show improved long-term patency rates. Regardless, the beneficial effects of resection of the involved segment resulting in direct sympathectomy are significant. Unfortunately, other causes of thrombosis such as the collagen-vascular diseases or Buerger's disease are not usually amenable to direct vascular reconstruction.

Upper extremity aneurysms are typically the result of either blunt or penetrating trauma. Atherosclerotic aneurysms are very rare in the upper extremity. The presence of an aneurysm is suggested by a (usually) nonpainful pulsatile mass, with or without distal vascular symptoms. A bruit may be present over the mass. Treatment is resection, with either arterial ligation (if sufficient collateral circulation exists) or reconstruction with a vein graft, if necessary.

Arteriovenous fistulas (AVF) are also typically the result of trauma (gunshot or stab wound). Certain congenital arteriovenous malformations with AVF may be associated with extremity overgrowth. Resection of the bulk of the vascular malformation may be the only definitive treatment for AVF. Traumatically derived AVF may have sufficient flow to be hemodynamically significant. The diagnosis is usually verified by palpation, the appearance of venous distension, a bruit, and Branham's sign (slowing of the pulse associated with fistula compression). A confirmatory arteriogram is generally indicated if surgical intervention is contemplated. Treatment of AVF obeys the tenets of Holman: quadripolar ligation. However, recent reports cite reconstitution of arterial as well as venous integrity. Occasionally, simple surgical division with closure of the arteriotomy or venotomy is sufficient.

The predominant source of emboli to the upper extremity is the heart, usually associated with arrhythmia or infarction. Approximately 15% of emboli travel to the upper extremity. Large emboli may lodge proximally in the limb and cause sudden and global symptoms of ischemia (pain, pallor, pulselessness, paresthesia, and paralysis). Emboli may also arise from an arterial source (such as an atherosclerotic plaque) and may have distal symptoms or occasionally be manifested as showers of microemboli with less dramatic symptoms. Treatment is surgical embolectomy or the use of thrombolytic agents (streptokinase, urokinase) if surgery is otherwise contraindicated. Anticoagulation with heparin may be indicated.

Vasospastic disorders may occur in collagen diseases, following frostbite, and probably in reflex sympathetic dystrophy (RDS). Raynaud's phenomenon is most classic. It is a vasospastic pallor of the fingers (with or without cyanosis) after exposure to cold, frequently with paresthesia, and followed by hyperemia. The diagnosis is typically made clinically by reproducing the symptoms with cold exposure. Raynaud's *disease* is the term used when these symptoms occur without identified collagen disease or other etiology. It characteristically occurs in young women (4:1) and usually involves progressively severe episodes with eventual trophic and ischemic changes. Raynaud's *phenomenon* refers to these symptoms in association with another identified disease, most commonly the collagen diseases. Scleroderma and Raynaud's phenomenon coexist in the "CREST" syndrome, which is characterized by calcinosis, Raynaud's phenomenon, esophageal stricture, scleroderma, and telangiectasia.

Nicotine, if used, must be eliminated. Intra-arterial reserpine, guanethidine, calcium channel blockers, as well as regional sympathetic blockade have moderate success. Avoidance of cold exposure may require geographic relocation. Cervicodorsal sympathectomy has also been only moderately successful, but digital sympathectomy has been more effective (although more difficult to perform). Unfortunately, with progression of the basic disease, vascular occlusion may become permanent, and ischemia may eventually result in amputations.

While atherosclerosis frequently spares the upper extremity, it will occasionally have a segmental nature that lends itself to vascular repair or bypass. Treatment of Buerger's disease (which appears to be an accelerated form of atherosclerosis occurring primarily in males who abuse nicotine) is particularly difficult. Cessation of nicotine exposure is *the* most important therapeutic intervention.

Upper extremity lymphedema is most commonly associated with surgical axillary lymphadenectomy or radiation to this area. Primary lymphedema of the upper extremity is rare. The fundamental problem is the interference with lymph egress. While primary and secondary (obstructive) lymphedema is classically discussed, the pathophysiology is probably similar. Indeed, one theory holds that the basic flaw is a failure of the regenerative ability of the lymphatics in both processes. This theory could explain phenomena such as a primary lymphedema occurring at a later point in life (the praecox or tarda forms) and may well explain why postmastectomy lymphedema develops in some patients and not in others (having had virtually the same operative procedures).

The diagnosis is generally made on a clinical basis, and a history of axillary lymphadenectomy is the most significant historical fact. Lymphangiography is of no diagnostic value and may indeed be harmful to existing lymphatics. Treatment is fundamentally conservative and consists first of patient education. The hallmarks of therapy are elevation and elastic compression. These simple maneuvers will manage the vast majority of cases. Most efficient compression is with a custom-constructed elastic compressive sleeve; nighttime elevation will frequently help to "empty" the extremity. Because the lymphatics are compromised, any infection is dangerous, and a failure to expeditiously treat patients may result in progression of the lymphedema. Therefore, antibiotics should be used at the first sign of any lymphangitis and probably with most minor skin violations. In addition, meticulous hygiene should be encouraged to avoid infection. Occasionally, diuretics and the benzopirones as well as weight reduction in obese patients have shown some value. Recalcitrant edema may require one of the automatic intermittent compression devices. Those providing a peristaltic-like compression of the extremity seem most effective.

Surgical treatment of upper extremity lymphedema should be rare. Although a variety of ingenious surgical applications either ablating the lymphedematous tissue or augmenting lymph flow have been suggested, most long-term results are disappointing. Although conceptually most sound, the construction of lymphovenous anastomoses has not provided the success originally suggested. At present, the most effective treatment for a massively swollen and dysfunctional upper extremity is probably surgical ablation, which consists of the elevation of relatively thin flaps and resection of the lymphedematous subcutaneous tissue. The operation can be performed on the lateral surface and subsequently repeated on the medial surface if necessary.

AESTHETIC DEFORMITIES OF THE UPPER EXTREMITY

Although functional considerations are paramount in the hand and upper extremity, aesthetic concerns are also important and may assume a significant role in certain patients. Acquired or perceived variations from normal may result from trauma (scarring and/or deletion of parts), disease (arthritides producing obvious deformity), congenital disorders (polydactyly, syndactyly, etc.), variations in size (lipodystrophy and lymphedema), and age (skin laxity and pigmentation problems). Nail deformities may be particularly distressing. Frequently, treatment of the underlying disorder will concomitantly improve hand appearance, but certain conditions such as amputations may simply have to be accepted by the patient (aesthetically acceptable prostheses are available).

Flaccidity, particularly of the arm in its proximal aspect, may follow significant weight loss or can simply occur with loss of muscle tone and advancing age. Dermolipectomy with a "rocket-shaped" excision on the medial aspect of the arm offers the only option for tightening and smoothing of this skin. While the results can be quite satisfying, the patient must accept the necessary incision scar.

Skin laxity and pigmentation changes are other common complaints associated with aging skin, particularly after excessive sun exposure. If abnormal pigmentation is the primary complaint, there are limited applications for either trichloracetic acid (TCA) or phenol-based chemical peel procedures. However, the subsequent bleaching is dramatic (with phenol particularly) and may make the skin look less normal than the original appearance. Skin tightening procedures, although rarely utilized, may solve specific problems. Dorsal wrist incisions have been employed for skin tightening of the dorsum of the hand and distal part of the forearm, occasionally with gratifying results.

Aesthetic surgery for nail deformities is most typically required for reconstruction of a posttraumatic (acquired) defect. Since the eponychial fold is responsible for the shiny surface of the nail, injury here may result in blemishes. Loss of a section of the germinal matrix may result in a split nail or an absent nail distally. Loss of a section of the nail bed (sterile matrix) may also result in a split nail or in nonadherence of the nail distal to the scar, possibly with curvature and distortion.

Nail ridges are frequently caused by irregularities in the underlying nail bed. A smooth nail bed is necessary for regrowth of a normal nail, and resection of the nail bed scar or smoothing of the underlying bone may be necessary to create a flat nail. A split nail may be the result of a ridge or scar in the germinal matrix or the nail bed because nail is not produced by scar tissue. Conceivably, if the scar is in the sterile matrix (bed), direct excision of the scar and reapproximation of the normal matrix edges will restore nail continuity. In practice, however, a scar large enough to cause a split nail is often too wide to reapproximate without tension. Excision of the scar and replacement with a split-thickness graft from the adjacent nail bed or a toe may correct the deformity. If a nail bed scar is wide, the nail distal to it may be nonadherant. This can also occasionally be corrected by excising the scar and replacing it with a split-thickness nail bed graft.

Complete absence of the nail is a difficult problem. Some patients, especially children, may be candidates for composite nail grafts (using a toe as the donor site), but the results are rarely satisfactory. In adults where a free microvascular graft is an option, the result is rarely normal, but if a growing nail can be accomplished, shaping and synthetic bonding may provide a more normal appearance.

The hooked nail deformity ("parrot beak deformity") is most typically produced by the nail bed being pulled over the distal phalanx to help close a distal fingertip amputation or by loss of phalanx support for the nail bed. This deformity can be at least partially corrected by replacing the soft tissue of the tip. This can be accomplished with either a V-Y advancement flap, cross-finger flap, or occasionally a full-thickness skin graft. Adding bone length with the graft is an alternative, although long-term maintenance of the graft volume is a problem. Correction of nail deformities is often less than satisfying to surgeon and patient.

CONTRACTURES

Contractures are fundamentally limitations of joint movement. They may be mild, such as a limited contracture produced by a longitudinal skin scar, or severe, totally preventing joint motion. Mechanically contractures are either intrinsic to the joint (affecting collateral ligaments or the volar plate) or extrinsic (involving soft tissues other than the immediate periarticular tissues) (see Fig 24–3). An extrinsic contracture significantly limiting joint excursion could ultimately cause collateral ligament shortening or volar plate fixation and thus result in an intrinsic contracture. From an etiologic standpoint, contractures may be congenital (arthrogryposis, trigger digits, camptodactyly) or acquired. Scar tissue is generally the cause of acquired joint contractures.

Prevention of contraction (and subse-

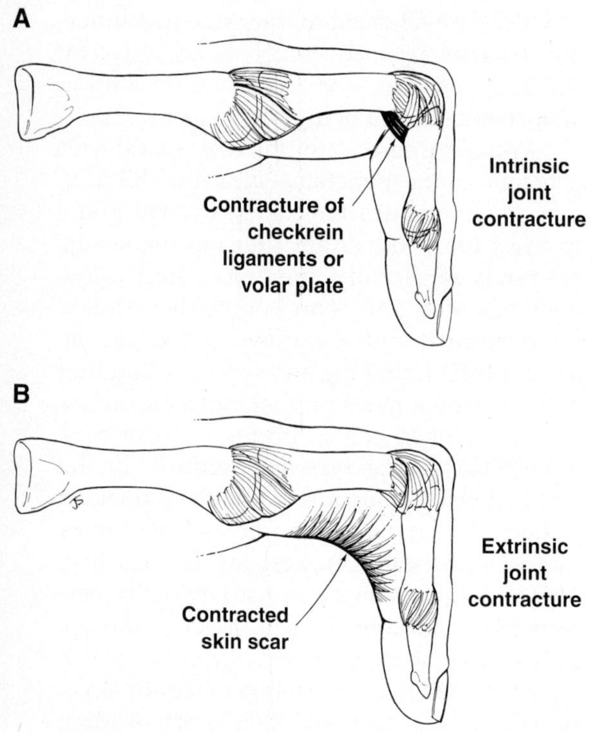

FIG 24–3.
Mechanism of intrinsic joint contracture *(top)* vs. extrinsic joint contracture *(bottom).*

quent contracture) is the key to avoidance of acquired contractures. Measures include proper timing and correction of the underlying problem, patient education, splinting, and appropriate therapy. While some existing contractures can be modified and improved with the above methods, prevention is obviously desirable. When conservative measures (rarely helpful in congenital contracture) fail to improve joint motion or when progress has halted for 2 months, surgical intervention is indicated for disabling contractures.

Among the congenital contractures, flexor tendon triggering is among the most common. If persistent beyond the third year (approximately a third will resolve spontaneously), it is corrected by tenovaginotomy of the A1 pulley (similar to acquired triggering in adults). Camptodactyly, finger contracture commonly affecting the PIP joint, is probably related to an anomaly of the superficialis tendon. It will not respond to extensor splinting, and correction (by release of the constricting band or superficialis tendon), if done late, may be unsuccessful.

Extrinsic contractures result from burns; skin loss with scarring; diseases such as RA, cerebral palsy, or acquired spastic disorders; and Dupuytren's contracture. These extrinsic contractures should be released prior to the formation of irreversible intrinsic joint contractures. Similarly, adhesions following flexor tendon repair that limit IP joint extension may require tenolysis and should be timed to prevent IP intrinsic contractures. When intrinsic joint contracture occurs and is recalcitrant to splinting measures, surgical release is indicated. In the IP joints, the collateral ligament arrangement is such that ligaments are least stressed in the flexed position. Thus any ligamentous shortening, particularly of the so-called checkreign ligaments in the PIP joints (found at the proximal lateral edges of the volar plate at the proximal phalanx), will prevent joint extension. Surgical release of IP joint contractures frequently requires division of these checkreign ligaments as well as additional portions of the accessory collateral ligaments until the joint comes easily into full extension. Additional release of volar plate adhesions may be necessary.

In the MP joints the collateral ligaments are tightest in the flexed position because of the cam configuration of the joint; thus intrinsic contractures with collateral ligament shortening result in an extended position of the MP joint. Release of the MP joint collateral ligaments is begun dorsally and usually requires complete division of these collateral ligaments. The MP joints should be splinted in the flexed position following contracture release. Intrinsic joint contracture should be carefully distinguished from intrinsic contracture, which is commonly used to refer to contracture of the intrinsic muscles of the hand and is, indeed, a contracture force that is extrinsic to the actual joint.

Dupuytren's contracture is a classic example of an extrinsic process resulting in intrinsic joint contracture. It is particularly common in Caucasians of eastern European extraction. The pathophysiology seems to involve abnormal fibroblast activity (probably involving the myofibroblast) of the palmar fascia (or aponeurosis) and may extend into the fingers as well as involve the pretendinous bands, the natatory ligaments, the superficial transverse ligaments, the lateral digital sheath, and Grayson's ligaments. Interestingly, Cleland's ligaments are spared. This process usually results in one or more contracted longitudinal bands, which may limit extension of the MP joints and/or the PIP joints. Involvement of the pretendinous bands appears to result in MP joint contracture, while involvement of the spiral cords results in PIP joint contracture. Spiral cord involvement may also result in central and volar displacement of the neurovascular structures and thus subject them to potential injury during surgery. Conservative therapy appears to have no role in treating this disorder. Simple observation is generally indicated in the absence of significant joint contracture. The only other surgical indication is significant pain in the scar. Although there is variation in opinion regarding the degree of MP joint contracture that should be allowed prior to surgery, most surgeons agree that any degree of PIP joint contracture is an indication for surgical intervention.

Controversy exists regarding adequate surgical therapy, but most agree that all obviously involved fascial tissue should be removed. Full joint extension should be achieved at the end of the procedure. Capsulectomy of the PIP joint may occasionally be required. However, this generally foretells a lack of total success. Postoperative hematoma (which has been related to more aggressive recurrence) is the most dreaded complication. The "open" vs. the closed approach to the palm skin, the indication for Z-plasties or other lengthening procedures, the choice of skin grafting, etc., vary with the case and the surgeon's preference.

HAND AND UPPER EXTREMITY REHABILITATION

It has been wisely stated that well-done surgical correction of disorders in the hand provides only half of what is necessary for full recovery. That other half is rehabilitation. It is inappropriate for the surgeon to simply refer his patient postoperatively to the rehabilitation expert or therapist; the sophistication and variety of techniques employed in this area require close coordination between the surgeon and the hand therapist.

Early postoperative goals are optimal wound healing, control of edema, and appropriately timed mobilization to properly allow healing and yet minimize adhesions and subsequent stiffness. The balance between immobilization (splinting) and mobilization is perhaps the most delicate consideration.

Splints are generally used for immobilization (static) or controlled mobilization (dynamic). Principles of common sense generally abide. Splinting following flexor tendon repair should prevent excessive or inappropriate extension and might therefore be designed to maintain some joint flexion. Following extensor repair, protection in the opposite direction is important. Dynamic splinting either specifically applies force to obtain movement or allows limited movement under controlled parameters. Static or blocking splints may simply protect the wound from movement to optimize healing or prevent sudden or violent movement as in the later phases of fracture healing.

Many additional tools or modalities are available, including active motion, active assisted motion, passive motion, compression, massage, biofeedback, heat, ultrasound, and transcutaneous electrical nerve stimulation (TENS). Each must be applied in proper sequence. Trauma to nerves and particularly amputations are prone to hypersensitivity. Various desensitization techniques including rubbing, tapping, gentle abrasion with various roughened surfaces, etc., often result in diminished unpleasant sensations. Sensory reeducation is a useful tool following nerve repair. Even following optimal nerve reconstruction the potential for sensory recovery is probably always less than 100%, except perhaps in the very young. Sensory reeducation can improve sensory capability much as one relearns motor functions following musculotendinous or motor nerve injury. This technique employs repetitive identification of various objects by palpation with the affected part and visual confirmation. In this manner altered neuro-pathways and/or receptors may be used to reidentify previously familiar sensations.

From time to time the surgeon must evaluate and provide determinations of permanent impairment or disability. This process should be as objective as possible, but in the final analysis it always assumes some subjective interpretation. The publication *Guides to the Evaluation of Permanent Impairment* by the American Medical Association allows some standardization of evaluation. Various measurements of joint motion restriction, amputation length, sensation, etc., correspond to a relatively objective and standard rating. Pain is probably the most difficult to evaluate, but muscle strength may be similarly subjective. The influence of potential monetary gain or pending litigation is difficult if not impossible to factor into an evaluation.

DIAGNOSIS AND MANAGEMENT OF PAIN SYNDROMES, REFLEX SYMPATHETIC DYSTROPHY

Pain is the least definable symptom associated with upper extremity disorders. Since it cannot be measured, its significance is difficult to evaluate. However, it can clearly be disabling in certain chronic hand conditions. Posttraumatic persistent pain may fit into one of the dystrophy syndromes. Unfortunately, these diagnoses can be abused by the patient in circumstances such as compensation claims. Most pain syndromes will respond to appropriate medication, skillfully applied occupational and physical therapy, and concerned interest on the part of the surgeon and therapist.

As defined by the American Association for Hand Surgery committee on reflex sympathetic dystrophy, RSD is a pain syndrome in which there is also loss of function and evidence of autonomic dysfunction. Current theory suggests that three conditions must be fulfilled before RSD develops: a persistent painful lesion, a predisposition to the development of RSD (often personality related), and an abnormal sympathetic reflex. The normal sympathetic reflex following an injury produces vasoconstriction, which prevents excessive blood loss or swelling. In patients with RSD, this sympathetic response continues beyond the appropriate time limit. The intense vasoconstriction produces ischemia, which causes pain. The sympathetic discharge is perpetuated by a pathologic positive-feedback mechanism sustaining the ischemia and further pain.

Three criteria have been suggested for the diagnosis of RSD: diffuse pain, loss of hand function, and sympathetic dysfunction. Four chief symptoms are usually presented: pain, swelling, stiffness, and discoloration. Secondary signs (which are variable but often present) include osteoporosis, sudomotor changes, temperature changes, trophic changes (such as alteration in hair growth), vasomotor instability, and palmar fibrosis. These signs and symptoms are frequently much more severe than would be expected by the original disease or trauma that precipitated them. In general, a presumptive diagnosis is made.

The best outcome can be expected with early diagnosis and treatment, the primary therapy being some type of interruption of the sympathetic nerve reflex. Oral sympatholytic agents include α-blockers (phenoxybenzamine, phentolamine, propranolol), reserpine, and guanethidine. In general, these agents are limited by the nonspecificity of their action and side effects. They are most useful very early in the course of the disease.

Sympathetic blockade by infiltration of local anesthetic into the stellate and upper two or three dorsal sympathetic ganglia will temporarily block the efferent sympathetic activity of the extremity. The effectiveness of the block can be judged by the amount of warming and flushing of the skin as well as the presence of Horner's syndrome. Somatic nerve blocks (such as an axillary block) interrupt the sensory afferent signals as well as the efferent signals and prevent feedback of the pain reflex. Although not as long lasting as the stellate blocks, they can be given more frequently. The somatic block may be indicated for patients with less severe symptoms or for relief of recurrent symptoms between stellate blocks.

Surgical intervention (sympathectomy) is indicated when at least four stellate blocks have been successful but have failed to eliminate the abnormal sympathetic reflex, if the disease has lasted for 6 months or more, or if the symptoms are so severe that stellate blocks are ineffective. Although not without significant morbidity, surgery typically produces some improvement and may avoid further complications of RSD. Severe cases and especially those diagnosed late may result in a totally dysfunctional and chronically painful hand.

SUGGESTED READING

Amadio PC, Mackinnon SE, Merritt WH, et al: Reflex sympathetic dystrophy syndrome: Consensus report of an ad hoc committee of the American Association for Hand Surgery on the definition of reflex sympathetic dystrophy syndrome. *Plast Reconstr Surg* 1991; 87:371–375.

Engelberg AL: *Guides to the Evaluation of Permanent Impairment,* ed 3. Chicago, American Medical Association, 1989.

Puckett CL: Lymphedema in the upper extremity, in McCarthy JG (ed): *Plastic Surgery.* Philadelphia, WB Saunders, 1990.

Tenney CG, Lisak JM: *Atlas of Hand Splinting,* ed 1. Boston, Little, Brown, 1986.

Zook EG: Injuries of the fingernail, in Green DP (ed): *Operative Hand Surgery,* New York, Churchill Livingstone, 1982.

Chapter 25

Reconstruction

Robert C. Russell, M.D., F.R.A.C.S., F.A.C.S.
William A. Zamboni, M.D.

CONTENTS

CHAPTER OBJECTIVE

At the end of this chapter the resident understands the principles and techniques of hand and upper extremity reconstruction and applies these to a variety of developmental, traumatic, and other problems.

LEARNER OBJECTIVES

On completion of this chapter the resident

1. **Knows the principles, indications, and techniques of tendon reconstruction in the hand, including tendon grafting (sources, methods, indications) and the use of prostheses (indications, timing, techniques).**
2. **Has a thorough understanding of functional deficits resulting from loss of segments of the anatomic system.**
3. **Has familiarity with the diagnostic techniques for evaluation of functional loss, including EMG and conduction studies, arteriography, conventional radiographs, CT scan, and MRI evaluation.**
4. **Has an understanding of the management of nerve injuries of the upper extremity, including primary, delayed primary, and secondary repair.**
5. **Has knowledge of the techniques of grouped interfascicular nerve grafting and of nerve graft harvesting (including use of vascularized nerve grafts).**
6. **Has knowledge of the indications and techniques for reconstruction of the amputated thumb, including lengthening, pollicization, free whole-toe transfer, and free wrap-around techniques.**
7. **Has knowledge of the indications for and specific technical methods of skin and soft-tissue coverage, including skin grafts, local flaps, distant flaps, and free tissue transfers.**
8. **Has knowledge of the specific requirements and resurfacing techniques for areas of critical innervation in the hand.**
9. Understands the use of tendon transfer and pedicled muscle/tendon substitution (including use of free muscle transfer) to redistribute functional activities in the upper extremity.
10. Has knowledge of the indications and techniques (including joint replacement) for treatment of digital dysfunction and joint deformities secondary to trauma or disease.
11. Understands the consequences of derangement of the bony architec-

ture of the hand and the methods and techniques for bone stabilization.

12. Understands the indications and techniques for correction of bony deficits of the hand, including lengthening, free nonvascularized bone grafting, and free microvascular bone transfer techniques.
13. Understands the principles of management of patients with brachial plexus injuries, including radiologic and electrical evaluation and surgical treatment (early and late).

CLINICAL PRACTICE ACTIVITIES

During the course of the training program, the resident

1. **Evaluates and surgically treats patients with tendon injuries requiring the use of primary and secondary tendon repair techniques (including tendon grafting).**
2. **Evaluates and surgically treats patients with nerve injuries of the upper extremity requiring early and late repair (excluding brachial plexus injuries).**
3. **Evaluates and surgically treats patients requiring restoration of functional cutaneous coverage of the hands and fingers (including free tissue transfer).**
4. Evaluates and surgically treats patients requiring musculotendon transfer or substitution techniques.
5. Evaluates and surgically treats patients requiring restoration of digi-

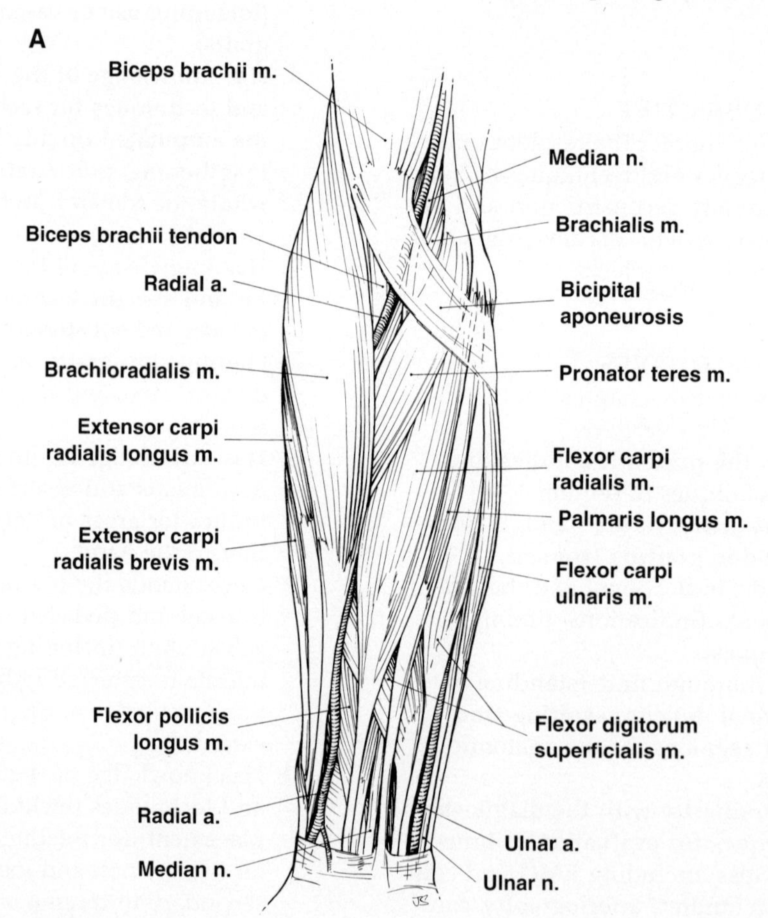

FIG 25–1.
Extrinsic flexor and extensor tendons.

tal function (including reconstruction of an absent thumb and joint replacement).
6. Evaluates and surgically treats patients requiring bony stabilization, including the addition of bone to manage hand defects.
7. Evaluates and treats patients with established brachial plexus injuries.

TENDON RECONSTRUCTION

The *extrinsic* flexor and extensor tendons of the upper extremity originate from the medial and lateral epicondyles in the forearm and insert into the hand to provide voluntary movement of the wrist and digits (Fig 25–1). There are two wrist flexor tendons, the flexor carpi ulnaris, which inserts into the pisiform, and the flexor carpi radialis, which inserts into the second metacarpal. All digital flexor tendons including the four flexor digitorum superficialis, four flexor digitorum profundus, and the flexor pollicis longus tendons travel into the hand with the median nerve through the carpal tunnel. All digital flexor tendons pass through a tight fibrous tunnel that includes a system of pulleys for each finger beginning at the distal palmar crease over the base of the proximal phalanx and extending along the volar aspect of the finger to the distal interphalangeal (DIP) joint flexion crease. All extrinsic flexor muscles are innervated by the median nerve except the flexor carpi ulnaris and flexor digitorum profundus muscles to the ring and small fingers, which are supplied by the ulnar nerve. The ulnar nerve and artery lie beneath the flexor carpi ulnaris muscle in the forearm and enter the hand just radial to the pisiform bone within the canal of Guyon.

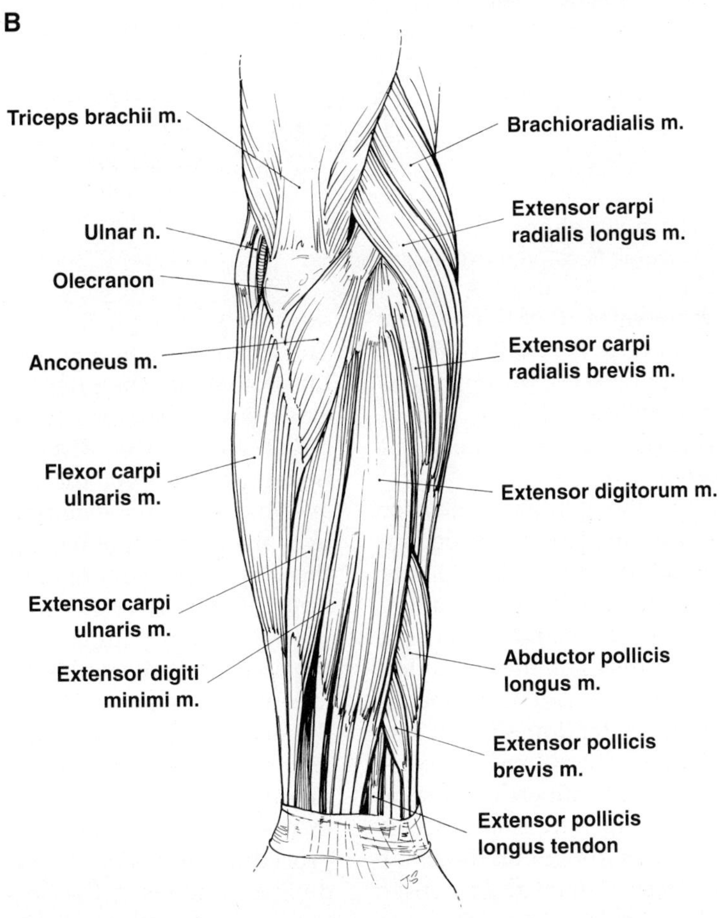

FIG 25–1 (cont.).
Extrinsic flexor and extensor tendons.

(Continued.)

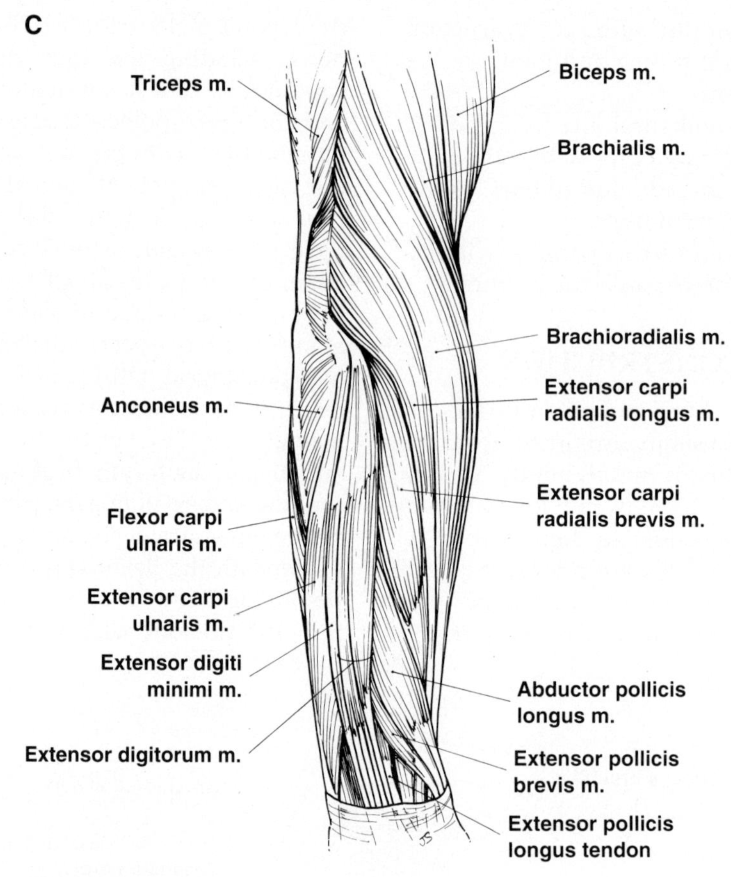

FIG 25–1 (cont.).
Extrinsic flexor and extensor tendons.

The ulnar nerve innervates all of the *intrinsic* muscles of the hand except for "half a LOAF," the first two *l*umbrical muscles, the *o*pponens pollicis, the *a*bductor pollicis brevis, and half of the *f*lexor pollicis brevis, which are innervated by the median nerve.

The tendons of the extrinsic extensor muscles originate from the lateral epicondyle and pass into the hand within six separate compartments across the dorsal surface of the wrist beneath the extensor retinaculum (Fig 25–2). The first compartment on the radial side of the wrist contains the extensor pollicis brevis and the multiple tendon slips of the abductor pollicis longus. The second compartment just radial to Lister's tubercle contains the extensor carpi radialis longus and brevis tendons. The third compartment on the ulnar side of Lister's tubercle contains the extensor pollicis longus. The extensor indicis proprius and the extensor digitorum communis tendons pass through the fourth compartment. The extensor digiti quinti is in the fifth, while in the sixth lies the extensor carpi ulnaris. All extrinsic extensor muscles are supplied by the radial nerve. The distal extensor tendons become flatter over the dorsal hand surface and insert into the extensor hood mechanism over the metacarpophalangeal (MP) joints of the digits. (For a more detailed discussion of upper extremity anatomy, see Chapter 20.)

All tendon injuries, if possible, should be repaired primarily within the first 7 to 10 days following injury. Occasionally other life-threatening injuries preclude early repair; this results in shortening of divided musculotendinous units, which then require less satisfactory secondary tendon grafting or transfer procedures to restore hand function. Sharply divided tendons in the hand or distal end of the forearm are best repaired primarily with 4-0 nylon or Prolene sutures and must be

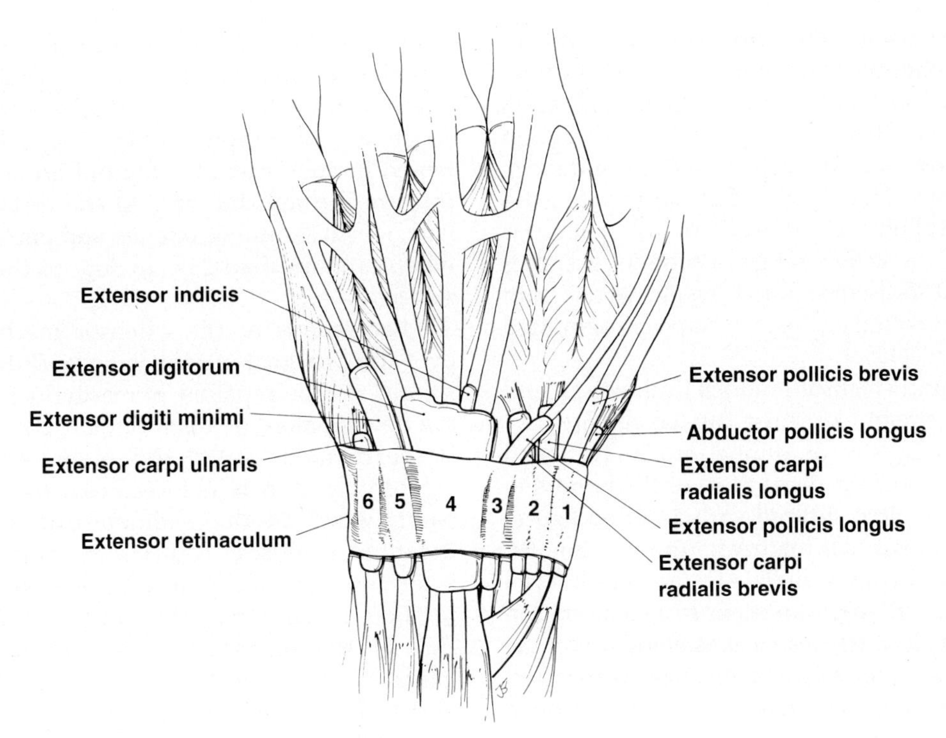

FIG 25–2.
Extensor retinaculum compartments.

repaired anatomically to restore their gliding function after surgery. Flexor tendons are best repaired by using a modified Kessler or Bunnel suture technique with precise approximation of the tendon ends (Fig 25–3). This creates a smooth uniform tendon repair that can be moved passively without resistance through a full range of digital motion at the time of repair. Flexor tendons repaired within the fibro-osseous tunnels of the digital flexor sheath (zone II) are especially prone to the development of adhesions with resultant decreased excursion after repair. Partial division of the fibro-osseous pulley mechanism is indicated after repair if full tendon excursion is not possible during passive digital flexion

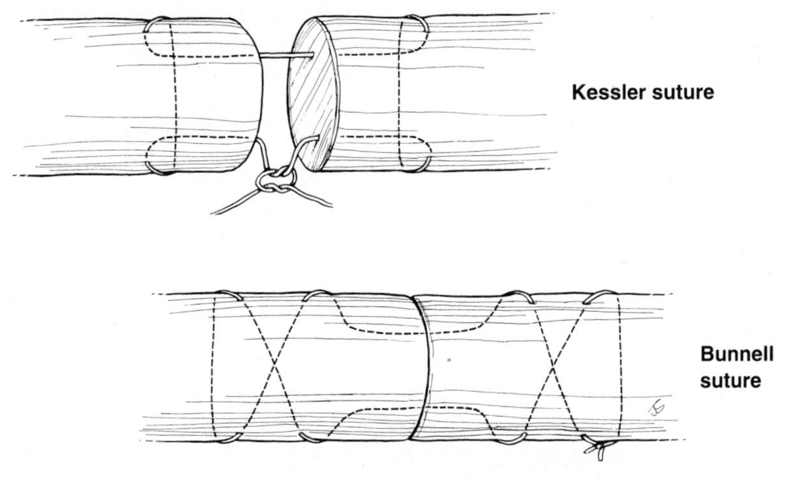

FIG 25–3.
Bunnel's and Kessler's sutures.

and extension. Protective dynamic rubber band splinting maintained for 4 to 5 weeks after surgery allows active digital extension and passive flexion and permits some tendon movement at the repair site to minimize adhesions. Five weeks after surgery the dynamic splints are removed, and the patient is started on active range-of-motion exercises without resistance for 1 week. Active and passive motion against resistance is permitted after 6 weeks.

Round extensor tendons in the distal end of the forearm or wrist can be repaired by using a Kessler or Bunnel stitch. Flattened tendons over the distal third of the hand and digits are often sutured with a buried figure-of-8 or horizontal mattress suture technique. Transection of the digital extensor mechanism over the DIP joint can occur from a laceration or from blunt trauma such as being hit on the tip of the finger with a baseball. Such an injury is termed a mallet finger (Fig 25–4). An open injury should be repaired primarily, while a closed injury may be splinted in extension for 8 weeks and will heal without an open repair. A lateral radiograph should always be obtained in such cases to rule out an articular fracture through the base of the distal phalanx, which should be opened and pinned if it involves more than 25% to 30% of the joint surface.

Lacerations of the extensor mechanism over the proximal interphalangeal (PIP) joint should also be repaired primarily to prevent the development of a boutonniere deformity. If the divided central slip of the extrinsic extensor tendon is not repaired, the lateral bands, which are the tendinous extensions of the intrinsic muscles contributing to PIP joint extension, may fall volar to the axis of digital rotation and become active PIP joint flexors. Pull of the intrinsic muscles through the lateral bands causes the injured finger to flex at the PIP joint when the patient attempts to extend the finger with secondary hyperextension of the DIP joint (Fig 25–5). Tendon repairs over the PIP joint should be splinted either internally or externally for 6 to 8 weeks in extension. More proximal extensor tendon repairs over the MP joints or dorsal hand surface should be splinted for 4 weeks with the wrist in extension and the MP joints in 30 to 45 degrees of flexion to prevent shortening of the collateral ligaments and residual joint stiffness. Some dynamic splinting programs are now available to improve tendon gliding after repair of distal forearm or dorsal hand extensor tendons. (For additional discussion

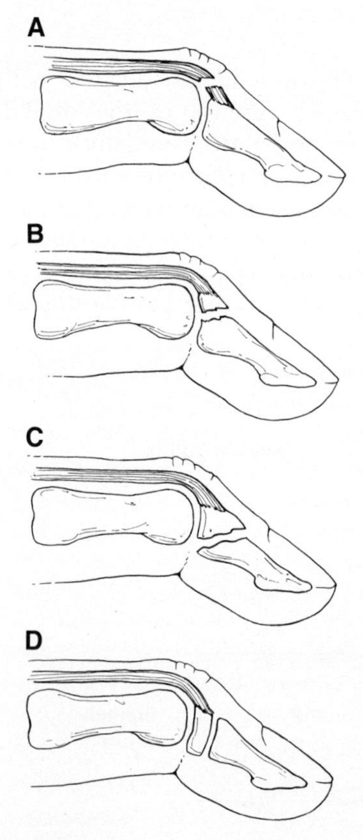

FIG 25–4.
Mallet finger.

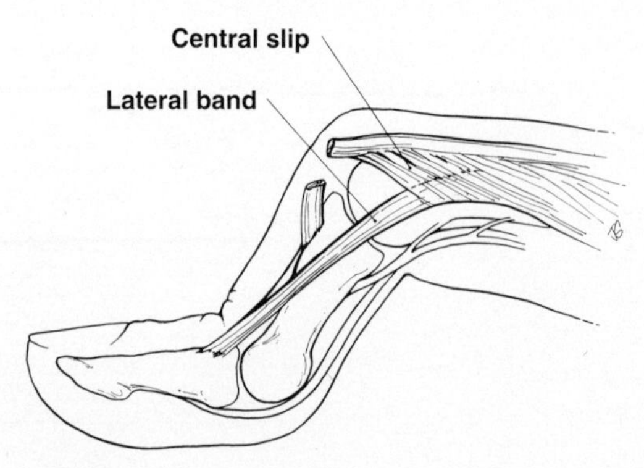

FIG 25–5.
Boutonniere deformity.

of tendon repair and reconstruction, see Chapter 23.)

Occasionally primary tendon repair is not possible, or the patient is referred several weeks or months after injury. Divided tendon ends undergo atrophy and proximal shortening, often making delayed primary repair impossible. Severe injuries over the flexor or extensor surface of the hand and forearm with extensive soft-tissue damage or loss may result in extensive scarring and/or require reconstruction with the use of a pedicle flap or microvascular free tissue transfer. Such patients may also require tendon reconstruction after adequate soft-tissue coverage has been restored. If primary repair is not possible at the time of the initial surgical procedure, the proximal divided tendon ends should be held to their proper length by suturing them to surrounding structures such as the fibro-osseous tendon sheath, the transverse carpal ligament, or the extensor retinaculum. A two-stage tendon reconstruction may then be possible by placing a silicone tendon replacement along the course of the missing tendon segment across the back of the hand or on the volar surface from the base of the distal phalanx through the digital sheath into the palm or wrist. Missing annular pulleys, especially A2 and A4, should be reconstructed at this stage by using segments of the discarded tendons or a strip of extensor retinaculum. A pseudosynovial sheath forms around the silicone rod over the next 3 months as the scar matures and the wound softens. Proximal and distal skin incisions are then made over the ends of the Silastic rod at a secondary procedure. A suitable tendon graft using an expendable tendon such as the palmaris longus, extensor indicis proprius, plantaris tendon from the calf, or a foot/toe extensor is used to replace the silicone rod. The tendon graft is sutured to the end of the silicone rod, which is then pulled through the previously created pseudosheath. The distal end of the tendon graft is sutured first into bone at the base of the distal phalanx by using a wire pullout suture on the flexor side or into the extensor hood mechanism over the MP joint on the extensor surface of the hand. The proximal tendon end is then identified, freed of surrounding scar, and pulled to its normal resting length. The tendon is checked for normal excursion by placing distal traction on the cut tendon end. The proximal end of the tendon graft is woven (Pulvertaft weave) two or three times through the end and sides of the proximally divided tendon end and the correct tension determined by sliding the graft back and forth through the weave. The proximal repair is held with a single suture and the correct tension checked by flexing and extending the wrist to determine whether the proper tension has been applied to the graft. The tendon weave is secured by several 4-0 mattress nonabsorbable sutures. Protective splinting is used after surgery to allow passive motion of the reconstructed musculotendinous units so as to minimize peritendinous adhesions. Unguarded active and passive motion is usually begun at about 6 weeks.

RECONSTRUCTION OF NERVE AND MUSCLE DEFICITS

Functional nerve and muscle loss usually results from trauma or surgical resection for malignancy. Patients with acute upper extremity injuries should have a thorough muscle function and sensory examination performed in the emergency room. Routine radiographs are indicated to rule out fractures or the presence of foreign bodies such as glass, gravel, or metal fragments. Wood splinters or thorns are poorly visualized on routine radiography and require more detailed evaluation with computed tomography (CT) or magnetic resonance imaging (MRI) for identification. Suspected vascular injuries can be identified by using angiography and are surgical emergencies when arterial disruption has produced distal extremity ischemia. Extremity CT and MRI are also useful to identify the extent of soft-tissue malignancies such as sarcomas.

Loss of muscle function can be secondary to nerve injury or transection of musculotendinous units. The surgeon must first properly identify the etiology of the problem by evaluating nerve and muscle function of the entire upper extremity before formulating a treatment plan. Muscle function for each musculotendinous unit in the upper extremity can be tested and graded on a scale of 0 to 5. When muscle function is in question, a follow-up examination with electromyography (EMG) and nerve conduction studies may be indicated to determine the presence or absence of muscle neurotization. Denervated muscles can be clearly identified 2 weeks following nerve transection by a lack of insertional activity or motor unit action potentials. An EMG and nerve conduction study can help identify the area of nerve trauma and differentiate a nerve injury that will recover spontaneously (neurapraxia) from a nerve transection (neurotmesis) that requires surgical exploration and repair.

Transection of a mixed motor and sensory nerve such as the median or ulnar nerve at the wrist will produce both a motor and a sensory deficit easily confirmed by physical examination. Most traumatic nerve lacerations should be repaired primarily by using either an epineurial or grouped fascicular microsurgical repair. The guiding principle for nerve repair is accurate fascicular alignment to permit axon sprouts to reenter the proper distal fascicles. This is particularly difficult when segments of nerve have been destroyed or resected during tumor ablation. Divided nerves should be repaired without tension by proximal and distal mobilization of the nerve ends or by use of interpositional nerve grafts or conduits when end-to-end repair is not possible. The composition and position of fascicles relative to each other change along the course of a nerve from the brachial plexus to the fingertip. Detailed maps of the fascicular anatomy have been created by Sunderland, Jabalay, Terzis, and others and are useful to the reconstructive surgeon when grafting large nerve defects. A useful technique for smaller defects is to map the size and position of fascicular groups in the proximal and distal nerve stumps and then connect the proximal fascicular groups to similar fascicular groups in the distal nerve stump. Conventional grafts are obtained from cutaneous nerves such as the sural nerve in the leg or, for smaller digital nerve reconstructions, the medial or lateral antebrachial cutaneous nerves in the forearm. Several smaller-diameter nerve cable grafts are often necessary to reconstruct a single larger-diameter peripheral nerve deficit and therefore require a longer donor nerve segment that is cut into appropriate lengths to bridge the nerve defect. Harvesting a sensory nerve produces an area of donor site anesthesia that should be discussed with the patient prior to surgery. Conventional nerve grafts provide devascularized collagen scaffolding containing Schwann cells through which axon sprouts travel to the distal nerve stump. They are best placed in a well-vascularized bed to ensure survival of their cellular elements by plasma imbibition and vascular ingrowth. Recently, larger-diameter nerve grafts revascularized by microsurgical technique have been employed in special circumstances to reconstruct large mixed nerve defects, especially across areas of poor vascularity. Vascularized nerve grafts from the sural and ulnar nerves have been used to reconstruct the median nerve but are technically difficult to carry out and result in increased donor site morbidity.

Occasionally, primary nerve repair is not possible because of other life-threatening injuries or an inability to determine the proximal and distal extent of nerve injury. Massive extremity trauma with soft-tissue crushing or avulsion may require delayed nerve repair after primary wound healing has been achieved. Such patients usually require multiple debridements and eventual graft or flap coverage. The divided nerve ends in such cases should be held to length by suturing to adjacent structures, with secondary nerve reconstruction done later by delayed primary repair or nerve grafting procedures. (For additional discussion of nerve repair, see Chapter 23.)

When nerve repair is not possible or has failed to restore muscle function, tendon transfer procedures may be used to regain lost function. A functioning musculotendinous unit is divided from its normal insertion and transferred into the tendon of the nonfunctioning muscle. Loss of radial nerve–innervated forearm muscles, for example, with loss of thumb, digital, and wrist extension, can be corrected by transferring median nerve–innervated musculotendinous units to the extensor surface. The traditional transfers include the palmaris longus to the extensor pollicis longus, the pronator teres to the extensor carpi radialis brevis, and the flexor carpi ulnaris to the extensor digitorum communis. Transfers from the extensor surface can be used to restore extrinsic forearm flexors: the brachioradialis to the flexor pollicis longus and the extensor carpi radialis longus to the flexor digitorum profundus of the index and long fingers. The flexor digitorum superficialis to the ring finger can be used to restore thumb opposition in patients with low median nerve injury and loss of thenar muscle function or to prevent digital MP joint hyperextension (clawing) in patients with low ulnar and/or median nerve loss. The transfers are done by rerouting the transferred muscles in a direct line to the paralyzed or lost muscles and weaving the donor tendons into the recipient tendons. Following sufficient immobilization after surgery the patient must then relearn to activate the transferred muscles to produce the desired hand function. Biofeedback programs are especially helpful for this purpose.

Occasionally extremity crush injuries or compartment syndromes can cause extrinsic muscle loss or ischemia and fibrosis. Such patients have frequently been treated by using a free gracilis muscle transfer to the volar or dorsal aspect of the forearm to replace lost or fibrotic flexor or extensor muscles. The gracilis is revascularized and then reinnervated by connecting the gracilis motor nerve to a branch of the normal motor nerve of the muscles whose function has been lost.

Before proceeding with any tendon transfer or a free muscle flap reconstruction, the total function of all muscles remaining in the extremity must be evaluated and the possibility of later improvement following nerve repair considered. Transferred muscles must have adequate muscle strength of at least grade 4 prior to transfer and should not produce a functional loss in the donor area. Patients who undergo major peripheral nerve repairs, tendon transfers, or free muscle flap techniques should be followed after surgery by experienced hand therapists to obtain optimal functional results.

RECONSTRUCTION OF MISSING PARTS

A partial or complete digital amputation results in varying degrees of functional loss. Efforts to reconstruct missing parts should be based on the individual functional needs of each patient.

The thumb is vital to proper hand function, especially when accompanied by congenital or traumatic deficits of other digits. Approximately 50% of normal hand function is lost when the thumb is missing.

The method chosen for thumb reconstruction is determined after a complete evaluation of hand function. The level of amputation and the length of the remaining stump are the most important elements in determining reconstruction, for example, metacarpal lengthening and web space deepening are appropriate with a thumb amputated near the interphalangeal (IP) joint, but not for one proximal to the MP joint. Several other factors must also be considered in deciding which surgical technique is best in a particular case, including the patient's age, occupation, and level of activity; the condition of other fingers; whether the deficit is congenital or acquired; and the sensibility and strength of the thumb stump. It is important to review the advantages and disadvantages of each surgical option with the patient, including any donor site morbidity, and to outline specific goals so that realistic expectations can be achieved after surgery.

Matev thumb metacarpal lengthening is useful in patients who desire increased length to improve pinch and power grasp. This procedure is also preferable for patients who do not want a donor site defect such as results from a toe-to-hand transfer. Three prerequisites are necessary for a successful outcome from metacarpal thumb lengthening. The skin on the stump tip must be durable and have satisfactory sensibility. At least two thirds and preferably the entire metacarpal must be present. There should be an adequate first web space with good skin quality. Patients who desire a thumbnail or require IP joint motion are not candidates. A surgical osteotomy of the metacarpal is performed after an external fixation device has been applied to the proximal and distal ends of the metacarpal. The thumb is gradually lengthened by distracting the external fixation device over a period of several weeks. In children the metacarpal deficit created by lengthening may ossify by itself but usually requires a secondary bone graft in adults. Deepening of the first web space may functionally lengthen the thumb in patients with more proximal amputations. This can be accomplished after thumb length has been restored by Z-plasties, a local flap, or a skin graft. The complications of distraction lengthening include pin tract infection, angulation, and nonunion of the metacarpal.

Microsurgical toe-to-hand transfer, initially reported by Cobett and later popularized by Buncke, O'Brien, May, and Morrison, is now the mainstay of thumb reconstruction. The great toe has many similarities to the thumb and is preferred over second toe transfer. The toe may be transferred in toto, including the IP joint and flexor and extensor tendons, or as a partial-toe transfer, which more closely resembles a normal thumb as described by Morrison. Complete toe-to-hand transfer is the procedure of choice for deficits at or proximal to the MP joint. The main disadvantage of this procedure is that it requires microsurgical technique with a 5% failure rate and produces a donor defect that may be unacceptable to some patients.

Prior to transfer, the blood supply to the foot, including the dorsalis pedis, first dorsal metatarsal artery, and plantar vessels, must be evaluated to determine the dominant blood supply to the toe. This can usually be accomplished by physical examination or by the use of a Doppler flow probe but may require angiography in some cases. The transferred toe is dissected to the desired length and may include the distal phalanx, proximal phalanx, and portions of the metacarpal, depending on the length necessary for thumb reconstruction. The toe is dissected free on its dominant vascular pedicle, transferred to the hand, and revascularized by microsurgical technique, usually to the radial artery in the snuffbox and to the cephalic vein. The digital nerves to the thumb should be connected to the digital nerves in the toe to provide transfer sensibility. A whole-toe transfer has the advantage of including the IP and sometimes the MP joint, while the great toe wraparound procedure takes only a portion of the circumference of the great toe soft tissue and nail. The Morrison procedure produces a much more aesthetic thumb but requires the use of a cortical cancellous bone graft to maintain length and does not transfer joint function. Several modifications of this procedure have been described that permit versatility in tailoring the flap to more closely resemble the opposite normal thumb.

Pollicization procedures that involve transfer of a digit (usually the index finger) to the thumb position are most useful in congenital thumb absence. This method may also be used for traumatic thumb loss when the index finger has been amputated through the middle phalanx. Pollicization of the index finger has the added advantage, in congenital cases, of transferring normal sensibility from the index finger to the thumb position. In congenital absences surgery, is usually done in the first 12 to 18 months of life to allow the patient to gain normal thumb use patterns. The index finger is usually divided through the metacarpal, with the MP joint serving as the carpometacarpal joint for the new thumb. The digit is rotated approximately 120 degrees into a palmar plane to permit opposition to the remaining fingers.

Finally, patients with amputations of multiple digits may be candidates for digital reconstruction using second and/or third toe transfers. The techniques and principles involved in digital reconstruction are similar to those used for the thumb. Single or bilateral second toe-to-hand transfers are indicated in patients with amputations of two or more fingers, especially to the radial digits to restore pinch and power grasp function. Sacrifice of a single second toe usually produces minimal cosmetic or functional loss. Transfer of two adjacent toes, however, may significantly narrow the foot and can compromise foot function. Second toe transfers are best used in patients with distal amputations through the proximal or middle phalanx. A small portion of the great or second toe pulp and/or toenail bed may be used to reconstruct fingertip nail bed injuries. This is technically demanding microsurgery and should be performed only by experienced surgeons in selected cases.

RECONSTRUCTION OF SOFT-TISSUE DEFICITS

Soft-tissue loss in the hand and upper extremity usually occurs following trauma. The glabrous skin on the volar hand surface is specially suited for pinch and grasp function and contains special sensory receptor sites, the pacinian corpuscles, Meissner corpuscles, and Merkel cell neurite disks, that are not found in other types of skin. Volar soft-tissue loss is best replaced with similar tissue whenever possible. The skin on the dorsal hand surface is thinner, mobile, and more easily avulsed. Exposed extensor tendons without peritenon cannot be skin-grafted and may require flap coverage. More extensive soft-tissue loss is best treated by serial debridements at 2- to 3-day intervals followed by split-thickness skin grafting or flap closure.

Superficial skin loss from the volar surface of the fingertip without exposed bone may be closed with a split-thickness skin graft from the hypothenar eminence. More proximal injuries with exposed bone usually require flap coverage. Dorsally directed amputations with loss of the sterile nail bed may be treated by removing the remaining nail plate and reconstructing the nail bed with a split nail bed graft from uninjured sterile nail bed or, for larger areas, with a split nail bed graft from the great toe. Transverse midnail amputations are best repaired by using a V-Y or volar surface advancement flap (Fig 25–6). These flaps are cut in a V from the volar surface as described by Atasoy or bilaterally from the sides of the digit as described by Cutler. The fibrous septa connecting palmar skin to the underlying bone are freed while preserving digital nerve and artery branches. The flap over the tip defect is advanced to form a Y closure at the donor site. The flap is sutured without tension to prevent vascular compromise. A volar advancement flap is useful for thumb tip amputations (Moberg flap) and is elevated by bilateral incisions in the midlateral lines and elevation of the flap from the flexor tendon sheath while preserving the digital nerve and arterial connections to the flap. The thumb is flexed to allow flap advancement over the tip defect. This method is less satisfactory for fingertip amputations because the flexed position of the digit may cause digital stiffness. Volarly directed digital tip amputations with exposed bone are usually treated by using a cross-finger flap from the dorsal surface of the middle phalanx of an adjacent digit. The flap is elevated at the level of the extensor tendon peritenon and based along the midlateral line on the lateral side of the donor digit. The injured finger is flexed and the flap turned over like a book page to close the tip defect (Fig 25–7). The donor site is closed with a full-thickness skin graft usually from the groin. The flap is divided and inset approximately 2 weeks later.

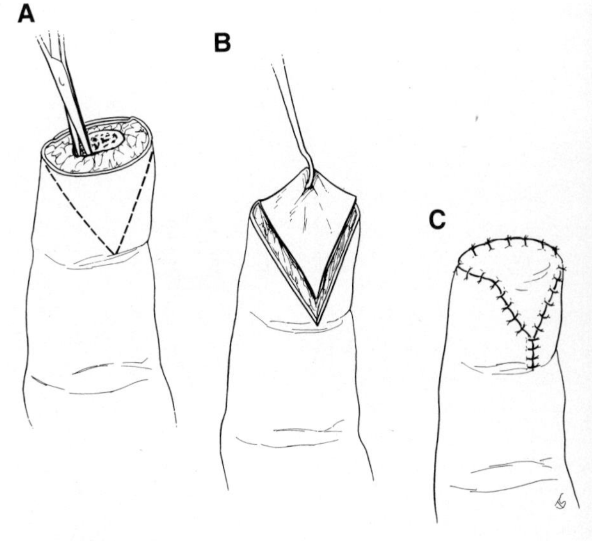

FIG 25–6.
V-Y flap.

Loss of the volar thumb tip pad is usually treated by using an innervated island flap either based on the first dorsal metacarpal artery and a superficial branch of the radial nerve from the dorsal surface of the index finger or less commonly based on a single digital artery and nerve from the ring or long finger. Island flaps are more difficult to dissect and require care to preserve flap blood supply. (For additional discussion of fingertip injuries, see Chapter 23.)

Larger areas of soft-tissue loss involving

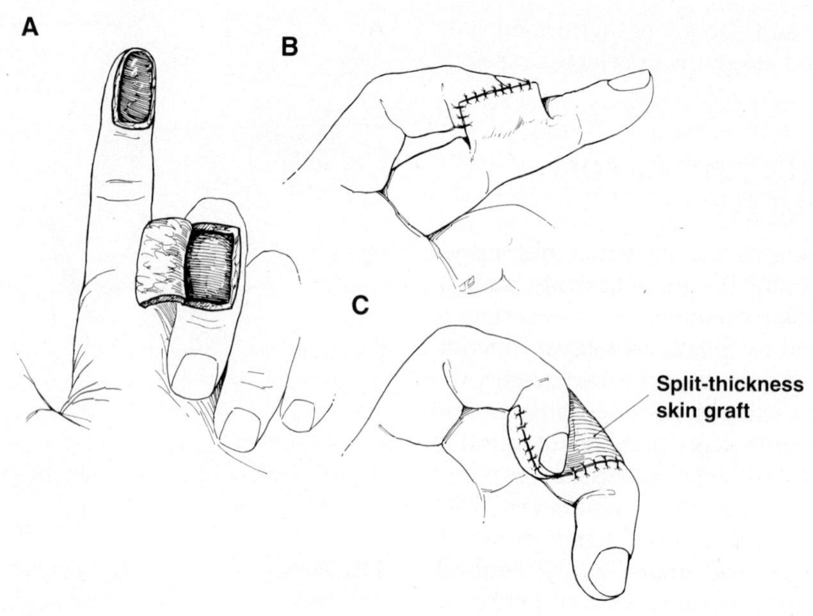

FIG 25–7.
Cross finger flap.

the dorsal or palmar hand surface are commonly seen following thermal trauma or more severe crush or avulsion injuries. Thermal injuries are usually treated by early tangential or full-thickness eschar excision and split-skin grafting within the first week following injury. Severe crush or avulsion injuries are often associated with injury to underlying tendons, nerves, and bones, which are usually repaired at the initial surgical debridement. The timing and choice of flap coverage depend on many factors, including the site, the size of the area to be covered, the thickness of tissue required for reconstruction, and the ability to perform later secondary reconstructive procedures beneath the flap. Flap coverage can be performed at the time of the initial debridement if all devitalized tissue has been removed, but coverage must often be delayed until serial debridements have produced a surgically clean wound.

The most commonly used flap for larger soft-tissue defects of the hand is the pedicle groin flap described by McGregor and based on the superficial circumflex iliac vessels. The flap is elevated from the groin, tubed at its base, and attached to the injured hand. This flap has the disadvantage of placing the hand in a dependent position, which can allow edema formation and requires a secondary procedure for division of the pedicle 2 to 3 weeks following the initial procedure. Recently, microsurgical free tissue transfer has allowed reconstruction of large soft-tissue hand defects with more suitable tissue. The deltoid and lateral arm fasciocutaneous flaps allow reinnervation of the flap after transfer to provide some return of sensibility to the injured hand. The temporalis fascia flap covered with a split-thickness skin graft provides a thin well-vascularized flap to cover dorsal hand injuries and has little donor site morbidity. Free tissue transfers have the added advantage of allowing the hand to be kept in an elevated position after surgery, decreasing edema, and allowing early mobilization of injured tendons. They can be tailored more precisely to fit the dimensions of the defect and often require fewer revisions than standard pedicle flaps. All flaps can be partially elevated at a secondary procedure to allow later tendon or nerve reconstruction beneath the flap. Larger areas of soft-tissue loss in the forearm may require the use of larger flaps such as the latissimus dorsi or scapular fasciocutaneous flap.

JOINT DEFORMITY

Joint deformity may result from traumatic injury, infection, or diseases such as rheumatoid arthritis, osteoarthritis, or Dupuytren's disease. Scarring and contracture of the supporting joint tissues, including the volar plate, collateral ligaments, and joint capsule, can create digital stiffness. Adhesions of extrinsic flexor or extensor tendons may also result in digital stiffness. Persistent joint pain usually implies bony destruction, as is often seen with osteoarthritis. A thorough patient history, complete hand examination, and x-ray study are necessary to formulate an accurate diagnosis that will ultimately determine the surgical treatment plan.

Preventive splinting is an important adjunct to repair and/or replacement techniques. Distal joints can be protected by splinting in a safe position with the IP joints extended and the MP joints flexed at 45 to 90 degrees. This keeps the collateral ligaments stretched, minimizes edema formation within the joint space, and ultimately reduces the likelihood of stiffness and contracture.

Flexion contractures are more common at the PIP joint, while extension contractures are more common at the MP joints. Minimal PIP flexion contractures seen early after injury or surgery can often be corrected by dynamic splinting in extension with a joint jack or wire foam spring splint. More severe or long-standing contractures often do not respond to splinting and require surgical correction.

Shortening of the checkrein ligaments is usually present in digits with a PIP joint flexion contracture. The checkrein ligaments form proximal to the volar plate and become shortened and contracted when the PIP joint is held in a flexed position (Fig 25–8). Surgical correction through a volar approach requires division of the checkrein ligaments, which allows the volar plate to slide distally and the PIP joint to extend. An ulnar-based Brunner incision and retraction of the flexor sheath and tendons provide good exposure to the volar plate and checkrein ligaments. A Z- or Y-V–plasty may be necessary to provide skin lengthening to allow full extension of the joint with long-standing contracture. Early active range of motion is encouraged postoperatively.

Extension contractures of the PIP joint are rare and usually result from extrinsic conditions such as extensor or flexor tendon adhesions. Painful PIP joint extension contractures may follow volar plate avulsion injuries. If range-of-motion therapy and splinting do not help, a dorsal capsulotomy may be indicated. This can be accomplished through a dorsolateral approach involving elevation of the lateral bands, incision of the capsule, and passive flexion of the joint. Concomitant tenolysis or surgical reattachment of the distal volar plate is carried out when indicated. Pulling on the flexor digitorum profundus tendon through a counter incision at the wrist confirms full PIP joint flexion, especially following tenolysis.

Extension contractures more commonly occur at the MP joint and are usually secondary to fibrosis of the capsule and collateral ligaments. Long-standing contractures generally do not respond to splinting and necessitate surgical release of the dorsal capsule. A dorsal transverse incision is made over the MP joint, and the capsule is exposed by division of the ulnar sagittal band and retraction of the extensor mechanism. An incision is made through the capsule, and the joint is passively flexed. It may be necessary to partially divide

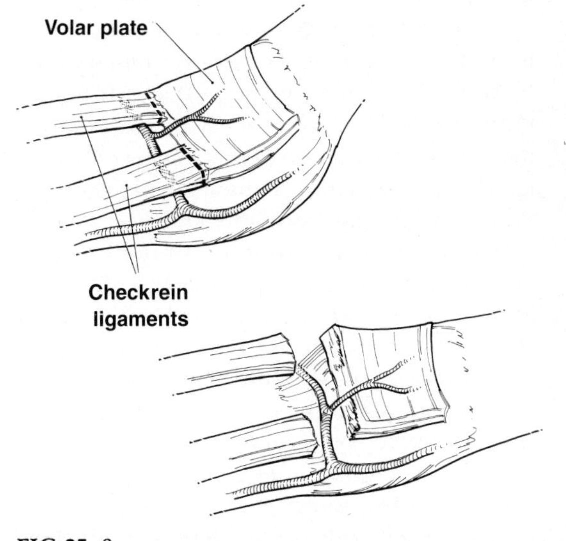

FIG 25–8.
Checkrein ligaments.

the collateral ligaments near their attachment to the metacarpal head in order to achieve full passive flexion. Early mobilization and night splinting in flexion are begun postoperatively.

Bony degeneration of the joint may be secondary to trauma such as crushing or severe articular fracture or to synovitis associated with rheumatoid arthritis or osteoarthritis. Treatment for a painful degenerative joint depends on the etiology and location of the disease as well as the age and occupation of the patient. Surgical options for treatment include arthrodesis, soft-tissue arthroplasty, or joint replacement with a silicone prosthesis or free joint transfer from the toe. Prosthetic joint replacement is usually reserved for patients with isolated PIP or multiple MP joint involvement who desire pain-free motion. Young patients in heavy labor occupations are best treated with nonprosthetic techniques because of the limited life span and susceptibility to wear and tear of present-day silicone implants. The prosthesis most commonly used is the Swanson silicone joint, which is surgically inserted following joint resection by inserting the limbs of the implant into the cored-out proximal and distal marrow cavities. This is accomplished by a volar or lateral approach at the PIP joint or by a dorsal approach over the MP joints. Use of cemented prostheses has fallen out of favor because of long-term problems with loosening and material failure.

Arthrodesis in a position of function is indicated in patients who desire stability over motion, particularly at the DIP and PIP joint locations. Arthrodesis at the MP level is rarely indicated since motion at this joint is critical to good hand function. Patients with rheumatoid arthritis and both PIP and MP disease may be treated by arthrodesis of the PIP joint and Swanson silicone arthroplasties of the MP joints. It is important to remember that wrist stabilization procedures are a prerequisite to the treatment of MP and IP joint disease in rheumatoid patients.

Soft-tissue arthroplasty using the volar plate or a tendon interposition should be considered in young patients with isolated posttraumatic MP joint destruction. Soft-tissue arthroplasty following trapezium resection as described by Burton and others is the preferred technique to treat degenerative arthritis of the thumb carpometacarpal joint; however, silicone arthroplasty or basilar joint fusion procedures are still used in selected cases.

Vascularized free joint transfer is an option for joint replacement in young patients. This technique is best suited for the MP joint since results from PIP joint replacement have been disappointing because of the limited motion obtained after surgery. The MP joint of the second toe may be transferred by microvascular technique because of its good lateral stability in addition to the presence of two growth plates. This microvascular transfer is based on the first dorsal metatarsal artery, which is sutured to the radial artery. The advantages of free joint transfer include durability and growth potential in young patients, satisfactory motion of 30 to 65 degrees, and the ability to transfer composite tissues such as bone, tendon, and/or skin to the hand.

RECONSTRUCTION OF BONY DEFICITS

Bony defects of the upper extremity range from simple fracture nonunions to segmental bone loss, usually following trauma, tumor resection, or osteomyelitis. Reconstructive options include the use of autogenous or allograft bone or vascularized bone transfer. The first consideration in bone reconstruction is the condition of the recipient bed and soft tissues. Unstable traumatized or irradiated tissue must be replaced with vascularized tissue in the form of local or distant flaps. Bony reconstruction is carried out once soft-tissue coverage is obtained. Most bone defects in the hand such as a fracture nonunion are relatively small and can be treated by resecting the nonunion back to bleeding bone and placing an autogenous cortical cancellous bone graft from the distal end of the radius or iliac crest with K-wire fixation. Defects in the wrist should be treated by partial or total carpal arthrodesis with cancellous bone. Free vascularized bone transfer using the fibula provides a good option for reconstructing large defects of the radius or ulna, particularly if the vascularity of the surrounding tissues is compromised.

RECONSTRUCTION FOLLOWING BRACHIAL PLEXUS INJURY

Disruption of the brachial plexus in adults usually occurs following high-energy trauma in motor vehicle or motorcycle accidents. In infants it is most commonly seen as obstetric palsy associated with traumatic injuries that occur during delivery. Management of such proximal nerve injuries is a reconstructive challenge that is demanding.

The brachial plexus is formed from nerve roots that exit the spinal cord in the neck above the fifth, sixth, and seventh cervical vertebrae (C5–7) and below the seventh cervical (C8) and first thoracic vertebrae (T1) (Fig 25–9). Roots C5 and C6 combine to form the upper trunk, C7 continues as the middle trunk, and C8 and T1 combine to form the lower trunk and emerge between the anterior and posterior scalene muscles in the lower part of the posterior cervical triangle. The three trunks divide into the anterior and posterior divisions as they pass beneath the clavicle. The three posterior divisions unite to form the posterior cord (C5–8, T1) behind the axillary artery. The anterior divisions of the upper and middle trunks combine to form the lateral cord (C5–7) lateral to the axillary artery, and the anterior division of the lower trunk continues as the medial cord (C8–T1). Most major peripheral nerves in the upper extremity arise from the cords, including the axillary and radial nerves from the posterior cord, the ulnar nerve as a continuation of the medial cord, the musculocutaneous nerve as a continuation of the lateral cord, and the median nerve as a combination of branches from the medial and lateral cords. The long thoracic nerve originates from the fifth, sixth, and seventh cervical roots and innervates the serratus anterior muscle. The dorsal scapular nerve to the levator scapulae and rhomboid muscles arises from the fifth cervical root. When these muscles are not functioning after injury, it suggests a more proximal plexus injury or root avulsion and diminishes the chances for successful reconstruction; this contrasts with more distal injuries, which can often be repaired or grafted. Similarly, the presence of Horner's syndrome suggests C8–T1 root avulsion. The suprascapular nerve (C5–6) is a branch of the upper trunk above the clavicle and innervates the supraspinatus

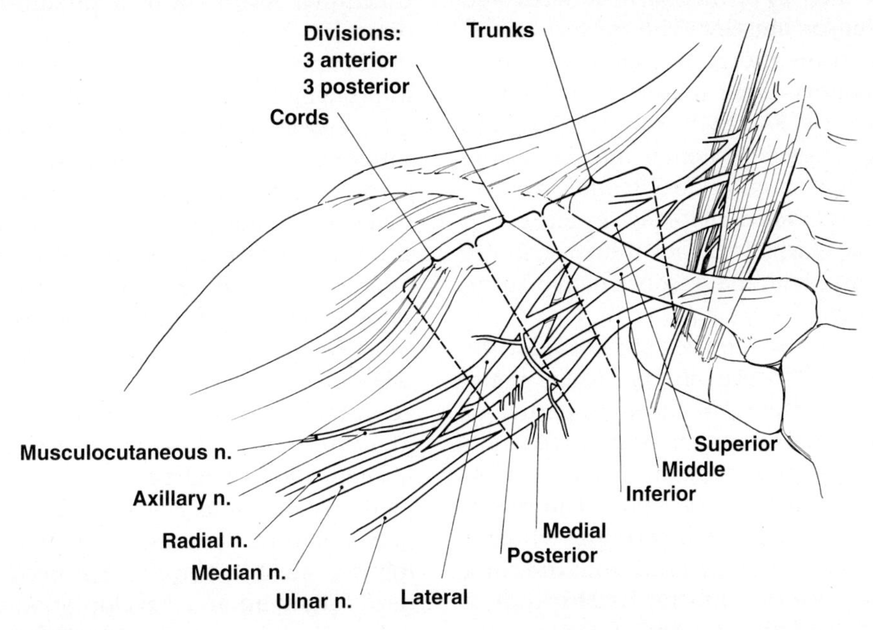

FIG 25–9.
Brachial plexus.

and infraspinatus muscles. These muscles will be spared in injuries distal to the upper trunk. The lateral pectoral nerve (C5–6) emerges from the lateral cord beneath the head of the pectoralis minor muscle to innervate the clavicular head of the pectoralis major muscle. The medial pectoral nerve originates from the medial cord and along with branches from the lateral pectoral nerve supplies the sternal head of the pectoralis muscle. Paralysis of the clavicular head of the pectoralis muscle suggests injury to the lateral pectoral nerve or lateral cord, while loss of the sternal head implies injury to both the lateral and medial pectoral nerves or medial and lateral cords. The musculocutaneous nerve arises from the lateral cord and passes through the coracobrachialis muscle to innervate that muscle as well as the brachialis and biceps muscles. Paralysis of these muscles suggests musculocutaneous nerve or lateral cord injury. The axillary nerve originates from the posterior cord, passes behind the humerus, and exits with the posterior humeral circumflex artery through the quadrangular space to innervate the deltoid muscle and supply sensation to the posterior shoulder skin above the deltoid triceps grove. The posterior cord continues into the arm as the radial nerve innervating the triceps and all of the extrinsic wrist and digital extensor muscles. The posterior cord also gives off the thoracodorsal nerve (C6–8) to the latissimus dorsi muscle and the subscapular nerve (C5–7) to the subscapularis and teres major muscles. Manual muscle testing and individual muscle EMG studies are important to determine the exact location and extent of a brachial plexus injury prior to initiating any definitive reconstructive surgical treatment.

Brachial plexus injuries are classified by the degree of nerve injury from nerve contusion (neurapraxia), through partial or complete internal disruption of axons (axonotmesis) to complete nerve transection (neurotmesis), and by the level of injury. The reconstructive surgeon must determine whether nerve roots have been avulsed from the cord, completely transected, or stretched to produce axonotmesis and an incontinuity lesion.

When nerve roots have been avulsed from the cord, motor and sensory function is lost, but wallerian degeneration of sensory axons does not occur because they originate in the dorsal sensory ganglion, which is still intact and results in normal sensory fiber conduction studies. Root avulsion injury cannot be repaired but may be treated in selected cases with neurotization procedures, usually by using the intercostal nerves. Management of open injuries to the brachial plexus are uncommon and are usually treated by direct epineural repair. If the level of nerve injury cannot be determined at the time of the initial surgical exploration, delayed primary nerve repair or nerve grafting may be indicated. The longitudinal extent of nerve injury can usually be determined by the third week after injury, and because little scar has formed, this may be an ideal time for exploration and/or reconstruction.

The most common type of plexus injury is produced by a closed traction mechanism that results in an incontinuity lesion or root avulsion. Patients with incontinuity lesions are usually observed for 3 to 6 months for clinical patterns of recovery. Physical therapy programs should be initiated to provide passive digital, wrist, elbow, and shoulder motion. Patients who show an orderly progression of functional return from a proximal to distal direction along the nerve course are observed until improvement ceases. If there is no improvement in 3 to 6 months or improvement ceases, surgical exploration is indicated. Intraoperative nerve stimulation is useful to identify nerves with intact axons or fascicles that can sometimes be improved by neurolysis. When there is loss of nerve substance, cable nerve grafting procedures may restore some degree of function. Return of nerve function after brachial plexus repair usually takes several months and is never normal. Occasionally secondary procedures such as joint fusions or tendon transfers are performed after all nerve regeneration is complete, usually 2 to 3 years after repair. Surgeons that treat patients with brachial plexus injuries must anticipate the need for long-term follow-up and develop good physician/patient relationships to ensure the best possible functional results.

SUGGESTED READING

Beckenbaugh RD, Linscheid RL: Arthroplasty in the hand and wrist, in *Operative Hand Surgery,* ed 2. New York, Churchill Livingstone, 1988.

Burkhalter WE: Median nerve palsy, in *Operative Hand Surgery,* ed 2. New York, Churchill Livingstone, 1988.

Ellis PR, Tsai TM: Management of the traumatized joint of the finger. *Clin Plast Surg* 1989; 16:457–473.

Green DP: Radial nerve palsy, in *Operative Hand Surgery,* ed 2. New York, Churchill Livingstone, 1988.

Leffert RD: Brachial plexus, in *Operative Hand Surgery,* ed 2. New York, Churchill Livingstone, 1988.

MacKinnon SE, Dellon AL: Brachial plexus injuries, in *Surgery of the Peripheral Nerve.* New York, Thieme Medical Publishers, 1988.

Manktelow RT: Free muscle transfers, in *Operative Hand Surgery,* ed 2. New York, Churchill Livingstone, 1988.

May JW: Microvascular great toe to hand transfer for reconstruction of the amputated thumb, in McCarthy JG, May JW, Littler JW (eds): *Plastic Surgery.* Philadelphia, WB Saunders, 1990.

Omer GE Jr: Ulnar nerve palsy, in *Operative Hand Surgery,* ed 2. New York, Churchill Livingstone, 1988.

Russell RC: Management of soft tissue injuries of the upper extremity, including hands and digits, in *Textbook of Plastic, Maxillofacial and Reconstructive Surgery,* ed 2. Baltimore, Williams & Wilkins, 1992.

Weiland AJ: Small joint arthrodesis and bony defect reconstruction, in McCarthy JG, May JW, Littler JW (eds): *Plastic Surgery.* Philadelphia, WB Saunders, 1990.

PART VI

Plastic Surgery of the Trunk and Breast

Chapter 26

Anatomy/Physiology/Embryology

David A. Janssen, M.D.
Mary H. McGrath, M.D.

CONTENTS

NOTE: The material in this chapter is frequently covered during the prerequisite training period of many plastic surgery residents. This chapter should serve as a valuable review of important material in such cases. For residents who have not mastered this material previously, this chapter is essential.

CHAPTER OBJECTIVE

At the end of this chapter the resident has a thorough knowledge of the anatomy, physiology, and embryology of the trunk and breast and applies this information to the comprehensive management of a variety of problems in these anatomic areas.

LEARNER OBJECTIVES

On completion of this chapter the resident

1. **Demonstrates knowledge of the musculature, blood supply, lymphatic drainage, and innervation of the trunk, abdominal wall, and breast.**
2. **Demonstrates knowledge of the glandular structure and function of the breasts and understands hormonal influence on breast development and function.**
3. **Recognizes differences in breast structure and function in adolescence, the reproductive years, pregnancy, lactation, and menopause.**
4. **Understands the relationships between breast diseases and breast physiology.**
5. Is familiar with embryonic development of the trunk, abdominal wall, and breast.
6. Is familiar with the structure and function of the male as well as female breast.

CLINICAL PRACTICE ACTIVITIES

During the training program, the resident **performs aesthetic and reconstructive surgery on the trunk, breast, and abdomen.**

EMBRYOLOGY OF THE TRUNK AND ABDOMINAL WALL

Cutaneous innervation over the trunk is provided in dermatomes, which are defined as the area of skin supplied by a single spinal nerve and its spinal ganglion distributed in segmental bands supplying the chest and abdominal wall. Dermatomes are derived from lateral somite migration of dermal, lateral plate mesodermal, and neural crest cells. On the chest wall, the intercostal nerves are direct continuations of the anterior primary rami of the upper 11 thoracic spinal nerves. The intercostal nerves supply the intercostal muscles and give anterior and lateral branches that supply the overlying skin, including that of the breast. The lower six intercostal nerves continue past the costal margin into the anterior abdominal wall and are therefore identified as thoracoabdominal nerves. Dermatomes and cutaneous nerve areas, the area of skin supplied by a peripheral nerve, have considerable overlap on the trunk. This is because there may be significant mixing of innervation between adjacent dorsal nerve roots; thus a dorsal root segmental nerve can be cut, and there may be only a slight deficit in the associated dermatome.

During development, the skeletal musculature of the chest wall is derived from myotomes, with the exception of certain neck muscles derived from branchial mesenchyme and certain of the limb muscles. Each myotome divides into dorsal and ventral regions, the former innervated by the dorsal ramus of the corresponding spinal nerve and the latter migrating ventrally in the body wall. The myogenic masses derived from the myotomes may divide and remain separate, or they may fuse to form sheets of muscles such as the external abdominal oblique or the transversus abdominis muscles. Some muscles may also migrate in a rostrocaudal direction, as in the case of the latissimus dorsi, which is derived from the lower cervical myotomes and is innervated accordingly.

The intercostal arteries originate in two groups, anterior and posterior, and all except those to the first two costal spaces are branches of the thoracic aorta (Fig 26–1). The anterosuperior intercostal arteries extend to

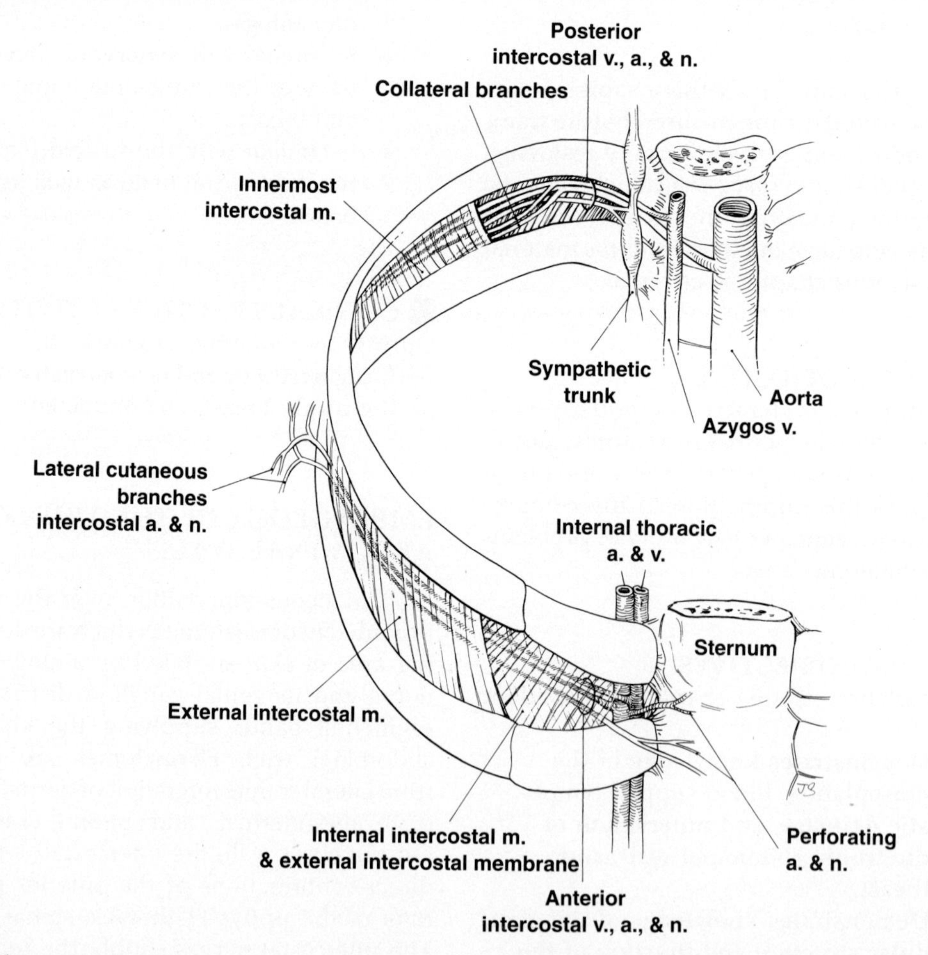

FIG 26–1.
Diagram of a segment of the chest wall showing the relationship of structures to the ribs. (From Bland KI, Copeland EM: The Breast: *Comprehensive Management of Benign and Malignant Disease.* Philadelphia, WB Saunders, 1991, p 26. Used by permission.)

the region of the costochondral junction from the internal mammary artery. The superior epigastric artery arises as a branch of the internal mammary artery at the lateral aspect of the xiphoid. The deep inferior epigastric artery arises from the common femoral artery and is the dominant vascular supply for the rectus abdominis muscle.

The lymphatic vessels of the thoracic wall include the more superficial lymphatic channels that drain the skin and superficial fascia and the deeper lymphatic vessels that drain the muscles of the thorax, the intercostal spaces, and the diaphragm. The superficial lymphatic channels drain the back region superficial to the trapezius and latissimus dorsi and course anteriorly to form 10 to 12 trunks that terminate in the subscapular group of axillary lymph nodes. The vessels that drain the pectoral region, including the periphery of the mammary gland, course dorsally to the pectoral group of nodes. Others near the lateral aspect of the sternum pass inward beneath the rib cartilages and end in the parasternal nodes. The lymphatic drainage of the anterior of the abdomen is divided by Sappey's line, a 5-cm band-like area extending from just above the umbilicus toward the L2–3 level. Above this line, lymphatic drainage is to the axillary nodes, while drainage below this line is to the superficial inguinal lymph nodes.

INTERNAL ANATOMY OF THE TRUNK

The thoracic wall is composed of skeletal and muscular components. Eleven pairs of external and internal intercostal muscles provide motor function between the ribs and are superficial to the subcostal and transverse thoracic muscles on the internal surface of the thoracic wall. All of these muscles are innervated by the intercostal nerves that are associated with them; these nerves also supply sensibility to the overlying skin. The anterior abdominal wall is considered to have two parts. The anterolateral portion is composed of the external oblique, internal oblique, and the transverse abdominal muscles, and the midline portion is composed of the rectus abdominis and pyramidalis muscles. The anterolateral muscles are roughly parallel as they approach their insertion on the rectus sheath and are perpendicular to the rectus abdominis muscle. The rectus abdominis originates from the sixth, seventh, and eighth costal cartilages and inserts into the superior ramus of the pubis, the symphysis pubis, and the linea alba below. The pyramidalis muscle is absent in one or both sides in 10% to 20% of subjects.

The rectus abdominis muscle is enclosed in a sheath that is the aponeurosis of the anterolateral abdominal muscles passing anterior and posterior to the muscle and attaching medially to the linea alba (Fig 26–2). The linea semilunaris corresponds to the lateral aspect of the rectus sheath. In the lower fourth of the abdomen, the aponeurosis of the internal oblique and transversus abdominis passes anterior to the muscle, which is then bound posteriorly by the internal lamina of the transversalis fascia only. The dividing line is the linea semicircularis, the arcuate line or line of Douglas, which marks the level at which the rectus sheath loses its thick posterior wall. Thus, excisions of the rectus sheath with muscle removal, as in transverse rectus abdominis myocutaneous (TRAM) flap development, result in loss of support below the semicircular line and require special closure methods to avoid abdominal wall weakness. Blood supply to the rectus abdominis is primarily from the deep inferior epigastric vessel of the common femoral artery. The superior epigastric artery is a nondominant vascular supply to the rectus abdominis in humans. Innervation to the rectus abdominis is a segmental one, through the 5th to the 12th intercostal nerves.

The latissimus dorsi muscle originates from the spinous processes of the lower six vertebrae and the iliac crest. It inserts on the lower aspect of the intertubercular groove of the humerus and is supplied by the thoracodorsal nerve. The thoracodorsal artery, a 2.5-mm-diameter branch of the subscapular artery, is the dominant blood supply. Injury or resection of the latissimus results in weakness of medial rotation and adduction of the shoulder.

The serratus anterior muscle originates

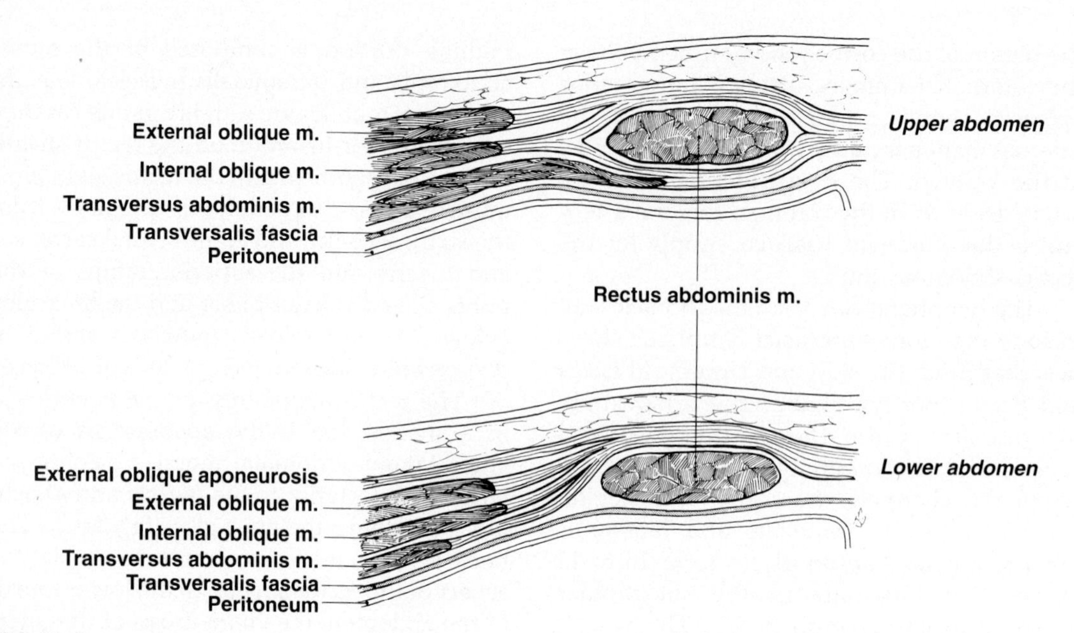

FIG 26–2.
Transverse sections of the anterior abdominal wall above and below the umbilicus.

from the seventh through tenth ribs anteriorly and inserts on the costal surface of the vertebral border of the scapula. It has a dual blood supply from the lateral thoracic artery and a branch of the thoracodorsal artery. Motor innervation is by the long thoracic nerve; injury to this nerve or use of this muscle as a flap results in "winging" of the scapula.

The pectoralis major muscle takes origin from the sternum, the medial half of the clavicle, and the first five ribs and inserts on the intertubercular groove of the humerus. Its blood supply is from the thoracoacromial branch of the axillary artery. Innervation is provided by the medial and lateral pectoral nerves from the brachial plexus.

The trapezius muscle originates from a broad aponeurosis from the occiput to the cervical and all thoracic vertebral spines. It inserts on an area from the spine of the scapula to the tip of the clavicle. The dominant blood supply is from the transverse cervical artery, a branch of the thyrocervical trunk, and it is innervated by the 11th cranial nerve. Each of the above-named muscles plays a critical role in flap reconstructive procedures. Each may be designed as either isolated muscle or myocutaneous (except for the serratus) flaps in reconstructive procedures.

SURFACE ANATOMY OF THE TRUNK

Fat cells in the newborn are about one fourth the size of adipose cells in the adult. Lipid is stored by hypertrophy of these adipocytes, and once approximately 40 kg of adult lipid body weight is stored, new fat cells will form to accommodate further excess lipid stores. Distribution of fat is different in men and women. In women with moderate weight gain, adipocyte hypertrophy will occur primarily in the lower part of the trunk, hips, buttocks, and thighs. With marked weight gain, new cells form in all regions. In men, moderate weight gain is characterized by increased abdominal girth with excess fat accumulation in the torso, upper part of the abdomen, and the nape of the neck. With marked weight gain, men accumulate fat by initial hypertrophy and subsequent hyperplasia of the cells in subcutaneous and visceral depots.

The skin of the trunk, including the breast, is subject to hormonal, expansible weight, and gravitational influences as well as the effects of diminished elasticity with age. Striae, tears in the dermis with thinning of the overlying epidermis, are often seen in the abdominal skin as well as the upper quadrants and periareolar skin regions of the breast. It is felt that this is because the nipple-areolar skin has thinner dermis than the remainder of the skin on the breast.

The escutcheon, or the pubic hair distribution, differs between the sexes. In the male, it is dispersed in a diamond-shaped area and extends from the pubis to the umbilicus, while in the female it is triangular with the base of the triangle at the superior margin of the mons pubis.

ANATOMY OF THE BREAST

The breast is a group of large glands derived from the epidermis and lying in a fascial network derived from the dermis and superficial fascia. The connective tissue stroma of the breast forms from the mesoderm. The nipple is a local proliferation of the stratum spinosum of the epidermis. During the second month of gestation, bands of thickened ectoderm appear on the ventral body wall from the axilla to below the groin and represent potential mammary gland tissue. From this thickened ectoderm, 16 to 24 buds of ectodermal cells grow into the underlying dermal mesoderm during the 12th week of gestation. These solid buds will become canalized near term to form the lactiferous ducts. The base of these ducts gives rise to the secretory apparatus during lactation. The nipple, at first a shallow pit, usually becomes everted at term. The areola is the darkened skin surrounding the nipple. It contains glands that are transitional between sweat and lactiferous glands; these are known as the areolar glands of Montgomery.

The breast is located within the superficial fascia of the anterior chest wall, with its base extending from the second rib superiorly to the sixth or seventh rib inferiorly and from the costal border medially to the midaxillary line laterally. The deep aspect of the breast lies anterior to the pectoralis major and serratus anterior muscles, and a small part may lie over the aponeurosis of the external abdominal oblique muscle or over the uppermost part of the rectus sheath. In approximately 95% of women, there is extension of the upper lateral quadrant breast tissue toward the axilla. This tissue (the tail of Spence) enters a hiatus in the deep fascia of the medial axillary wall. This is the only breast tissue found deep to the deep fascia.

Each breast is composed of 15 to 20 lobules. Each lobule of the mammary gland ends in a lactiferous duct that opens through a constricted orifice onto the nipple. Although these lobules together with their ducts are anatomic units, they are not surgical units. In the fat-free area under the areola, each duct has a dilated portion known as the lactiferous sinus; these sinuses are the site of milk storage. The suspensory ligaments of Cooper form a network of strong connective tissue fibers passing between the lobules of parenchyma, and they connect the dermis of the skin with the deep layer of superficial fascia.

Histologically, the lactiferous sinuses and ducts opening onto the nipple and areola are lined with stratified squamous epithelium. Deeper in the parenchyma, the lining of the lactiferous ducts undergoes a gradual transition to cuboidal cells, with cuboidal or columnar cells throughout the remainder of the ductal system. Myoepithelial cells of ectodermal origin lie within the epithelium between the surface epithelial cells and the basal lamina. These myoepithelial cells, arranged in a basket-like network, are present in the secretory portion of the gland but are more apparent in the larger ducts that contain myofibers and are strikingly similar to smooth muscle cells histologically. The morphology of the secretory portion of the mammary gland varies greatly with age and during pregnancy and lactation.

The epidermis of the nipple and areola is covered by a keratinized stratified squamous epithelium. Deep to the nipple and areola, bundles of smooth muscle fibers are arranged radially and circumferentially in the dense connective tissue and longitudinally along the lactiferous ducts that extend up into the nipple, and these bundles are responsible for erection of the nipple occurring in response to stimuli. The areola contains sebaceous glands, sweat glands, and accessory areolar glands (of Montgomery) that are intermediate in their structure between true mammary glands and sweat glands. The distal end of the nipple contains numerous free sensory nerve cell endings and Meissner's corpuscles in the dermal papillae; the areola contains fewer of these structures.

Absence of the breast (amastia) is rare and may result from absence of the milk lines or from their excessive obliteration later, whereas the presence of an areola without a nipple or glandular tissue implies that a fragment of the milk line was present but insufficient to induce an entire breast. When breast tissue is present but a nipple is not, the condition is termed athelia. Unusual at the normal site, athelia is not infrequent in accessory mammary structures at other locations. Polymastia occurs when more than two breasts are found; they are said to be accessory if they lie on the embryonic milk line that runs on the ventrolateral aspect of the trunk from the axilla to the groin. Breast tissue found outside of this milk line is said to be ectopic. The great majority of supernumerary breasts are accessory and are nearly always axillary or thoracic. In Caucasians, approximately 95% of accessory breasts are found just inferior to the normal breast, 5% are axillary, and fewer than 5% are abdominal. However, among Japanese, accessory breasts are found above the normal breast in 95% of female cases. Ectopic breasts have been reported in a variety of sites outside the milk line, and these cases may represent displacement of the milk line anlage or may be true ectopia. Polythelia, the presence of extra nipples, is common and may be seen in normal breasts or within the areola of a normal breast. Gynecomastia, or excessive development of the male breast, commonly develops without any pathologic basis during periods of physiologic change such as puberty or senescence. It has been reported to occur in 64% of adolescent boys, with a peak incidence at 14 to 14.5 years and an average duration of 1 to 2 years. Bilateral enlargement to a mean diameter of 2.0 to 2.5 cm and subareolar tenderness are the rule. Gynecomastia may also accompany a wide variety of systemic and metabolic diseases and serves in some cases as the first sign of the underlying disorder. The breast enlargement in gynecomastia results from variable degrees of ductal proliferation and stromal hyperplasia. Pseudogynecomastia is an increase in male breast size that results from fat deposition and is bilateral with no true hyperplasia of the breast tissue.

There are three main arterial sources supplying the breast. The internal thoracic distribution lies just lateral but in close proximity to the sternum with perforators through the intercostal spaces and provides 60% of the total breast blood flow. The axillary artery supplies the breast through three branches. They include the supreme thoracic artery, the pectoral branch of the thoracoacromial artery, and the lateral thoracic artery. These branches supply approximately 30% of the blood flow to the breast, mostly to the lateral aspect of the breast. Arterial supply to the lower lateral aspect of the breast is through branches of the third, fourth, and fifth posterior intercostal arteries.

The venous drainage of the breast is via a superficial drainage system that has transverse and long networks and via a deep drainage system located within the chest wall in the intercostal veins. The largest vessels consist of the perforating branches of the internal thoracic vein, which drains into the innominate vein (Fig 26–3).

The sensory innervation of the upper part of the breast is provided by the supraclavicular nerves in the third and fourth branches of the cervical plexus. The remainder of the sensory innervation is provided by the lateral and anterior cutaneous branches of the second through the sixth intercostal nerves. All of these nerves also carry sympathetic fibers to the breast and overlying skin, thereby influencing the flow of blood as well as the secretory function of the breast. While the secretory activity of the breast is chiefly under ovarian and hypophyseal hormonal control, the sympathetics influence secretory function of the cutaneous sweat glands and cause contraction of the smooth muscle of the nipple and blood vessels. Specialized receptors, including Krause end bulbs, Ruffini-like temperature sensors, and multibranched free nerve endings, are located in the dermis of the areola and nipple and provide sensitivity to touch, stretch, and warmth.

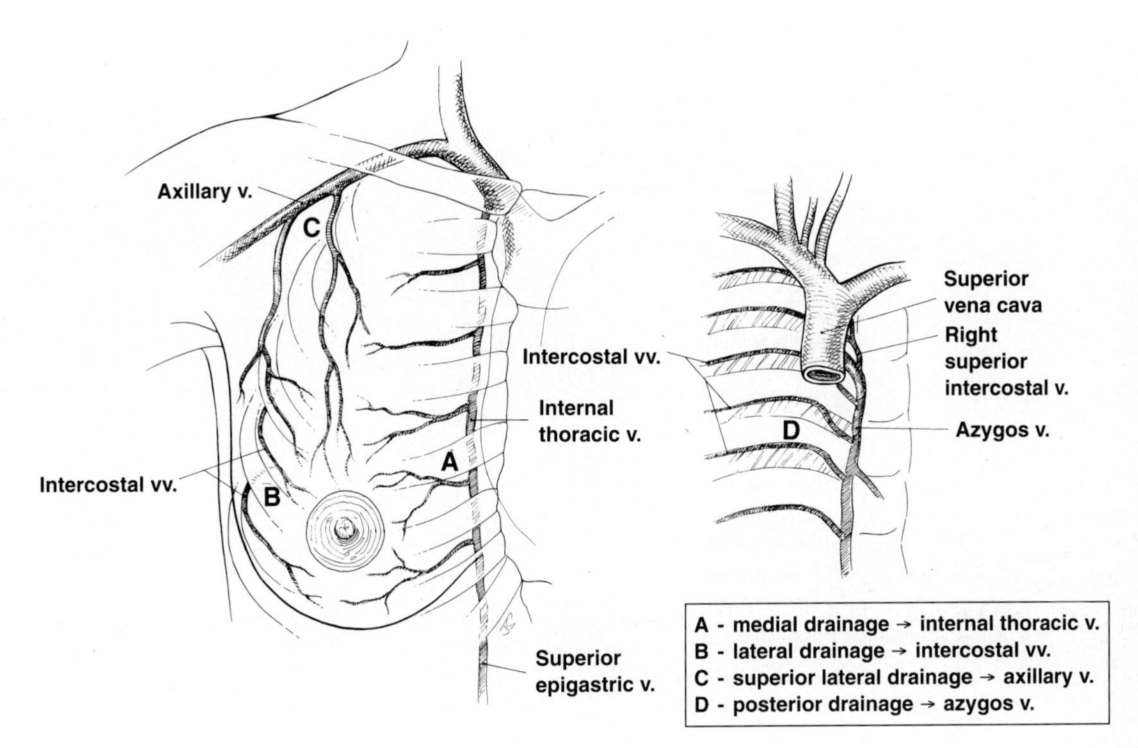

FIG 26–3.
Diagram of the venous drainage of the breast.

Lymphatic routes in the breast are rich and arborize in multiple directions through skin and mesenchymal lymphatic vessels. Lymphatic channels flow into inconsistent groups of lymph nodes with varying numbers and sizes of nodes. In general, lymphatic drainage of the breast accompanies the venous drainage, and there are valves to direct the flow. The major groups of lymph nodes include the axillary group, which handles about 75% of the lymph, and the internal thoracic group, which handles the remaining 25%. The groups average 35.3 and 8.5 nodes respectively. Surgeons have identified six primary groups of axillary lymph nodes: (1) the external mammary group along the lower border of the pectoralis minor, which follows the lateral thoracic vessels; (2) the scapular group along the posterior wall of the axilla, which is associated with the subscapular vessels; (3) the axillary vein group, which lies medial or posterior to the axillary vein; (4) the central group in the fat of the axilla, which receives lymph from the three preceding groups; (5) the intrapectoral or Rotter's nodes between the pectoralis major and minor, which are usually inaccessible until the pectoral major muscle is removed; and (6) the subclavicular or apical group along the medial aspect of the axillary vein, which receives lymph from all the other groups of axillary lymph nodes. The efferent channels from the subclavicular group unite to form the subclavian trunk, which may flow directly into the internal jugular or subclavian veins, into the thoracic duct, or into the deep cervical lymph nodes (Fig 26–4).

BREAST PHYSIOLOGY

The development and function of breast tissue are influenced by a variety of hormones. Estrogen has its effect on mammary epithelium and initiates ductal development, while progesterone is responsible for differentiation of the epithelial cells and lobular development. Pituitary steroids including prolactin are responsible for the growth and development of the adipose tissue and are a

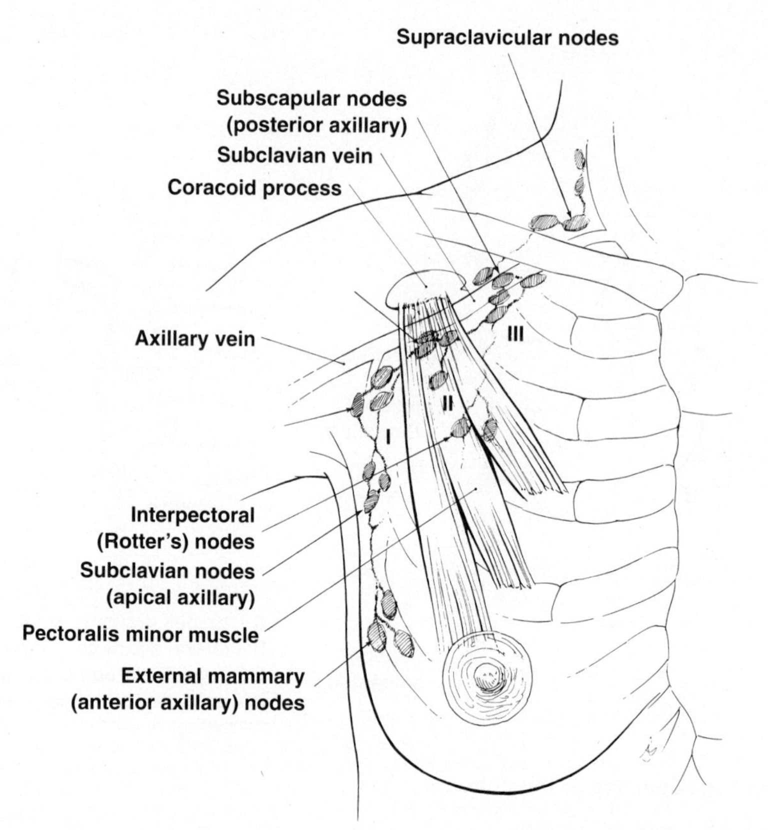

FIG 26–4.
Diagram of the major lymph node groups associated with the lymphatic drainage of the breast.-

primary stimulus for lactogenesis. The precise role for other hormones, including growth hormone, adrenocorticotropic hormone (ACTH), thyroid-stimulating hormone (TSH), and insulin-like growth factor 1 (IGF-1), is less clear. Growth of the breast in human females correlates closely with the change in plasma estradiol levels. Treatment of normal prepubertal human females with estrogen stimulates breast development with proliferation of ductal epithelium, myoepithelial cells, and stromal cells of the breast parenchyma. Progesterone, together with estrogen, initiates formation of the secretory acinar components at the distalmost aspect of the ductules. With the onset of menarche, the cyclic increases in estrogen and progesterone cause further ductal development and the formation of lobules. With pregnancy, the ductular structures of the breast begin to enlarge and branch by the end of the first month of the pregnancy. Proliferating glandular epithelium replaces connective tissue and adipose components of the breast under the influence of estrogen and progesterone from the corpus luteum. Later in pregnancy, prolactin and placentally derived hormones cause differentiation into a presecretory architecture. In the last weeks of pregnancy, limited synthesis of milk fats and proteins is initiated under the effect of prolactin on breast lobules. Following parturition, prolactin further induces secretion and is involved in the neuroreflex response with oxytocin in milk letdown. In the postmenopausal state there is a decrease in the number and size of glandular elements along with hypoplasia and atrophy of the epithelial and lobular elements of the breast.

Galactorrhea is defined as persistent discharge of milk or milk-like secretions from the breast in the absence of parturition, that is, discharge in a nonnursing mother. When galactorrhea is associated with hyperprolactinemia, a pituitary adenoma must be suspected. However, in the majority of patients it is considered idiopathic. Lactational deficiency of endocrine origin is expressed as Sheehan's syndrome, a result of postpartum hemorrhage and pituitary infarction. Other hormonal deficiencies can affect breast development to varying degrees. Pubertal disorders with premature sexual development are caused by either iatrogenic exposure to estrogens, estrogen-secreting neoplasms, ovarian cysts, or true precocious puberty. True precocious puberty may occur with central nervous system (CNS) tumors or other CNS disorders, but it is usually idiopathic in origin.

SUGGESTED READING

Bland KI, Copeland EM: *The Breast: Comprehensive Management of Benign and Malignant Disease.* Philadelphia, WB Saunders, 1991.

Gray SW, Skandalakis JE: *Embryology for Surgeons.* Philadelphia, WB Saunders, 1972.

Markman B: Anatomy and physiology of adipose tissue. *Clin Plast Surg* 1989; 16:235.

McCraw JB, Arnold PG: *Atlas of Muscle and Musculocutaneous Flaps.* Norfolk, Va, Hampton Press, 1986.

Skandalakis JE, Gray SW, Rowe JS: *Anatomical Complications in General Surgery.* New York, McGraw-Hill, 1983.

Williams PL (ed): *Gray's Anatomy.* Edinburgh, Churchill Livingstone, 1989.

Chapter 27

Congenital Disorders

Susan D. Vasko, M.D.
Robert L. Ruberg, M.D.

CONTENTS

CHAPTER OBJECTIVE

At the end of this chapter the resident has a thorough working knowledge of congenital disorders of the trunk, breast, and abdomen and performs complete plastic surgical management of such problems.

LEARNER OBJECTIVES

On completion of this chapter the resident

1. **Demonstrates knowledge of normal male and female breast growth and development and understands the general physiologic principles of systemic disease in which breast abnormalities may be but one manifestation.**
2. **Understands the basic principles and techniques of the surgical treatment of common developmental breast anomalies, including amastia, Poland's syndrome, ectopic mammary tissue, virginal hypertrophy, gynecomastia, etc.**
3. **Is familiar with chest wall embryology and anatomy as applied to developmental chest wall deformities.**
4. **Recognizes the physiologic consequences of developmental chest wall deformities.**
5. Has detailed knowledge of the surgical aspects of treatment of patients with developmental chest wall deformities such as pectus carinatum and pectus excavatum.
6. Demonstrates knowledge of the common deformities of the posterior aspect of the trunk.
7. Has a detailed knowledge of reconstructive surgery of posterior trunk defects such as meningomyelocele, sacrococcygeal teratomas, etc., and recognizes the need for multiple-team approaches to these problems.
8. Understands the embryology and developmental anatomy of congenital abdominal wall deformities.
9. Is familiar with the reconstructive surgical management of congenital abdominal wall deformities.

CLINICAL PRACTICE ACTIVITIES:

During the course of the training program, the resident

1. Evaluates patients with developmental breast abnormalities, performs appropriate diagnostic studies, and

interacts with appropriate consultants in allied areas of expertise.
2. Performs perioperative care and surgery on patients with developmental breast abnormalities.
3. Critically analyzes patients with developmental chest wall deformities from both an aesthetic and functional point of view.
4. Performs reconstructive surgery on patients with developmental chest wall deformities.
5. Evaluates and participates in the multispecialty surgical evaluation of patients with congenital deformities of the posterior of the trunk.
6. Participates in the reconstruction of posterior trunk congenital defects.
7. Participates in the evaluation and surgical planning (in concert with other surgical specialists) of congenital abdominal wall deformities.
8. Performs reconstructive surgery on patients with abdominal wall deformities of a congenital nature.

BREAST

Embryology

Breast development begins at 6 weeks of gestation with the formation of mammary ridges from the axilla to the inguinal region. These subsequently disappear except in the pectoral region, where at 4 months a downward thickening of ectoderm grows into the underlying mesenchyme. Fifteen to 20 solid cords fan out beneath the skin with club-shaped dilatations at the ends (primary milk ducts). At the seventh to eighth month of development, the ducts hollow to develop lumina, and small depressions form on the chest wall (mammary pits) that will become the nipples. The surrounding mesenchyme develops into connective tissue and fat. In the perinatal period, the nipple forms as mesenchyme proliferates underneath the areola.

Development

Shortly after birth, the surrounding connective tissue proliferates, and the nipples become raised and pigmented. There is little further development of the breast in males.

Only the main mammary ducts exist at birth. In adolescent females, a prepubertal "bud" develops, the areola elevates, and the nipple becomes more prominent. Histologically, one sees formation of lobules as well as elongation and terminal branching of primary ducts. By adulthood, each lobe is a compound tuboalveolar gland with a separate excretory duct.

During pregnancy, there may be a two- to threefold enlargement of the breast. The nipple and areola become more prominent and more pigmented. Montgomery's tubercles form as openings of Montgomery's glands on the areola. There is histologic evidence of an increased number of lobules and the production of secretory tubules and alveoli.

At menopause the gland involutes. Lobules disappear and are replaced by fat. The vestigial ductal system is then similar to the prepubescent breast.

Congenital Disorders

Congenital breast anomalies include athelia (absent nipple), amastia (absent breast), polythelia (supernumerary nipples), and polymastia (extra breasts). The latter two can occur anywhere along the mammary ridge but will usually be found just inferior to the normal breast. The deformity can be unilateral or bilateral.

Treatment for polymastia and polythelia is excision of the redundant structures. Athelia is treated by nipple construction. Breast construction, as described below for Poland's syndrome, is the approach to amastia.

Poland's syndrome, described in 1841 by Alfred Poland, is based on an anatomic dissection. His original description included absent pectoralis major and minor muscles and syndactyly but did not mention the breast. The full spectrum was first summarized by Thompson in 1895 and may include absent pectoralis major and minor muscles, brachysyndactyly, absent ribs, chest wall depression, athelia or amastia, absent axillary hair, and limited subcutaneous chest wall fat.

The breast deformity in females with Poland's syndrome can be corrected through a variety of methods, depending on the individual's subcutaneous fat, chest wall musculature, and rib deformities. For minor asymmetry, a breast implant may be adequate. For a moderate deformity, a tissue expander may be required to expand the chest wall skin. For larger tissue requirements, a latissimus dorsi muscle or myocutaneous flap can be used to provide bulk and coverage over a breast implant. Correction of chest wall deformities in males will be addressed below.

Prepubertal hypertrophy is usually bilateral and requires a workup for functioning ovarian, adrenal, or pituitary tumors, although there may be no identifiable cause. Hypermastia is excessive breast development after puberty, sometimes called "virginal" hypertrophy or, after pregnancy, persistent breast enlargement. The enlargement is usually due to hypertrophied fat and fibrous tissue. Gigantomastia is massive enlargement that often occurs rapidly and may recur after reduction mammaplasty. It is probably the result of increased end-organ response to hormonal stimulation. The above conditions are usually amenable to reduction mammaplasty techniques.

Tuberous breast deformity, sometimes called tubular breast deformity, is characterized by breasts that may be deficient vertically and/or horizontally and have a constricted base, large areola, and herniation of breast tissue into the areola. Patients with tuberous breasts often have breast asymmetry. The deformity is accentuated by standard augmentation mammaplasty or mastopexy tech-

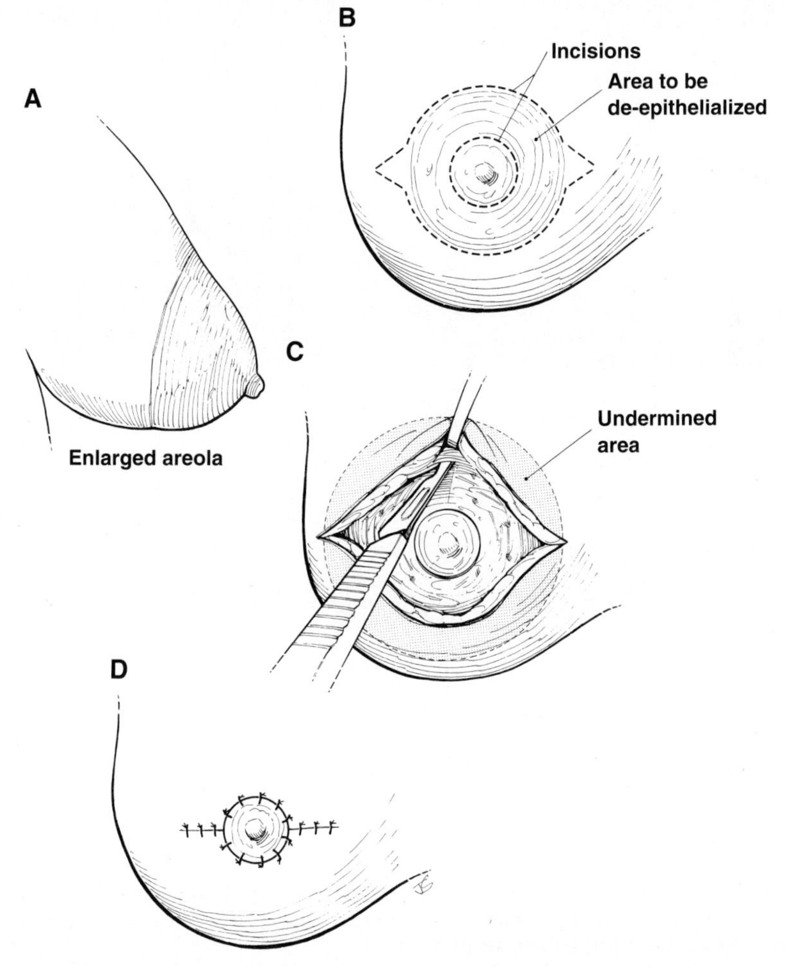

FIG 27–1.
Correction of tuberous deformity with breast tissue herniated into the areola. **A,** the deformity with herniation of breast tissue. **B,** incisions. **C,** undermined tissue to be advanced. **D,** position of implant, if needed. **D,** use of expander implant if desired.

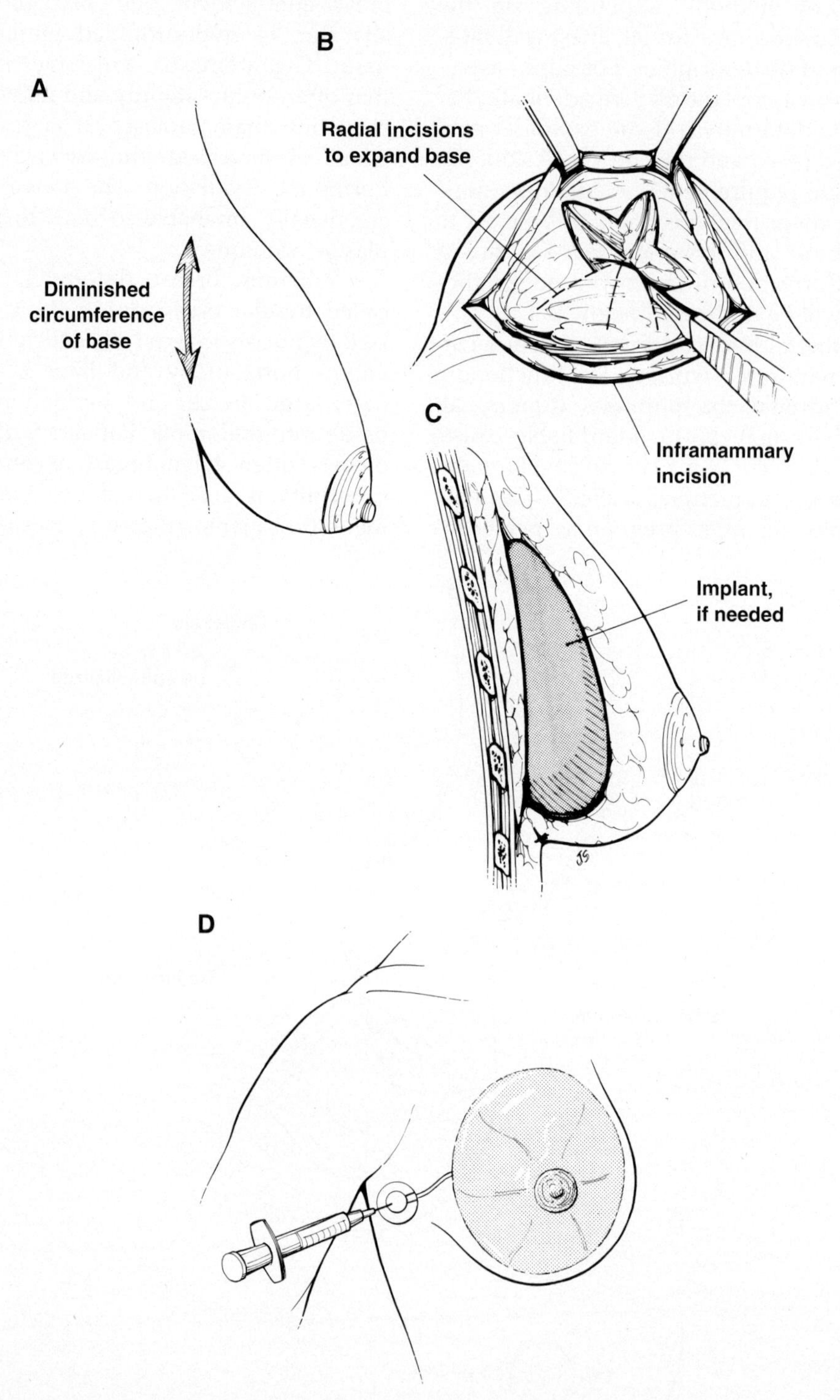

FIG 27–2.
Correction of tuberous deformity without herniation of tissue into the areola. **A,** the deformity without herniation of breast tissue. **B,** radial incisions to expand the base of the breast. **C,** position of implant, if needed. **D,** use of expander implant if desired.

niques. Treatment may include combinations of the following steps: radial incisions in the breast tissue to release the constriction, areola reduction, and breast augmentation with attention to correction of the asymmetry (Figs. 27–1 and 27–2). (For additional discussion of tuberous breast deformity, see Chapter 30.)

Gynecomastia (abnormal male breast development) is common in pubertal males and usually regresses spontaneously. Sixty-five percent of males aged 14 to 15 years have gynecomastia. Regression occurs in almost all cases within about 2 years. The tissue is usually glandular in this age group as opposed to the fatty tissue seen in older men with gynecomastia.

Although most cases of gynecomastia are idiopathic, the patient should be evaluated for other possible, more significant causes. These are listed in Table 27–1.

Gynecomastia can be divided into three types: (1) a localized button of breast tissue beneath the areola in an otherwise thin individual, which is easily removed by surgical excision; (2) diffuse gynecomastia with ill-defined edges on a fatty chest, which is best treated by a combination of excision and suction lipectomy; and (3) diffuse gynecomastia plus excess skin, which requires excision of excess tissue and skin with or without nipple repositioning. (For additional discussion of gynecomastia, see Chapter 28.)

TABLE 27–1.
Causes of Gynecomastia

Causes of Gynecomastia
Testicular tumors (Leydig and Sertoli cell, choriocarcinoma)
Hyperthyroidism, hypothyroidism
Pituitary adenomas
Acromegaly
Adrenal tumors
Cirrhosis of the liver, hepatitis
Drugs (digitalis, estrogen, cimetidine, cannabis, anabolic steroids, heroin)
Klinefelter's syndrome

Nipple inversion can be corrected through a variety of techniques. Through a periareolar approach the nipple can be freed from the underlying tissue, everted, and held in place with a purse-string suture. Another option is to retract the nipple with traction sutures, incise around the base of the nipple, and then undermine the surrounding areola. The areola is then advanced and closed around the nipple with a purse-string suture. Figures 27–3, 27–4, and 27–5 illustrate options available to correct nipple inversion. (For ad-

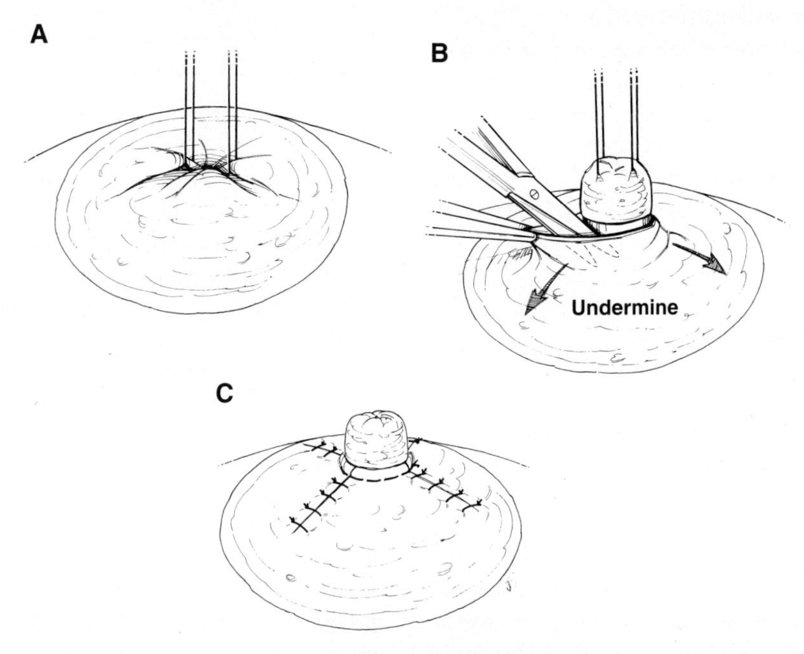

FIG 27–3.
Correction of nipple inversion. **A,** eversion of the nipple with sutures (common to all techniques). **B** and **C,** technique I—purse-string suture at the base of the nipple.

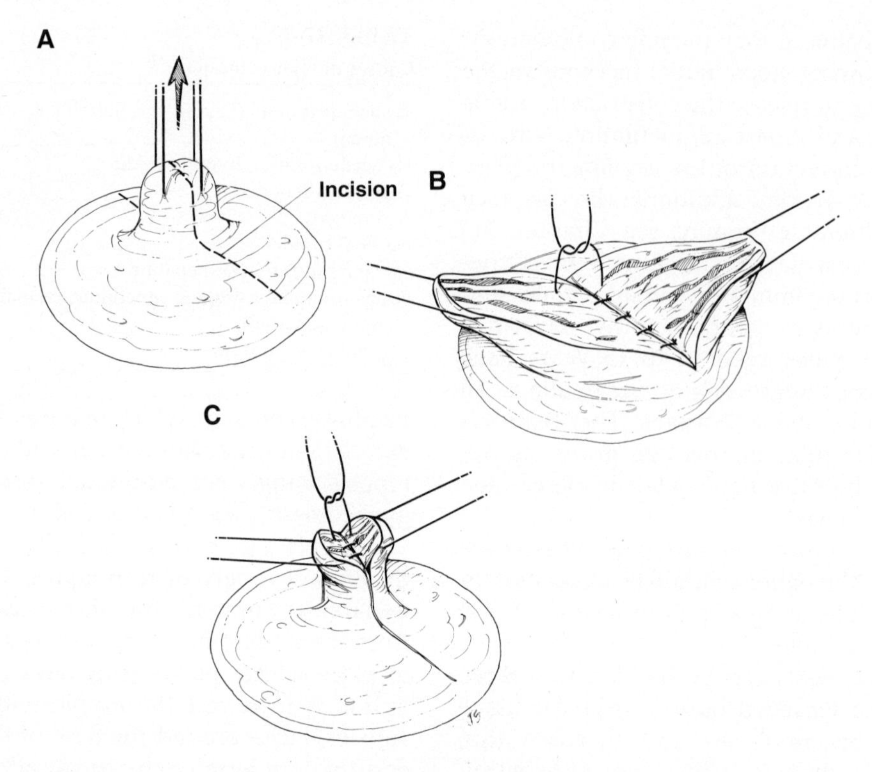

FIG 27–4.
Correction of nipple inversion by technique II—incision of fibrous and muscular tissue between the ducts.

ditional discussion of the treatment of inverted nipples, see Chapter 30.)

Nipple hypertrophy can be corrected by circumferential deepithelialization of a segment, imbrication of this segment, and closure (Regnault technique). Excess nipple length can also corrected with a wedge excision and closure, among other options. Care must be taken to not block the lactiferous ducts.

CHEST WALL

Embryology

Ribs develop from thoracic vertebrae as mesenchymal costal processes during the fifth week of gestation. They first become cartilaginous in the embryonic periods and then ossify. The sternum is formed independently from the ribs as a pair of mesenchymal sternal bands. Sternal plates are formed as these bands chondrify. The plates fuse in the midline in a cranial-to-caudad fashion, and the uppermost costal cartilages attach to them. Ossification centers form craniocaudally before birth.

Congenital Disorders

Sternal clefts can vary from simple to complex. Clefts involving only the sternum may include the entire sternum or variable amounts of clefting beginning at the lower aspect. In *ectopia cordis,* the heart is outside of the chest with variable degrees of sternal clefting. Cantrell's pentology includes (1) lower sternal cleft, (2) defect of the ventral diaphragm, (3) abdominal wall defect or omphalocele, (4) apical pericardial defect communicating with the peritoneum, and (5) ventricular aneurysm or septal defect.

Operative repair is usually done in early infancy to reduce the chance of injury to the mediastinal structures. Sternal clefts are usually treated by approximation of the two bony halves and closure of the defect. In cases where the cardiopulmonary status will not tolerate closure of the cleft, coverage with mesh and muscle flaps is a surgical option.

The chest wall deformities of Poland's syndrome (described above) are rarely physiologically significant but may pose an aesthetic problem. Small chest wall defects can often be corrected with a custom silicone implant. Areas with absent ribs or rib anomalies can be corrected with autogenous rib struts, synthetic mesh, or rib osteotomies and recontouring. The latissimus dorsi muscle can provide bulk to the area as well as establish an anterior axillary fold. When the latissimus dorsi muscle is hypoplastic or absent, a free flap may be used to correct contour abnormalities. (For additional discussion of Poland's syndrome, see Chapter 29.)

Pectus excavatum ("funnel chest") is characterized by depression of the sternum and anterior chest wall, often asymmetrically. The deepest depression is usually at the inferior aspect of the sternum. Physiologic compromise in either cardiac or pulmonary functions, especially at rest, is rare except in the most severe deformities. Symptomatic pectus excavatum is usually manifested as exercise intolerance.

Minor chest wall defects can be treated by implantation of custom implants; however, extrusion, palpable borders, and movement of the implants have been described in many cases. The incidence of complications can be decreased by placing the implant in a subpectoral position. The most common surgical approach for pectus excavatum repair is the Ravitch procedure, which includes midline incision, elevation of musculocutaneous flaps, perichondrial elevation, excision of deformed cartilages, sternal osteotomy and elevation, and "tripod fixation" of the sternum.

Another option, the sternal turnover technique, is accomplished by division of the costal cartilages or ribs at the costal arches, ligation of the internal mammary vessels, transection of the superior aspect of the sternum, and turnover of the sternum en bloc. The cartilage is contoured via wedge resections.

Pectus carinatum ("pigeon chest"), is characterized by convexity of the anterior of the chest at either the inferior aspect (chondroglandular) or superior aspect (chondromanubrial). Surgical treatment is similar to pectus excavatum, i.e., recontouring of abnormal costal cartilages and sternal osteotomies with realignment.

THE BACK

Embryology

During the fourth week of development, mesenchymal sclerotomes surround the noto-

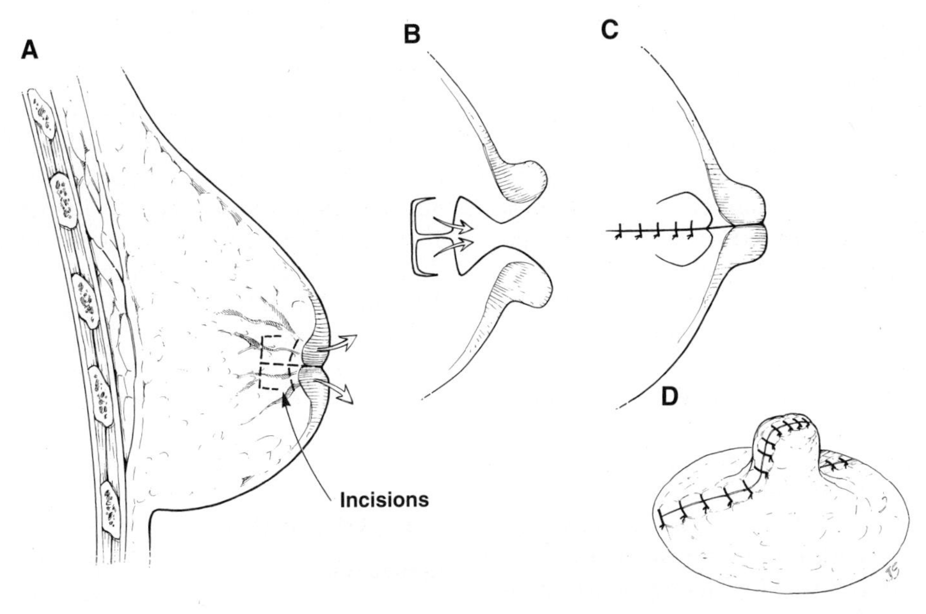

FIG 27–5.
Correction of nipple inversion by technique III—internal flap eversion.

cord to form the vertebral bodies and surround the neural tube to form the vertebral arches. Chondrification centers appear during the sixth week, and ossification begins about week 8. At birth, three bony segments connected by cartilage exist for each vertebra. Ossification continues into adulthood. The neural tube begins to develop during the third week. The caudal aspect becomes the spinal cord.

Spina Bifida

Spina bifida is a congenital anomaly characterized by defective closure of the bony encasement of the spinal cord. It is caused by a failure of closure of the caudal neuropore at the fourth week of development. With *open* neural tube defects, α-fetoprotein levels are increased in the amnionic fluid. Spina bifida can occur anywhere along the vertebral axis but is usually in the lumbar area.

In *spina bifida occulta,* there is a bony defect without protrusion of the cord or meninges. Neurologic abnormalities are rare. Physical characteristics may include hair, a nevoid patch, or a dimple on the skin overlying the vertebral defect. A child with a sacral dimple should be evaluated with spinal radiographs before surgical excision is planned. If spina bifida occulta is present, the surgeon should recognize that a dermal sinus may connect to the dura mater.

Spina bifida cystica has protrusion of meninges (meningocele), spinal cord elements (myelocele), or both (meningomyelocele) through the bony defect. Meningomyelocele is the most common variant. *Syringomyelocele* is a meningomyelocele with dilatation of the central canal of the spinal cord.

The incidence of spina bifida is 1:1,000 live births. The etiology is unknown. The incidence among siblings increases to 1:25 after 1 child is affected. Most patients (75%) have normal intelligence, with mental retardation usually secondary to meningitis or hydrocephalus. Meningocele (10% to 15% of the total) has the associated risk of neurologic contamination through rupture of the atrophic skin covering. Meningomyelocele is associated with hydrocephalus (80% to 90%), bowel and bladder incontinence, and orthopedic problems. Eighty-five percent of patients with meningomyelocele can ambulate.

Surgical Repair

The goals of surgical repair are to protect the spinal cord and prevent contamination of the cerebrospinal fluid. Although many defects are repaired by neurosurgeons, larger defects requiring complex closure often benefit from a multidisciplinary team approach.

Myelocele defects with intact skin can have repair delayed until several weeks of life, but most surgeons treat myelocele defects with poor skin quality or meningomyelocele defects within 24 hours after birth. Small defects can often be closed with skin undermining and then primary closure, skin grafts, or simple rotation flaps. There are several options for closure of large defects. Local skin flaps can be designed with various configurations (e.g., rhomboid, double Z-plasty, bipedical flaps). The latissimus dorsi muscle can be advanced with or without relaxing incisions. Ramirez has described the latissimus dorsi–gluteus maximus advancement method of closure, which preserves muscle attachments and function (Fig 27–6). Another option is to turn the gluteus maximus or latissimus dorsi muscles over and cover them with split-thickness skin grafts.

Sacrococcygeal Teratoma

Sacrococcygeal teratomas are characterized by a mass overlying the buttocks that ranges in size from a few centimeters to massive proportions. The incidence is 1 in 40,000 live births. Most lesions are benign, but there is a high malignant potential after about 2 months of life. Cure rates are high when the lesion is completely excised during the first few days of life. Closure of the resultant wound is usually accomplished with local skin flaps.

THE ABDOMEN

Embryology

During the sixth week of development, the midgut loop projects into the umbilical

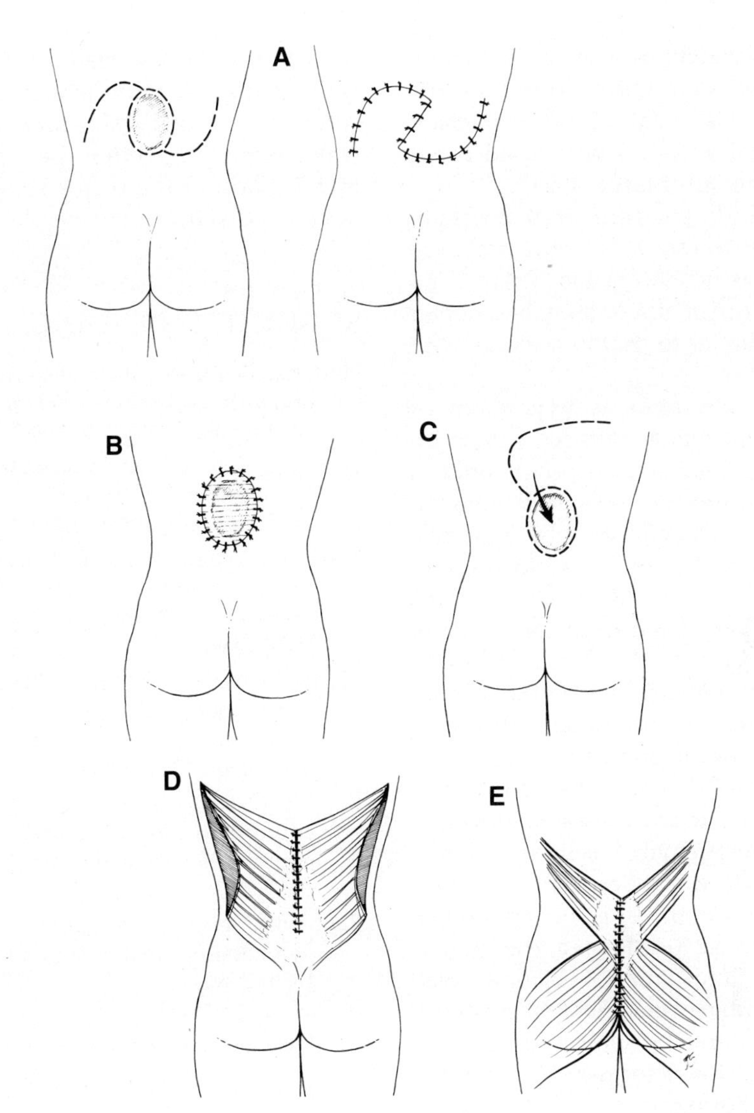

FIG 27–6.
Techniques for closure of a myelomeningocele defect. **A,** transposition flaps, bilateral. **B,** split-thickness skin graft, delayed, on dura. **C,** lumbosacral flap. **D,** bilateral latissimus dorsi myocutaneous flaps with relaxing incisions. **E,** bilateral double myocutaneous flaps (latissimus dorsi and gluteus maximus).

cord and begins to return to the abdomen during the tenth week. The abdominal wall forms as the umbilical ring contracts. Umbilical hernias occur when this ring fails to close. Small defects (<1 cm) usually close spontaneously by the age of 2 years. Larger defects can take longer to close or require operative repair. Surgical closure is through primary repair of the fascial defect.

An omphalocele is caused by failure of the midgut to return to the abdominal cavity. The defect usually has a hernia sac and can be over 4 cm in diameter. Two thirds of those children affected will have other associated anomalies. Correction of the abnormality is undertaken when the patient is stable and nutritionally repleted. For smaller defects, skin undermining and fascial closure may be adequate. For larger defects, a "silo" is constructed by attaching prosthetic mesh to the margins of the defect. Over a 1- to 2-week course, the midgut structures are gradually pushed into the abdominal cavity and the size of the silo reduced. If the viscera are returned to the abdominal cavity too quickly, respiratory compromise or impaired venous return may occur. Once the gut is reduced into the abdominal cavity, the fascial defect is repaired. Another alternative is to widely undermine and close the surrounding skin with closure of the ventral hernia at a later date. Tissue expansion of the abdominal wall has been used as an adjunct to the repair of large defects.

Gastroschisis differs from omphalocele in that the defect is to the right of the umbilical cord and there is no hernia sac. There is no increased incidence of other anomalies. Repair is undertaken similar to that in patients with omphalocele.

Prune-belly syndrome is hypoplasia or aplasia of the abdominal muscles and wrinkled lower abdominal skin. It occurs only in males and has associated urogenital anomalies. Correction is accomplished by wide dissection of the muscular remnants, closure, and excision of excess skin. Muscle flaps (e.g., rectus femoris) have been used for repair of this defect.

Failure of complete closure of the inferior aspect of the anterior abdominal wall results in exstrophy of the bladder; this occurs predominantly in males. Embryologically, it is a failure during the fourth week of development of the mesenchymal cells to migrate between the surface ectoderm and the urogenital sinus. Since there is no abdominal musculature formed in this area, the attenuated epidermis and anterior bladder wall rupture and result in exposure of the posterior wall of the bladder. The symphysis pubis is often separated. This deformity is commonly associated with epispadias.

Closure of the bladder and abdominal wall are done within the first few days of life. After closure of the bladder, the abdominal wall defect can often be closed through mobilization of the rectus abdominis muscle, fascia, and skin.

SUGGESTED READING

Hester R, Bostwick J: Poland's syndrome: Correction with latissimus muscle transposition. *Plast Reconstr Surg* 1982; 69:226–233.

Hirayama T, Nozaki M, Wakamatsu S: A new surgical method for repair of funnel chest. *Ann Plast Surg* 1985; 14:213–223.

Marks M, Argenta L, Lee D: Silicone implant correction of pectus excavatum: Indications and refinement in technique. *Plast Reconstr Surg* 1984; 74:52–58.

Moore T, Dreyer T, Bevin G: Closure of large spina bifida cystica defects with bilateral bipedicled musculocutaneous flaps. *Plast Reconstr Surg* 1984; 73:288–292.

Ramirez O, Ramasastry S, et al: A new surgical approach to closure of large lumbosacral meningomyelocele defects. *Plast Reconstr Surg* 1987; 80:799–807.

Regnault P: Nipple hypertrophy. A physiologic reduction by circumcision. *Clin Plast Surg* 1975; 2:391.

Shamberger R, Welch K: Surgical repair of pectus excavatum. *J Pediatr Surg* 1988; 23:615–622.

Chapter 28

Benign and Malignant Tumors

John Woods, M.D.

CONTENTS

NOTE: Some of the material in this chapter is frequently covered during the prerequisite training period of many plastic surgery residents. This chapter should serve as a valuable review of important material in such cases. For residents who have not mastered this material previously, this chapter is essential.

CHAPTER OBJECTIVE

At the end of this chapter the resident is familiar with the biological behavior, histologic characteristics, and management principles of benign and malignant processes of the breast and trunk and carries out comprehensive medical and surgical management of such problems.

LEARNER OBJECTIVES

On completion of this chapter the resident

1. **Understands the biological behavior, histologic characteristics, and clinical manifestations of malignancies of the breast.**
2. **Is familiar with plastic surgical options for management of the opposite breast after mastectomy for carcinoma and the principles of long-term management of patients with breast carcinoma.**
3. **Is familiar with diagnostic techniques and treatment methods (surgical and nonsurgical) for management of premalignant disease and other pathologic processes of the breast.**
4. **Has a thorough knowledge of breast reconstruction (see Chapter 29).**
5. **Understands the etiology of gynecomastia and is familiar with the various surgical options for treatment.**
6. Knows the various treatment protocols (including surgery, radiation, and chemotherapy, plus combinations) for management of carcinoma of the breast.
7. Is familiar with the principles of management of benign and malignant tumors of the trunk, including the thoracic cage and abdominal wall.

■ CLINICAL PRACTICE ACTIVITIES

During the course of the training program, the resident

1. **Performs reconstructive surgery after breast carcinoma, including procedures on the opposite breast, and participates in the long-term management of these patients.**
2. Evaluates and treats patients with premalignant disease of the breast and performs prophylactic mastectomy in selected patients.
3. Evaluates and surgically treats patients with gynecomastia.
4. Participates in the treatment of patients with malignancy of the trunk, thorax, and/or abdominal wall.

Although the primary concern of this discussion is benign and malignant tumors, other conditions of the breast will be briefly addressed. Essential to the assessment of any breast condition is an understanding of the appropriate diagnostic approaches.

PATIENT EVALUATION

History and Physical Examination

When there is any concern about malignancy, a detailed history of risk factors for cancer should be taken, with special emphasis on maternal family history. These factors will be discussed below.

Examination of the breast should be carried out in a well-lighted room with the patient initially in the upright position in order to ascertain any abnormalities of the nipple and areola and any skin retraction, color changes, or edema. After the initial inspection, the axillae are carefully palpated for adenopathy. Palpation of the breasts is then carried out with the patient supine so that breast tissue can be compressed against the chest wall and each quadrant and the tissue under the areolae carefully palpated. Although benign tumors may be firm, they are usually well circumscribed, while carcinomas are less well defined and in addition give the sense of attachment to surrounding tissue.

Breast Imaging and Other Diagnostic Modalities

Mammography has become an integral part of breast assessment and should be carried out whenever there is any question of malignancy. There is a general consensus that mammography should be carried out in all women, first at the age of 35 years and then at 40 and every 2 years thereafter, with yearly mammograms recommended for women 50 years of age or older. Ultrasound, magnetic resonance imaging (MRI), and computer-assisted tomography (CAT) are used when additional information is needed.

Fine-needle aspiration (FNA) is helpful in distinguishing solid from cystic masses. When cancer is suspected, cytologic examination of the aspirate may be useful but should not serve as the basis for definitive treatment without other confirmatory evidence.

Biopsy with careful histopathologic evaluation by a qualified histopathologist is the cornerstone of final diagnosis. Stereoscopically placed wires are extremely helpful in localizing nonpalpable lesions for biopsy.

BENIGN BREAST DISEASES

Gynecomastia

Hypertrophy of breast tissue in males may be divided into *pubertal,* which is seen between the ages of 13 and 17 years, and *senescent,* which occurs in males over 50 years of age. Known causes include the use of medications such as cimetidine, spironolactone, etc., although the etiology is frequently unidentifiable. The diagnosis is made by palpation of a disk of thickened breast tissue underlying the nipple.

In teenage boys the condition is common, may be bilateral or unilateral, and often passes unnoticed unless it is unilateral and painful. It usually regresses in adulthood. Surgical removal, sparing the nipple, is carried out only if the condition persists after adolescence or is cosmetically unacceptable.

Resection may be accomplished through a hemicircumareolar incision (with a small extension of the incision laterally if necessary). Liposuction has also been employed, but because of the density of breast tissue in adolescents, it is rarely successful.

In adults the hypertrophy may be extensive, diffuse, and again unilateral or bilateral. Tenderness or discomfort is common. The condition may be seen with the use of a number of common medications including digoxin, thiazides, estrogens, phenothiazines, and theophylline. It may also be a manifestation of hepatic cirrhosis, renal failure, and malnutrition.

Resection in adults may be carried out as for adolescent gynecomastia; liposuction serves quite well in many instances. In patients with extreme hypertrophy, subcutaneous mastectomy with some form of skin reduction may be appropriate. (For additional discussion of gynecomastia, see Chapter 27.)

Nipple Discharge

Nipple discharge is common and not usually associated with any underlying malignancy. The discharge may be unilateral or bilateral and arise from one or multiple ducts. Discharge that is truly milky (containing lactose, fat, and milk-specific proteins) is very rare.

Discharge from one nipple that is nonmilky and not associated with an underlying mass indicates cancer in approximately 5% of patients. Nipple discharge that contains blood and comes from a single duct should be investigated further.

Discharge from a single duct is most commonly due to a solitary intraductal papilloma in one of the large subareolar ductules. Biopsy is appropriate in this situation as with any bloody discharge. Bilateral nipple discharge that originates in multiple ducts is usually not a surgical problem.

Fibrocystic Mastopathy and Other Benign Tumors and Processes

Fibrocystic "disease" is a misnomer in that it is so general as to be meaningless. The changes that occur in the breast encompass a wide spectrum of clinical and histologic findings, including cyst formation, breast nodularity, stromal proliferation, and epithelial hyperplasia. It is probably an exaggerated response of epithelial and stromal elements to hormones and growth factors.

The diagnosis is made clinically by palpation of firm breast tissue with nodularity and frequently palpable gross cysts. Mammography may be helpful in patients when there is concern about possible malignant change or as a routine in patients over 40 years of age. The breasts are often painful and tender to touch.

Histologically the changes with fibrocystic mastopathy include microcysts and macrocysts, stromal fibrosis, adenosis, and epithelial metaplasia and hyperplasia to varying degrees. These changes may all be found to some extent in virtually every female breast. No increased risk for breast malignancy has been associated with fibrocystic mastopathy. When epithelial hyperplasia with atypia is noted, however, the risk of cancer is increased to about 25%; some surgeons may consider this to be an indication for some form of prophylactic or risk reduction surgery.

Medical treatment of fibrocystic mastopathy is largely limited to the use of danazol in patients with severe mastodynia, with some response in the occasional patient to the avoidance of all forms of caffeine and cessation of smoking when the habit is present.

Aspiration of macrocysts that are tense and painful may be appropriate. For suspicious masses, biopsy is carried out when mammography is not diagnostic. In the occasional patient with pain so severe that it interferes with a normal life-style, subcutaneous mastectomy may be considered after a thorough discussion of the risks and complications and repeated emphasis that complete pain relief may not be afforded.

In some patients who have undergone multiple biopsies for extensive mastopathy and when there is the prospect of further biopsies and significant patient and surgeon anxiety, subcutaneous or simple mastectomy may be an option, especially in instances where extremely dense breast tissue makes interpretation of mammograms difficult or impossible.

TABLE 28–1.
Indications for Prophylactic Subcutaneous or Simple Mastectomy

High or increased risk for breast cancer
Previous cancer of the opposite breast with a high incidence of bilaterality, (e.g., lobular carcinoma)
Extensive multimacronodular cystic mastopathy with difficulty in examination and interpretation of mammograms
Previous multiple breast biopsy specimens with histopathologic findings of premalignant disease (e.g., intraductal or lobular hyperplasia with atypia or florid intraductal papillomatosis)
Severe disabling mastodynia in a patient willing to accept no promise of complete relief
Chronic suppurative mastitis unresponsive to more conservative therapy
Overwhelming cancerophobia not responding to psychiatric counseling
In situ or intraductal carcinoma

Prophylactic or Risk Reduction Mastectomy

Surgery to prevent or reduce the risk of cancer or to obviate further problems falls into two categories: simple (or "total") mastectomy, which removes essentially all breast tissue, and subcutaneous mastectomy, which leaves approximately 5% to 10% of breast tissue (in the subareolar area). The other differences are that subcutaneous mastectomy preserves the nipple-areolar complex and may be combined with skin tailoring or mastopexy so that the skin envelope conforms nicely to implants that may be placed for reconstruction at the time of mastectomy. The indications for these procedures are shown above in Table 28–1.

There are many factors that increase the risk of breast cancer. Table 28–2 presents a summary of these factors.

Prior to undertaking prophylactic mastectomy, patient expectations are explored and the risks and complications thoroughly discussed. For simple mastectomy the complications include infection, bleeding, and flap loss, as well as complications relating to the use of implants or tissue expanders if they are employed in reconstruction.

Complications of subcutaneous mastec-

TABLE 28–2.
Breast Cancer Risk Factors*

Factor	Increase in Risk†
Family history	
Primary relative with breast cancer	1.2–3.0
Premenopausal	3.1
Premenopausal and bilaterality	8.5–9.0
Postmenopausal	1.5
Postmenopausal and bilaterality	4.0–5.4
Menstrual history	
Age at menarche: 12 yr	1.3
Age at menopause: 55 with 40 menstrual years	1.48–2.0
Pregnancy	
First child after 35 yr of age	2.0–3.0
Nulliparous	3.0
Other neoplasms	
Contralateral breast cancer	5.0
Cancer of a major salivary gland	4.0
Cancer of the uterus	2.0
Benign breast disease	
Atypical lobular hyperplasia	4.0
Lobular carcinoma in situ	7.2
Previous biopsy	1.86–2.13

* From Love SM, Gelman RS, Sien W: *N Engl J Med* 1982; 307:1010. Used by permission. The risk of cancer in the general population at time of publication was 1 in 5 or 6.
† General population risk, 1.0.

tomy, in addition to those noted for simple mastectomy, include nipple-areolar necrosis and, as with any type of implant, the possibility of implant failure or leak as well as capsular contracture. The patient should also be aware that a natural consequence of any type of mastectomy is a loss of sensation in the skin of the breast and in the nipple and areola if preserved.

One other alternative form of prophylactic mastectomy combines aspects of simple and subcutaneous mastectomies. In this procedure a total mastectomy is first done, and then the nipple is replaced as a free full-thickness skin graft. The complications of this procedure include a failure of graft take plus all of the complications described for the previous procedures. The choice between the various prophylactic mastectomy procedures largely depends on the surgeon's preference. Simple mastectomy produces the best aesthetic result but removes only about 95% of the breast tissue. There have been cases of breast cancer reported in patients who have undergone prophylactic subcutaneous mastectomy, but the incidence is quite low (<1% of cases). The total mastectomy and total mastectomy plus nipple graft procedures remove virtually all of the breast tissue but produce a result that is often much less aesthetically pleasing than the subcutaneous method. At times it may be appropriate to have the patient participate in the choice between these two approaches.

Technique of Subcutaneous Mastectomy

Considerable skill is required to carry out subcutaneous mastectomy with a minimum of complications such as loss of the nipple-areolar complex or skin from ischemic necrosis. If there is a significant degree of ptosis, concomitant mastopexy may be appropriate to achieve an optimal result, although the risk of necrosis is somewhat higher when simultaneous mastopexy is carried out.

A detailed description of the technique of subcutaneous mastectomy will be found in the Suggested Reading list. The technique for subcutaneous mastectomy without mastopexy is illustrated in Figures 28–1 and 28–2.

Subcutaneous mastectomy is usually accomplished through a generous inframammary incision. Fascia is left on the pectoralis major muscle. The entire breast is removed except for a 1-cm disk of tissue below the areola and nipple. Immediate reconstruction is achieved with an implant or tissue expander placed in a submuscular pocket.

In patients with minimal to moderate ptosis, a "doughnut" mastopexy may be used in conjunction with the subcutaneous mastectomy. If the ptosis is more severe, a formal mastopexy using the vertical pedicle of McKissock can be employed to reduce the skin envelope covering the implants or expander. This technique is illustrated in Figure 28–3.

Technique of Simple Mastectomy

Simple (or total) mastectomy is usually performed through transverse incisions encompassing the entire nipple-areola complex. Thin skin flaps are developed, and all of the breast tissue is removed, usually with preservation of the underlying pectoralis major fascia. When simple mastectomy is combined with a free nipple graft, a circumareolar incision is often employed with lateral and, if needed, medial extension. The nipple-areola complex is removed from the breast, thinned, and replaced at an appropriate site after "de-epithelialization" of the underlying skin. An implant or tissue expander is placed in a submuscular pocket prior to closure (Fig 28–4).

Breast Cyst

Cysts are common, may be single or multiple, and are fluid-filled, epithelial-lined cavities within the breast tissue that vary greatly in size. They are almost certainly influenced by ovarian hormones, which accounts for their variation in size during the menstrual cycle. Current consensus holds that cystic mastopathy is not associated with an increased risk of the development of breast cancer. Treatment is usually by observation or by aspiration if the mass is large and uncomfortable. Biopsy is carried out when there is concern about malignancy. Ultrasound may be helpful in distinguishing between fluid-filled and solid masses.

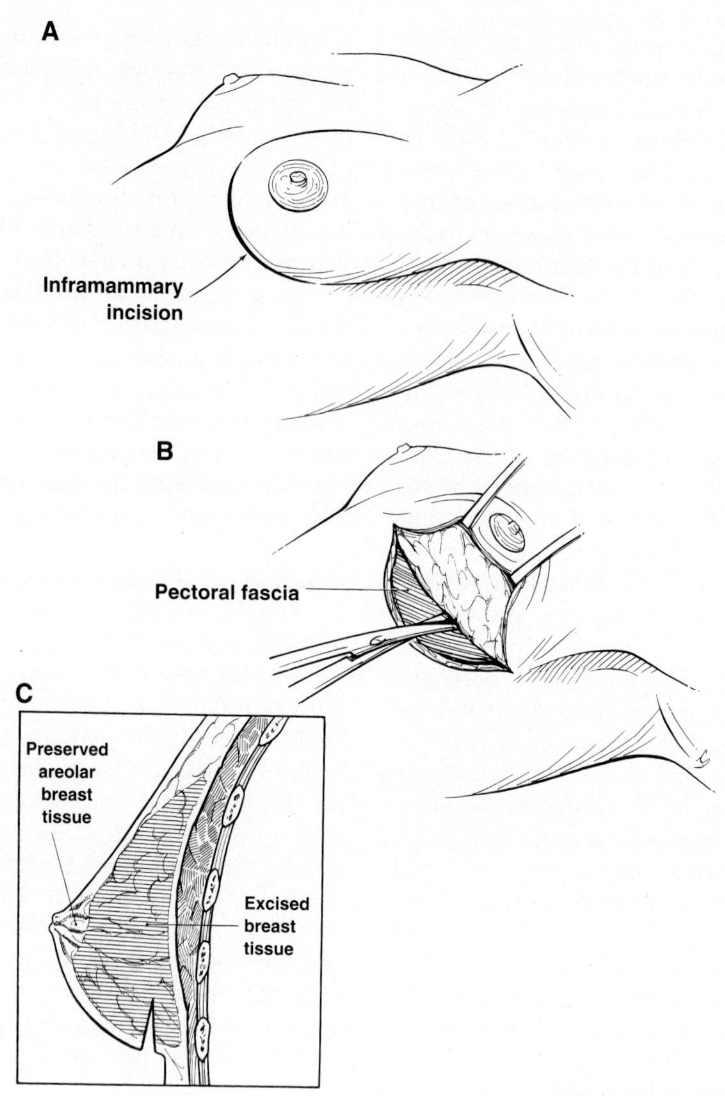

FIG 28–1.
A, a generous inframammary incision is made. For patients with mild to moderate ptosis, a "donut"-type mastopexy procedure may be added. **B,** the breast is dissected from the chest wall and the prepectoral fascia preserved wherever possible. **C,** completion of the breast removal. In the area of the areola a 1-cm-thick disk of breast tissue is left behind to preserve viability of the nipple.

Fibroadenomas and Related Tumors

This group, in addition to fibroadenoma, includes such processes as giant or juvenile fibroadenoma, hamartoma, and adenoma. Fibroadenoma is the second most common tumor of the breast (after carcinoma), is most common in women under 30 years of age, and is composed of both stromal and epithelial elements of the breast. These lesions are most commonly firm, solitary tumors that gradually increase in size. When a fibroadenoma achieves a size greater than 5 cm, the term giant or juvenile fibroadenoma is applied. Adenomas and hamartomas consisting of varying amounts of epithelium and stromal supporting tissue are clinically indistinguishable from fibroadenomas. The treatment of all of these tumors is excisional biopsy. Some form of breast reconstruction may be needed after resection of a giant fibroadenoma.

Papillomas and Other Ductal Tumors

Located under the areola in a majority of patients, solitary intraductal papillomas are true polyps of epithelium-lined breast ducts. In contrast, multiple intraductal papillomas are often more peripherally located and have been associated with an increased risk of cancer.

Papillomas, which are generally less than 1 cm in size, may on occasion grow to 4 to 5 cm in diameter. They are most commonly accompanied by a bloody nipple discharge, although they may sometimes be found as a palpable mass under the areola. Treatment is total excision through a circumareolar incision.

These conditions are to be distinguished from a condition known as papillomatosis, which is actually epithelial hyperplasia and may be of premalignant portent in the presence of atypical epithelial proliferation.

Sclerosing Disorders

This group includes sclerosing adenosis, which is important primarily for its simulation of carcinoma, both grossly and histologically. It is frequently seen in association with fibrocystic changes and has no malignant potential.

Other conditions that may simulate carcinoma either mammographically or with skin dimpling include radial scarring and fat necrosis. When there is any doubt whatsoever, biopsy should be carried out.

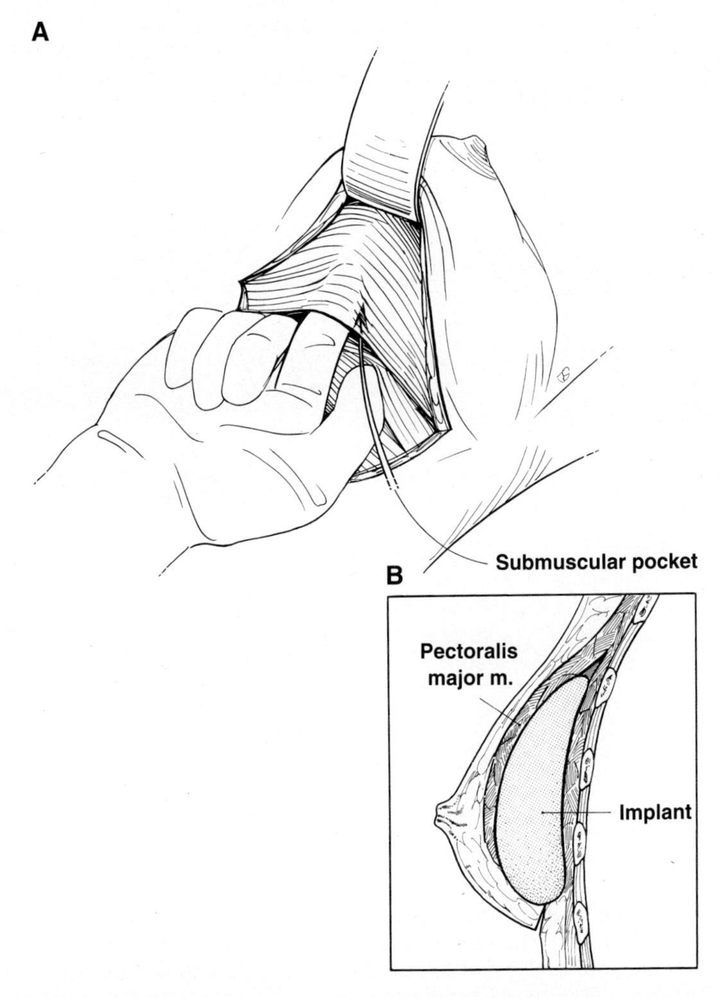

FIG 28–2.
A, once the breast is removed, a submuscular pocket is created. **B,** a prosthesis or tissue expander is inserted into the pocket, and total muscle coverage is achieved if possible.

Breast Abscess and Infections

An abscess is most commonly seen in the subareolar area. When obstruction of major ducts occurs, infection may proliferate, and a fistulous tract may occur. The treatment is preferentially conservative: antibiotics initially in conjunction with hot compresses. Intravenous antibiotics may be necessary in more severe infections. Incision and drainage are employed when antibiotics fail; when infection is recurrent, excision of the infected subareolar ducts may be necessary.

Generalized mastitis or cellulitis may be associated with menstrual cycle irregularity or more commonly with lactation and should be treated conservatively with heat or ice packs and, in lactation, with the use of a breast pump. When these measures fail, broad-spectrum antibiotics may be appropriate.

When mastitis fails to resolve completely, the possibility of inflammatory carcinoma must be entertained and ruled out.

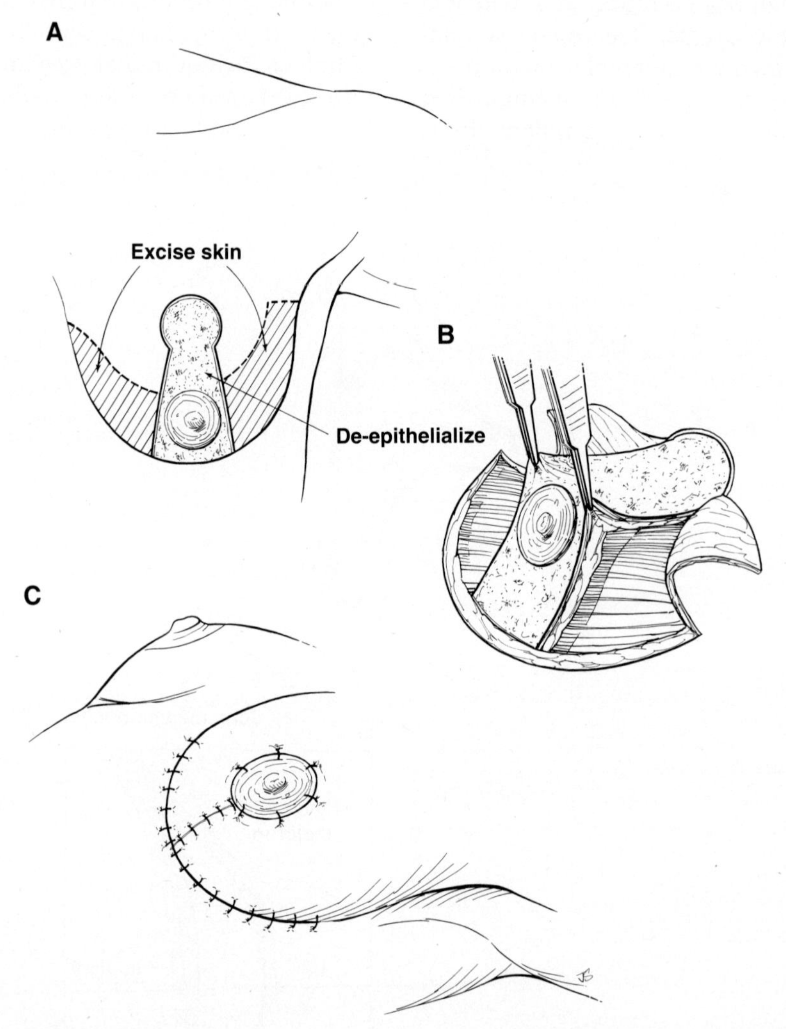

FIG 28–3.
A, pattern for mastopexy combined with subcutaneous mastectomy. The vertical pedicle is deepithelialized to provide a vascular bridge to the nipple. **B,** the breast is removed with preservation of the vertical pedicle. In the subareolar area, 1 cm of breast tissue is left behind on the pedicle to preserve viability of the nipple. **C,** the completed mastectomy/mastopexy after submuscular insertion of an implant or expander.

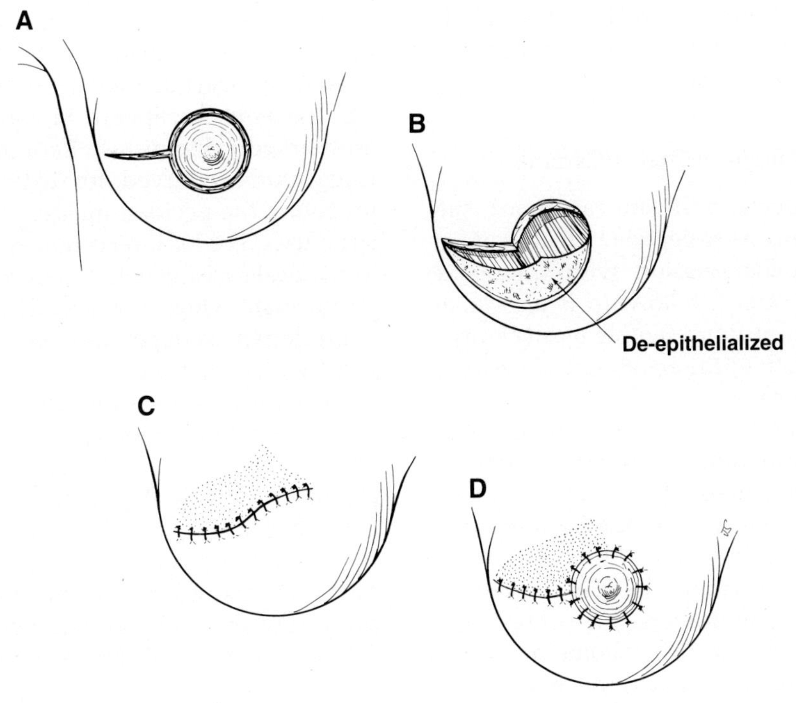

FIG 28–4.
A, incisions for simple (or total) mastectomy—circumareolar, with lateral extension if needed. **B,** mastectomy is completed. An implant or tissue expander can be inserted into a submuscular pocket. The lower skin edge can be deepithelialized for advancement under the upper edge. **C,** the closure is completed. **D,** the nipple-areola complex is replaced at an appropriate site as a free full-thickness graft.

MALIGNANT BREAST DISEASE

Incidence of Breast Cancer

Breast cancer is the most common malignancy in women, with an estimated 180,000 new cases in 1992 and approximately 46,000 deaths in the same year. In women it is exceeded only by lung cancer as a cause of death. It appears that the incidence of breast cancer is increasing, with a current incidence of about 10% of women or perhaps slightly higher.

Pathology of Breast Cancer

Malignant tumors of the breast may be classified into noninvasive and invasive. Noninvasive tumors include intraductal carcinoma and lobular carcinoma in situ. Theoretically these tumors have no potential for metastasis, although they may be precursors of invasive tumors.

Invasive tumors include invasive ductal carcinoma, invasive lobular carcinoma, and mucinous, medullary, papillary, tubular, adenoid cystic, secretory, and apocrine carcinomas in addition to carcinoma with metaplasia of various types and Paget's disease of the nipple (according to the World Health Organization [WHO] classification of breast tumors). Malignant mixed connective tissue and epithelial tumors include phylloides tumor (cystosarcoma phylloides) and carcinosarcoma. The most common of the invasive tumors is infiltrating ductal carcinoma, while invasive lobular carcinoma constitutes about 10% of breast cancers. The remaining variants are seen less frequently.

Diagnosis of Breast Cancer

As noted previously, the history and physical examination, FNA results, and imaging all play an important part in the diagnosis of breast cancer. Definitive treatment should be planned, however, only on the basis of a clear histopathologic diagnosis.

Primary Treatment of Breast Carcinoma

For intraductal or in situ carcinoma, simple mastectomy is acceptable treatment, although complete excision with tumor-free margins and careful follow-up is also advocated by many authors. Simple mastectomy is also appropriate in the treatment of cystosarcoma phylloides.

Invasive breast cancer is currently managed either by modified radical mastectomy or by conservation therapy, which usually consists of local resection or lumpectomy plus radiation, most commonly with axillary node sampling or dissection. There is still controversy as to the indications for conservation therapy, but most surgeons would agree that for large tumors (<4 cm) or multicentric cancers, modified radical mastectomy is the preferred approach.

Since the primary indication for conservation therapy is cosmetic, any procedure that will distort breast contour or *significantly alter symmetry* should be contraindicated. Two normal-appearing breasts that are not symmetrical do not constitute an aesthetically acceptable result. This principle has been largely overlooked by enthusiasts for conservation therapy.

While survival rates for modified radical mastectomy and conservation therapy are similar, the local recurrence rate is higher with the latter. Good salvage rates after recurrence are achieved with mastectomy and, if appropriate, further radiation. The prospects of satisfactory reconstruction with tissue expanders after therapeutic radiation, however, are markedly diminished. Radical mastectomy is currently reserved for extensive tumors involving the pectoral muscles or contiguous structures. For local recurrences after mastectomy, local excision with tumor-free margins is appropriate where possible. The use of radiation therapy is dependent on previous treatment with radiation.

For massive recurrences with tumor necrosis, debridement for hygiene may be essential. On occasion, reconstruction with skin grafting or muscle flaps (or rarely an omental flap) may be indicated to provide a closed wound for improved quality of life despite the near certainty of further recurrence. Any such procedure should be undertaken only after a full discussion of all factors with the patient.

Adjuvant Therapy for Breast Carcinoma

Adjuvant therapy, with respect to which there is no universal agreement, is summarized in Table 28–3.

Management of the Opposite Breast After Mastectomy

Management of the opposite breast depends on a number of factors and is again an area of controversy. Factors to be considered as favoring contralateral prophylactic mastectomy include a young age at mastectomy, a cancer with a known relatively high incidence

TABLE 28–3.

1985 National Institutes of Health Consensus Development Conference Conclusion: Adjuvant Therapy for State I and II Breast Cancer*

Menopausal Status	Axillary Nodes	Hormone Receptors	Recommended Treatment
Pre	Positive	+ or −	Combination
Pre	Negative	+ or −	Further clinical trials (combination chemotherapy considered)
Post	Positive	+	Tamoxifen
Post	Positive	−	Further clinical trials (combination chemotherapy considered)
Post	Negative	+ or −	Further clinical trials

* From Iglehart JD: The diagnosis and management of breast cancer: An update, in Sabiston DC Jr (ed): *Textbook of Surgery: The Biological Basis of Modern Surgical Practice, Update 1.* Philadelphia, WB Saunders, 1988. (Used by permission.)

of bilaterality such as invasive lobular carcinoma, the desire for reconstruction of the breast, and the importance of symmetry to the patient. Multicentricity of the original tumor may be an additional factor. A large, pendulous contralateral breast that causes postural problems or imbalance may also be an indication for contralateral simple mastectomy. The various techniques for prophylactic mastectomy, as discussed earlier in this chapter, would be applicable to the "opposite breast."

The alternative is monthly self-examination of the breast, physician examination twice yearly, and yearly mammography. The role of the surgeon is to fully present all appropriate information and to support the patient in her decision.

OTHER TUMORS

Since skin and soft-tissue tumors are dealt with elsewhere in this book (see Chapter 11), only those of special interest in the chest wall and abdomen will be addressed here.

Desmoid tumors are more commonly seen in the musculoaponeurotic system of the abdominal wall. They are fibrous in nature and histopathologically benign but have a strong propensity for recurrence. Their treatment is excision with margins widely free of tumor to avoid recurrence.

Soft-tissue sarcomas, while they are not common, may occur in both the abdomen and chest wall. They include the following in their approximate order of frequency of occurrence: malignant fibrous histiocytoma, liposarcoma, fibrosarcoma, rhabdomyosarcoma, leiomyosarcoma, synovial sarcoma, malignant neurilemoma, mesenchymoma, Kaposi's sarcoma, angiosarcoma, and extraskeletal osteogenic sarcoma and chondrosarcoma. Although nodal metastases are not a common feature of these tumors, the incidence in some such as rhabdomyosarcoma and synovial sarcoma may be as high as 10% to 20%.

The primary treatment of sarcomas is wide excision. For recurrences, reasonably good results have been achieved in patients without metastases by using preoperative doxorubicin, radiation therapy, and wide resection of the recurrence.

SUGGESTED READING

Donegan Sprat (eds): *Cancer of the Breast,* ed 3. Philadelphia, WB Saunders, 1988.

Patrick MG (ed): Plastic and reconstructive breast surgery. *Clin Plast Surg* 1988; 15:655–665, 667–675, 677–685.

Sabiston DC Jr (ed): *Textbook of Surgery, the Biological Basis of Surgical Practice,* ed 14. Philadelphia, WB Saunders, 1991.

Woods JE: Detailed technique of subcutaneous mastectomy with and without mastopexy. *Ann Plast Surg* 1987; 18:51–61.

Chapter 29

Trauma and Reconstruction

Carl I. Price, M.D.
Foad Nahai, M.D.

■ CONTENTS

■ CHAPTER OBJECTIVE

At the end of this chapter the resident understands the principles of management of trauma-related problems of the breast and trunk and carries out surgical management, including complex reconstruction for such disorders.

■ LEARNER OBJECTIVES

On completion of this chapter the resident

1. **Understands the basic principles of medical and surgical management of common acute traumatic trunk and breast injuries.**
2. **Has detailed knowledge of the surgical aspects of breast reconstruction, including the rationale for choices between different methods and recognizes the complications of reconstruction and their prevention and treatment.**
3. **Is familiar with the prosthetic devices used in breast reconstruction, including implants and tissue expanders.**
4. **Understands the psychosocial aspects of postmastectomy reconstruction.**
5. **Understands the etiology and nonsurgical management of pressure sores (including preventive measures).**
6. **Has detailed knowledge of the surgical aspects of pressure sore reconstruction.**
7. Demonstrates knowledge of the common posttraumatic deformities of the trunk and breast.
8. Has detailed knowledge of the surgical aspects of trunk reconstruction.

■ CLINICAL PRACTICE ACTIVITIES

During the course of the training program, the resident

1. **Evaluates and treats patients with postsurgical breast deformities.**
2. **Performs breast reconstruction with various techniques such as implants, tissue expanders, and flaps.**
3. **Performs nipple reconstruction.**
4. **Evaluates and treats patients with pressure sores.**
5. **Performs reconstructive procedures on patients with pressure sores.**
6. **Performs reconstructive procedures for posttraumatic thoracic deformities.**
7. Performs reconstructive procedures for posttraumatic breast deformities.
8. Performs reconstruction of sternal wound dehiscence.
9. Performs abdominal wall reconstruction with fascial flaps or grafts.
10. Performs reconstruction of radiation injury of the trunk and/or breast.
11. Evaluates and manages complications arising from reconstructive procedures of the trunk and breast.
12. *Manages patients with acute thoracic and/or abdominal visceral injury.*

Plastic surgery of the trunk and breast presents reconstructive challenges that require not only intimate knowledge of anatomy and technical skill but an aesthetic sense as well to produce favorable results. The goal is to safely combine the restoration of function with the achievement of an aesthetically acceptable result.

CHEST WALL RECONSTRUCTION

Chest wall defects result from trauma, infection, or tumor extirpation. Reconstructions should provide appropriate soft-tissue coverage while replacing the underlying supportive structures when necessary. (For reconstruction of congenital anomalies such as Poland's syndrome and pectus excavatum, see Chapter 27.)

All defects involving the rigid support of the chest case do not require structural reconstruction. If a large defect will adversely affect pulmonary function, rigid replacement should be considered, but even large resections can be tolerated well without rigid reconstruction. The choice of material for rigid reconstruction varies, but we prefer either autologous bone (most commonly rib) or Prolene mesh. For massive defects the combination of methyl methacrylate with mesh has been advocated but is not usually necessary. Stable soft-tissue coverage of rigid reconstruction is important to prevent future implant extrusion, infection, or exposure.

Soft-tissue defects of the anterior aspect of the chest can be closed with either local or distant tissue. First consideration is given to primary closure or skin grafting. When the underlying process or size of the defect precludes this, a number of local flaps are available. The pectoralis, latissimus, and rectus muscles are all available as either muscle or musculocutaneous flaps to cover defects. Radiation to the chest may affect the choice of flap, but radiation to the pedicle area of a particular flap does not necessarily preclude its use. Of the locally available flaps, the latissimus is the most versatile and can be mobilized to reach the contralateral hemithorax. The serratus anterior muscle can be used for smaller defects, and use of the triceps brachii has been described for upper thoracic defects. When other muscle flaps are not available or inadequate, the omental flap is an excellent option to fill large complex defects. Free flaps are rarely needed.

STERNAL AND INTRATHORACIC INFECTIONS

Infections involving the sternum and mediastinum are a serious complication of cardiothoracic surgery. Prior to the application of muscle flaps, treatment of these infections involved open packing or irrigation and resulted in both high morbidity and mortality. Wide debridement combined with vascularized tissue coverage has evolved into the primary treatment of sternal and mediastinal infections and has significantly improved the clinical outcome of these patients. A one-stage procedure is most often indicated. Usually the sternal wound is opened, debrided, and covered with well-vascularized tissue early. A two-stage procedure with debridement and flap coverage at separate settings is reserved for more severe infections or complicated situations. Patients who are seen late (usually more than 6 weeks after the initial surgery) are treated with caution, and preoperative computed tomography (CT) may be used to determine the extent of retrosternal involvement.

The primary muscles available for sternal coverage include the pectoralis, rectus, and (to a lesser extent) the latissimus muscles (Fig 29–1). Removal of involved sternal wires and complete debridement of all infected bone and cartilage are necessary before flap coverage. Bacterial control of the wound results from adequate debridement. Well-vascularized flaps should obliterate the dead space, and suction drains should be liberally employed. The first choice is the pectoralis muscle, which can be rotated into the wound and supplied by the thoracoacromial vessels or turned over and supplied by the internal mammary perforators. The pectoralis muscle will cover most of the widespread sternal defect; however, occasionally the rectus muscle is also needed for lower sternal wounds. The widespread use of the internal mammary vessel in cardiac revascularization may prevent the use of the ipsilateral rectus or the turnover pectoralis flap, and variations of these flaps may be necessary (Table 29–1). The skin is usually easily closed over the flaps, and skin grafts are rarely necessary. Musculocutaneous flaps are rarely used. The omentum is reserved for severe infections requiring a large amount of tissue or situations when the

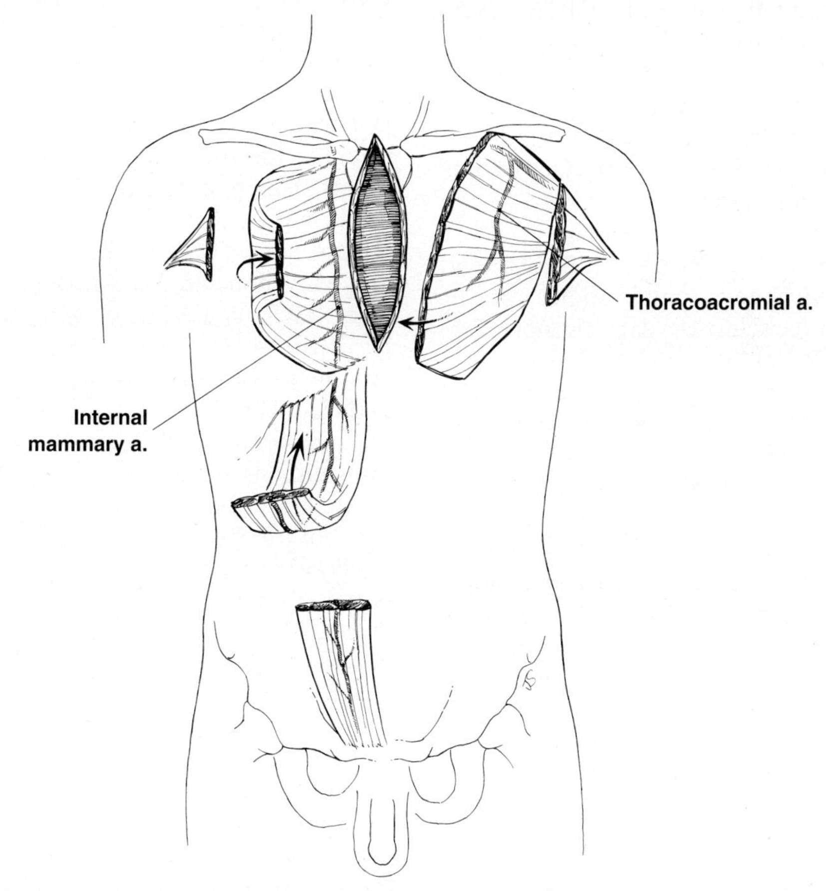

FIG 29–1.
Muscle flaps available for sternal wound coverage primarily include the pectoralis major and the rectus abdominis. The pectoralis major based on the thoracoacromial artery can be transposed or turned over and based on the medial perforators arising from the internal mammary artery and intercostals.

TABLE 29–1.
Local Flap Selection for Sternal Wound Closure Following Coronary Artery Bypass Procedures

If vein grafts alone used:
- Unilateral split pectoralis turnover
- Unilateral rectus abdominis
- Pectoralis rotation-advancement
- Combined flaps

If unilateral IMA used*:
- Contralateral split pectoralis turnover
- Contralateral rectus abdominis
- Pectoralis rotation-advancement
- Combined flaps

If bilateral IMA used:
- Segmental pectoralis flap
- Rectus abdominis (intercostal blood supply)
- Pectoralis rotation-advancement
- Bipedicle pectoralis-rectus
- Omentum
- Latissimus dorsi

* IMA = internal mammary artery.

pectoralis and rectus are not available. Pediatric patients are managed in a similar manner except that less radical cartilage debridement is done because of concern for subsequent growth abnormalities; in addition, the rectus muscle is preferred because of the lack of bulk in the pectoralis muscles.

Other intrathoracic problems, refractory empyema cavity, bronchopleural fistulas, and postpneumonectomy complications can be treated with local muscle flap transfers. Empyema cavities can be successfully obliterated with transposition of the latissimus, serratus, rectus, or pectoralis muscles or various combinations of these muscles (Fig. 29–2). Even after thoracotomy there is usually sufficient muscle for intrathoracic transfer, so the omental flap is rarely needed. Obliteration of empyema cavities is usually done in a single stage with minimal morbidity. The need to completely obliterate an empyema space, with thoracoplasty if necessary, is debatable. Care must be taken in the decision to harvest the rectus in patients who have marginal pulmonary reserve since it can be an important accessory respiratory muscle.

ABDOMINAL RECONSTRUCTION

Abdominal defects requiring complex closure result from trauma, tumor extirpation, or infectious processes. The defect must be assessed in terms of both soft-tissue and structural support. The presence of underlying bowel contamination or a fistula will have an influence on the timing and type of reconstruction. Situations that involve extensive lysis of adhesions or extensive manipulation of the abdominal viscera are best handled in staged procedures. When definitive abdominal reconstruction is not indicated or possible, the defect can be closed with mesh, which is allowed to granulate and is subsequently skin-grafted. Smaller wounds may be treated with local care alone.

For structural reconstruction of the abdominal wall, alloplastic material is most often used; free fascia lata grafts are also available. There is considerable debate as to the best material, with Marlex (Bard), Prolene (Ethicon), Vicryl (Ethicon), Dexon (Davis and Geck), and Gore-Tex all having been used successfully. Generally there is insufficient fibrous ingrowth into the absorbable products (Vicryl, Dexon) to result in abdominal wall stability. The ingrowth of tissue into Gore-Tex is less than that of either Prolene or Marlex mesh, which may account for the ease with which Gore-Tex can be subsequently removed. When alloplastic material is not desirable, fascia lata is used as a free graft or pedicled on the tensor fasciae latae (TFL) muscle to provide vascularized tissue. The pedicled TFL fascia will seldom reach above the midabdomen. Care must be taken when insetting fascia lata to orient the lines of maximal wound tension with the longitudinal fibers of the fascia. Two overlapping layers of fascia oriented at 90 degrees provide bidirectional strength. The need for short-term abdominal wall integrity in complicated situations may dictate less-than-optimal soft-tissue coverage of mesh reconstructions; in these situations vascularized fascia lata on a TFL pedicle flap should be considered. When possible, stable soft-tissue cover is mandatory to minimize the subsequent extrusion of mesh. Flaps may be necessary for stable coverage, and classification of the defect by location into upper, mid, and lower abdominal defects aids in selection among flap options (Table 29–2).

For a midline structural defect primary

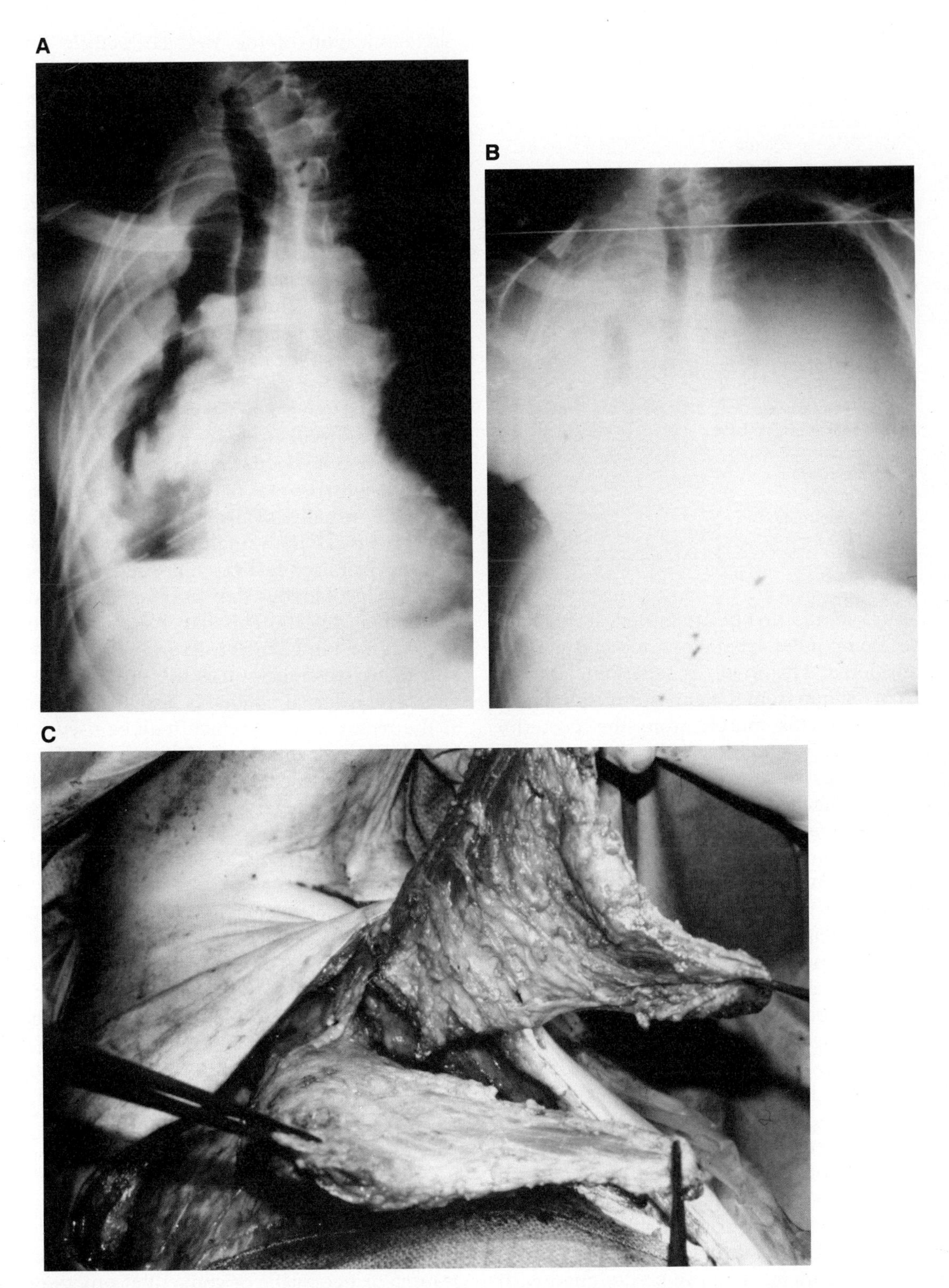

FIG 29–2.
Fifty-six-year-old male after lobectomy for small-cell carcinoma of the lung **(A)**. A refractory empyema developed and was treated with latissimus and serratus muscle transposition into the empyema space **(B)**. Note the amount of muscle still available after a thoracotomy incision **(C)**.

TABLE 29–2.
Abdominal Reconstruction: Flap Choices

Upper abdomen
Rectus abdominis
External oblique
Latissimus dorsi
Rectus femoris
Omentum
Free flap
Midabdomen
Tensor fasciae latae
Rectus abdominis
External oblique
Rectus femoris
Omentum
Free flap
Lower abdomen
Tensor fasciae latae
Rectus abdominis
Rectus femoris
Gracilis
Omentum
Free flap

closure should first be attempted. If this fails, the "component separation" method may be considered. This involves separating the external oblique from the anterior rectus sheath and the rectus muscle from the posterior rectus sheath and then advancing the anterior rectus sheath, underlying rectus muscle, and attached internal oblique and transversalis muscle toward the midline. This dynamic muscle transposition may be advanced 5 cm in the epigastrium, 10 cm at the waist, and 3 cm in the suprapubic area. Bilateral flaps would theoretically double these distances.

Upper abdominal defects are difficult to manage, especially when large amounts of soft tissue are needed. Local flaps, although often inadequate, should be considered first. The rectus muscle or musculocutaneous flap can be fashioned to cover most moderate-sized defects of the upper part of the abdomen, but consideration must be given to the potential donor morbidity in an already compromised abdominal wall. The external oblique flap is an alternative for some defects. The latissimus musculocutaneous flap can be designed with an extended fasciocutaneous portion to cover some areas of the upper portion of the abdomen. Disinsertion of the muscle and skeletonization of the vascular pedicle can extend the reach of the latissimus; alternatively, the vascular pedicle can be extended with microvascular techniques and vein grafts. Omental flaps with skin grafts can also be used. The omentum has the advantage of covering extremely large defects; however, since it provides no structural support, its use usually necessitates underlying support, and it is often unavailable because of the process that produced the abdominal defect. The rectus femoris can be used for defects up to the costal margin if the flap is turned over on itself rather than rotated, but it provides only muscle that must remain innervated to provide any support.

Mid and lower abdominal defects may be covered with several flaps. The rectus abdominis is usually available, but donor site concerns make it an unattractive option. The TFL can be raised as a vascularized fascial flap or a fasciocutaneous flap to cover most midabdominal defects. This flap has the advantage of providing both structural support and soft-tissue coverage and is the preferred option. The external oblique is also available, as is the rectus femoris, which may be used for midabdominal defects. Groin and superficial interior epigastric artery flaps can provide soft-tissue coverage. The lower part of the abdomen can be reconstructed with TFL, rectus femoris, rectus abdominis, or gracilis flaps.

Free tissue transfer for abdominal reconstruction may require vein grafting to establish inflow. This is best provided with a long vascular loop from the femoral vessels. The vascular pedicle of the latissimus can also be extended with vein grafts to reach most defects. Free tissue transfer is reserved for those situations that are otherwise unsolvable.

POSTERIOR TRUNK RECONSTRUCTION

Posterior trunk defects may result from trauma or neoplastic or congenital processes. These often include infected orthopedic hardware or complicated wounds after spinal surgery that require stable soft-tissue coverage. Effective bacterial control of the infected wound by debridement is a prerequisite for successful soft-tissue coverage. Adequate surgical debridement may include removal of infected hardware. The posterior of the trunk can be divided into thirds for flap selection purposes. Upper-third back wounds may be reconstructed with either latissimus dorsi or trapezius muscle flaps. Both will cover scapular or cervical wounds. The latissimus offers more flexibility in designing skin islands and is generally preferred. The latissimus may be based on either the thoracodorsal pedicle laterally or on the intercostal perforators medially. When based medially, the flap can be turned over on the inferior perforating vessels to cover midthoracic and upper lumbar defects. Lower defects can also be covered with a transverse lumbar flap. These lower defects can also be covered with a microvascularly extended pedicled latissimus flap (Fig 29–3).

For coverage of meningomyelocele defects the latissimus can be mobilized to cover defects as low as L4. Bipedicle flaps can be used, but grafting of the donor sites is necessary, and the cutaneous suture line may lie over the dural repair. Alternatively, a latissimus and gluteal musculocutaneous flap can be advanced in an en bloc fashion to close even larger defects.

PRESSURE SORES

Pressure ulcers are a common malady among immobile, hospitalized, and neurologically impaired patients. They are often inaccurately referred to as "decubitus ulcers," a term correctly applied only to ulcers resulting from recumbency. The preferred term "pressure sore" includes ulcerations resulting from other positions. It has been estimated that pressure ulcers occur in 3% to 4% of all hospital admissions and may be present in 45% of all admissions to chronic care facilities. Pressure sores develop in paraplegics at a rate of 5% to 8% per year, while quadraplegics have an even higher rate. The cost of care for these patients is staggering. It has been suggested that 25% of the cost of care for patients with spinal cord injury results from pressure ulcer treatment. Death rates are increased

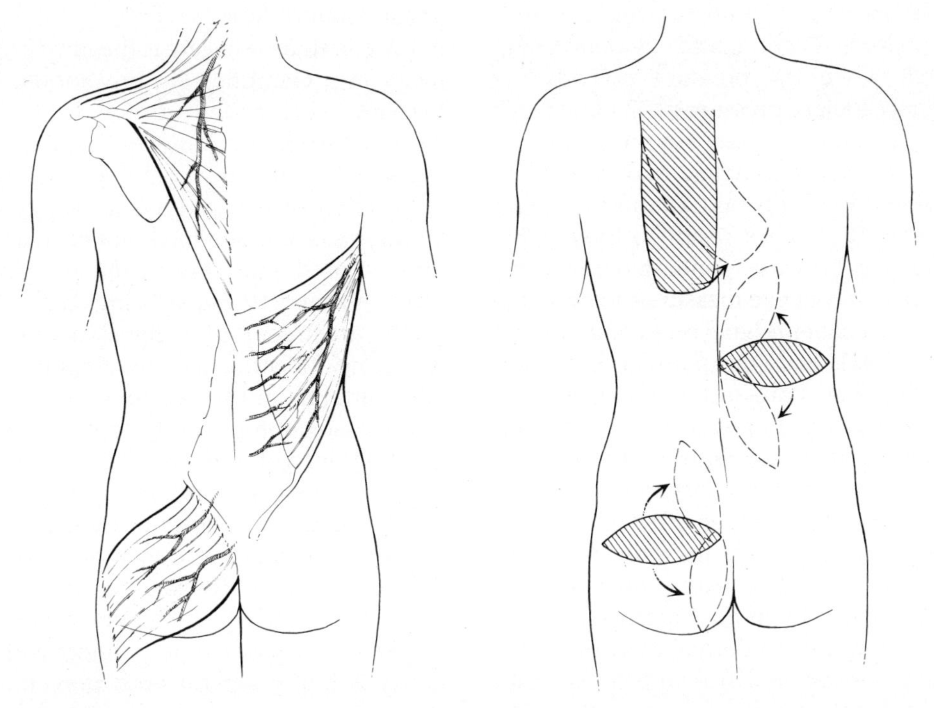

FIG 29–3.
Options available for closure of posterior trunk defects.

fourfold in geriatric populations with pressure ulcers; pressure ulcers also account for 8% of paraplegic deaths. The areas particularly susceptible to ulceration are those overlying bony prominences. In bedridden, nonparalyzed patients the sacrum and trochanteric areas are most commonly involved. Paraplegic patients ulcerate in the ischial, trochanteric, sacral, and heel areas in decreasing order of frequency. Correspondingly, 90% of all pressure ulcers occur in the lower half of the body, with a third of these occurring in the lower extremity and two thirds in the hips and buttocks.

Pathogenesis

While a deficit of trophic substances such as growth factors and the loss of normal innervation may contribute to pressure ulcers, those are not the main etiologic factors. Pressure ulcer skin breakdown results, as the name clearly implies, from sustained pressure. Shear forces, friction, and moisture can initiate the ulcer process, while nutritional and infectious considerations contribute to the progression and persistence of ulcers.

Prolonged skin pressure exceeding capillary pressure usually initiates the development of ulcers. Experimental evidence suggests that when the pressure exceeds the endarterial capillary pressure of 32 mm Hg for extended periods or 70 mm Hg for as short as 2 hours, irreversible ischemia may result. On the other hand, short periods of pressure of up to 240 mm Hg may *not* result in irreversible tissue damage. Pressures generated over bony prominences have been measured to be 100 to 150 mm Hg in patients lying on a conventional mattress. Muscle and subcutaneous tissue are more susceptible to pressure-induced necrosis than dermis is, which accounts for the deep undermining often seen with pressure ulcers. Shear forces magnify the ischemic effects of pressure on these deeper tissues through stretch and angulation of the nutrient blood vessels. Friction and moisture, on the other hand, contribute to more superficial breakdown through intraepidermal blistering, erosions, and maceration. Once an ulcer is established, bacterial counts of greater than 10^5 colony-forming units per gram of tissue delay or impair healing, as does malnutrition.

Prevention

Prevention is the key in dealing with pressure sores. Prevention entails pressure relief, identification of at-risk patients, and the early detection of impending ulceration. Early physical signs of pressure sore development are erythema and hyperemia, which resolve within an hour of pressure relief. If pressure persists for 2 to 6 hours, then ischemia will be evidenced by erythema that may take up to 36 hours to resolve. Pressure for longer than 6 hours usually results in irreversible tissue necrosis or ulceration. It has been suggested that immobility combined with hypoalbuminemia, fecal incontinence, and the presence of a fracture in elderly patients are risk factors for the development of pressure sores. If identified, these factors may help to designate patients who require aggressive preventive measures. In patients with spinal cord injury, spasticity, poor nutrition, and unstable social situations place patients at high risk for ulceration. Once the early lesion or at-risk patient has been identified, skin care, relief of spasticity, weight dispersion, local wound care, infection control, and nutrition support are important in preventing ulceration or the progression of lesions.

Meticulous skin care is the most important factor in preventing skin breakdown. Simple measures such as talcum powder to prevent friction, turning the patient every 2 hours, and massage of pressure points are helpful. The application of barrier-type dressings such as Duoderm or Op Site have not been as important as good skin care in the prevention of ulcers, although these dressings can be helpful in the treatment of early skin breakdown. Reducing moisture and eliminating particulate matter from the bedding are also important measures to prevent ulceration. Keeping bedding clean of urine may require indwelling urinary catheters. Condom catheters in males are discouraged because of their higher incidence of infectious and local wound complications. Intestinal diversion may be indicated to keep the bedding and wound clean of feces.

Relief of spasticity in patients with spinal injury is important for both prevention and postoperative care. The degree of severity dictates the treatment. Pharmacologic treatment with agents like benzodiazepams, baclofen, and dantrolene can be useful, but care must be taken to avoid dependence. Spinal cord interventions such as anterior rhizotomy or alcohol injections can be helpful, although the loss of reflex sexual activity and bladder control can devastate these patients' sometimes fragile sense of adequacy and worth. Careful and frank discussions are mandatory before embarking on an irreversible treatment path, although a difficult choice may have to be made between a permanently disabling operation and a large chronic pressure sore that may lead to continued sepsis and death.

Many methods are available to aid in the dispersion of pressure. Pressure awareness education should be mandatory in all cooperative patients and should include routine examination of pressure areas, with a mirror if necessary. Capable wheelchair-bound patients so able should lift themselves every 10 to 15 minutes for 10 seconds. Wheelchair seat cushions that alleviate pressure should be mandatory; however, these cushions do not obviate patient responsibility for pressure relief by lifting, adequate pressure awareness, and nursing care. The low air loss cushion and the air-fluidized bed are important devices for pressure relief in bedridden patients. These can be useful adjuncts in both the prevention and the treatment of pressure ulcers. However, pressure awareness, patient compliance, and good nursing care are far and away more important than any mechanical aid!

Treatment

Once a pressure sore is established, local wound care is important in the initial management. This care may be all that is necessary in debilitated or terminally ill patients to avoid life-threatening sepsis from their pressure sores. The wound can be classified according to depth (Table 29–3), but it should be recognized that pressure ulcers are usually more extensive than they first appear because of the sensitivity of subcutaneous fat and muscle to pressure necrosis and the relative resistance of dermal elements to the same pressure. Surgical debridement is necessary to remove necrotic debris and to gain initial bacterial control. Clinical and experimental evidence suggests that bacterial counts of greater than 10^5 organisms per gram will inhibit healing. Initial debridement can often be done at the bedside even when large amounts of necrotic tissue are present. Pressure dressings may be necessary to control persistent oozing immediately after debridement. Enzymatic debridement has at best a minor role. Topical antimicrobials such as silver sulfadiazine are helpful in controlling bacterial counts in more heavily contaminated wounds, but no amount of antimicrobial agent can substitute for good surgical debridement!

TABLE 29–3.
Pressure Sore Grading

Grade	Description
Grade I	Epidermal-dermal damage
Grade II	Extension into subcutaneous tissue
Grade III	Underlying muscle involvement
Grade IV	Bone and joint exposure

After the initial debridement a decision is made concerning surgical closure. Not all patients are candidates for surgical closure. Many pressure sores, given adequate local treatment and time, will close spontaneously. However, a long-standing nonhealing ulcer should raise concern for squamous cell carcinoma (Marjolin's ulcer). A patient who is critically ill, unstable, debilitated with organic brain syndrome, or unsuitable for any rehabilitation beyond the vegetative state or refuses to cooperate with the demands of operative and postoperative management is not a candidate for surgical closure. On the other hand, indications for surgery may include ulcers too large to expect spontaneous closure in a reasonable period of time, ulcers with underlying bursae, ulcers with thin unstable scar over bony prominence, and ulcers with areas of heterotrophic calcification. Other indications for surgical closure may be ulcers associated with chronic pyarthrosis or those associated with enteric or urinary fistulas. Unfortunately, surgery is often not the definitive solution. Recividism rates may be greater than 50%. This is especially true of young patients with traumatic spinal cord injury because these individuals are more likely to have an unstable social situation and poor home care.

The goal of surgical treatment is to achieve a stable closed wound. The surgeon must have a well–thought out reconstructive plan that leaves other reconstructive options open for future procedures should they become necessary. Basic principles include complete excision of the ulcer, adjacent scar, and bursae. Instilling methylene blue and hydrogen peroxide into the wound will stain the tissues and aid in bursal identification for excision. Excision of the ulcer can be quite bloody, especially in patients with spinal injury who lack sympathetic tone; therefore, blood should always be available. Suction drainage should be liberally used in all pressure sore reconstructions. Excision of the underlying bone and obliteration of dead space with well-vascularized tissue are important surgical steps. Total ischiectomy has been advocated in the past, but this procedure may cause significant redistribution of pressure and subsequent ulceration at other sites. The authors' preferences for flap closure at various sites are outlined in Table 29–4. Avoidance of tight closures and placement of sutures away from pressure points contribute to success. Sensate flaps should be considered if available. Postoperatively patients should be maintained on pressure-relieving beds for at least 3 weeks. Wheelchair-bound patients should be kept recumbent for 3 weeks and then slowly allowed to sit. It is important during this period to intensively reeducate patients whose behavior patterns contributed to ulcer formation.

Sacral Ulcers

A variety of flaps are available to close sacral sores. An initial choice for smaller ulcers is the transverse lumbosacral flap. The main advantage of this flap is that it leaves the buttocks unscarred for subsequent reconstructions. Next is the gluteus fasciocutaneous flap as a unilateral or bilateral "V-Y" advancement. A rotational fasciocutaneous flap is also possible. Finally, a gluteus musculocutaneous flap is reserved for major defects or recurrences. This may be advanced as a V-Y flap, with additional mobility obtained by detaching the trochanteric insertion. In ambulatory patients there is a significant negative impact on the ability to ambulate when the insertion of the gluteal muscles is mobilized. The posterior thigh flap can be used to close smaller defects, although this is not generally a first choice (Fig 29–4).

TABLE 29–4.
Flap Choices for Pressure Sores

Sacral
Transverse lumbar flap
Gluteal fasciocutaneous flap
Gluteal musculocutaneous flap
Trochanteric
Posterior thigh flap
Rectus femoris flap
Tensor fasciae latae flap
Vastus lateralis flap
Ischial
Posterior thigh flap
Gracilis muscle flap
Gluteal musculocutaneous flap
Hamstring flap

Trochanteric Ulcers

Trochanteric sores can be initially closed with the posterior thigh flap (see Fig 29–4). This flap is easy to raise and leaves most subsequent flap options open. The next choice may be the rectus femoris flap. This flap has a fairly reliable skin island and is raised with relative ease. The easy arc of rotation allows for tension-free closures. The next option is the TFL fasciocutaneous flap. This myocutaneous flap has a significant fasciocutaneous portion that can be extended with delay. It can provide sensibility in the low-level paraplegic since it has cutaneous innervation from T12 to L3 and can be used to close combined trochanteric and ischial ulcers. The vastus lateralis muscle can also be used in its proximal two thirds to close trochanteric sores. The distal third is not reliably elevated. A large skin island can be taken, and the arc of rotation is similar to the TFL flap. The dissection is tedious and often bloody.

Ischial Ulcers

Any flap closure of the ischium should allow tension-free closure with the hips flexed as in the sitting position. While relatively uncommon, bowel or bladder fistulas do occur in these ulcers. When fistulas are present, they must be controlled by appropriate proximal urinary or fecal diversion prior to closure of the ulcer.

Good first choices for closure are the posterior thigh flap or gracilis muscle flap. A

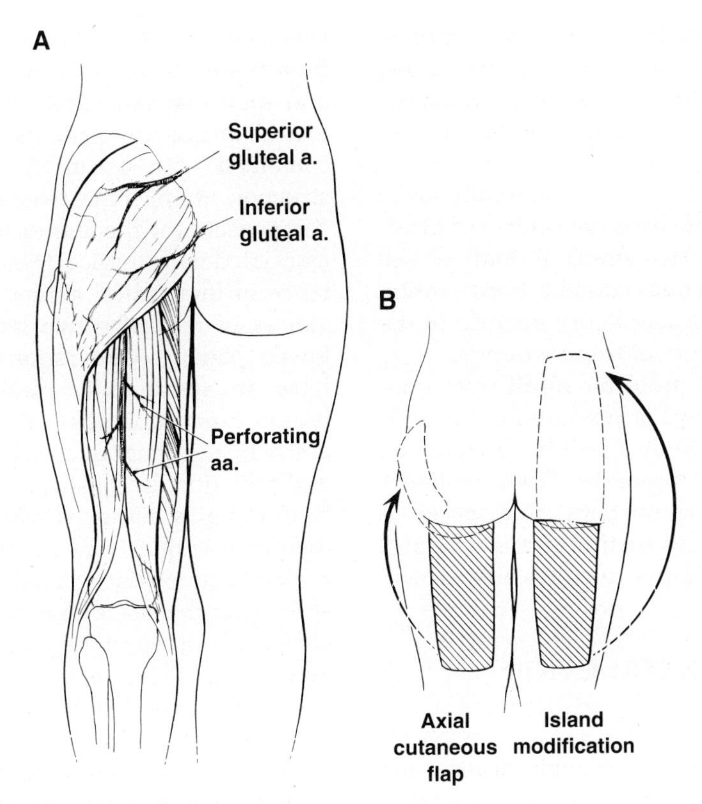

FIG 29–4.
A posterior thigh flap is a good initial option for ischial and trochanteric ulcers; it may also be used for sacral pressure sores.

skin island can be taken with the gracilis muscle, although it is not always reliable. Another initial option is the hamstring V-Y advancement flap. Even large defects can be closed with this flap, but care must be taken to flex the hips when insetting so as to avoid undue tension when the patient sits in a wheelchair. Additional mobilization can be obtained by dividing the biceps femoris tendon. This flap can be readvanced to treat recurrences. A previous posterior thigh flap precludes use of the hamstring flap. Ischial sores can also be closed by using the inferior portion of the gluteus maximus as an island flap supplied by the inferior gluteal vessels. This does leave the superior portion available for sacral ulcers.

Other Options

With massive ulcers or multiple recurrent ulcers, amputation of the lower extremity and a total thigh fillet flap may be necessary. This flap provides a large amount of well-vascularized tissue that can increase patient mobility and ease transfers in some situations. Free tissue transfer is an option but is reserved for desperate situations.

Complications

Complications of major flap reconstructions are related to the magnitude of the operation and the condition of the patient. Preoperative nutritional and medical support are often necessary. Flap necrosis is rare given sound flap design based on an understanding of the regional blood supply. Hematomas are the most common complication and can have an impact on subsequent ulcer recurrence and infection. Aggressive use of suction drainage and staged reconstruction in particularly bloody debridements can reduce hematoma formation. Significant hematomas should be surgically drained.

Seromas are a common but usually insignificant complication. Incomplete dead space obliteration and inadequate patient immobilization postoperatively with resultant shear forces can contribute to seroma formation. Prolonged suction drainage may be preventive.

Infections occur most commonly as a result of inadequate bacterial control of ulcers by debridement. Hematoma formation will contribute to infectious complications. Antibiotic prophylaxis is mandatory because of the contaminated nature of these wounds.

Other wound problems result from poor operative planning or execution. Wounds closed with tension or a poorly vascularized flap will not heal properly. Postoperatively, prolonged pressure on flaps predisposes to problems. Shear and friction forces may also result in postoperative wound breakdown.

BREAST RECONSTRUCTION

Breast Cancer

Breast cancer is a major public health issue that affects 1 in 8 or 9 women in the United States. There will be as many as 140,000 new breast cancers diagnosed per year. Reconstructive surgeons are often involved in early treatment options presented to a patient and therefore should be familiar with the current oncologic management of breast cancer.

It is interesting to note that breast cancer therapy over the last 30 years has not had a significant impact on the long-term survival. Recent emphasis on screening and education may eventually result in improved outcomes. Mammography and regular examination by a trained health professional are the keys to screening. Routine plain-film mammography should be performed on a biannual basis after the age of 40 years and yearly after the age of 50. High-risk patients, such as those with a strong family history or an atypical proliferative lesion on biopsy, should have more aggressive early screening. Other imaging techniques such as CT or magnetic resonance imaging (MRI) have limited value in screening. (For additional discussion of the management of malignant breast disease, see Chapter 28.)

The major thrust of conservative surgical treatment is preservation of breast aesthetics. Breasts are a focus of femininity in our society, and their loss can have a profound psychological impact on patients, especially when combined with a cancer diagnosis. Reconstruction offers some patients the chance to compensate for the loss of body image often associated with surgical treatment. The acceptance of less radical surgery along with advances in reconstructive technique have allowed patients who require mastectomy to have an aesthetically pleasing breast after tumor extirpation that often surpasses the aesthetic result obtained with limited surgery and radiation. Reconstructive options should be thoroughly discussed with patients prior to definitive surgical oncologic treatment with the realization that reconstruction is not desired by or the best option for all patients. For some, the prospect of multiple procedures, financial hardship, or a complex reconstruction is far worse than the resultant deformity; in these patients, reconstruction is not indicated. Often patients contemplating their oncologic treatment options are simply overwhelmed by the prospect of choosing among reconstructive options and cannot effectively choose. Patient satisfaction is high in those who choose reconstruction even when the surgeon feels that less than an aesthetic triumph has been achieved.

The only true contraindication to breast reconstruction after mastectomy is a medical condition that precludes the safe performance of reconstructive surgery. Advanced age and the presence of systemic disease should not exclude a patient from consideration for reconstruction, especially if a patient feels that reconstruction is important and reconstruction can be safely performed. It must be remembered, however, that reconstruction is an elective procedure and should not interfere with oncologic therapy. Complications or slow healing after a reconstructive procedure that delays adjunctive therapy may have an adverse effect on the long-term oncologic outcome. Therefore, in patients with advanced disease careful selection and frank discussions are mandatory. Local recurrence may be hidden by reconstruction, so obsessive follow-up is necessary in such patients. Any suspicious area in a reconstructed breast should have tissue diagnosis by fine-needle aspiration or biopsy.

Reconstructive Options

Selection of reconstructive options is dependent on several factors. Will the reconstruction be done as an immediate or delayed procedure? Is the opposite breast easily matched, or will it require surgical modification to match the reconstructed breast? What is the medical condition and prognosis of the patient? Will a lengthy procedure be tolerated, or should a more limited procedure be considered? What are the patient's desires? Does she wish to have an autologous reconstruction, or will she accept an implant? Does she have the body habitus to support autologous reconstruction? What is the skill and track record of the oncologic surgeon? Long bloody extirpative surgery, after which one is left with tenuous mastectomy flaps, limits reconstructive options.

Immediate vs. Delayed Reconstruction

The first decision is whether reconstruction will be immediate or delayed. This should be decided jointly between the patient and the reconstructive and oncologic surgeons. Psychological, oncologic, and aesthetic considerations all have an influence on the reconstructive decision. Patients who are overwhelmed by oncologic decisions may be better served by delayed reconstruction even when immediate reconstruction is available. Alternatively, patients who have a strong body image dependence upon their breasts should be encouraged to consider immediate reconstruction.

Immediate reconstruction is appealing for several reasons. The psychological trauma that is involved in the disfiguring extirpative surgery can be obviated with immediate reconstruction. The resultant reconstruction in the immediate setting is generally superior to delayed reconstruction since there may be part of the breast skin envelope remaining to help shape the reconstruction, especially when a skin-sparing type of mastectomy is performed.

Immediate reconstruction has complications that are a result of both the oncologic and reconstructive procedures and therefore are partially out of the reconstructive surgeon's control. Extirpation time, blood loss, and mastectomy skin flap thickness are important issues that can have an influence on reconstructive choices and outcome. If there are thin, tenuous mastectomy flaps, reconstruction with implants or expanders carries more risk, and autologous tissue coverage or autologous reconstruction may be necessary. Immediate reconstruction also demands that the reconstructive surgeon realistically assess complication rates and tailor the reconstructive methods to achieve the most reliable healing. Flap problems or delayed healing may result in delay of adjunctive therapy, which may in turn jeopardize the oncologic outcome in patients with more advanced disease. Reconstructions with available tissue and implants can be less likely to delay adjunctive therapy, but the trade-off may be a more reliably healed reconstruction that is less likely aesthetic. Patients who receive postoperative adjunctive therapy may have a prolonged reconstructive course because of interruptions from oncologic treatments. In the patient having postoperative irradiation, immediate reconstructions may be a problem unless extremely hardy tissues are used; even then the final result may be less than satisfactory. Immediate reconstruction should generally be approached with caution in patients who are to receive postoperative radiation.

Delayed reconstruction has advantages. The complication rate is a result of the reconstructive procedure alone, and from an oncologic standpoint, the delay allows for the completion of any adjunctive therapy and detection of recurrences. Delayed reconstruction also allows the reconstructive process to proceed through to completion without interruption by oncologic concerns. However, some patients who opt for delayed reconstruction prolong the length of their mastectomy recovery by delaying resumption of their usual activities because of body image concerns. Patients forced to live with the deformity may suffer significant psychological trauma. Conversely, some patients eventually adjust to their deformity and may not desire reconstruction. From a technical standpoint, delayed reconstructions, especially those involving microsurgery, are more difficult and tedious.

Expander/Implant Reconstruction

The major preoperative issue with expander/implant reconstruction is whether an aesthetically acceptable reconstruction can be achieved with an implant and local tissues. Other clinical factors include whether adequate skin and muscle are available for coverage and whether the opposite breast can be matched with expander/implant techniques. Reconstructions with implants or expanders placed under the mastectomy flaps can produce good results, although they may have complications including implant/expander infection and extrusion. Placing the expander or implant under muscular cover will reduce these complications and perhaps lower the incidence of capsular contracture. Silicone concerns and the reduced number of implant options has led to reduced demand for this type of reconstruction. Saline implants are less satisfactory in breast reconstruction from an aesthetic and "feel" standpoint than are gel implants. Capsular contractures were seen in as many as 30% of all implant patients prior to the introduction of polyurethane implants. With the unavailability of the polyurethane-covered implant, capsular contracture may again become a significant problem. The final aesthetic result can be unpredictable, and the time to completion of the reconstruction may be up to 7 or 8 months with an average of greater than two operations. The predictability of the results may be improved with the use of newer anatomic implants and expanders (Fig 29–5).

Latissimus Dorsi Flap

When local tissues are inadequate, the latissimus dorsi muscle can be used either as a muscle flap to cover an implant/expander or as a musculocutaneous flap to restore a skin deficit. Latissimus reconstructions can be done as a single-stage procedure. Occasionally there will be sufficient back tissue present for an all-autologous reconstruction using a latissimus musculocutaneous flap. Skin islands are reliable and can be designed to fill most defects. If only muscle is needed for coverage, it may be harvested through the mastectomy incision. Even with a separate incision the donor defect is usually minimal, and there is no significant morbidity from loss of the latissimus. The complication rate for latissimus reconstructions is low, but there is a propensity for long-term seroma formation at the donor site. Ideally, the thoracodorsal pedicle or at least the crossing branch to the serratus anterior muscle is intact for safe flap elevation. With most conservative mastectomies there is little risk to the pedicle (Fig 29–6).

Transverse Rectus Abdominis Musculocutaneous Flap

The transverse rectus abdominis musculocutaneous (TRAM) flap has significantly advanced autologous breast reconstruction. It allows a completely autologous reconstruction with an excellent aesthetic result and the added benefit of an abdominoplasty at the donor site. The flap may be raised as a unipedicle flap using one rectus muscle, a bipedicle flap using both rectus muscles, or a free flap. Two unipedicle flaps can be raised to support each "hemiabdomen" when bilateral reconstruction is needed. When pedicled, the flap is based on the superior epigastric vessel. When designed as a free flap, it is supplied by the deep inferior epigastric vessel. Bilateral free flaps can also be fashioned for bilateral reconstruction, although this is a major undertaking. Laboratory studies and experience have demonstrated the importance of the periumbilical perforators in flap perfusion. Flap design has evolved so that at least a centimeter of supraumbilical skin is included to capture these perforators. It is also important to realize the zones of perfusion so that the most tenuous portions of the flap may be removed first when insetting (Fig 29–7).

The abdominal donor site has the potential for herniation, weakness, and bulging. The free TRAM flap may have fewer abdominal complications, although some claim that there is little difference in the incidence of abdominal hernias between free and pedicled TRAM flaps. Reviews have shown that the morbidity of pedicled TRAM flap harvest was

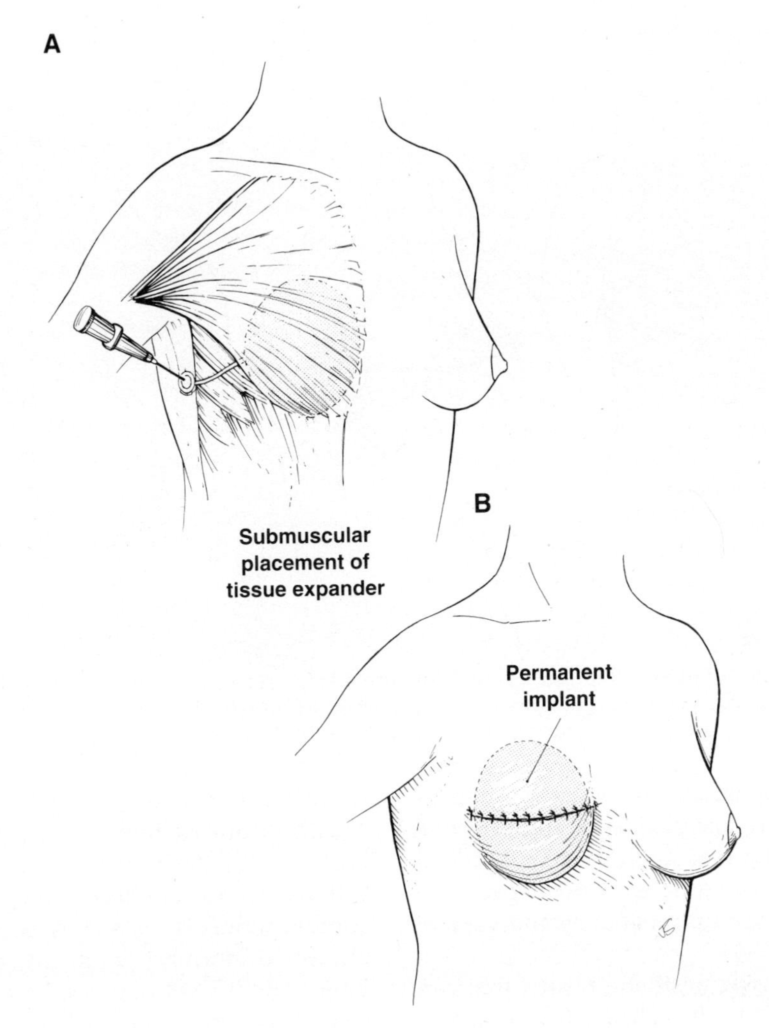

FIG 29–5.
A, expander/implant reconstruction is best done by placing the device under good muscle cover with the pectoralis, serratus, and rectus fascia. Occasionally the latissimus must be used to get good coverage. **B,** the expander is filled with saline. **C,** the expander is replaced with a "permanent" implant.

mild, with many patients being able to return to their preoperative activities even when these included aerobics and tennis.

Pedicled TRAM flaps have a low incidence of flap loss. In over 500 pedicled TRAM flaps, most of which were bipedicled, our experience shows only 1 complete flap loss, although there is a 15% incidence of fat necrosis. Surprisingly, the incidence of fat necrosis with the better-vascularized free TRAM flap based on the dominant inferior vessels is not different from pedicled flaps based on the secondary superior blood supply. The indications for unipedicle, bipedicle, or free TRAM flaps vary, but generally unipedicle flaps should be avoided in all but the best-risk patients. Bipedicle TRAM flaps are most reliably done by harvesting the entire muscle since any muscle left behind is of questionable benefit and thin muscle pedicles can compromise the vascular supply. In high-risk situations such as the obese patient, smokers, or patients with previous radiation or previous upper abdominal transverse incisions, delay or free flap should be considered. In patients in whom there is a concern about abdominal integrity, free TRAM flaps should theoretically have less long-term abdominal morbidity because of the preservation of most of the rectus muscle. Regardless of whether a free or pedicled flap

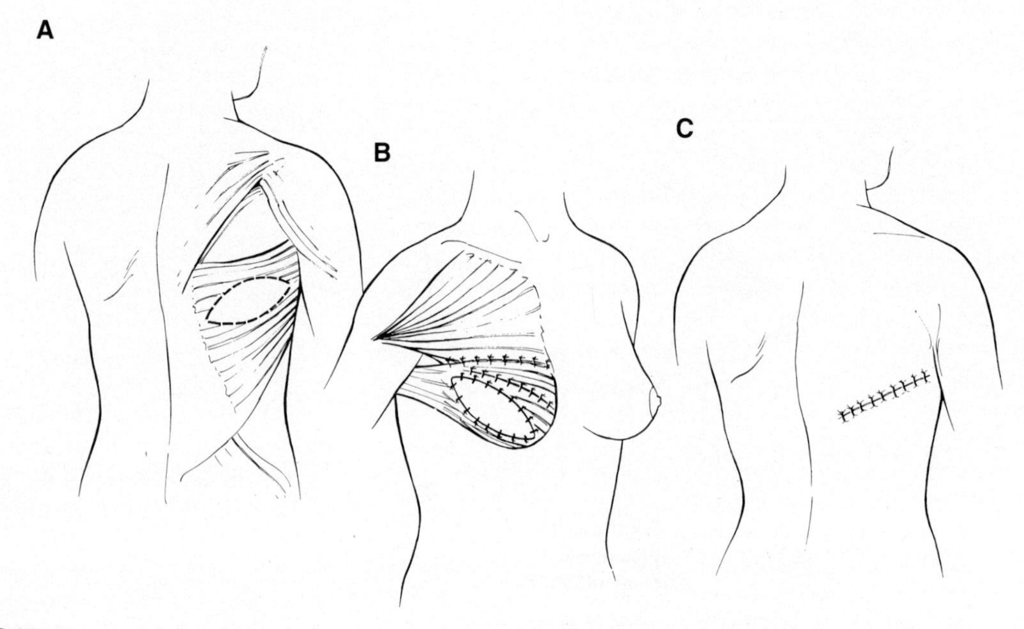

FIG 29–6.
The latissimus myocutaneous flap can be used for single-stage reconstruction. Occasionally an all-autologous reconstruction can be done, but most often an implant is required. **A,** flap located on the back. **B,** flap transferred to the anterior of the chest. **C,** the back wound after closure.

is done, abdominal closure must be meticulous, with secure fascial closure and selective use of mesh reinforcement to avoid abdominal complications. A TRAM flap does not preclude subsequent successful pregnancy and vaginal delivery.

The impressive aesthetic results that can be achieved with the TRAM flap must be tempered by the magnitude of the procedure. The patient, the oncologic surgeon, and the reconstructive surgeon must realize that a TRAM reconstruction is a major surgical procedure with the potential for major complications. In experienced hands the rate of complications is very low and the results almost uniformly good. In inexperienced hands the TRAM flap can be a long complicated procedure jeopardizing the patient's well-being and the final results of reconstruction (Fig 29–8).

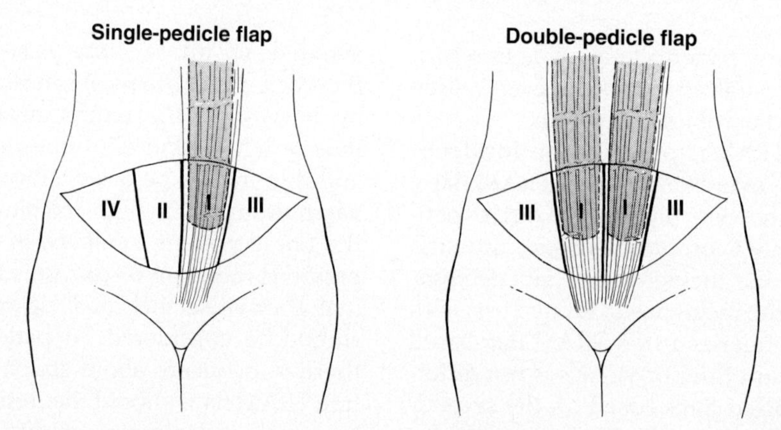

FIG 29–7.
Zones of perfusion of the TRAM flap with a single and double superior pedicle. The free flap based on the inferior vessels is not shown but is generally regarded as the most vascularized of the TRAM flaps.

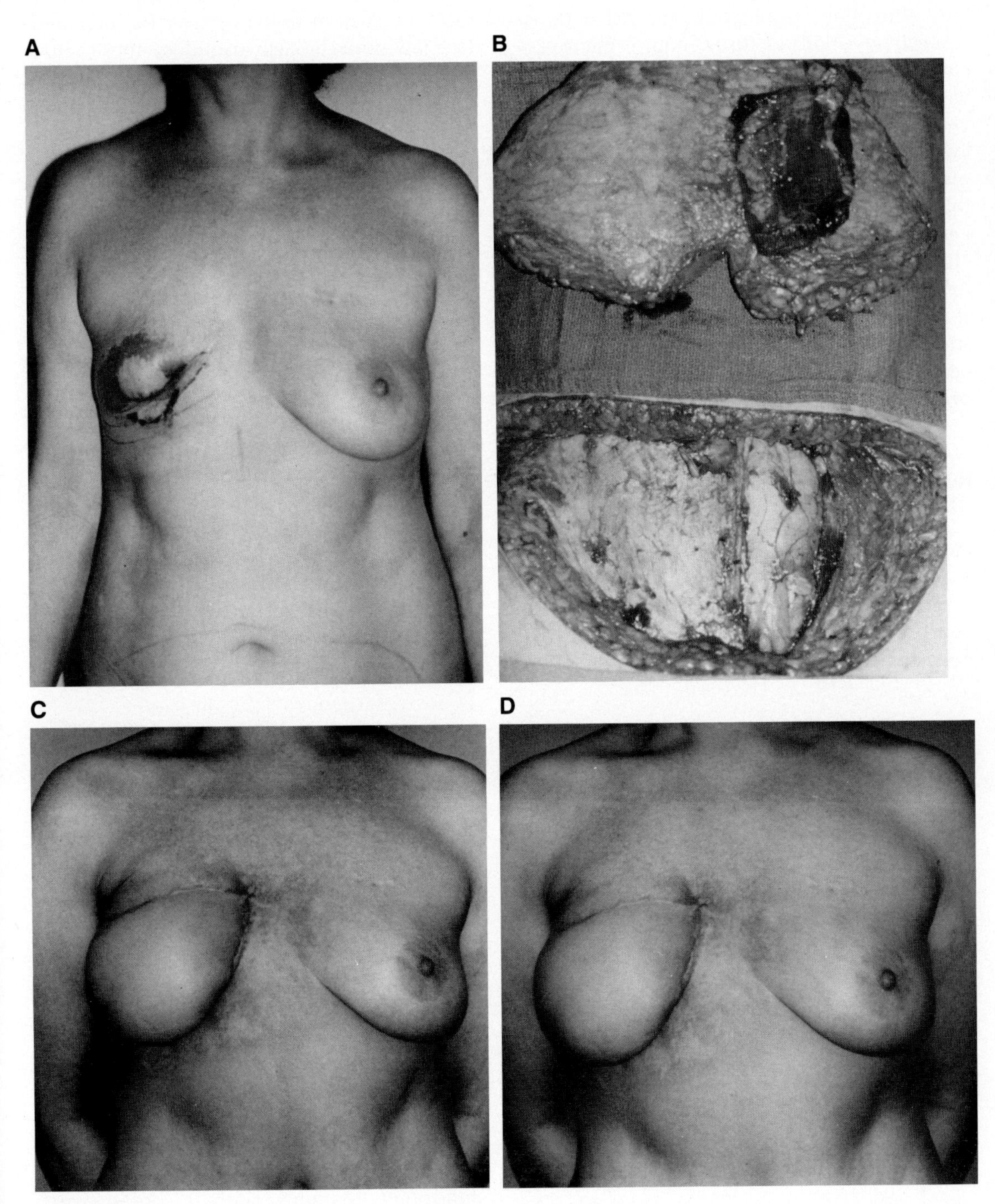

FIG 29–8.
A, Preoperative view (note markings). **B,** clinical picture of the transverse rectus abdominis myocutaneous flap. **C, D,** postoperative views.

Gluteal Flap and Tensor Fasciae Latae Flap

The gluteal and TFL flaps are second- and third-line autologous reconstructions, respectively; both of these require microvascular anastomosis. The gluteal flap can be based on the superior or inferior gluteal vessels. The inferiorly based flap results in a longer pedicle and a more aesthetically placed donor defect in the inferior gluteal fold (Fig 29–9). The TFL flap can be harvested as a transverse or longitudinal flap, although the donor defect is generally poor. Adequate tissue can be obtained from either source for most reconstructions. Omental tissue has been used for reconstruction but is best considered as a salvage procedure at present.

Reconstruction After Limited Surgery

Breast conservation surgery has become more common in recent years in certain regions of the country. The results of limited surgery followed by radiation can be quite good aesthetically, and no reconstruction is normally needed. In smaller breasts or when larger local resections are needed, reconstruction with either local flaps of breast tissue or custom implants may be indicated. The latissimus is also useful in these situations. The effect of reconstruction on the ability to follow the breast has not been determined. When faced with a large defect from a local excision, consideration should be given to a skin-sparing mastectomy with reconstruction, which will produce a better result.

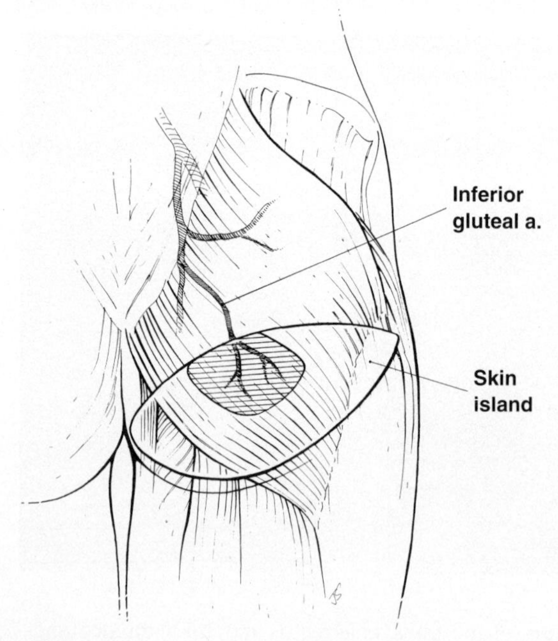

FIG 29–9.
The gluteal flap is a second-line reconstructive technique.

Nipple-Areola Reconstruction

Nipple-areola reconstruction is usually done at least 6 weeks after completion of the breast reconstruction to ensure accurate placement. There are many different local flaps for construction of the nipple. When a larger projecting nipple is needed, the skate flap is a good choice, while smaller nipples can be satisfactorily constructed with a "C-D" flap (Fig 29–10). Areola reconstruction is most often done with a tattoo, although full-thickness skin grafts can be done when a projecting areola is needed.

Contralateral Breast

Often when reconstruction is done the contralateral breast must be addressed in order to achieve symmetry. Initial attempts should be directed toward making the reconstructed breast closely match the opposite breast. When this is not possible or the aesthetics of the contralateral breast dictate, a simultaneous procedure should be considered on the unreconstructed breast. This may include a mastopexy to correct ptosis or a reduction mammoplasty to achieve size match. Sometimes augmentation mammoplasty must also be used for size match. The contralateral breast must also be addressed from an oncologic as well as an aesthetic standpoint. Patients with a breast carcinoma have an approximate risk of 1% per year for a tumor developing in the contralateral breast and must be carefully followed.

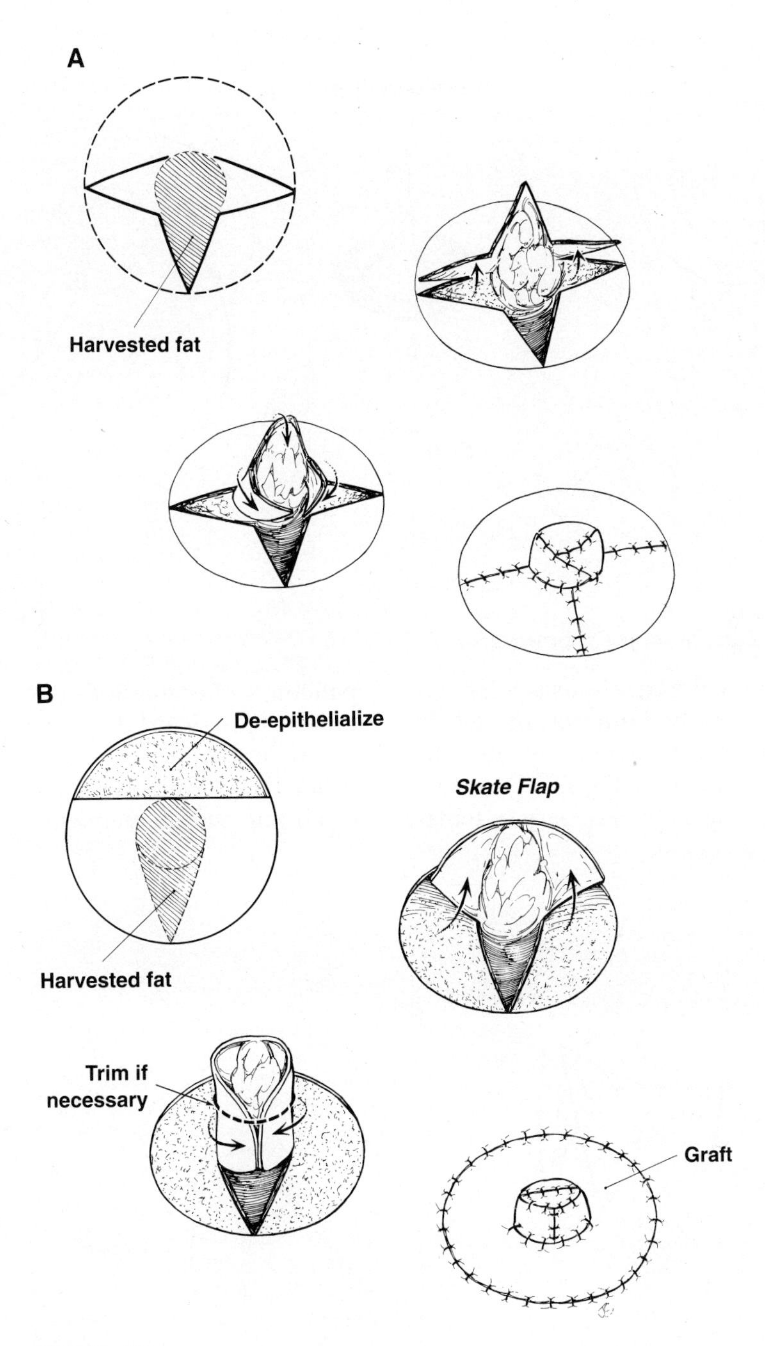

FIG 29–10.
Various local flaps for nipple reconstruction. *(Continued.)*

Poland's Syndrome

Poland's syndrome describes the complex thoracic wall deformity that includes absence of the sternal head of the pectoralis muscle, hypoplasia or aplasia of the breast or nipple, deficiency of subcutaneous fat and axillary hair, abnormalities of costal cartilage and anterior ribs, along with abnormalities of the ipsilateral upper extremity including brachysyndactyly and shortening. If the latissimus muscle is available and uninvolved, it provides the best reconstruction of the anterior chest wall.

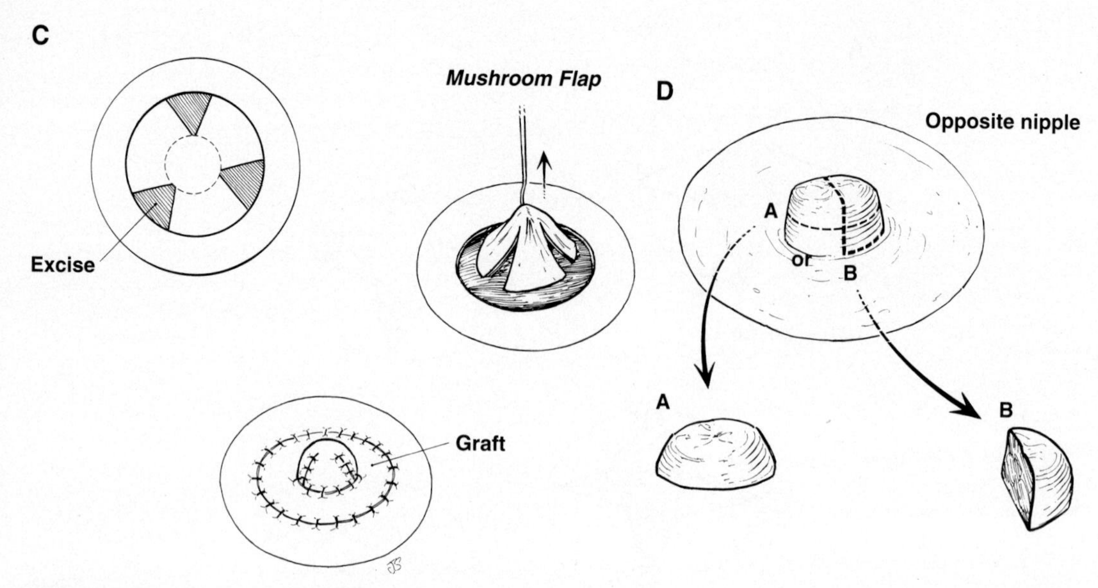

FIG 29–10 (cont.).
Various local flaps for nipple reconstruction.

When the origin of the latissimus is reinserted into the anterior of the humerus and left innervated, it can be made to replace some of the pectoralis muscle function (Fig 29–11). A mammary prothesis is usually necessary in female patients. Other methods of breast reconstruction such as TRAM flaps or implants may also be applicable in patients with Poland's syndrome. (For additional discussion of Poland's syndrome, see Chapter 27.)

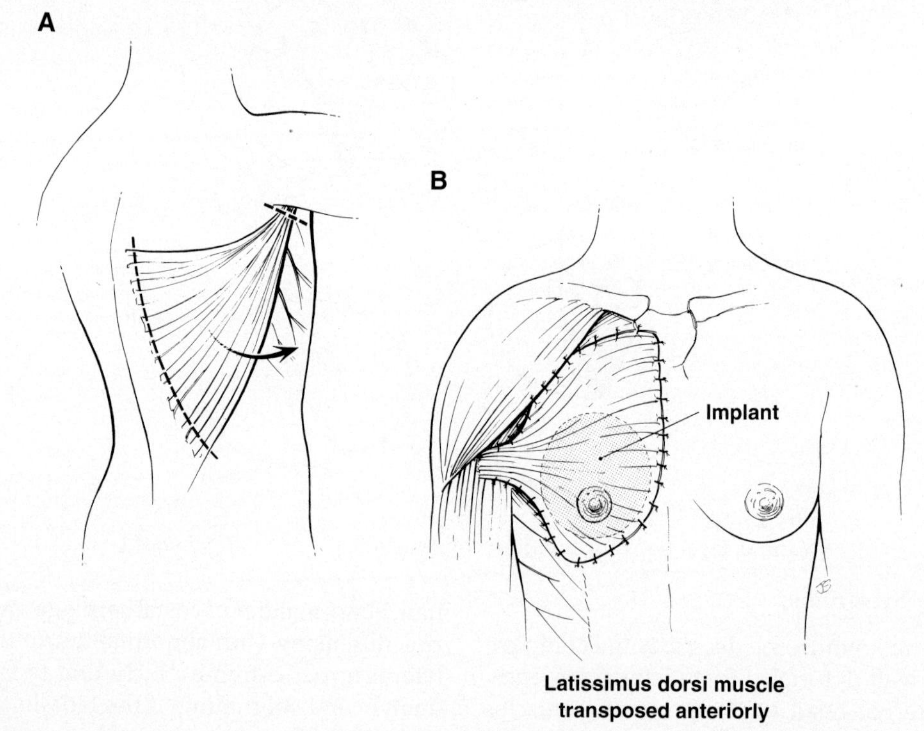

FIG 29–11.
Functional reconstruction of a patient with Poland's syndrome by using the latissimus muscle with the muscle insertion transposed anteriorly. An implant is placed in a female patient.

SUGGESTED READING

Bostwick J III: *Plastic and Reconstructive Surgery of the Breast.* St Louis, Quality Medical Publishing, 1990.

Harris JR, Lippman ME, Veronesi U, et al: Breast cancer (part 1). *N Engl J Med* 1992; 327:319–328.

Harris J, Lippman ME, Veronesi U, et al: Breast cancer (part 2). *N Engl J Med* 1992; 327:390–398.

Harris J, Lippman ME, Veronesi U, et al: Breast cancer (part 3). *N Engl J Med* 1992; 327:473–480.

Jones G, Nahai F: Pressure ulcers. *Adv Plast Surg* 1989; 6:209–229.

Jurkiewicz MJ, et al: Infected median sternotomy wound: Successful treatment by muscle flaps. *Ann Surg* 1980; 191:738–744.

Mathes SJ, Nahai F: *Clinical Applications for Muscle and Musculocutaneous Flaps.* St Louis, Mosby–Year Book, 1982.

Miller JI, Mansour KA, et al: Single stage complete muscle flap closure of the postpneumonectomy empyema space: A new method and possible solution to a disturbing complication. *Ann Thorac Surg* 1984; 38:227–231.

Nahai F, Rand RP, et al: Primary treatment of the infected sternotomy wound with muscle flaps: A review of 211 consecutive cases. *Plast Reconstr Surg* 1989; 84:433–441.

Seyfer AE, Graeber GM: Chest wall reconstruction. *Surg Clin North Am* 1989; 65.

Chapter 30

Aesthetic and Functional Problems

R. Barrett Noone, M.D.
Ronald A. Lohner, M.D.

CONTENTS

CHAPTER OBJECTIVE

At the end of this chapter the resident is thoroughly familiar with aesthetic and functional problems of the trunk and breast and undertakes comprehensive surgical management of such problems.

LEARNER OBJECTIVES

On completion of this chapter the resident

1. **Knows the normal anatomy of the breast, including common measurements.**
2. **Knows the pathologic anatomy and histology of the breast as related to mammary hyperplasia, hypoplasia, and ptosis.**
3. **Is familiar with the various surgical techniques for breast reduction, the indications for and contraindications to the procedures, and the complications of breast reduction and their prevention and management.**
4. **Knows the various surgical techniques for breast augmentation, the indications for and contraindications to the procedures, and the complications of augmentation**

mammoplasty and their prevention and management.

5. **Is familiar with the different types of breast implants and the reasons for selection of a particular type for a particular problem.**
6. **Knows the basic techniques for mastopexy, the indications for and contraindications to these procedures, and the complications of mastopexy and their prevention and management.**
7. **Understands the techniques for the treatment of aesthetic deformity of the abdomen (including panniculectomy and abdominoplasty), the indications for and contraindications to the procedures, and the complications of the procedures and their prevention and management.**
8. **Knows the techniques of suction lipectomy as applied to aesthetic deformities of the trunk.**
9. **Understands the principles of selection of procedures for specific deformities, e.g., mastopexy vs. augmentation mammoplasty, abdominoplasty vs. abdominal liposuction.**
10. **Knows the basic principles and techniques for treating other aesthetic deformities of the breast and trunk such as inverted nipples, localized lipodystrophy, tubular breast, etc.**
11. **Recognizes the long-term consequences of augmentation mammoplasty and the methods for follow-up, including special techniques for mammography.**

■ CLINICAL PRACTICE ACTIVITIES

During the course of the training program, the resident

1. **Evaluates patients with mammary hypertrophy, marks and operates upon them, and performs postoperative care.**
2. **Evaluates and treats patients with mammary hypoplasia, including both acute management and the care of patients with late problems (such as capsular contracture).**
3. **Evaluates and treats patients with mammary ptosis.**
4. **Evaluates and treats patients with aesthetic deformity of the abdomen and the trunk and performs abdominoplasty, panniculectomy, and/or abdominal suction lipectomy.**
5. Evaluates and treats patients with other aesthetic deformities of the breast such as inverted nipples and tubular breast.

MAMMARY HYPERTROPHY

It is difficult to precisely define mammary hypertrophy. The etiology of the condition is unclear and is most likely multifactorial. Although patients usually have physical signs and symptoms, the psychosocial and psychosexual implications are far-reaching. Fortunately, the success rate of improving both the patient's symptoms and social well-being is high. A number of techniques have been devised to reduce breast volume, provide safe transposition of the nipple, and yield acceptable aesthetic results.

Historical Aspects

Initial nonsurgical attempts to treat hypertrophy of the breast were unsuccessful and included the application of topical agents and methodical compression. Early surgical treatment in the late 1890s developed with the introduction of partial- and total-breast amputations. Subsequent advances focused on the placement of incisions and the location of breast parenchymal resections. These pioneering procedures, however, provided for only marginal resections of tissue volume and did not address the issue of ptosis deformities.

In the early 20th century, the evolution of anesthesia, the treatment of patients with less severe glandular hypertrophy, and improvements in planning and surgical technique all contributed to better results. The aesthetic outcome of Lexer's bilateral mammectomy was improved with Thorek's introduction of free nipple grafting in 1922. A significant contribution was the introduction of pedicled nipple-areolar transposition, which not only improved nipple survival but also provided for the correction of ptosis. Wide undermining of the skin with resection of the underlying parenchyma and reshaping with a new skin brassiere were popularized by Axhausen and Biesenberger. Because of the superior aesthetic results, these techniques remained popular for a long time despite the relatively high incidence of nipple-areolar necrosis. One of the major contributions in this early era was understanding the importance of maintaining the dermal attachments to the nipple as a means of preserving or protecting its blood supply. Schwarzmann introduced this concept in 1937. It has since been incorporated into most current modifications of reduction mammaplasty techniques.

Subsequent innovations included refinements to minimize ischemia of the nipple-areolar complex and improve the overall aesthetics of the procedure. After extensive study of the blood supply to the breast, new procedures were introduced to improve and protect nipple-areolar viability. As reduction techniques were further refined, concerns of improved postoperative nipple sensation and retention of the ability to breast-feed received greater attention. The role of preoperative planning was elucidated by Bames in the late 1940s. Wise emphasized the need for accurate preoperative marking and provided a pattern to minimize postoperative complications and improve overall breast shape.

Currently, the most popular procedures performed for reduction mammaplasty are combinations of previous innovations. Most benefit from a Wise pattern of skin and breast parenchymal resection followed by transposition of the nipple-areolar complex on a local dermoglandular flap.

Blood Supply

The breast receives its blood supply from four major sources: the lateral thoracic artery, branches of the thorocoacromial artery, perforators of the internal mammary arteries, and branches of the intercostal arteries. Although there is not a clearly dominant source, the internal mammary perforators are often considered the chief blood supply. The presence of a nondominant, densely anastomotic blood supply is further supported by the success of numerous dermal and parenchymal pedicle flaps. Sufficient blood supply is available to the nipple-areola complex when flaps are properly designed from any direction.

Developmentally, breast enlargement occurs within the envelope of the superficial fascia beneath the deep subcutaneous plexus. This results in a dense vascular network running superficial to the breast parenchyma and below the dermal margin of the skin. The presence of this subdermal plexus enables nipple-areolar survival in techniques based solely on dermal pedicles.

Innervation

The superior skin of the breast is innervated by the supraclavicular branch of the cervical plexus. Innervation of the lateral aspect of the breast is by means of the anterior rami of the lateral cutaneous nerve branches of the third through the sixth intercostal nerves. Medially, the skin receives its sensation from the anterior branches of the second through the sixth intercostal nerves. The sensibility of the nipple and areola appears to be derived from the depths of the breast and not from nerves running in superficial planes. Although reports are contradictory, nipple sensation appears not to arise from a single nerve. The third, fourth, and fifth anterior cutaneous nerves and the fourth and fifth lateral cutaneous nerves all appear to be contributory. Of note, the lateral branches of the intercostal nerves emerge at the lateral border of the pectoralis major and enter the breast posteriorly 2 cm from its lateral edge. Although a rich nerve supply to the nipple with overlapping distributions likely exists, preservation of these lateral nerves should be attempted in all techniques of dermal or parenchymal reduction mammaplasties.

Patient Selection

From the plastic surgeon's standpoint, the goal of reduction mammaplasty is to create smaller, aesthetically appealing breasts with minimal scarring while preserving nipple viability, nipple sensation, and the ability to lactate. However, the specific motivations and expectations of each patient must be addressed during consultation. A significant percentage of patients seeking consultation suffer from obesity as well as mammary hypertrophy. Since there is an increased incidence of postoperative complications in obese patients (hematoma formation, infection, nipple-areolar ischemia, and fat necrosis), preoperative weight loss should be discussed with these patients.

Patients most often have physical complaints. Frequently described signs or symptoms include the persistence of neck and back discomfort, headaches, upper extremity neurologic manifestations, shoulder grooving and pain, poor posture, and inframammary dermatologic concerns such as intertrigo. Anatomic correlations have been described for these symptoms, which often improve with reduction mammaplasty. Physical examination of the patient should include an assessment of breast volume, planned areas of tissue resection, and the presence of asymmetry. Asymmetrical findings should be identified and discussed with the patient preoperatively to potentially avoid any unrealistic expectations of postoperative perfect symmetry. Evaluation of the nipple-areolar size and location can influence the choice of technique for safe and uncomplicated transposition of the nipple-areolar complex or the need for a free nipple grafting procedure. A thorough examination includes a complete search for breast masses or other stigmata of breast pathology. Mammography should be included for all patients over the age of 30 years.

Preoperative Concerns

Preoperative counseling should include a full disclosure of the potential pitfalls and complications of the procedure. Patients must understand that although some women have been able to lactate or successfully breast-feed postoperatively, many patients are unable to do so. There may be an association between the amount of breast parenchyma retained between the level of the nipple and the midhumeral point and the ability to lactate (a landmark used previously by some surgeons to determine appropriate nipple height). Aesthetic goals for reduction mammaplasty, however, should not be the creation of breasts conforming to a set of standard measurements and dimensions. Breast shape and size should be optimal for each patient and her body habitus. Attempts to recreate a virginal contour and uniform radius of the breast will be limited by the preoperative size, degree of ptosis, composition of breast tissue, and elasticity of the skin.

Preoperative marking can be performed either the day prior to or the day of surgery (Fig 30–1). Patients should be marked prior to the administration of sedation because marking while the patient is in the sitting or standing position allows more accuracy. We have preferred same-day marking performed in the holding area prior to sedation with the patient in the erect sitting or standing position.

Straight lines are drawn from the midclavicular point through the breast meridians. Next, after positioning the nipple in the horizontal plane, one establishes the vertical nipple height. This step is the most critical aspect of preoperative marking. The key element is to prevent a "high-riding" nipple deformity, a common cause of postoperative dissatisfaction. Correction of the deformity is a problem in that prominent and unsightly supra-areolar scarring often results. The position may worsen from its immediate postoperative orientation because inferior breast skin relaxes and "bottoming out" of the breast results. This not only affects breast contour but may also result in an even higher nipple position accentuated by exaggerated superior projection. Vertical nipple height is most accurately determined as related to the existing inframammary fold. Anterior transposition of the inframammary fold can be performed visually with the aid of the thumb and index finger to facilitate nipple positioning. A more technically sound and reproducible

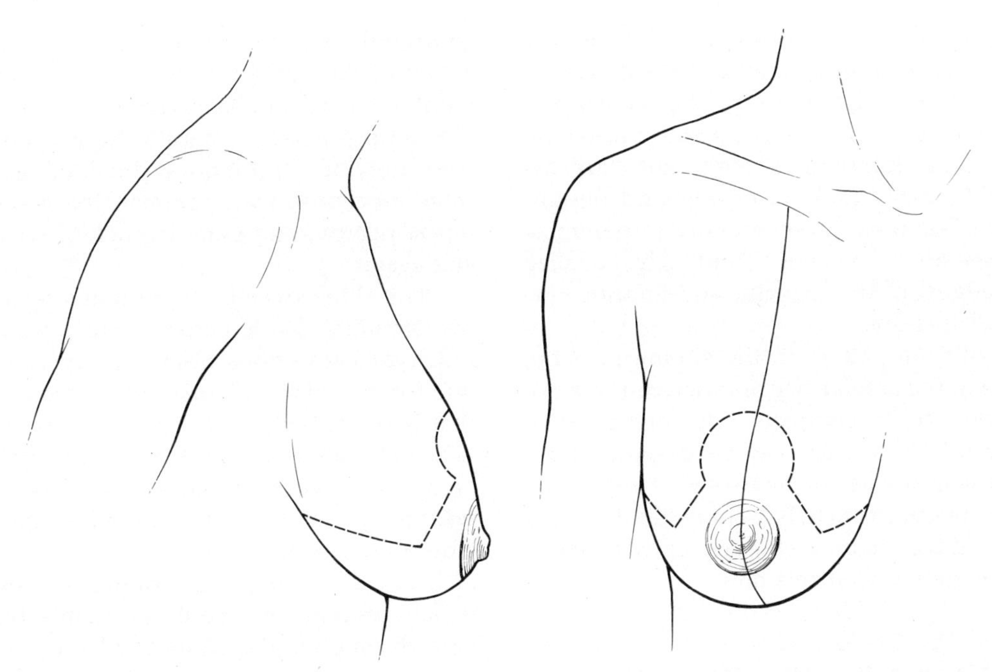

FIG 30–1.
Preoperative marking. Careful planning and accurate marking are crucial to a successful reduction mammaplasty. Nipple position is determined as the anterior projection of the infra-mammary fold. A Wise pattern is the standard template for nipple outline and skin excision.

method employs the use of obstetric calipers. After measuring the distance from the mid-clavicular point to the inframammary fold, the calipers are positioned anteriorly to determine nipple height. Accuracy of the planned nipple position can be confirmed by measuring the nipple-to-midsternal distance and comparing it with the contralateral side.

Determining the position of the inframammary fold is also facilitated by supporting the weight of the breast. This places the incision for the planned fold slightly up on the breast. The medial and lateral aspects of skin resection should be marked even higher on the breast and not extend beyond the breast itself. The lateral limit is the anterior axillary line and medially should fall short of the midline. Encroachment on the sternum leaves more visible scarring in an area that has a tendency for hypertrophic scar formation. Confluence of this incision with the contralateral side may result in hooding or a web deformity.

The Wise pattern of skin resection is used for most of the commonly performed reduction mammaplasty techniques. Either a template or freehand marking may be used, depending on the surgeon's preference. Lateral rotation of the keyhole equalizes the medial and lateral horizontal incisions and minimizes the postoperative "boxy" appearance. The vertical limbs of the keyhole should be maintained in close proximity to the areolar border. This positioning provides a skin brassiere of maximum volume that may be decreased during closure of the skin. Outlining the planned position of the nipple-areola in the keyhole pattern may be performed preoperatively or delayed until closure as the final step in the procedure. Delaying this step allows for fine adjustments of nipple position but adds the problem of locating the nipple while the patient is recumbent or semisitting on the operating table.

The length of the vertical limbs depends on the anticipated shape and size of the final result. The average length measures 5 or 6 cm from the inferior aspect of the areola to the inframammary fold. If nipple position is to be determined at final closure, the vertical limb from the nipple center to the inframammary fold should measure approximately 7 cm, depending on the final breast size.

The superior horizontal incisions are subsequently drawn between the inferior extent of the vertical limbs to the medial and lateral extents of the proposed inframammary fold. Although straight lines are acceptable, many authors recommend designing an S-shaped curve laterally to minimize postoperative "boxiness" and help equalize the lengths of the superior and inferior horizontal incisions.

With the patient in the supine position, marking the areolar size and determining the pedicle width complete the preoperative marking. The areola may be designed freehand with a ruler or by using a template. A radius of approximately 2 cm is standard. If a pedicled technique is chosen, the pedicle can also be designed at this time.

Techniques of Reduction Mammaplasty

Horizontal Bipedicle Technique

Strombeck designed a horizontal two-pedicle procedure based on Ragnell's previously reported technique. The blood supply of the pedicle is based on the internal mammary and lateral thoracic arteries. The important contributions of the procedure were minimization of skin undermining and the development of medial and lateral pedicles to support the nipple-areolar complex. Improvements over previous techniques provided a one-stage procedure with minimal risk of skin or nipple necrosis and a safe, cosmetically acceptable result.

The skin envelope is designed by using the standard Wise pattern (Fig 30–2). Parenchymal resections from the superior and inferior poles yield a horizontal bipedicle flap that is deepithelialized. Upon closure of the skin incisions, Strombeck reported that the areola is automatically transposed to its new position as outlined by the Wise pattern. However, dissatisfaction with the technique included difficulty in positioning the pedicle, which resulted in significant nipple distortion. Strombeck also introduced the concept of lateral pedicle division when traction or inversion of the nipple resulted. He is therefore credited with the medially based unipedicle technique of reduction mammaplasty (Fig 30–3).

The horizontal bipedicle technique is applicable to a range of breast sizes and degrees

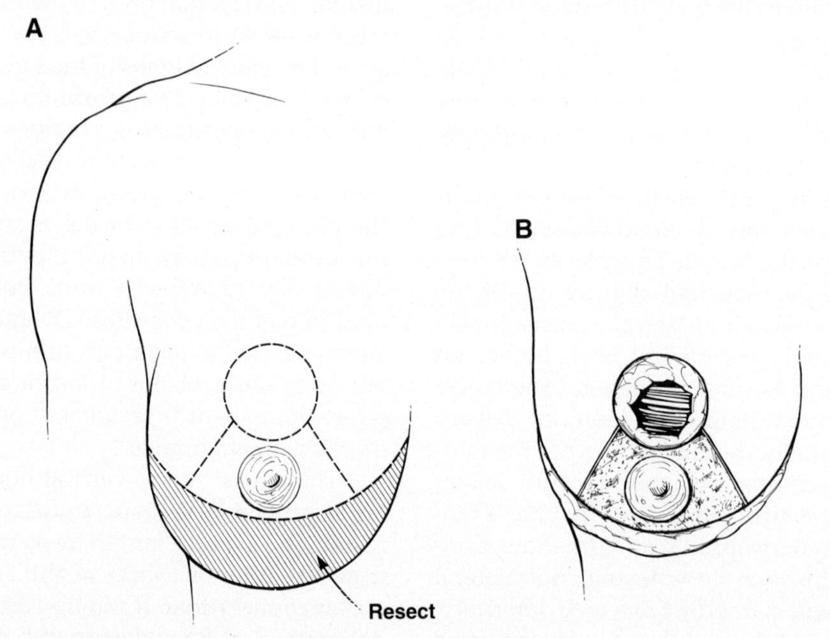

FIG 30–2.
Horizontal bipedicle technique. Significant improvement in nipple survival was introduced by Strombeck with a one-stage technique and minimal skin undermining. **A,** the bulk of breast resection is from the lower pole of the breast. **B,** the nipple areolar complex is supported on a horizontal bipedicle.

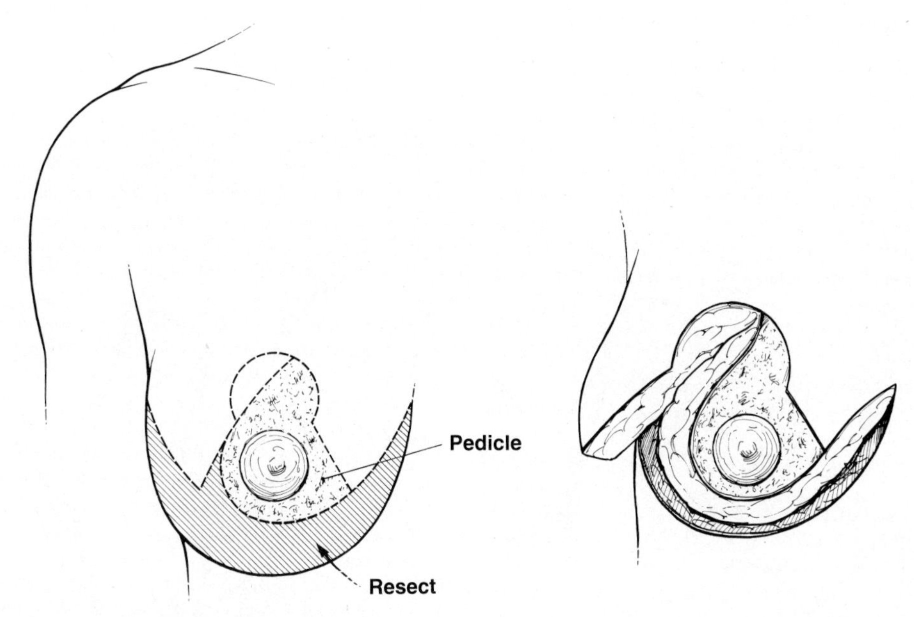

FIG 30–3.
Medial unipedicle technique. Preserving the nipple areolar complex on a medially based pedicle was a later modification of Strombeck's technique.

of ptosis. The best results are described in patients with moderate hypertrophy and moderate ptosis.

Vertical Bipedicle Technique

A likely outgrowth of the horizontal bipedicle technique was the development of McKissock's vertical bipedicle reduction mammaplasty (Fig 30–4). The sites of parenchymal resection were changed from the superior and inferior poles to medial and lateral locations. These resections are performed with a more extensive lateral excision because of the axillary extension of the breast and to minimize inferior "boxiness." Only the supra-areolar portion of the vertical bipedicle flap undergoes folding, which minimizes distortion upon closure of the skin flaps. The blood and nerve supply to the nipple-areola complex is protected since the inferior pedicle harbors the cutaneous nerve supply and the subdermal plexus. The superior pedicle may also serve to supplement vascularity and sensation, although the contribution is probably minimal.

The planning steps of the technique are similar to that of the Strombeck procedure with the use of a conventional Wise pattern. McKissock emphasizes the need to maintain a narrow keyhole to provide a generous skin brassiere and to avoid the common postoperative flat-bottomed appearance. The vertical limbs should be designed to closely approximate the areola. The vertical flap is deepithelialized from the new nipple position to the inframammary fold. The glandular excision is performed medially and laterally with care taken to not undermine the inferior aspect of the pedicle. Extreme caution must be exercised to prevent beveling into the vascular pedicle when performing the resection to the chest wall. Resection of breast tissue from beneath the superior aspect of the pedicle decreases breast volume and creates a true bipedicled flap allowing greater mobility of the nipple-areolar complex. Limiting deep dissection to a plane above the pectoralis fascia preserves integrity of the nerve supply and diminishes postoperative nipple numbness. After preparing the central pedicle, the skin flaps are developed superiorly to permit redraping of the remaining breast tissue. Insetting of the nipple-areola complex includes folding of the pedicle and may necessitate back-cutting the superior pedicle to ensure acceptable nipple-areolar position and

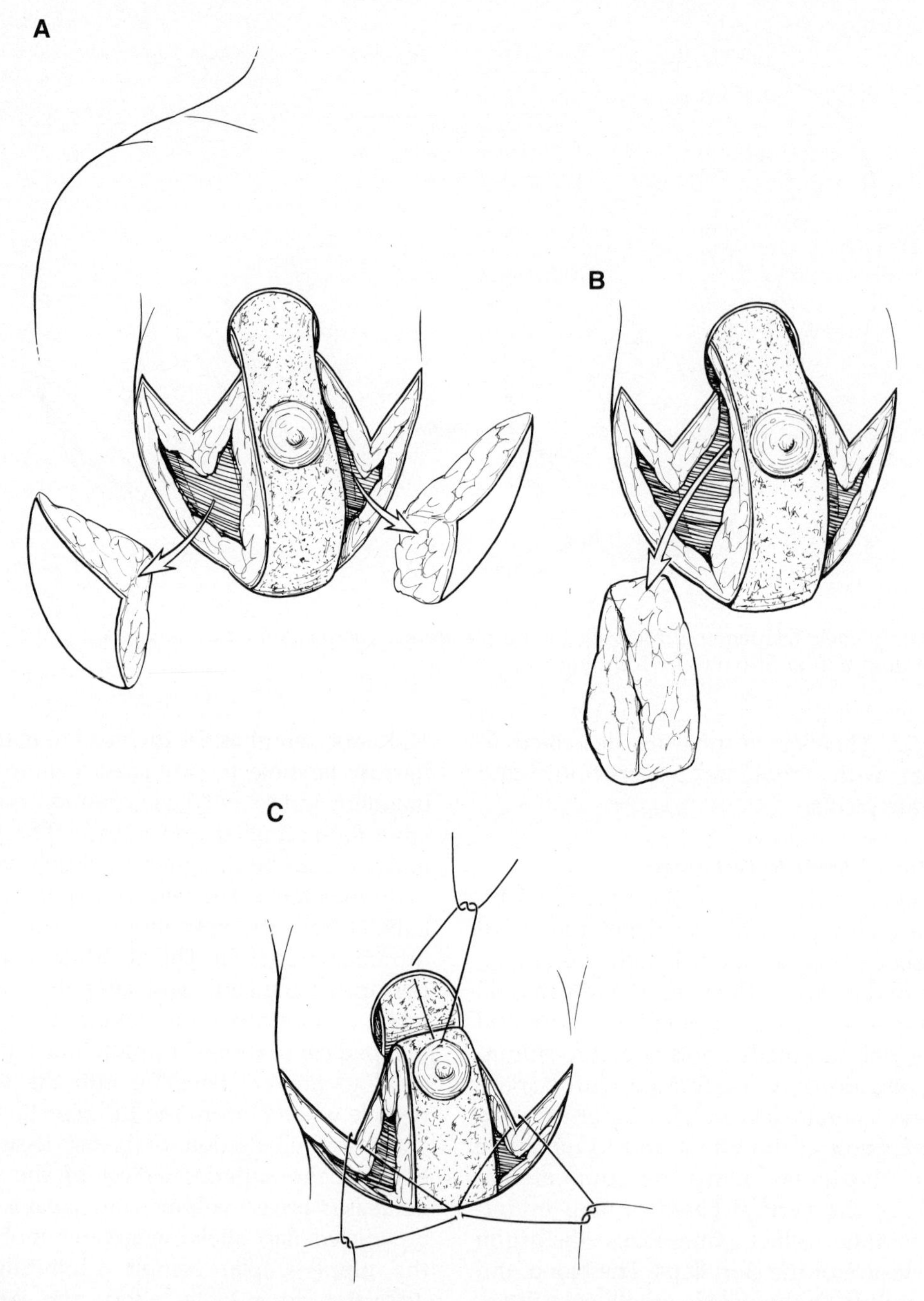

FIG 30–4.
McKissock vertical bipedicle technique. **A,** after deepithelialization of the vertical bipedicle, medial, and lateral resections of skin and parenchyma are performed. **B,** excision of breast tissue from under the pedicle improves mobility of the nipple areolar complex and folding of the pedicle. **C,** the nipple-areolar complex is secured superficially to the folded pedicle.

projection. The standard closure is performed so as to minimize tension at the T junction and approximate the wound edges in a two-layered fashion.

The vertical bipedicle technique yields good aesthetic results with an acceptable margin of safety. Overly aggressive resection or undermining of the pedicle can compromise nipple-areolar vascularity and must be avoided. Similar to other pedicle techniques, it is a safe and predictable technique of reduction mammaplasty suitable to a range of breast deformities.

Superior Pedicle Technique

The development of the superiorly based dermal pedicle technique by Weiner was based on Schwarzmann's description of the subdermal plexus and cutaneous circulation complex; Weiner found that an adequately designed pedicle provided a safe technique for transposition on the cutaneous circulation alone. A simple en bloc amputation of the inferior pole is performed from the standard preoperative markings, and closure of the skin is without vascular compromise to the pedicle (Fig 30–5).

The superior pedicle technique is most effective when the nipple transposition distance is short. After standard preoperative marking, the planned superior pedicle contained within a keyhole and vertical limbs of the Wise pattern is deepithelialized. After developing the superior pedicle, the dermal attachments may be either severed or maintained. Isolating the pedicle creates a free nipple-areola complex supported by dermis alone. Maintaining the underlying attachments produces a composite dermoglandular pedicle. The nipple is then transposed to its new location by folding the superior pedicle and placing tacking sutures. An en bloc resection is performed on skin and breast tissue between the planned and existing inframammary lines. Planes of resection should be perpendicular to the chest wall. Closure of the skin and final insetting of the nipple complete the procedure, with backcutting of the pedicle if necessary to improve any nipple distortion or circulatory embarrassment.

This technique is suitable to a wide range of ptoses and hypertrophies. Safety is enhanced because parenchymal resection occurs only after the development of the pedicle and transposition of the nipple have been completed. Sensation often remains adequate, and with minimal undermining of the soft tissues, dead space is limited.

The broad suitability, simplicity of design, and inherent safety of the procedure all contribute to the success of this widely employed technique of reduction mammaplasty.

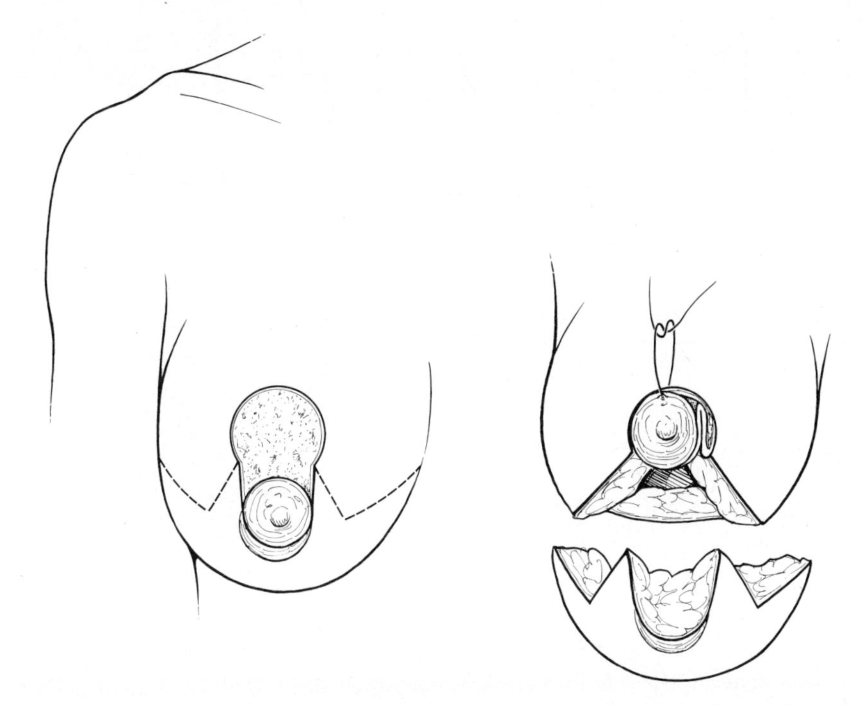

FIG 30–5.
Superior pedicle technique. After developing a superiorly based pedicle, an en bloc resection of the inferior pole is performed, based on a Wise pattern.

Inferior Pedicle Technique

Unlike the superior technique, which employs minimal undermining and an inferior amputation, the inferior pedicle technique requires wide skin elevation, with subsequent breast shape and bulk provided by the retained inferior segment of the breast (Fig 30–6). Similarly, however, this technique may be performed as either a dermal pedicle or composite dermoglandular pedicle. A distinct advantage of the technique is mobility of the nipple-areolar complex, which allows for a much greater transposition than with other techniques.

The first operative step is deepithelialization of the inferior pedicle. Approximately 1 to 2 cm of dermis and parenchyma should be maintained around the superior, medial, and lateral aspects of the retained areola. Next, the skin flap is developed and a thickness of 1 to 2 cm maintained. Some surgeons develop the natural plane that exists between the subcutaneous fat and breast tissue, while others opt to leave some breast parenchyma on the flap to maintain adequate thickness. The medial and lateral aspects of the pedicle are resected, with most of the parenchymal excision laterally.

The inferior pedicle approach is the most commonly performed contemporary technique of reduction mammaplasty. It safely protects the vascularity of the nipple-areola and provides acceptable nipple sensation. The

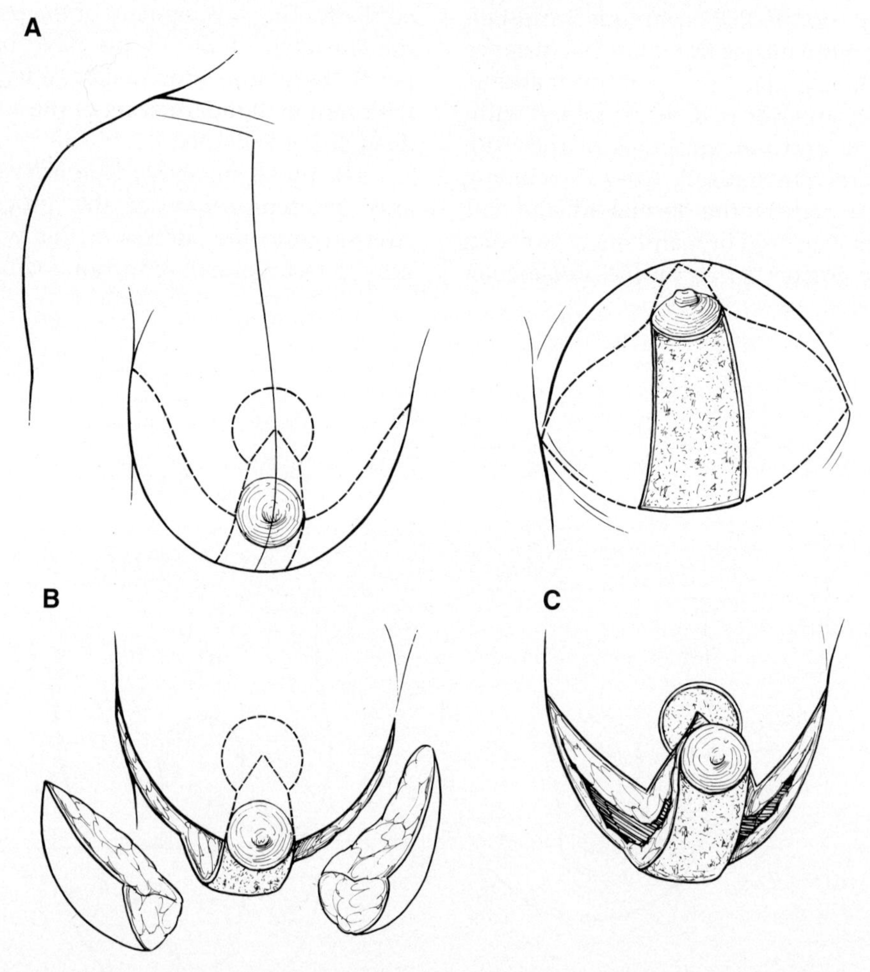

FIG 30–6.
Inferior pedicle technique. **A,** the inferior pedicle is deepithelialized. **B,** development of the superior skin flap is followed by resections of the medial and lateral aspects of the breast. **C,** after the dermal or dermoglandular pedicle is completed, transposition of the nipple and skin closure are performed.

flexibility afforded is due to the independent control of parenchymal volume and the position of the nipple. The procedure can be executed by either retaining or discarding the overlying dermis of the inferior pedicle. Retaining the dermis not only offers protection to the subdermal plexus but also provides a healthy base for granulation or grafting if necrosis at the T junction should occur. It may also serve as a healthy graft bed should poor nipple viability require free nipple transposition and grafting.

Symmetry may be more difficult to achieve because the procedure requires separate tangential parenchymal excisions from the skin flap and from the breast mound. Operating time may also be somewhat longer with this approach.

Reduction mammaplasty based on an inferior dermal or composite pedicle is useful for virtually all patients with hypertrophy or ptosis. It is the pedicle procedure of choice for large reductions requiring significant transposition of the nipple-areolar complex.

Free Nipple Grafting Technique

The indications for choosing free nipple grafting over transpositional pedicled techniques are not clearly defined. Most surgeons reserve this approach for patients requiring parenchymal resection of 1,500 to 2,000 g per breast or greater. Virtually all authors agree that pleasurable nipple sensation and the ability to retain lactation function postoperatively are best maintained with a pedicle technique. Proponents of free nipple grafting cite the ease of breast shaping without regard for pedicle length, folding, or torsion, essentially eliminating the risk of nipple loss. Those in favor of nipple transposition techniques have reported excellent success with pedicle lengths of up to 30 cm. They also note complications of free nipple grafting, including hypopigmentation of the nipple-areolar complex, the potential for graft failure, and insufficient nipple-areolar projection, in addition to changes in lactation and sensation.

The procedure commences with a full-thickness excision of the nipple-areolar complex. The composite graft should include a portion of the underlying smooth muscle. The resectional component of the procedure is similar to that of the superior pedicle technique: amputation of the inferior segment of the breast below the markings of the standard Wise pattern. Horizontal and vertical incisions are closed in standard fashion after ensuring symmetry and acceptable hemostasis. Nipple positioning with securing of the free nipple graft and placement of a tie-over bolster completes the procedure.

In general, partial breast amputation with free nipple grafting can be recommended in obese patients with severe ptosis, in elderly women for whom shorter anesthesia is desirable, and for massive reductions of 1,500 to 2,000 g per breast or greater.

Complications

Although most contemporary techniques of reduction mammaplasty are considered safe procedures, complications do occur. These are usually related to wound healing or to the presence of unacceptable aesthetic results. Postoperative infections and hematoma may occur following any surgical procedures and are related to surgical technique and meticulous hemostasis.

Necrosis of skin flaps and the nipple-areolar complex was more prevalent with older techniques. Tissue loss is often related to procedure design and the extent of soft-tissue resection. Skin loss is usually minor and often occurs at the T junction of the horizontal and vertical limbs. Proper planning of the skin brassiere and execution of a multilayered wound closure help to minimize tension on skin edges. Compromise of the microcirculation may also be contributory to the development of necrosis, especially in patients with diabetes or collagen vascular disease or those who continue to smoke perioperatively. Conservative management is usually sufficient in the treatment of superficial skin loss. Significant soft-tissue necrosis requires debridement after demarcation occurs. Most defects will heal by secondary intention, although skin grafting will be required for major skin loss. Fat necrosis may also develop as a result of ischemic injury with or without superficial tissue loss. It most often results in the formation of hard lumps within the breast parenchyma and without significant volume loss.

Loss of the nipple-areolar complex is fortunately rare. Ischemic tissue should be discovered prior to the onset of irreversible injury. Intraoperatively, periareolar epinephrine injections and the creation of tension or twisting of the pedicle must be avoided. If the nipple appears to be jeopardized immediately postoperatively, repeat surgery is indicated to explore for hematoma and verify pedicle position and tension. If ischemia cannot be reversed, the nipple should be removed from the pedicle and replaced as a free graft. Complete nipple loss will require nipple-areolar reconstruction with conventional postmastectomy techniques.

Hypertrophic scarring is frequent in reduction mammaplasty, especially at the ends of the inframammary incision and around the areola. Patient satisfaction pertaining to scarring depends most on preoperative expectations. Patients should therefore be made aware of the unpredictable nature of wound healing and apprised of the potential for hypertrophic scar formation. New techniques to minimize inframammary incisional length and eliminate the vertical limb are promising. However, they tend to yield inferior projection and contour when compared with the standard Wise-pattern skin brassiere. Compression techniques, steroid injections, silicone gel applications, or scar revisions may be attempted to minimize hypertrophic scarring.

The exact incidence of patient dissatisfaction from changes in nipple-areolar sensation is unknown. Studies have documented a wide range of temporary and permanent loss of sensation as well as discrepancies between subjective and objective findings. Nipple-areolar anesthesia will improve over time for either pedicled or free nipple grafting techniques but improves to a lesser extent with free grafting procedures. Intraoperatively an attempt to limit dissection to a plane above the pectoralis fascia is felt to spare lateral cutaneous sensory nerves and maintain nipple sensation to a greater degree.

Even though reduction mammaplasty is a plastic surgical procedure designed to relieve symptoms related to large uncomfortable breasts, unattractive shape, projection, and asymmetries may result. Preoperative discussions should include the surgeon's and patient's expectations for postoperative size to avoid inadequate reduction or overreduction. Late postoperative changes in breast contour continue to occur despite numerous creative attempts to prevent caudal migration of parenchyma and relaxation of skin. This phenomenon is referred to as "bottoming out" or "dropping out." Contour changes cause superior projection of a high-appearing nipple in association with inferior fullness of the breast. These deformities do not appear immediately but rather in a delayed fashion with insidious lengthening of the vertical limb. Adequate correction can usually be achieved with resection of additional skin above the inferior mammary fold. Bottoming out of the breast secondary to skin relaxation and parenchymal migration is a late postoperative sequela. Other aesthetic concerns include improper nipple placement, nipple inversion, and incisional dog-ears. These occur secondary to errors in planning or technique and may require revisional surgery.

MAMMARY HYPOPLASIA

Through the ages, the female breast has been a symbol of both sexual attractiveness and fertility and has led to the 20th century emphasis on breast appearance as an integral part of the female body image. Although small breasts have occasionally been fashionable, such as in the United States in the 1920s, the dominant female image in this century has included an appropriately sized and proportioned breast. Interest in achieving this ideal self-image has stimulated approximately 2 million women to undergo breast enlargement surgery.

History of Augmentation Mammaplasty

The earliest attempts at augmentation mammaplasty date to 1895, when Czerny successfully transplanted a benign lipoma from the back of a patient to reconstruct a volume defect in her breast. Since then, multiple attempts at enlarging the breast have been introduced, including the use of percutaneous injections of paraffin by Gersuny in 1899, followed by other attempts at free fat grafts, dermal-fat grafts, and other foreign materials such as glass bead implants. The paraffin injections and glass bead implants led to predictable granulomatous reactions, unsightly breast contours, and ultimate disfavor. A small amount of success was seen with dermal-fat grafts and dermal-fat flaps. However, interest in autogenous tissue augmentation waned with the introduction by Pangman in 1951 of a synthetic implant consisting of polyvinyl, alcohol, and formaldehyde, known as the Ivalon sponge implant. Other alloplastic materials such as Teflon and Etheron were also introduced. Sustained use of these materials, however, was not seen because of poor aesthetic results and the high incidence of infection and seroma formation caused by the severe foreign-body reaction. Although some surgeons practiced the injection of liquid silicone beginning in the 1950s, a significant number of complications were seen, including migration of the silicone, persistent chronic edema and inflammation, the development of granulomas, and even silicone embolism. The search for a more ideal implantable material led to the development of a silicone elastomer envelope enclosing the gel form of the polydimethylsiloxane polymer. In 1962, Cronin and Gerow began the modern era of breast augmentation by implanting this new gel-filled silicone implant in the retromammary position. Although many modifications have been introduced, the basic silicone gel–filled implant has enjoyed a 30-year popularity as one of the most frequently implanted medical devices.

Numerous modifications in the implant have been introduced since the initial Cronin model. When the phenomenon of "gel bleed" was discovered and the permeability of the silicone shell to minute droplets of silicone was noticed, modifications in the shell envelope were made in order to reduce the rate of gel diffusion.

Types of Implants

A confusing array of mammary implants was introduced to the market during the 1970s and 1980s, with modifications primarily directed toward creating a solution for the foreign-body reaction that led to scar capsule contracture. The standard gel-filled, smooth-walled implant was modified with the addition of an outer lumen used for the introduction of saline in order to give the opportunity for size adjustment at surgery. Original reasons for the second lumen included the opportunity for percutaneous aspiration of saline in order to reduce the volume and thereby treat capsule contracture. However, because of the dynamic nature of the breast implant capsule, this earlier concept has not proved effective. This added reservoir, however, has provided some surgeons the opportunity to instill antibiotics or corticosteroids to take advantage of the slow diffusion properties of the silicone wall. In addition, the outer silicone shell adds an additional barrier to silicone "bleed." The standard double-lumen implant has evolved into a reverse double-lumen implant in which the silicone is in the outer compartment and the inner lumen can be expanded by the introduction of saline through a fill tube. The subcutaneously implanted filling tube is eventually removed and the permanently placed expansion device left as a mammary implant. Although used at times in augmentation mammaplasty, this form of implant has been more popular for breast reconstruction after mastectomy.

Because silicone gel "bleed" had been implicated as a possible cause of capsule contracture, saline inflatable implants were introduced. Initial enthusiasm for the silicone shell saline-filled implant was dampened by the less natural "feel" and appearance of the saline implant when compared with the best, noncontracted results of the silicone gel implant. In addition, there appeared to be a rather high leak rate with the early saline-filled implants. Loss of popularity of the saline implant was reversed with the Food and Drug Administration (FDA) restriction of the silicone gel implants in 1992.

Attempts to decrease the incidence of

capsule contracture led to the coating of the silicone gel implant with a polyurethane foam. This implant was first introduced in 1970 by Ashley. Although a clear explanation of the mechanism of action of polyurethane in preventing capsular contracture is not available, it appears that there is a disruption of the formation of the smooth linear periprosthetic capsule that leads to lower contracture rates. Concerns about the effects of the breakdown product of polyurethane, toluene-diamine, led the FDA to request a voluntary moratorium in production and sales in 1991. Soon after this moratorium, the single manufacturer of this implant announced its withdrawal from the production of plastic surgery products and ceased its business activities. However, many patients still have this type of implant in place.

In recent years, texturing of the outer surface of silicone devices has been aimed at achieving the low capsular contracture rates of the polyurethane implants without exposure to potential health risks from polyurethane.

Issues of Regulation

The Medical Device Amendment to the Food, Drug and Cosmetic Act was enacted by Congress in 1976. This law provided for the classification of medical devices into three categories and gave the FDA additional authority to regulate all medical devices, including breast implants. The categories were class I, those devices for which no regulation other than sound manufacturing practices were necessary; class II, those devices requiring performance standards; and class III, those life-sustaining or implantable devices that did not fall within classes I or II. Because breast implants were already in widespread use when the law was enacted, they were judged on the basis of performance, were accepted as safe and effective, and were provisionally left without reclassification. Since they were class II devices, the manufacturers were not required to provide scientific evidence to the FDA regarding the safety and efficacy of the devices. In June 1988, the FDA reclassified breast implants as class III devices and required each manufacturer to provide scientific proof that the implants were safe and effective. The manufacturers provided this evidence to the FDA in 1991. The scientific data were evaluated by the FDA scientific staff and its advisory panel of consultants. A final rule from the FDA was promulgated in April 1992 and restricted the gel-filled implant to those women who needed completion of a mastectomy reconstruction and were undergoing soft-tissue expansion, to those who had need of implant replacement because of complications such as symptomatic scar capsular contracture and implant rupture, and to those women who were to have immediate reconstruction following mastectomy. Further evaluation of the gel implant was to be done on carefully controlled, limited clinical trials under the direction of the FDA. Following the final rule on the gel-filled implant, the FDA indicated their plan to place premarket approval requirements on the manufacturers for their saline-filled implants. (For additional discussion of silicone implants, see Chapter 4.)

Preoperative Consultation and Informed Consent

History taking from the breast augmentation candidate must include a personal as well as family history regarding benign and malignant breast disease, a knowledge of the patient's mammography history, a general medical history including medications and allergies, and occupational and recreational discussions. For example, female weight lifters and body builders would not be candidates for submuscular augmentation. A strong family history of breast cancer and/or previous biopsies of premalignant breast disease may be strong indicators to defer an augmentation because of the potential difficulties in following the patient mammographically. On physical examination, attention must be paid to the symmetry of both the breasts and the thoracic skeleton. Developmental deformities of the breast (such as the tubular breast) should be noted. The location of the inframammary fold, an important landmark in judging implant placement, should be recorded, especially with regard to its relation to the nipple position. The presence and degree of ptosis will determine the anatomic placement of the implant and may also indicate the need for a simultaneous mastopexy with the augmentation. A complete breast examination should be performed with the patient in a recumbent position, and any abnormalities must be studied and diagnosed conclusively before augmentation is performed.

Proper informed consent for the breast augmentation patient must include a detailed discussion about the most frequent sequela to the operation, namely, capsular contracture. Although the etiology is not clear, certain contributory factors, as noted later in this chapter, should be discussed with the patient. Some fair estimate of the frequency of appearance of contracture in the submammary and submuscular positions should be made. Of course, the complications described later in this section should be discussed. The manufacturer's product information brochure should be given to the patient, and the informed consent form specific to the implant suggested for use must be signed by the patient and given to her, with a duplicate copy kept in the patient's clinical record.

Surgical Techniques

Augmentation mammaplasty is most often done as an outpatient procedure, depending on the local facilities available. General or local anesthesia may be used, the selection based on the preferences of the patient and surgeon. If local anesthesia is selected, intravenous sedation with full monitoring is important. Supplemental intercostal block anesthesia may be used with local anesthesia.

Three incisions are useful in approaching the dissection preliminary to implant placement. The original inframammary incision first used by Cronin and Gerow is still in widespread practice because it offers the advantage that the entire operative field may be more completely visualized and thus lead to a more accurate and more easily performed procedure. However, the noticeable scar is less aesthetic than that from either the axillary incision or the periareolar incision. The transaxillary approach was described by Hoehler in 1973. This incision is followed by dissection in either the submammary or subpectoral plane. The advantage to this approach is the avoidance of a scar on the breast area. Disadvantages include difficulties in achieving symmetry at the inframammary fold level because of its distance from the incision, the need for blunt dissection, and poor visualization. The inability to visualize the operative field is also a disadvantage when secondary procedures are required for treatment of hematoma, capsular contracture, or implant malposition. Incisions in the periareolar area became popular in the late 1970s. With the periareolar approach, the final scar is frequently more aesthetic than the inframammary incision. Better control of symmetry can be achieved than with the transaxillary approach because of better visualization. However, dissection either through or around breast tissue is needed, and the periareolar approach encroaches more on the mammary gland, with more possibility of postoperative glandular scarring than with the other two approaches.

The three locations for implant placement include submammary, subpectoral, or submuscular. The subglandular, or submammary, method is the oldest placement method and still retains popularity. The gland is dissected from the surface of the pectoral muscles with blunt, sharp, or cautery dissection. Pocket size is controlled as desired for the patient's anatomy, and this provides the most natural result in some patients with slight degrees of mammary ptosis. Concerns about scar capsule contracture in the submammary position led to the development of first the subpectoral and then total submuscular pocket development in an attempt to reduce the incidence of capsular contracture. In the subpectoral approach, the implant is placed behind the pectoralis major muscle superiorly and in either a subglandular, subfascial, or subcutaneous plane at the inferior aspect of the pocket. The submuscular pocket is beneath portions of the pectoralis major, pectoralis minor, serratus anterior, rectus abdominis, and external abdominal oblique muscles. This complete coverage with muscle produces less of a problem with scar capsule contracture when smooth-walled implants are used and allows for more complete, although not total mammographic surveillance of the breast. However, aesthetic results are less natural, especially at the inframammary fold area in women who have a looser skin envelope with mammary ptosis of a degree not sufficient to require mastopexy.

Complications

Capsular Contracture

The development of a periprosthetic fibrotic capsule around the breast implant is the natural process expected with the implantation of any foreign material. This attempt by the human organism to enclose and extrude the foreign body results in a contraction of the fibrous envelope. Compression on the liquid- or gel-filled implant converts it from a flat or oval form into the smallest surface area per volume, namely, a sphere. The more compression generated, the firmer and more symptomatic the capsule becomes. The classification described by Baker has become the most universally used in describing the severity of capsular contracture: in class I, the augmented breast is as soft as the unoperated one; in class II, the breast is less soft, and the implant can be palpated but is not visible; in class III, the breast is firm, the implant can be palpated easily, and its distortion can be visualized; and in class IV, the breast is hard, tender, and painful, and distortion is pronounced. The frequency of capsular contracture varies widely in the surgical literature, with studies suffering from a lack of scientific control because of the variety of techniques and the ever-changing variety of implants that have been generated. Generally, it is accepted that smooth-walled implants placed in the submammary space have higher contracture rates (probably in the range of 20% to 40% of patients) than those placed in the submuscular position. Also, texturing of the implants, such as with a polyurethane cover or with the use of silicone textured devices, appears to have lower contracture rates than smooth-walled implants do (perhaps fewer than 5% of patients). Capsular contracture is most common within the first 6 months after surgery but can occur at any time after the operation. Late contracture may be preceded by a viral or bacterial infection elsewhere. Long-standing contractures may often be associated with "bleed" on the surface of the gel-filled implant and can contain calcifications; this makes the capsule even more rigid and leads to more difficulty with breast examination and mammography. Histologically, the capsule consists of layered collagen interspersed with flattened fibroblasts. Under the electron microscope, myofibroblasts are seen in recently contracted capsules or capsules postsurgically. These cells are probably the contractile mechanism of capsular contraction. The initiating cause of capsule contracture is not clear in the majority of contractures. If caused by a hematoma or frank infection, capsular contracture may be obvious. However, the great majority of contractures do not have an obvious cause and lead to conclusions of multifactorial etiologies, perhaps some related to the silicone material itself.

Treatment of the capsule contracture depends on the severity of the process and the concern of the patient about appearance and symptoms. Many patients are unconcerned about the firmness of the implant and do not have symptoms, thus requiring no treatment of the contracture. The more severe forms of contracture may be treated by capsulotomy or capsulectomy. Manual or closed compression capsulotomy, which involves the use of external force on the breast to rupture the capsule around the implant, enjoyed popularity in the 1970s and 1980s. However, because of the fear of implant rupture, especially in the devices that have been implanted for longer periods of time, this procedure has fallen into disfavor. Open capsulotomy or capsulectomy usually requires general anesthesia since the operation is technically more difficult than the original placement of the implant. If muscle scarring is not too significant, conversion of a submammary implant to the submuscular position may be done at the time of capsulectomy.

Unfavorable Shape or Position

Asymmetries following augmentation mammaplasty may require secondary procedures for correction. Discrepancies in the inframammary fold position of the implant or possible contracture may distort the implant on one side and require correction by unilateral capsulorrhaphy or capsulotomy.

Permanent Sensory Changes

Temporary sensation loss in the lower portion of the breast is commonly seen and generally abates within 6 to 12 months. Major loss of nipple sensation is less common and may occur if the sensory nerve to the nipple is divided with lateral dissection.

Hematoma

Any surgical procedure that produces dissection of a large space can lead to excess bleeding and the development of a hematoma, generally seen in approximately 2% of augmentation mammaplasties. Recognized hematomas should be surgically drained.

Hypertrophic Scars

These can be seen, especially with the inframammary approach. Excision and resuturing or the intralesional use of triamcinolone may be helpful.

Device Failure

Leakage from the implant may occur whether a saline-filled or gel-filled implant is used. Although past concepts have included the lack of "biodegradability" of the device, evidence is mounting that some implants may not last the lifetime of the patient without device failure such as leak or rupture. Leakage from the saline-filled implant caused by failure of the device is generally precipitous and produces an obvious loss of volume. Treatment is by replacement of the device. Rupture of the gel-filled implant is more difficult to detect. This may occur spontaneously or after manual capsulotomy. Many asymptomatic ruptures may occur and be detected only by imaging techniques. Occasionally, an asymmetrical shape or chronic pain can result from rupture, as can local gel migration producing extramammary silicone granulomas. It seems reasonable to assume that the duration of an implant may be based on both its physical properties and the lapsed time since its placement. Therefore, the longer the implant has been in position, the more likely the incidence of device failure.

Infection

True clinical infection of a smooth-walled silicone implant is fortunately rare. *Staphylococcus epidermidis* is usually the implicated organism, with symptoms manifested as erythema, pain, swelling, and asymmetry. Such infection is a true surgical emergency and can lead to the rarely reported complication of toxic shock syndrome.

Implant Exposure and Extrusion

This is a rare complication that can occur through a nonhealing incision and had been seen in the past when corticosteroids were placed in surgical pockets in an attempt to decrease capsular contracture.

Galactorrhea

The surgical technique of breast augmentation itself or pressure of the implant may stimulate the production of prolactin from the pituitary gland and result in galactorrhea.

Mondor's Disease

This is the spontaneous occurrence of breast vein thrombosis beneath the surface of the skin and is manifested by firm, tortuous, and slightly tender cords. This is usually slightly below the inframammary fold and resolves with warm compresses and salicylates.

Autoimmune Disease

Silicone breast implants have been linked with the development of a constellation of different symptoms mimicking diseases such as scleroderma, systemic lupus erythematosus, rheumatoid arthritis, and progressive systemic sclerosis. Symptoms of such autoimmune diseases and related symptoms of joint pain, musculoskeletal aching, chronic fatigue, etc., are seen in other ill-defined rheumatologic constellations in nonimplanted women in the same age group. Although isolated reports of the above symptom complexes associated with breast implantation are in the literature, a well-controlled scientific study has yet to demonstrate a cause-and-effect relationship.

Patient Follow-Up

Patients should be seen at appropriate intervals following surgery for wound care and should be evaluated at intervals during the first year. Since capsular contracture generally occurs within the first year, at least 1-year follow-up for the early postoperative period is required. Long-term follow-up is needed for breast examination and for evaluation of the integrity and long-term effects of the implanted device. Examination on an annual basis is recommended. Mammography should be performed according to the guidelines of the American College of Radiology and should include the compression technique of mammography to displace the implant.

MAMMARY PTOSIS

The surgical management of nonhypertrophic breast ptosis stems from a common origin and parallels the development of reduction mammaplasty techniques. Superior pole excisions and suspension procedures were the first methods introduced. Placement of internal sutures, dermal and fascial strips, and nonabsorbable meshes met with varying degrees of success. Preservation of the skin-parenchymal interface with limited skin undermining is practiced in many contemporary techniques of mastopexy. In general, limited excisions are performed for minor deformity, with major transpositions reserved for patients with severe ptosis.

Patients seeking plastic surgical consultation regarding breast ptosis usually voice aesthetic concerns. Only rarely will patients complain of excessive sweating and other dermatologic manifestations. The pathophysiology is relaxation of the skin envelope and caudal displacement of breast parenchyma. The etiology is multifactorial and related to dermochalasis, volume changes of pregnancy and cyclic hormonal responses, weight loss, and the results of aging. Although breast skin becomes thinner and less elastic, histologic evaluation demonstrates normal parenchymal involution.

In evaluating a patient for potential mastopexy, the degree of ptosis must be determined. A classification was developed and based on the relationship between the position of the nipple and the inframammary fold (Fig 30–7). Minor ptosis exists when the nipple lies on or just below the level of the inframammary fold and above the lower contour of the gland. Moderate ptosis is defined as nipple position below the inframammary fold but above the lower contour of the gland. A major

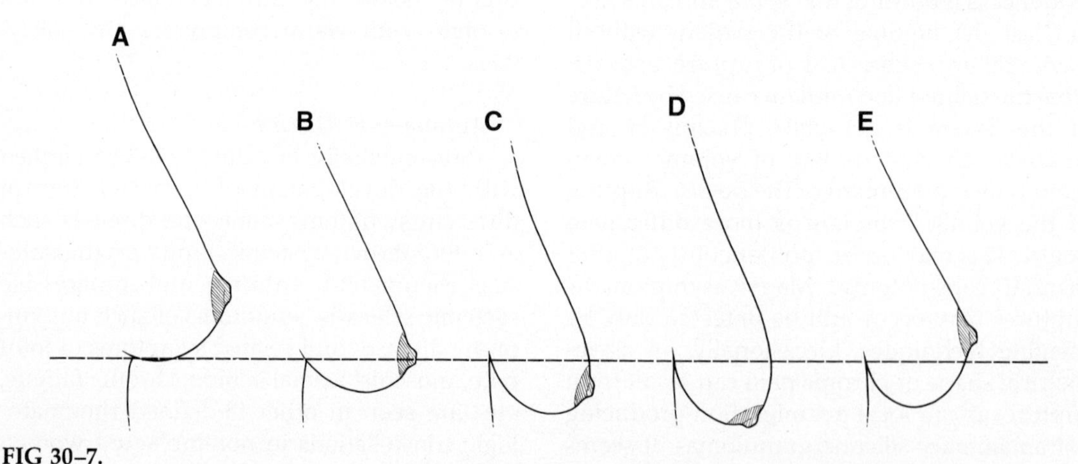

FIG 30–7.
Classification of ptosis deformities. Degree of ptosis is determined by the relationship of the nipple to the inframammary fold as well as the nipple position along the breast contour. **A,** normal breast. **B,** minor ptosis. **C,** moderate ptosis. **D,** major ptosis. **E,** glandular ptosis (pseudoptosis).

ptosis deformity exists when the nipple lies below the fold at the lower contour of the breast. These deformities must be differentiated from glandular ptosis in which the nipple remains at the inframammary fold despite caudal migration of breast parenchyma. Similar to other soft-tissue "pexy" procedures, simple mastopexy does not provide a permanent improvement, and the patient should be so informed.

No single procedure corrects all forms of breast ptosis. Planning should depend upon the type and degree of ptosis present.

Patients with minimal ptosis are candidates for either a simple soft-tissue procedure or augmentation, depending on the breast volume and desires. Mastopexy without augmentation is most commonly performed as either a circumareolar "donut" mastopexy or soft-tissue repositioning and skin redraping similar to reduction mammaplasty. Maintaining the fibrous attachments between the skin and breast tissue may retard the recurrence of ptosis. If the patient is unwilling to accept periareolar or subareolar scarring, augmentation alone can be offered with minimal scarring if larger breasts are desired. A mastopexy with or without augmentation is the treatment of moderate or major ptosis. Often there is superior flattening of the gland that is difficult to augment by using the simple mastopexy technique of soft-tissue transposition. The standard technique is similar to those for reduction mammaplasty. The addition of a subglandular prosthesis improves superior contour and achieves longer-lasting results.

DERMATOCHALASIS AND POSTOBESITY DEFORMITY

Functional and aesthetic reconstruction of the trunk includes those operations requiring skin excision for the relief of cutaneous laxity and those for removal of adipose tissue only by suction lipectomy. Resection of excess skin and fat of the abdomen has its roots as a combination procedure when done with repair of massive umbilical hernias. As with suction lipectomy, French surgeons appear to have initiated dermolipectomy in approximately 1890. The procedure was begun in the United States about one decade later and has gained in popularity as surgical techniques have improved and adjunctive procedures such as improved anesthetics and autotransfusion have been developed. Three basic techniques are used for treatment of the abdominal contour deformity: (1) suction lipectomy alone; (2) miniabdominoplasty, with or without suction lipectomy; and (3) classic abdominoplasty. Selection of the patient for the appropriate technique is the most important step in preoperative planning.

Suction Lipectomy Alone

The ideal candidates for suction lipectomy as an isolated procedure include individuals who are usually relatively young, have a localized deformity and satisfactory skin turgor, and have a definite potential for the skin to contract after suctioning. Even with proper patient selection, the patient must be informed during preoperative discussions that secondary procedures such as miniabdominoplasty or even full abdominoplasty may be required for the treatment of skin laxity. The incidence of secondary procedures in order to achieve the most ideal result may be as high as 20% to 30%.

The cannulas used for suction lipectomy of the abdomen are generally smaller in diameter than those used for major suctioning in thicker-skinned areas such as the lateral aspect of the thigh and hips. The use of smaller cannulas tends to decrease the postoperative contour irregularities of the skin. For example, cannulas between 3.7 and 5 mm in diameter can be used very effectively for suction lipectomy of the abdomen if multiple introductory sites are used.

Epidural or general anesthesia is usually required for abdominal suction lipectomy. Very small areas with small quantities of fat may be done under local anesthesia with sedation. Appropriate preoperative fluid loading with crystalloid solutions is necessary and is particularly required when large volumes would be removed in the suction aspirate. Blood replacement may become a necessity when the volume of aspirate is greater than 1,500 ml. When this potential is expected, the patient should be prepared with the donation of an autotransfusion unit. Such volumes are unusual in abdominal suction cases, however.

Surgical access to the subcutaneous fat of the abdomen and flanks can be gained through small incisions in the groin, the inguinal crease, the suprapubic hairline, or the periumbilical area. Multiple approaches are usually used with abdominal suction in order to produce a grid-like pattern. Undesired sequelae such as contour irregularities, hypoesthesia in the area of suction, ecchymosis, edema, and pigmentary deposits are usually temporary and improve with time. The persistence of contour irregularities, especially with skin laxity, may require secondary revisional surgery as described below. The complications of blood loss, hematoma, seroma, cutaneous infection, pulmonary emboli, fat emboli, thrombophlebitis of the lower extremities, and skin slough should be seen very rarely with proper patient selection, preoperative preparation, and intraoperative technique. However, these potential complications, some with serious results, must be considered, prevented when possible, and treated appropriately.

Suction Lipectomy as an Adjunctive Procedure

The technique of suction lipectomy may be used in other contouring procedures of the trunk as an adjunct to major excisional therapies. For example, use of the technique in combination with reduction mammaplasty is common, especially in reducing adipose deformities of the lateral portion of the thorax and axillary tail of the breast. Supplemental suctioning in the treatment of gynecomastia is almost a routine procedure. Many forms of gynecomastia may even be treated by suction lipectomy alone, with minimal breast excision. Usually, however, a combination of excision of breast tissue in the retroareolar area with suction lipectomy in the periphery of the breast is preferred. The suction technique may be combined with either a miniabdominoplasty or as a supplement to full abdominoplasty as described below.

Miniabdominoplasty

"Mini" or modified abdominoplasty is usually reserved for the patient who has a deformity limited primarily to the area below the umbilicus. It can be done in combination with full suction lipectomy of the abdomen, when indicated. The incision for miniabdominoplasty is essentially in the same location as for full, classic abdominoplasty, although it is shorter and can often be limited to the suprapubic hair-bearing region alone. When the skin is retracted inferiorly for excision, an evaluation of the supraumbilical area is made. If fullness persists, further suction lipectomy can free the umbilical stalk. Often, undermining above the umbilical stalk for 3 to 4 cm may be necessary to release and elongate the stalk. Excision of skin is performed after appropriate judgments are made regarding tension. Closed suction drainage is necessary, and a higher incidence of seroma can be expected when a combination of suction and flap elevation is performed.

Classic Abdominoplasty

The ideal patient for a traditional abdominoplasty is one in whom the skin laxity deformity exists both above and below the umbilicus. Such deformities may contain skin only, as in a sequela to pregnancy. A large abdominal apron containing skin and fat may result in intertrigo, maceration, chronic edema, skin pigmentation changes, and skin turgor changes. The latter deformity is seen in the morbidly obese, usually after a major weight loss of greater than 100 lb. Informed consent should include a discussion of the most frequent complications caused by cutaneous nerve damage, including skin separation, hematoma, and permanent sensory loss. The more severe complications of thromboembolism and fat embolism must also be mentioned.

General anesthesia is the preferred

method. With major dermolipectomy, urine output monitoring with an intraoperative Foley catheter and lower extremity pneumatic compression stockings are recommended.

Incision design, done with the patient in the standing position preoperatively, depends on the patient's body type and desires and is generally dictated by bathing apparel (Fig 30–8). For example, high French cut bathing suits may require incision lines within the iliac crest. Patients undergoing major dermolipectomy are usually best treated by extension of the natural abdominal skin crease fold below the iliac crest and into the posterolateral hip areas. This incision is also preferred for males.

The panniculus is generally elevated with electrodissection, with a thin layer of fat preserved on the fascia, and is lifted to the costal margin or even above, depending on the extent of the deformity. The umbilicus is circumscribed. Plication of the rectus abdominis diastasis is done with either interrupted nonabsorbable sutures or continuous suturing. For skin excision and closure, the patient is placed in a flexed position. Vertical cuts in the panniculus are made for sequential fat and skin removal as the panniculus is retracted caudally. The umbilicus, having been premarked with a button or other identification device, is pulled through the abdominal flap through a vertical incision in the midline. Closure of the abdominal wound is done in layers with subcuticular suturing to avoid skin suture marks. Closed suction drainage, usually through stab incisions at the mons pubis, are used. Pressure taping or abdominal support garments complete the procedure.

Reverse Abdominoplasty

An occasional patient, particularly one in the post–weight loss obesity category, may be a candidate for an abdominoplasty confined to the upper part of the abdomen. The incision is then placed under the inframammary fold, and skin excision is performed in a cranial direction. Occasionally, this procedure may be done in combination with reduction mammaplasty.

Complications

Major and minor complications become more frequent when multiple procedures are performed and would be expected to have the highest frequency in formerly morbidly obese patients who have a combination of dermolipectomy and suction lipectomy. Individual complications are managed as with any other major abdominal surgical procedure. Special attention must be given to the problem of thromboembolism and fat embolism in major abdominal body contour surgery. A serious thromboembolic episode may be expected to develop in approximately 1% of abdominoplasty patients, and approximately 1 in 1,000 would be expected to die from the event. With regard to fat embolism syndrome, it is suspected that the breakdown of fat into free fatty acids and subsequent lodging of the free fatty acids in the lungs produce the pulmonary effects. Some surgeons have advocated the use of intravenous alcohol solutions during surgery for prophylaxis against fat embolism syndrome.

Postoperative Care

After major abdominoplasty, patients are maintained in a flexed position for the day of surgery. Ambulation is initiated 24 hours following surgery. Systemic perioperative antibiotic therapy is recommended by most surgeons. Normal activity can be resumed within 3 to 4 weeks, and strenuous exercise is limited until 6 weeks following classic abdominoplasty.

OTHER AESTHETIC DEFORMITIES

Tuberous Breast and Inverted Nipple Deformities

The tubular breast deformity was first described by Rees and Aston in 1976. Characteristic features include a small gland that is constricted at the base and has an excessively large areola. The narrow base results in both a horizontal and vertical deficiency and is responsible for its characteristic contour. Glandular hypoplasia is usually present. Other authors have postulated that a deficiency in the skin envelope is responsible for the tubular breast contour. The nondistensibility of the skin at the breast base leads to parenchymal herniation into the areola and results in the characteristic areolar deformity.

Proper management of the tuberous breast requires an accurate preoperative diagnosis of the deformity. Standard mastopexy or prosthetic implantation serves to accentuate the pre-existing irregularities. Two techniques have been popularized to improve tuberous breast syndrome. The first method requires wide undermining of the skin and reshaping of the breast mound. A periareolar incision the size of the desired areola is made, with the remainder deepithelialized as a donut. Circumferential dissection frees attachments between the skin and the underlying parenchyma to the base of the breast. After developing the subglandular plane, the undersurface of the breast may be scored in radial fashion to widen the base. Parenchymal resection or tailoring may be necessary to improve breast shape. The decision to insert prostheses depends on subsequent contour and the desired size. A period of overexpansion has been recommended by some authors, followed by prosthetic implantation at a second procedure (Fig 30–9). Closure requires inward telescoping of the deepithelialized dermis. Debulking of smooth muscle and parenchyma under the remaining areola may reduce areolar projection.

The second technique is based on the premise of an inadequate skin envelope causing constriction at the base. Dinner proposed an inframammary transposition flap of skin and subcutaneous tissue to increase the circumference of the breast base. Areolar reduction and inframammary prosthetic implantation complete the correction. (For additional discussion see Chapter 27.)

Correction of an inverted nipple is usually of aesthetic concern. Since nipple inversion typically precludes breast feeding, surgical techniques that divide nipple ducts do not alter pre-existing lactation function. The deformity is an inadequate height of the nipple

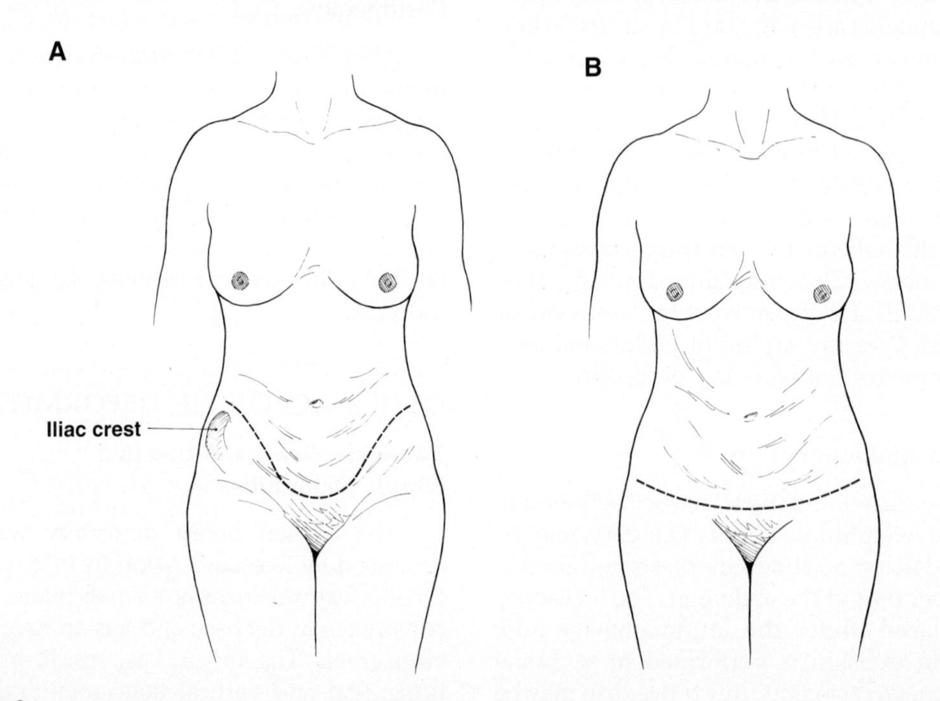

FIG 30–8.
Abdominoplasty incision. **A,** the incisions for patients who desire high "French cut" bathing apparel should be placed medial to the iliac crest. **B,** for major dermalipectomy, the incision is made in the natural abdominal skin crease fold below the iliac crest.

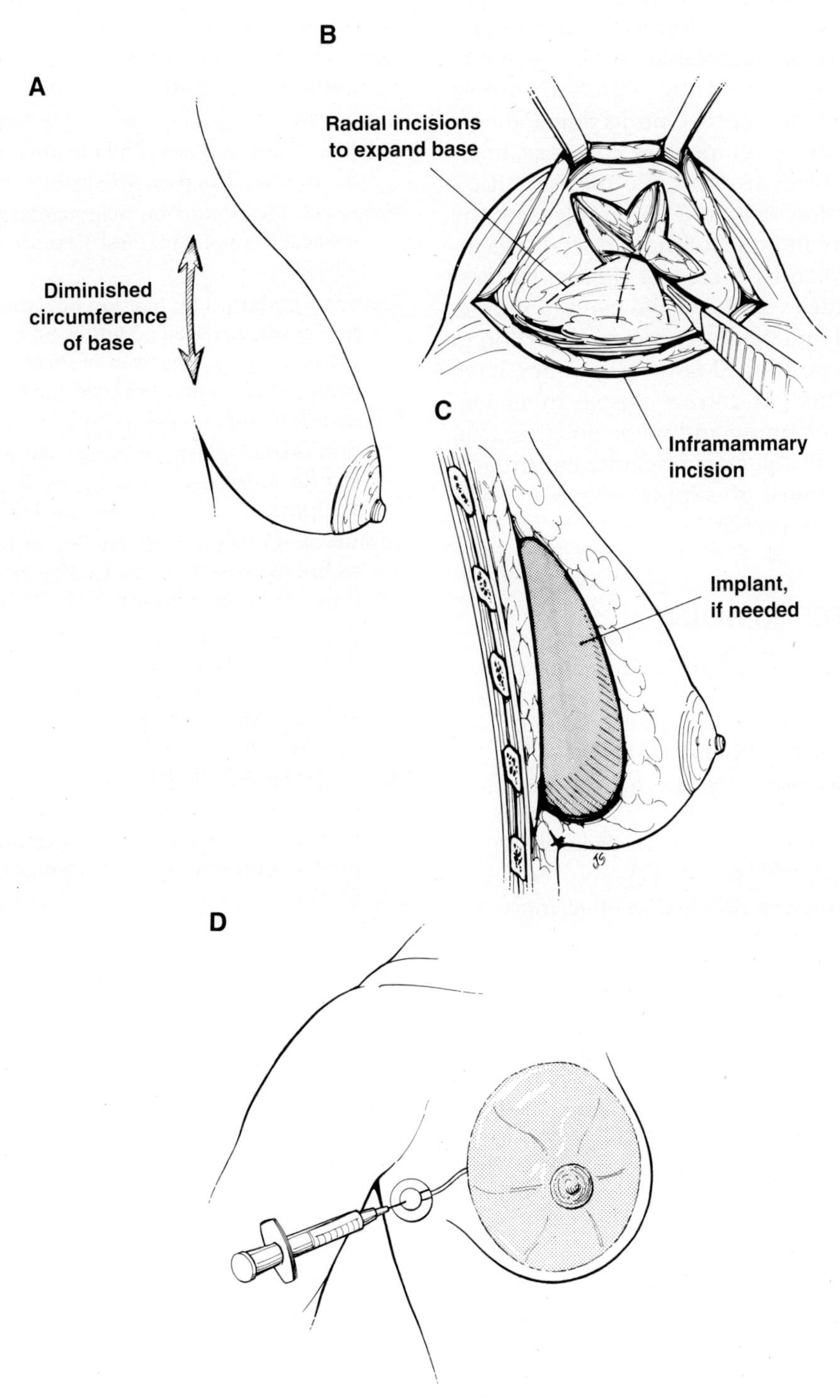

FIG 30–9.
Tuberous breast deformity. One technique of correction is radial scoring of the undersurface of the breast parenchyma followed by over-expansion postoperatively. A permanent expander implant may be used initially, or a temporary expander may be replaced with a permanent implant during a second procedure.

column. If coexistent with inadequate integumentary cover, most corrective techniques yield a less-than-acceptable result. This subgroup is best served by standard nipple reconstruction to improve projection. Patients with adequate integumentary coverage, however, will benefit from nipple release with a simple eversion technique. After releasing the nipple from its surrounding ductal attachments and bands, a core of adjacent breast tissue provides volume to the everted nipple. It is secured into place to prevent retraction to its original position. Many techniques have been described to correct nipple inversion. Thoughtful planning and meticulous surgical technique will safeguard against recurrence. (For illustrations of nipple eversion techniques, see Chapter 28.)

SUGGESTED READING

Biggs TM, Humphreys DH: Augmentation mammaplasty, in Smith JW, Aston SJ (eds): *Grabb and Smith's Plastic Surgery,* ed 4. Boston, Little, Brown, 1991, pp 1145–1156.

Brody GS: Overview of augmentation mammaplasty, in Noone RB (ed): *Plastic and Reconstructive Surgery of the Breast.* Philadelphia, BC Decker, 1991, pp 119–124.

Courtiss E, Goldwyn RM: Reduction mammaplasty by the inferior pedicle technique. *Plast Reconstr Surg* 1977; 50:500.

Goldwyn RM: *Reduction Mammaplasty.* Boston, Little, Brown, 1990.

Grazer FM: Abdominoplasty, in McCarthy JG (ed): *Plastic Surgery.* Philadelphia, WB Saunders, 1990, pp 3929–3963.

McKissock PK: Reduction mammaplasty with a vertical dermal flap, *Plast Reconstr Surg* 1972; 49:245.

Rohrich RJ, Mathes SJ: Suction lipectomy, in Jurkiewicz MJ, Krizek TJ, Mathes SJ, et al (eds): *Plastic Surgery: Principles in Practice.* St Louis, Mosby–Year Book, 1990, pp 1553–1572.

Rudolph RS: Unfavorable results of augmentation mammaplasty, in Noone RB (ed): *Plastic and Reconstructive Surgery of the Breast.* Philadelphia, BC Decker, 1991, pp 167–186.

Strombeck JO: Mammaplasty: Report of a new technique based on the two-pedicle procedure. *Br J Plast Surg* 1960; 12:79.

Wang T, Vasconez LO: Body contour surgery, in Jurkiewicz MJ, Krizek TJ, Mathes SJ, et al (eds): *Plastic Surgery: Principles in Practice.* St Louis, Mosby–Year Book, 1990, pp 1539–1550.

Weiner D, Aiache AE, Silver L, et al: A single dermal pedicle for nipple transposition in subcutaneous mastectomy, reduction mammaplasty or mastopexy. *Plast Reconstr Surg* 1973; 51:115.

PART VII

Plastic Surgery of the Lower Extremity

Chapter 31

Anatomy/Physiology/Embryology

William D. Morain, M.D.

CONTENTS

CHAPTER OBJECTIVE

At the end of this chapter the resident has comprehensive knowledge of the anatomy, physiology, and embryology of the lower extremity and uses this information in the management of a wide variety of surgical problems of the leg.

LEARNER OBJECTIVES

On completion of this chapter the resident

1. **Knows the vascular, neural, and osseous anatomy of the lower extremity.**
2. **Knows the muscular and vascular anatomy of specific flaps, including the tensor faciae latae, vastus lateralis, rectus femoris, sartorius, gracilis, and biceps femoris flaps.**
3. **Knows the boundaries of and vascular anatomy of specific cutaneous flaps, including the lateral thigh, medial thigh, posterior thigh, and groin flaps.**
4. **Knows the venous anatomy of the leg, including the saphenous vein.**
5. **Knows the muscular, cutaneous, and vascular anatomy of the medial and lateral gastrocnemius, the soleus, and the tibialis muscle flaps.**
6. **Understands the concept of fasciocutaneous flaps and can design them on the distal part of the lower extremity.**
7. **Knows the cutaneous margins and vascular anatomy of foot flaps, including the medial plantar–, lateral plantar–, V-Y plantar–, and dorsalis pedis–based flaps.**
8. **Understands the usefulness of the sural nerve as a graft based on its sensory distribution.**
9. **Knows the neuroanatomy of and boundaries of sensate flaps in the lower extremity.**
10. **Understands the physiology of arterial insufficiency, venous hypertension, and diabetes as they pertain to the lower extremity.**
11. Knows the detailed anatomy of the popliteal artery and its branches.
12. Knows the osseous and vascular anatomy of bone segments suitable as grafts.
13. Understands the function of the muscle groups of the lower extremity and how they compensate when one is injured or sacrificed.

14. Understands the normal plantar arch and the fundamentals of normal gait.
15. Understands the advantages and disadvantages of various levels of amputation.
16. Understands the basic lower extremity embryology, abnormal development, and sequelae (e.g., arteriovenous malformations and Klippel-Trenaunay syndrome).

CLINICAL PRACTICE ACTIVITIES

During the course of the training program, the resident

1. **Utilizes anatomic knowledge during the performance of surgical procedures on the lower extremity.**
2. Performs cadaver dissection of the lower extremity.
3. Applies anatomic and biomechanical knowledge to the choice of procedures for patients with lower extremity problems.

ANATOMY OF THE LOWER EXTREMITY

Surface Anatomy

Numerous bony prominences occur in the lower extremity. It is important to be familiar with them because of the role they play in the formation of pressure ulcerations. The superiormost prominences include the iliac crest and its terminations at the anterior superior spine and posterior superior spine. The ischial tuberosity lies vertically below the posterior superior spine and is covered by the gluteus maximus while standing but not during sitting. The greater trochanter is covered by the fascia lata. Deep in the depression between the greater trochanter and ischial tuberosity the sciatic nerve can be palpated. The patella is immediately subcutaneous at the knee and remains at a constant distance from the tibial tubercle as the knee flexes and extends. Whereas the medial femoral condyle is quite prominent to palpation, the lateral is obscured beneath the fascia lata and the bicipital tendon. Although the tibia is immediately subcutaneous along its entire anterior and medial border, the fibula is prominent only at its upper and lower ends. The prominent medial and lateral malleoli and calcaneus are so thinly covered that they are unusually susceptible to pressure injury. Weight-bearing prominences of the plantar surface, especially the calcaneus and metatarsal heads, are resistant to pressure ulceration unless trauma or neuropathy has destroyed the foot's natural arches.

Muscles

The muscles of the lower extremity are organized for the sole purposes of weight bearing and locomotion. At the proximal end the gluteus maximus, the largest muscle of the body, is a powerful extensor and external rotator of the thigh. Like the tensor fasciae latae, the other superficial muscle of this region, much of the gluteus maximus inserts into the iliotibial band, the distal portion of the fascia lata. The deep group of gluteal muscles is composed of the gluteus medius and minimus (powerful thigh abductors), and the piriformis, obturator internus, gemelli, and quadratus femoris (thigh lateral rotators).

In the obturator region, all of the thigh adductor muscles arise from a local area on the pubis. The largest and most posterior, the adductor magnus, contains the hiatus through which the femoral vessels pass. The adductor brevis and the more anterior adductor longus assist the magnus. They are augmented by the pectineus (also a thigh flexor) and the gracilis (an accessory knee flexor).

In the region of the femoral shaft are some of the muscles of greatest usefulness for reconstructive surgery. On the anterior surface the sartorius muscle forms the lateral boundary of the femoral trigone and the roof of the adductor canal. Its long, spiralling, downward and medial course makes it an abductor, flexor, and lateral rotator of the thigh and a flexor and medial rotator of the leg. The quadriceps femoris is the powerful knee extensor that inserts into the patella. While the rectus femoris takes origin from the anterior inferior iliac spine, the remaining three parts of the quadriceps (vastus lateralis, intermedius, and medialis) arise from the femur.

On the posterior surface of the thigh are three hamstring muscles arising from the ischial tuberosity and extending beyond the knee without any femoral attachments (except for the short head of the biceps). The biceps femoris inserts on the fibula, while the semimembranosus and semitendinosus insert into the tibia. All three extend the hip and flex the knee.

In the anterior compartment of the leg the tibialis anterior muscle passes downward to insert on the first metatarsal and first cuneiform. It dorsiflexes and inverts the foot. The extensor digitorum longus, extensor hallucis longus, and peroneus tertius insert into the terminal phalanges of the lesser toes, great toe, and fifth metatarsal base, respectively. All muscles of this compartment are supplied by the anterior tibial (deep peroneal) nerve.

In the lateral compartment of the leg the peroneus longus and brevis muscles are supplied by the superficial peroneal nerve. The peroneus brevis joins the peroneus tertius in inserting into the base of the fifth metatarsal, whereas the peroneus longus crosses the plantar aspect of the foot obliquely to insert into the base of the first metatarsal and first cuneiform. Both muscles aid in plantar flexion, abduction, and eversion of the foot.

The posterior compartment of the leg is in two segments. The more superficial contains the triceps surae (medial and lateral gastrocnemius and soleus) and plantaris muscles, while the deeper contains the flexor digitorum longus, flexor hallucis longus, and tibialis posterior muscles. Both gastrocnemius heads arise from the distal end of the femur, while the soleus has a more distal origin from the proximal end of the tibia and fibula. All of the triceps surae insert into the large Achilles tendon. The long, slender plantaris tendon inserts into the calcaneus at its medial edge, where it may be found surgically when needed as a tendon graft. In the deep compartment the tibialis posterior inserts into the navicular and acts as a powerful inverter of the foot. The flexor digitorum longus arises from the tibia and passes to the toes in parallel with the fibula-derived flexor hallucis longus.

In the foot the intrinsic muscles run generally in longitudinal fashion and assist in maintaining the horizontal and vertical arches. The surgically important intrinsic muscles include the abductor hallucis medially, the abductor digiti quinti laterally, and the flexor digitorum brevis centrally.

Nerves

The motor components of the major nerves to the lower extremity are distributed to well-defined muscle compartments, with the femoral nerve supplying the knee extensors, the obturator nerve supplying the hip adductors, the sciatic nerve supplying the knee flexors, the peroneal nerve supplying the peroneal compartment, and the tibial nerve supplying the ankle flexors and the foot intrinsics. The sensory distribution is demonstrated in Figure 31–1.

Some noteworthy anatomic relationships of these nerves are encountered in reconstructive surgery. The sciatic nerve lies lateral to the ischial tuberosity and can be injured when dissecting the inferior portion of the gluteus maximus flap. It can usually be identified by passing a finger into the areolar plane deep to the gluteus maximus muscle and just superficial to the nerve. The nerve can be palpated as a thick cord deep to this plane. More distally in the extremity, the peroneal nerve must be carefully identified and spared during transfer of a lateral gastrocnemius musculocutaneous flap.

The sural nerve is the preferred donor nerve for grafting. Arising from the peroneal nerve in the popliteal space, it passes subfascially between the two heads of the gastrocnemius muscle and emerges through the fascia in the midportion of the calf. It then passes distally around the posterior edge of the lateral malleolus to supply the lateral part of the dorsum of the foot. Although the sural nerve may be harvested surgically through a series of horizontal "ladder" incisions, it is less likely to be injured by approaching it directly through a vertical incision directly over the nerve.

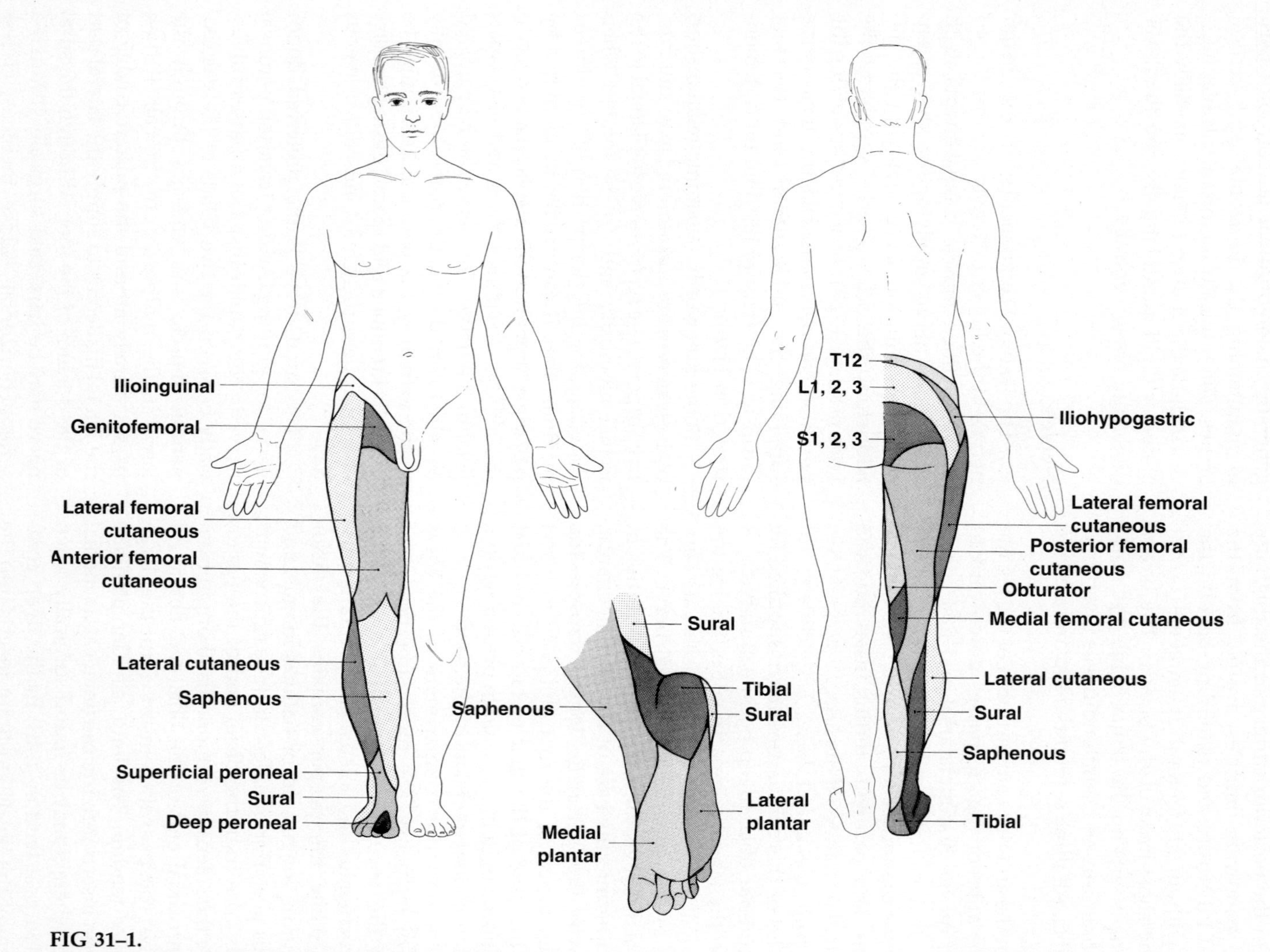

FIG 31–1.
Cutaneous nerve distribution to the lower extremity.

Vascular Supply

The lower extremities are predominantly supplied by branches of a single arterial system originating as the common femoral artery. After giving off a few superficial branches to inguinal and pubic cutaneous territories, it gives off its large profunda branch 4 cm below the inguinal ligament. The profunda femoris, in turn, branches in part into medial and lateral circumflex femoral arteries to supply the musculature of all compartments of the thigh. After giving off genicular branches the superficial femoral artery enters the popliteal space as the popliteal artery, hugs the posterior capsule of the knee joint, and gives off additional genicular branches.

Just below its point of penetration through the soleus muscle the popliteal artery divides into anterior and posterior tibial arteries. These vessels are in close apposition to the tibia and fibula, where they are vulnerable to injury in the event of fracture. The two arteries anastomose freely with each other, thereby ensuring the adequacy of distal circulation in the event of occlusion of either. About 2.5 cm distal to its origin the larger posterior tibial artery gives off the peroneal artery. Although the latter terminates at the ankle, the anterior and posterior tibial arteries continue as the dorsalis pedis and the plantar arteries, respectively. Whereas the medial plantar artery is small, the lateral plantar artery runs deeply to become the plantar arch and supplies digital arteries to most of the toes.

While much of the venous circulation of the lower extremity follows the deeply placed arterial circulation, a separate superficial system is an important supplement. The greater and lesser saphenous veins communicate with the deep veins through a system of valved vessels that prevent backflow of blood toward the feet. The valves favor flow toward the heart and from the superficial toward the deep venous system. Phlebitis and prolonged dependency may cause incompetence of the valves with subsequent stasis leading to edema, induration, and ulceration. This tendency toward tissue edema below the knee, with or without venous disease, is the greatest obstacle to healing in this region of the body and must be prophylactically counterbalanced by bed rest with elevation and by snug compression dressings when ambulatory.

Osteology

The femur is the longest and strongest bone of the human body. Its shaft inclines downward and medially toward the knee, with greater obliquity in females because of the relatively greater width of the female pelvis. Except at its ends the femoral shaft is fully enclosed with muscle. Its articulation with the tibia is complex through two weight-bearing facets and an elaborate mechanism of cartilaginous weight dispersion. The patella protects the knee joint in kneeling and provides a low-friction mechanism for load angulation. The knee joint is the largest and most complex in the body; it achieves stability and strength while permitting a wide range of motion, an unusual combination.

In the leg, the tibia bears most of the weight and is constructed accordingly. Unlike the femur, however, it is not centrally encased in muscle but is instead immediately subcutaneous over virtually its entire anteromedial surface. This produces a strong proclivity to exposure in the event of fracture, a source of challenging reconstructive tasks. The slender fibula, on the other hand, is deeply placed in the leg except at its proximal head and distal lateral malleolus. The distal ends of the tibia and fibula are inelastically united in a syndesmosis to form the unyielding ankle mortise for articulation with the talus. In turn, the ankle joint is spared considerable wear by the inversion and eversion taking place between the talus, navicular, and calcaneus.

The foot is able to accommodate large weight-bearing forces because of its large size and breadth, its perpendicularity to the leg, and its unique double-arch structure. The bones of the foot are short and solid and attached through thick ligaments and strong tendons. Motions in the foot are thus few and simple but rapidly accommodating. Most of the weight is borne through the medial bones of the foot (talus, navicular, three cuneiforms, three medial metatarsals and phalanges). The lateral group (calcaneus, cuboid, lateral two metatarsals and phalanges) are related to the fibula and primarily function in counterbalance. Because the toes are used more in balancing and running than in walking, their loss interferes only slightly with gait.

ANATOMY AS APPLIED TO SPECIFIC LOWER EXTREMITY FLAPS

The functional anatomy of the lower extremity creates both opportunity and limitation for arterialized flap transfer. Because of a certain redundancy among functioning muscle groups, this is the richest region in the body for musculocutaneous flap variety. In addition, defunctionalization of the lower extremities, as occurs with spinal cord injury, both induces greater need for flap transfer through pressure injury and releases more available muscle units for their coverage. However, the distal portion of the extremity demonstrates a paucity of available local arterialized flap units.

Axial Skin Flaps

A number of axial skin flaps may be reliably transferred on their intact vascular pedicles for lower extremity coverage. The *groin* (or *ilioinguinal*) *flap* is jointly supplied by the superficial circumflex iliac and the superficial inferior epigastric vessels, either of which will reliably carry the entire unit. Rotating about the takeoff point of these arteries from the femoral artery, the axis of the groin flap parallels the inguinal ligament and may extend superolaterally twice the distance from its origin to the anterior superior iliac spine. It is valuable for perineal, upper thigh, and scrotal coverage.

The *lateral thigh flap* is centered at the distalmost point of insertion of the gluteus maximus muscle into the iliotibial tract. It is at this point that the large septocutaneous artery from the profunda femoris emerges along the lateral intermuscular septum and passes forward and inferiorly. The flap may be pivoted superiorly to cover the trochanter or posteriorly to cover the ischium.

The *dorsalis pedis flap* is used for defects about the ankle. Customarily raised as an island flap, it is based on the dorsalis pedis artery. It is tedious to elevate, however, and may be associated with donor site problems of skin graft loss and sacrifice of the extensor hallucis longus tendon.

Muscle and Musculocutaneous Flaps

Numerous thigh muscles are valuable for extremity and lower trunk coverage because of their long arcs of rotation. The *tensor fasciae latae musculocutaneous flap* receives a single vascular pedicle from the lateral circumflex femoral artery. This musculofascial unit extends from the anterior superior spine and greater trochanter to the lateral aspect of the knee. With its lateral femoral cutaneous nerve, it can supply valuable sensibility to the sitting area in patients with myelomeningoceles. It may be otherwise used for groin coverage and for trochanteric pressure ulcers. Its use in an athlete, however, may cause a loss of lateral knee stability.

The *vastus lateralis muscle flap* is also supplied from the lateral circumflex femoral artery. This muscle, the largest in size below the gluteus maximus, takes origin from the proximal end of the femur and inserts into the patella along with the other three parts of the quadriceps mechanism. Having no appreciable cutaneous component, it is useful for defects of the trochanteric, ischial, groin, and hip areas, where well-vascularized muscle is essential for wound coverage. Its use is limited only by the technical difficulty in dissecting it cleanly from adjacent muscles.

The *rectus femoris muscle* or *musculocutaneous flap* is also supplied by a branch of the lateral femoral circumflex artery. The muscle extends from the anterior superior spine to the patella. It is preferred for lower abdominal wall reconstruction and is often used for hip and trochanteric defects. Its strong fascia and that contiguous with it make its structural integrity especially unyielding.

The *sartorius muscle* has limited usefulness as a flap because of its predominantly segmental blood supply. It takes origin from the anterior superior spine and spirals around the anterior thigh to insert on the posteromedial aspect of the tibia. It may be useful for limited defects in the region of the femoral triangle if only a short segment is transferred and minimal mobilization is required.

The *gracilis* may be transferred as a *muscle* or *musculocutaneous flap.* Extending from the pubic tubercle to the medial aspect of the knee, it is totally expendable as a functional unit. Its pedicle from the profunda femoris artery enters the muscle a hands-breadth below the pubic tubercle. Occasionally this entry site is more distal, however, and renders the flap too short to reach its proximal destination. When used for perineal or ischial coverage, as in vaginal reconstruction or ischial pressure ulcer defects, a middle-third skin paddle is usually carried with the muscle. The distal third of the overlying skin is a separate vascular territory and will not survive if taken with the flap. Practical disadvantages of the flap are the difficulty in placement of the skin paddle, troublesome vascular spasm with skin loss, and an unsightly donor scar.

The *biceps femoris musculocutaneous flap* has surprising usefulness despite its limited mobility. It is supplied by multiple deep, perforating, segmental vessels from the profunda femoris and popliteal vessels. The muscle extends from the ischial tuberosity (long head) and proximal end of the femur (short head) to the head of the fibula and lateral tibial condyle. This flap is used almost exclusively in a V-Y configuration for ischial pressure ulcers, and both its origin and insertion are divided to gain optimum proximal mobilization. The flap is sensate when taken with the posterior cutaneous nerve of the thigh.

The triceps surae muscle group is as much a resource for muscle flaps below the knee as the quadriceps is above. Either the *medial* or *lateral head* of the *gastrocnemius muscle* can be transferred with its respective branch of the sural artery without any functional loss. The two muscle bellies extend from their respective femoral condyles into the Achilles tendon midway between the knee and the ankle. The medial head is the larger of the two. The units are almost always transferred as muscle flaps with skin grafting because the musculocutaneous donor area is unsightly. The muscle flaps are used to cover defects about the knee and proximal third of the tibia and fibula. Care must be taken to avoid damage to the peroneal nerve when dissecting the lateral gastrocnemius muscle flap.

The *soleus muscle flap* is ideal for coverage of middle third pretibial defects. The muscle extends from the proximal ends of the tibia and fibula to a broad anterior insertion on the Achilles tendon. It is supplied directly from the popliteal artery at its proximal end. The appearance of the skin-grafted flap is quite satisfactory, and functional loss is negligible.

The *tibialis anterior muscle flap* may be used for small middle-third pretibial defects. However, because the muscle is essential for foot extension, its continuity must be preserved by transferring only a portion of it in muscle-splitting fashion. Skin grafting is required.

In the foot, flaps of the intrinsic muscles have limited usefulness for defects about the ankle and heel. The most reliable is a turnover flap of the *flexor digitorum brevis muscle* for defects of the plantar surface of the heel. The *abductor hallucis muscle flap* has some value for small defects of the medial aspect of the ankle. The *abductor digiti quinti muscle flap* is less reliable because of its small size and should be restricted to the smallest of lateral ankle defects. All three require skin grafting for wound closure.

Fascial and Fasciocutaneous Flaps

Random cutaneous flaps have empirically shown limited usefulness in the lower extremity because of the sparse skin capillary density of the region. However, laminating these flaps by adding the deep fascia to the undersurface typically creates a durable and well-perfused fasciocutaneous unit that can be transposed reliably in difficult reconstructive tasks. Although these flaps have occasionally been described as random-pattern units without regard to the fascial blood supply, they are best raised in careful relation to their arterial origins. The fascia's rich vascular plexus is supplied by perforating "septocutaneous" vessels that pass to the surface in the fascial septa between long thin muscles. Within the fascial plexus, the vascular orientation is predominantly longitudinal in the lower extremity, which permits useful flap orientation for planning most reconstructive tasks. Although fasciocutaneous flaps can be potentially raised in many areas of the lower extremity, they have shown greatest usefulness in the difficult distal third of the leg and the ankle.

The *medial thigh flap* is a superiorly based fasciocutaneous flap supplied by a large perforating vessel that exits the femoral artery at the apex of the femoral triangle. The flap may be rotated to reach the groin and may be sensate if the medial cutaneous nerve of the thigh is preserved in it. The saphenous vein is best dissected free of the flap and left in situ.

The *posterior thigh flap* is centered over the large terminal cutaneous branch of the inferior gluteal artery. It is usually raised as a long fasciocutaneous flap incorporating the posterior cutaneous nerve of the thigh for sensation. The posterior thigh flap is useful for defects in the ischial and perineal areas, even those that extend well onto the opposite thigh.

The *V-Y plantar advancement flap* is the procedure of choice for small- to medium-sized defects of the plantar surface. Because the plantar skin is supplied through numerous vessels that perforate the plantar fascia, considerable fasciocutaneous mobility can be achieved, provided that the plantar fascia is incised congruently with the skin incision. Because of the V-Y configuration, skin grafting is unnecessary.

Flaps That Include Bone

On occasion, lower extremity tissue transfers require incorporation of bone for an optimum result. Sizable interval defects of the tibia or femur, for example, are best treated by fibular transfer. This is usually best accomplished by microvascular means. Another donor region for vascularized bone transfer is the second metatarsal, which may be transferred along with the dorsalis pedis flap for complex upper extremity defects.

EMBRYOLOGY OF THE LOWER EXTREMITY

Embryologic development of the lower extremity parallels that of the upper extremity (Fig 31–2). Limb buds appear late in the fourth week as lateral swellings. The distal portion of each bud flattens into a paddle-like structure and segregates by a constriction from the more cylindrical proximal portion. Later, a second constriction begins to separate the cylindrical portion in two, thus defining the foot, leg, and thigh. Radial ridges appear and elongate as toes projecting beyond the original plates. The great and second toes separate early and widely.

Initially the lower extremity buds project caudad but shortly shift to project at right angles. The knee then shifts to a ventral angulation so that the sole faces the trunk with the great toe (tibial side) oriented in a cephalic direction. The entire lower extremity then rotates 90 degrees as a unit so that the knee points cephalad. The lower extremity lags behind the upper in early development, both in relative and absolute growth. Not until the second year after birth does lower extremity length catch up with that of the upper extremity. The leg continues to elongate relative to the rest of the body throughout the remainder of childhood.

A number of different vascular anomalies resulting from abnormalities of embryologic development may affect the lower extremity. These include hemangiomas, low-flow vascular malformations, high-flow vascular malformations, and combined vascular malformation and hypertrophy syndromes. (For information regarding hemagiomas and vascular malformations, please refer to Chapters 10 and 11.)

Combined vascular malformation and hypertrophy syndromes may be particularly difficult problems. The Klippel-Trenaunay syndrome is a combined capillary-lymphatic-venous malformation associated with limb hypertrophy. The Parkes-Weber syndrome is similar to the Klippel-Trenaunay syndrome except that in the former the vascular anomaly is primarily arteriovenous while in the latter the anomaly is venous alone. Mafucci's syndrome includes vascular malformations and

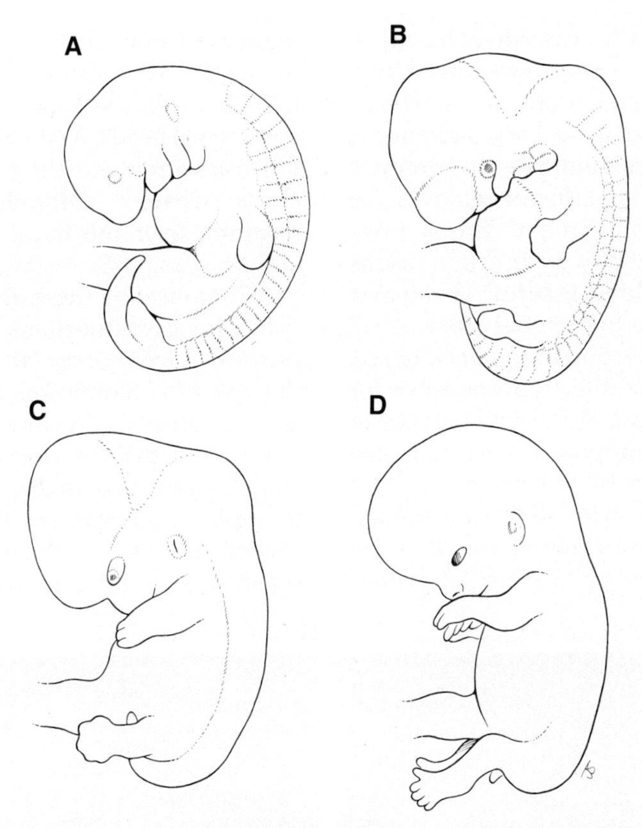

FIG 31–2.
A, rudimentary extremity limb buds at the fifth week. **B,** paddle-like extension of foot with proximal constriction. **C,** formation of a second constriction to segregate thigh from knee. **D,** rotation of lower extremity with knee pointing cephalad.

dyschondroplasia. Surgical treatment of these entities may require multiple stages and is often less than satisfactory in its outcome.

PATHOPHYSIOLOGY OF DIABETES MELLITUS IN THE LOWER EXTREMITY

The lower extremity is especially vulnerable to the pathophysiologic processes of diabetes mellitus, including alterations in circulatory, neurologic, and immunologic factors. However, the diabetic extremity is no less amenable to reconstructive surgical intervention than the nondiabetic extremity, provided that adequate arterial inflow is present.

One of the lingering controversies in diabetes is the role of "microvascular disease" in the etiology of diabetic foot problems. There is indeed a characteristic pattern of *large* vessel disease in infrapopliteal arteries with frequent sparing of foot vessels, thereby permitting successful distal bypass surgery to be performed by vascular surgeons. On the other hand, a substantial body of evidence exists to refute the notion of a characteristic diabetic lesion in the microvasculature. But regardless of whether or not an *anatomic* lesion can be identified in small vessels, it is established that microvascular flow is in fact sluggish in diabetic patients because of increased blood viscosity. This is in turn the result of stiffening of the red cell wall in response to hyperglycemia. At the same time, hyperglycemia induces a shift in the hemoglobin dissociation curve that results in less oxygen delivery to tissues. Ischemia may thus play a role in tissue catabolism in the diabetic foot.

A much greater etiologic factor in the formation of diabetic foot ulcers is neuropathy. As with the circulatory system, chronic hyperglycemia initiates a cascade of biochemical events resulting in nerve swelling, demyelination, and degeneration. As a consequence, abnormalities in sensory, sudomotor, and motor function summate to produce ulceration. Sensory impairment removes the warning signal from an area of chronic pressure overload. Sudomotor dysfunction results in dry, atrophic, cracking, fissuring skin that is especially vulnerable to bacterial entry.

It is motor dysfunction in the tibial nerve, however, that is most directly responsible for ulcer localization. Loss of the fine balance of intrinsic muscular support in the foot can result in destruction of the transverse and longitudinal arches with the unfortunate overexposure of bony prominences that are not well suited to weight bearing. Formation of the claw foot, directly homologous with the ulnar claw hand, causes pressure vulnerability initially over the tops of the toes and the metacarpal heads. As the remainder of the foot intrinsics attenuate, the midfoot falls into the classic Charcot deformity with ulceration resulting over the tarsal bones (Fig 31–3, A and B).

Complicating these ulcerations is the high risk of invasive infections in the foot. Since all pressure ulcers occur at bony prominences, the risk of osteomyelitis by direct contact is always present. Burrowing infections into tendon sheaths and deep spaces are an equivalent hazard. As with diabetic hand infections, multiple organisms are typically seen, with several species of both aerobic and anaerobic organisms present. Treatment must include

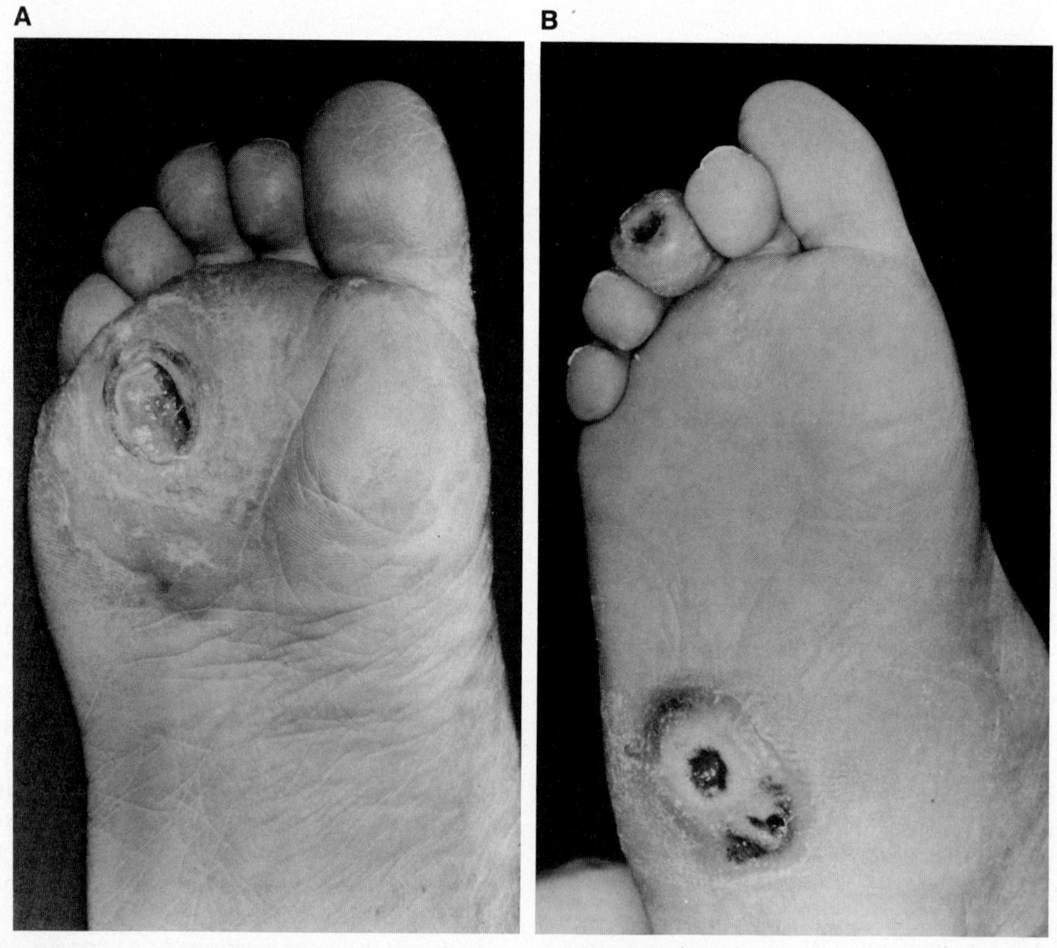

FIG 31–3.
A, an ulcer beneath the metatarsal head is an early manifestation of tibial neuropathy. **B,** the Charcot deformity results in ulceration at the midfoot level. A tip ulcer on the third hammer toe is also seen.

wide surgical drainage and debridement of all devitalized tissue and infected bone. In general, gram-positive organisms will predominate in conditions of hyperglycemia, whereas gram-negative organisms are more common in a hypoglycemic environment.

The weakest link in the bacteriologic defenses of a diabetic patient is the phagocyte. While breaks in the skin are frequent in the presence of diabetic neuropathy, the problem is compounded by the fact that the incompetent polymorphonuclear leukocyte and macrophage permit invading organisms to multiply unchecked. Impairment has been documented in all phases of phagocytic function, including luminal adherence, diapedesis, chemotaxis, and phagocytosis. These functions usually revert to normal with restoration of diabetic control. Less important abnormalities have also been documented in lymphocyte function and the humoral immune mechanisms of antibodies and complement.

Surgical correction of plantar and other distal defects of the lower extremity is an integral part of plastic surgery practice. The process must begin with the establishment of an anabolic, fully debrided wound. Adequate perfusion must be documented by noninvasive vascular studies. If insufficient, revascularization by surgical bypass must be completed before the foot is approached for reconstructive purposes. Toe ulcers are usually treated by amputation. Metatarsal head ulcers are readily closed by the use of V-Y advancement flaps or volar island toe flaps. The midfoot and hindfoot more typically require free flap transfer for adequate surface coverage. Podiatric assistance with pressure-redistributing footwear is essential in postoperative management, although consideration may be given to orthopedic fusions and other direct means of reestablishing the foot arches.

SUGGESTED READING

Anson BJ, Maddock WG: *Callander's Surgical Anatomy,* ed 4. Philadelphia, WB Saunders, 1958.

Arey LB: *Developmental Anatomy,* ed 6. Philadelphia, WB Saunders, 1954.

Cormack GC, Lamberty GH: *The Arterial Anatomy of Skin Flaps.* Edinburgh, Churchill Livingstone, 1986.

Hallock G: *Fasciocutaneous Flaps.* Boston, Little, Brown, 1991.

Mathes SJ, Nahai F: *Clinical Applications for Muscle and Musculocutaneous Flaps.* St Louis, Mosby–Year Book, 1982.

McCraw JB, Arnold PG: *McCraw and Arnold's Atlas of Muscle and Musculocutaneous Flaps.* Norfolk, Va, Hampton Press, 1986.

Chapter 32

Lower Extremity Trauma and Reconstruction

J. Daniel Labs, M.D.
James W. May, Jr., M.D.

CONTENTS

CHAPTER OBJECTIVE

At the end of this chapter the resident understands the principles of management of trauma and related problems of the lower extremity and carries out surgical management, including complex reconstruction of such problems.

LEARNER OBJECTIVES

On completion of this chapter the resident

1. **Understands the indications for and timing of closure of soft-tissue traumatic defects of the lower extremity.**
2. **Has thorough knowledge of coverage techniques (including skin grafts, local skin flaps, distant flaps, musculocutaneous flaps, and free flaps) for soft-tissue and bony closure of the lower extremity.**
3. **Understands the management of infectious processes (including osteomyelitis) related to traumatic injuries in the lower extremity.**
4. **Understands the pathophysiology of and techniques for nonoperative and operative management of traumatic, ischemic, venous stasis, hypertensive, diabetic, and infectious ulcers.**
5. **Knows the etiology and treatment of lymphedema (including nonoperative and operative measures).**
6. Understands the basis for classification of tibial fractures and the treatment modifications appropriate for injuries of varying severity.
7. Is familiar with orthopedic management of long-bone injuries, including internal and external fixation, leg lengthening, and standard techniques for replacement of bony defects.

8. Is familiar with common congenital deformities of the lower extremity (including ring constriction and syndactyly) and their management.
9. Understands the indications and techniques for replantation or revascularization of lower extremity devascularizing or amputative injuries.
10. Understands the principles and basic techniques of management of injuries to the peripheral nerves of the lower extremity.
11. Understands the principles and techniques of aesthetic contouring of the lower extremity (including excisional and liposuction techniques).

■ CLINICAL PRACTICE ACTIVITIES

During the course of the training program, the resident

1. **Undertakes perioperative management and surgical treatment of patients with major acute and chronic injuries of the lower extremities requiring reconstruction and resurfacing.**
2. **Evaluates and treats patients with lower extremity ulceration from a variety of origins.**
3. Undertakes perioperative management and surgical treatment of patients with major devascularizing injuries or conditions of the lower extremity.
4. Evaluates and treats patients with lymphedema of the lower extremity.
5. Performs aesthetic reconstruction and liposuction for body contouring of the lower extremity.

As man has evolved, the lower extremity has assumed the complete function of locomotion for bipedal ambulation. In the erect position, the lower extremity is in constant contact with the environment, and its structural integrity is essential. Likewise, sensory feedback from the lower extremity contributes significantly to limb preservation and the ability to ambulate. The plastic surgeon will most often be consulted about reconstruction of traumatic deformities of the lower extremity but increasingly is also called upon to participate in the treatment of disorders of the arteries, veins, and lymphatic system. Finally, aesthetic contouring of the lower extremity is often requested and can frequently be successfully accomplished.

TRAUMATIC DEFORMITY OF THE LOWER EXTREMITY

Evaluation of Injury

The evaluation and triage of a trauma victim proceeds in a systematic fashion. The airway, ventilation, and circulation are dealt with primarily, while control of hemorrhage is accomplished concomitantly. Next, a secondary evaluation is performed in order to identify all major injuries. As the lower extremity is examined, it is essential to determine the mechanism of injury, the energy of the injury, and the penetrating or blunt nature of the forces. To this end, an organized trauma team can often expedite patient evaluation, triage, and treatment. Lower extremity trauma must always be considered in the context of the overall status of the trauma victim, and decisions made in this context should be documented accurately.

The evaluation of the lower extremity proceeds from the secondary trauma evaluation through, in the case of extensive open trauma, the initial operative debridement. First and foremost, a determination of extremity viability must be made, along with some prediction of the possibility for meaningful salvage. A perspective of the patient's condition as well as the past medical history is essential in determining viability and salvageability. The decision for primary amputation is particularly difficult. The mangled extremity severity score (MESS) represents a classification scheme to consider various rankings of skeletal and soft-tissue damage, shock, ischemia, and age to predict need for amputation (Table 32–1). Ischemia is the most heavily weighted prognostic factor. Using MESS, the authors reviewed 25 patients retrospectively

TABLE 32–1.
Mangled Extremity Severity Score*

Type	Characteristics	Injuries	Points
Skeletal/soft-tissue group			
1	Low energy	Stab wounds, simple closed fractures, small-caliber gunshot wounds	1
2	Medium energy	Open or multiple-level fractures, dislocations, moderate crash injuries	2
3	High energy	Shotgun blast (close range), high-velocity gunshot wounds	3
4	Massive crush	Logging, railroad, oil rig accidents	4
Shock group			
1	Normotensive hemodynamics	BP† stable in field and in OR†	0
2	Transiently hypotensive	BP unstable in field but responsive to intravenous fluids	1
3	Prolonged hypotension	Systolic BP less than 90 mm Hg in field and responsive to intravenous fluid only in OR	2
Ischemia group			
1	None	A pulsatile limb without signs of ischemia	0
2	Mild	Diminished pulses without signs of ischemia	1‡
3	Moderate	No pulse by Doppler, sluggish capillary refill paresthesia, diminished motor activity	2‡
4	Advanced	Pulseless, cool, paralyzed, and numb without capillary refill	3‡
Age group			
1	<30 yr		0
2	>30, <50 yr		1
3	>50 yr		2

* From Helfet, et al: *Clin Orthop* 1990; 256:80. Used by permission.
† BP = blood pressure; OR = operating room.
‡ Points are multiplied by 2 if the ischemic time exceeds 6 hours.

and 26 patients prospectively. All salvaged limbs had scores less than or equal to 6, while all amputated limbs had scores 7 or higher. The score can be readily calculated in the emergency setting and is a useful statistical supplement to clinical judgment. The score, however, is only helpful in predicting the necessity of amputation and is not designed to determine functional outcome. Extremity viability and salvageability are separate questions, often answered at different stages of the postinjury course. If the extremity is viable and the patient's status allows, deferring the final decision on limb salvageability until completion of the first debridement when the intraoperative findings can be discussed with the patient is preferable.

Blood Vessels

The definitive examination of an injured lower extremity proceeds anatomically. An attempt is made to define the zone of injury. This is essential for identification of injury with respect to blood vessels, soft tissue, and nerves, as well as the bones and joints involved. Because significant vascular damage always adversely affects outcome, vessel injury must be diagnosed and treated efficiently. Initially, a severely injured extremity should be anatomically aligned to allow maximal distal circulation. Clinical examination includes color, temperature, capillary refill, and pulse examination as well as Doppler pulse and pressure checks. If the contralateral lower extremity is uninjured, it represents the best control for comparison. The status of the vasculature can change acutely with fracture manipulation or gradually with the onset of a compartment syndrome. Therefore, repeat examinations are a necessity. Additionally, the terminal segment of the extremity may appear viable, while an intercalary segment within the zone of injury may be relatively ischemic. This may be difficult to determine acutely but ultimately manifests itself as a nonhealing wound.

While standard x-ray studies diagnose fractures and dislocations, arteriography remains the gold standard for anatomic definition of arterial injury. The risks and benefits of a formal biplane radiologic study must be weighed against the limited but expeditious information obtained with a single-shot arteriogram in the operating room. Indications for arteriography are liberal (Table 32–2). Basically, the clinician obtains angiography for two reasons. First, arteriography is used to rule out vascular damage in the absence of ischemia when associated injuries are likely to produce intimal or subclinical injury. Distal femur fractures, proximal tibia fractures, and knee dislocation may disrupt the popliteal artery and should be considered indications for arteriography. Indeed, any fracture of the lower extremity that is severely displaced has the potential for arterial damage, and arteriography following reduction of the fracture is prudent. If fracture reduction results in or fails to relieve ischemia, arterial exploration is indicated, and arteriography may be bypassed or obtained following arterial reconstruction.

The second reason to obtain an angiogram is to confirm and localize arterial injury that is clinically suspected. Extremities that demonstrate terminal ischemia, i.e., a cold foot, require revascularization, and if the site of arterial disruption is not completely obvious from examination of the zone of injury, arteriography will provide anatomic information that is most useful. Intercalary segment ischemia is much more difficult to diagnose acutely but occurs in violent trauma that disrupts one or two of the tibial vessels so that the leg in the zone of injury is ischemic while the foot remains well perfused. Asymmetry in the vascular evaluation of an injured extremity as compared with the uninjured contralateral extremity, even in the absence of obvious ischemia, is an indication for arteriography, especially if the findings persist after fracture reduction and stabilization. Intimal injuries are likely to be missed with a single-shot intraoperative study, and therefore continued vascular surveillance is indicated because the possibility of delayed thrombosis is quite real. Venous injuries are not usually imaged but are seldom difficult to diagnose because of their profuse bleeding, swelling, and discoloration.

TABLE 32–2.
Indications for Angiography

Rule out arterial injury in the absence of ischemia
Distal femur fracture
Proximal tibia fracture
Knee dislocation
Any fracture with severe displacement
Confirm and localize arterial injury suspected from the clinical examination
Terminal ischemia
Intercalary ischemia
Asymmetry with an uninjured extremity
Color
Capillary refill
Temperature
Pulses
Doppler pressures

Soft Tissues

Following confirmation of vascular integrity, the particular order of structural evaluation is less important. Soft-tissue injuries of the lower extremity (including skin, subcutaneous fat, fascia, muscle, nerve, and tendons) are determined in large part by the mechanism of injury. Sharp trauma produces a limited zone of injury, while crush and avulsion mechanisms affect a much wider zone. The degree of contamination is also noted. Of importance, all four compartments in the leg must be evaluated for compartment syndrome since even large open injuries may contain nondecompressed fascial compartments. Even penetrating trauma that lacerates the deep fascia may create a hematoma within a compartment and lead to a compartment syndrome because of inadequate decompression through the entrance wound.

Nerves

Neurapraxia, axonotmesis, and neurotmesis may all produce similar clinical findings but may have differing treatments and prognoses. Therapeutic decisions are simplified by the knowledge of complete transection/avulsion of the posterior tibial nerve,

TABLE 32–3.
Classification of Open Tibial Fractures*

Type	Injury
I	Open fracture with cutaneous defect < 1 cm
II	Open fracture with extensive soft-tissue injury
IIIA	Open fracture with extensive soft-tissue lacerations; high-energy injury
IIIB	Open fracture with soft-tissue loss and periosteal stripping, usually with heavy contamination
IIIC	Open fracture with arterial injury requiring repair

* From Gustilo, et al: *J Bone Joint Surg [AM]* 1976; 58:453. Used by permission.

which in massive blunt lower extremity trauma usually precludes meaningful reconstruction. Often, however, the clinician is faced with traumatic peripheral neurapraxia or central alterations in the sensorium that preclude definitive early confirmation of the neurologic status. Every effort must be made to document the neurologic status as accurately as possible, and repeat examinations are essential.

On physical examination, certain autonomous sensory zones are important to investigate. First and foremost, the medial and lateral plantar nerves are both branches of the posterior tibial nerve and accompany their corresponding vessels in the foot. They provide sensation to the medial and lateral aspects of the plantar surface. The first web space is autonomously innervated by the terminal branch of the deep peroneal nerve, while the remaining sensory nerves have wide areas of overlap: the superficial peroneal nerve (dorsolateral aspect of the foot), the saphenous nerve (medial malleolus), the medial calcaneal nerve (heel), and the sural nerve (lateral malleolus).

Bones and Joints

Structural integrity is initially investigated by palpation. During the secondary examination, joints without obvious injury are put through a range of motion, and necessary radiographs are obtained. Definitive examination is performed in the operating room where the degree of comminution, periosteal stripping, contamination, and zone of injury are determined. The Gustilo classification of open tibial fractures (Table 32–3) has been important in predicting posttraumatic morbidity. It is the standard classification scheme and has implications for reconstructive treatment. Type I fractures have minimal soft-tissue injury with an open wound less than 1 cm long and minimal contamination, while type II fractures have a larger soft-tissue defect but no crush/avulsion component to the soft-tissue injury. Types I and II open fractures would most likely result from low-energy trauma.

In contradistinction, type III fractures are high-energy injuries. They are subdivided into type IIIA, where although extensive soft-tissue injury exists, it is predicted that coverage will be adequate without extensive reconstruction. Type IIIB fractures have extensive soft-tissue injury as well as significant periosteal stripping and heavy contamination. It is this class of fractures that the plastic surgeon is most often consulted for flap coverage. Type IIIC fractures are associated with ischemia and arterial injury requiring repair. Both the infection rate and the necessity for amputation increase up the scale from type I fractures to the type IIIC fracture, where amputation has been necessary in up to 87% of cases. A subgroup of patients increasingly recognized but still ill-defined includes patients who have sustained vascular trauma that does not initially appear to require reconstruction but in whom nonhealing bone and soft-tissue problems may appear in the postinjury period.

Principles of Treatment

The trauma team coordinates patient treatment priorities, but all teams should agree on prophylactic antibiotic coverage, individual operative consent, and tetanus toxoid or immune globulin administration. Three objectives are achieved by early operative intervention: (1) definitive evaluation of the zone of injury, (2) irrigation and debridement, and

(3) bony stabilization. Following these objectives, the blood supply to the lower extremity is reconfirmed. Open bony injuries are prone to infection if a delay in irrigation and debridement beyond 6 to 8 hours occurs. Large-volume (10 L or more) saline irrigation with jet pulse lavage is generally used. Injuries that were reduced and splinted in the field are recreated so that contaminated bone ends can be debrided and irrigated.

Blood Vessels

Vascular injuries elevate the priority of extremity treatment since muscle necrosis will begin within 6 hours of the warm ischemic time. Arterial failure may be caused by arterial laceration or transection, intramural hematoma, intimal injury with immediate or delayed thrombosis, or compression from fracture fragments or elevated compartment pressure (Fig 32–1). Penetrating injuries cause localized trauma, while avulsion-type injuries can damage the arterial wall over a wide zone. Intimal damage may contain "skip" areas and often extends to the next major arterial bifurcation. Major venous injuries commonly accompany arterial trauma but may occur in isolation. Venae comitantes can usually be ligated without morbidity, but major venous conduits such as the popliteal vein and femoral vein should be repaired if possible. It is also essential that the superficial venous sys-

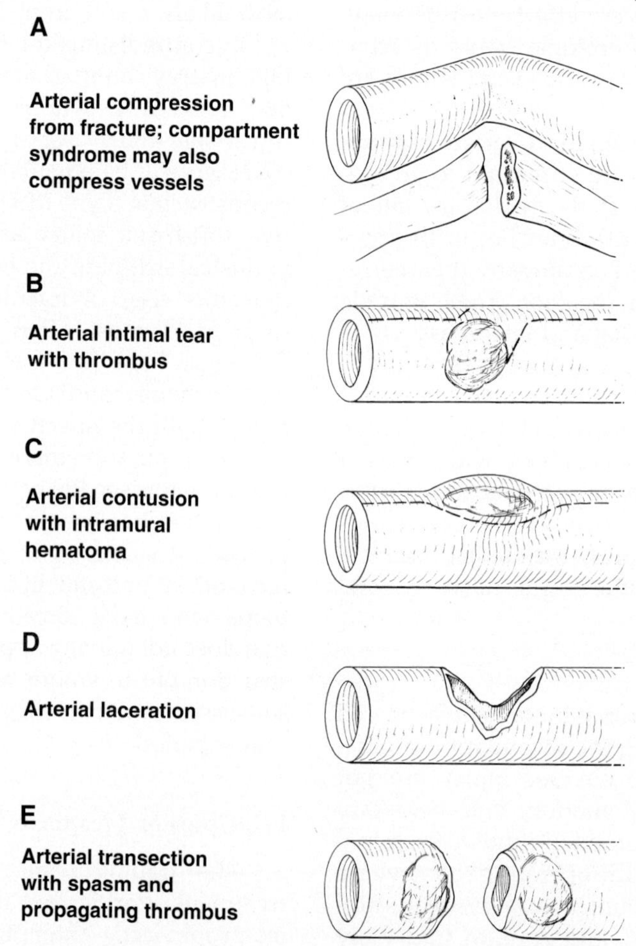

FIG 32–1.
Mechanisms of traumatic arterial failure. **A,** arterial compression from fracture; compartment syndrome may also compress vessels. **B,** arterial intimal tear with thrombus. **C,** arterial contusion with intramural hematoma. **D,** arterial laceration. **E,** arterial transection with spasm and a propagating thrombus.

tem be protected during surgical exploration because this may be the primary venous outflow when the deep system has been traumatized.

While vascular injuries in the iliofemoral system more often occur with penetrating trauma, the popliteal segment is frequently disrupted by bony injuries, especially knee dislocation. Traumatic occlusion of the iliofemoral-popliteal arterial circuit will inevitably lead to distal ischemia, and occlusion of the accompanying iliofemoral and popliteal veins increases the amputation rates dramatically. Significant late morbidity from chronic venous insufficiency may also occur.

Treatment of trifurcation injuries remains controversial. Extensive open lower extremity trauma will be accompanied by some vascular injury in up to 71% of cases. In addition, a "single-vessel" leg after trauma heals more poorly than an extremity where the anterior tibial and posterior tibial vessels have been reconstructed.

Soft Tissues

During intraoperative evaluation, soft tissues are debrided until only viable tissues remain. Dermal margins are freshened, and a combination of clinical factors including color, contractility, and bleeding are used to differentiate viable vs. nonviable muscle. A four-compartment fasciotomy is performed, if indicated, through limited medial and lateral exposures, but the fibula should rarely be sacrificed because it may be utilized later in bony reconstruction. Tendons that are sharply lacerated can be reapproximated provided that soft-tissue coverage is adequate. Operative reexamination is planned 48 to 72 hours after the initial exploration.

Nerves

All nonfunctioning nerves within the zone of injury should be explored. The fact that most major nerves in the lower extremity are mixed motor and sensory nerves, and the mechanism of injury is often avulsion, are both reasons for poor functional results from repair in this area. In addition long nerve regeneration distances lead to dubious results. Indeed, most classification systems suggest early amputation with an open tibial fracture and complete transection of the posterior tibial nerve. However, clinical circumstances such as the age of the patient, clean vs. an avulsion nerve injury, etc., should be considered. Clean nerve transections that can be covered with soft tissue should be repaired acutely, while major cutaneous sensory nerves should be either coapted or buried deeply within the soft tissue to avoid painful neuromas.

Bones and Joints

In treating bones and joints, injuries are recreated in the operating room to allow complete and thorough irrigation of all contaminants. Bone fragments that have been devascularized by fracture disruption of the endosteal blood supply as well as periosteal stripping should be debrided. Aggressive bony debridement increases the possibility that bone grafting or skeletal reconstruction will be required; however, the risk of posttraumatic osteomyelitis is decreased.

Fractures are reduced and stabilized and adjacent nerves and vessels protected. Acetabular and proximal femur fractures require open reduction and internal fixation, while mid and distal femur fractures can be treated with traction, plates, or intramedullary rod fixation. Traction is the simplest form of treatment but relegates the patient to bed rest with increased risks of thromboembolic disorders as well as pulmonary complications. Open reduction–internal fixation with plates is a time-honored method but requires extensive operative exposure. Although intramedullary rod fixation will sacrifice endosteal blood supply, in the femur the procedure requires limited exposure and provides excellent rigid fixation. The technique cannot be used for severely comminuted fractures.

External fixation is the safest method for initial stabilization of an open tibia fracture. Most often, the foot is included to maintain the ankle at 90 degrees to prevent concomitant shortening of the gastrocnemius-soleus mechanism. The external fixator also helps in the management of soft-tissue injuries since the extremity can be elevated and supported by this device. Once complete soft-tissue healing has been achieved, the leg can be casted, although intramedullary rod fixation or open reduction and internal fixation with plates and screws may be utilized. As with the soft tissues, serial debridement is the key to achieve complete resection of all nonviable bone prior to definitive soft-tissue closure.

Replantation

Replantation in the lower extremity remains limited. Traditionally, the necessity for significant shortening precluded a good functional result. Now, however, free fibular grafting and the Ilizarov technique allow skeletal expansion to solve this problem. However, crush/avulsion mechanisms still predominate, and nerve regeneration is always incomplete. Prosthetic devices, especially with below-knee amputations, provide excellent ambulation with a lower risk of blood transfusions, sepsis, and prolonged hospitalization. Replantation should be considered in traumatic amputations in children, in bilateral amputations, and when a sharp mechanism has resulted in a narrow zone of injury. Since virtually all lower extremity replants will contain significant muscle mass, arterial shunting to minimize the ischemic time should be strongly considered.

A more frequent occurrence with traumatic lower extremity amputation involves the microvascular salvage of "spare parts." Fillet flaps of large areas of undamaged soft tissue from the amputated part can be harvested under hypothermic conditions while the amputation stump is readied for free tissue reattachment. Preservation of an exposed tibial stump to fit a below-knee prosthesis is a common scenario of the strategy.

Reconstructive Surgery of the Lower Extremity

The success of lower extremity reconstruction is not a closed wound but rather a functional lower extremity with ambulation that must be compared with that possible from an amputation stump with a well-fitted prosthesis. In a recent review, a 93% limb salvage rate was accomplished, but 66% of the patients had a significant decrease in range of motion at the ankle, and 44% had edema requiring elastic support. While 50% of the patients did not require assist devices to ambulate, only 28% of the patients undergoing lengthy and complex lower extremity reconstructions returned to work. Sixty-eight percent of amputees during the same time interval did return to work. The lower extremity reconstructive surgeon should have an in-depth awareness of the pros and cons of various amputation levels associated with functional prosthesis use. This helps to determine when to reconstruct as well as how to make a functional stump.

Blood Vessels

Although most vascular reconstructions are performed for acute distal extremity ischemia, there appears to be a significant advantage in repairing both tibial vessels to a functional status in the first 48 hours following injury. Recently this treatment strategy has been compared with delayed vascular reconstruction performed for nonhealing chronic wounds resulting from trauma; the results clearly favored early vascular reconstruction. Arterial repair can be performed by removing damaged arterial intima, by patch angioplasty, or by bypass surgery using the contralateral saphenous vein. While autogenous material is advocated uniformly below the knee, short segments above the knee have successfully been replaced with polytetrafluoroethylene (PTFE) grafts without increased morbidity. In the trauma victim, regional heparinization is preferred over systemic anticoagulation, but thrombolytic therapy is absolutely contraindicated with significant head, chest, and abdominal injuries. Temporary shunts are advocated as a temporizing maneuver and are indicated if the 6-hour ischemic limit is being exceeded prior to revascularization. Increased blood loss can be expected from this maneuver since complete control of the vasculature within the wound is generally not obtained prior to shunt insertion.

Soft Tissues

The plastic surgeon is most often called upon for soft-tissue reconstruction of a traumatized lower extremity. It is axiomatic that a myocutaneous or fasciocutaneous envelope is very beneficial for bone healing. For this

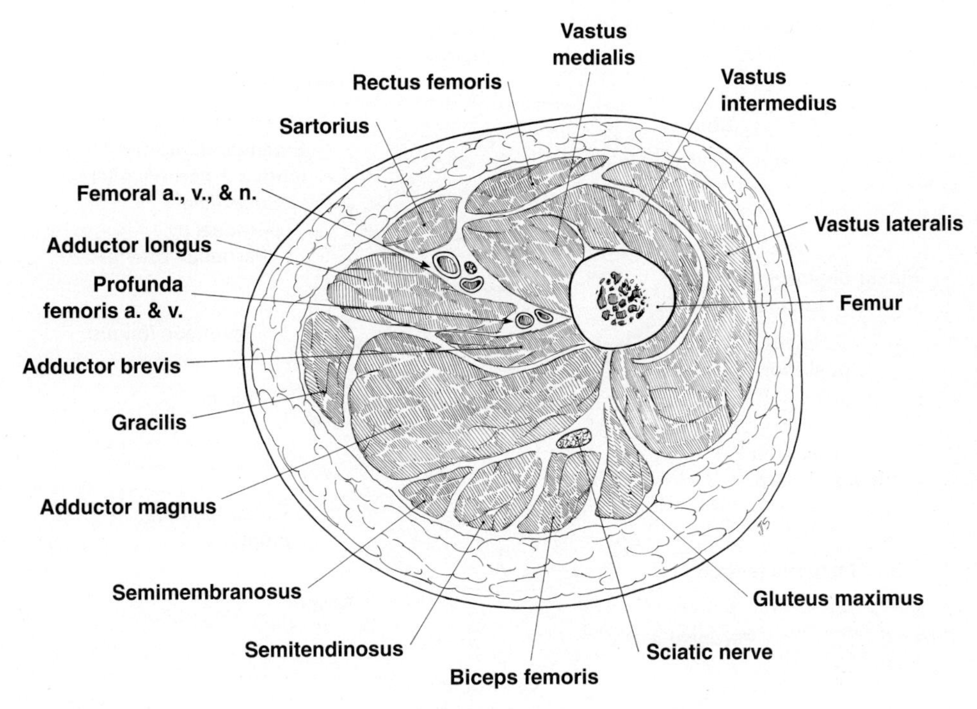

FIG 32–2.
Cross section of the thigh. Note circumferential muscle covering of the femur.

reason, soft-tissue transfer is seldom required in the thigh where a circumferential muscle layer exists around the femur (Fig 32–2). The knee, the anteromedial aspect of the tibia, and the tibia and fibula at the ankle are all subcutaneous structures (Fig 32–3). With extensive fractures, overlying skin and subcutaneous tissue are often lost in these regions, and replacement with muscle flaps has provided an effective strategy for bone healing. Although split-thickness skin grafts will survive on periosteum, they seldom provide stable coverage. Open joints and exposed tendons that have lost their peritenon also require flap coverage. In the leg, musculocutaneous and septocutaneous perforating vessels allow the design of fasciocutaneous transposition flaps to cover smaller defects (Fig 32–4). However, these flaps are difficult to contour to large bony defects and are frequently within the zone of injury, which makes their blood supply precarious. Muscle flaps remain the mainstay for coverage of exposed fracture sites in the leg because they can provide a large bulk of highly vascular soft tissue that is easily contoured. Additionally, it has been shown that the antibacterial properties of muscle flaps exceed that of other coverage modalities—a quality attributable to high blood flow.

Extensive data exist on the timing of coverage in lower extremity trauma. Immediate coverage including free tissue transfer is indicated in the case of an unprotected vascular reconstruction. For the remaining open wounds, it seems most prudent to debride the wound at 48-hour intervals until the zone of injury has been confidently defined. The surgeon must, at all times, maintain bacterial control of the wound. Then, an elective muscle transfer is scheduled at the earliest convenience. By using this strategy, a closed wound is routinely achieved within 14 days of injury. Delays beyond this can occur from a multitude of local and systemic factors and may be accompanied by decreased success of the reconstruction.

Orthopedic hardware exposure following attempted primary wound closure is a moderately urgent situation requiring soft-tissue reconstruction if the hardware cannot be removed. Provided that infection is not present or the cause of wound breakdown, early flap coverage can result in salvage of the

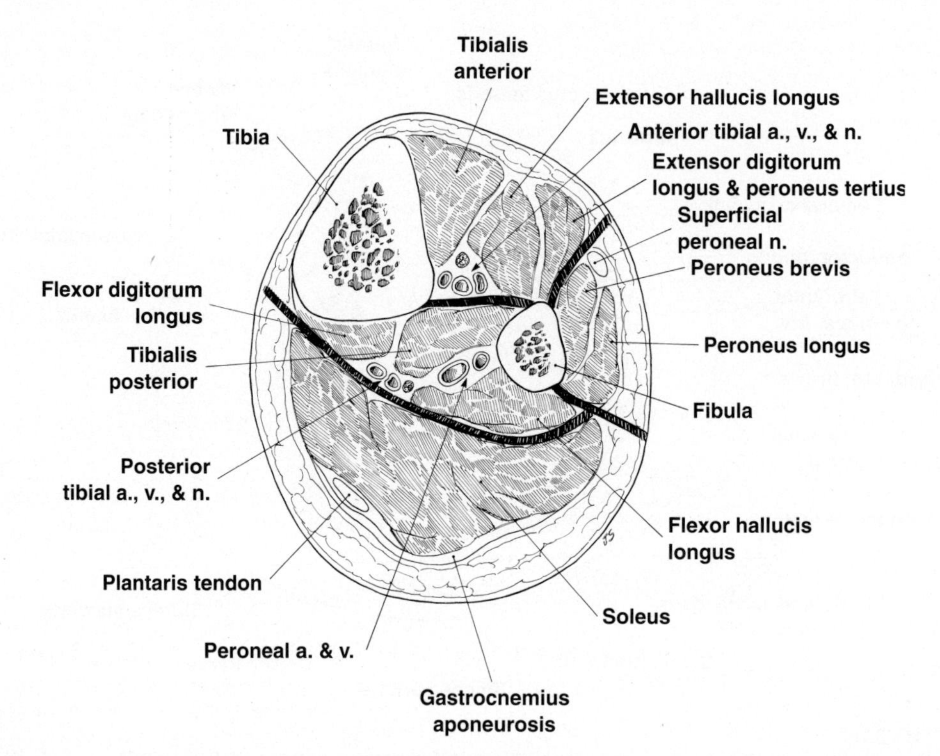

FIG 32–3.
Cross section of the leg. Note the subcutaneous position of the tibia and four muscle compartments: anterior, lateral, superficial posterior, and deep posterior *(heavy lines).*

orthopedic reconstruction. Ideally, however, hardware is removed and fixation established externally.

The necessity for angiography prior to free tissue transfer remains controversial. In the future, duplex scanning may prove to be adequately sensitive and specific. Indications for preoperative angiography may include 1, a suspicion of vascular injury from physical and Doppler examination; 2, a patient greater than 50 years old or in whom significant athero-sclerotic changes are likely; 3, and a patient who requires vascular reconstruction in the acute postinjury period. Many groups obtain angiography routinely under the rationaliza-tion that the low morbidity of this procedure

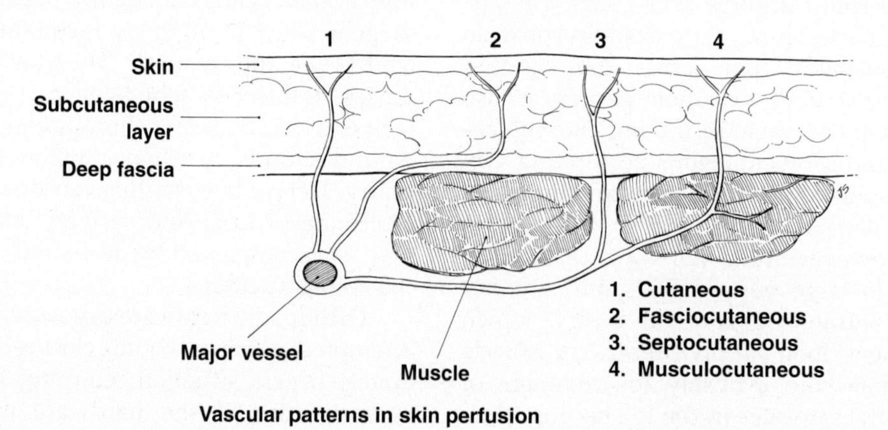

FIG 32–4.
Vascular patterns in skin perfusion: *(1)* cutaneous, *(2)* fasciocutaneous, *(3)* septocutaneous, *(4)* musculo-cutaneous.

is outweighed by the accurate diagnosis of unsuspected injuries and anomalies.

The level of injury dictates regional strategies in soft-tissue reconstruction. As always, the reconstructive ladder is respected, beginning with primary and secondary wound closures, skin grafting, local and regional solutions, and finally distant free tissue transfer. As with other areas of the body, manipulation of local anatomy can often result in effective reconstructive procedures for various segments of the injured lower extremity. The distal third of the leg, however, frequently requires distant tissue (Tables 32–4 and 32–5).

In the proximal third of the thigh, the circumferential muscle layer surrounding the femur often allows large skin defects to be closed with skin grafts. The groin, however, can present several difficult reconstructive scenarios when major lymphatics have been disrupted by trauma or radiation and when vascular reconstructions involving the femoral arterial circulation have become exposed. Muscle flaps transferred either as muscle flaps that are skin-grafted or as myocutaneous flaps can provide an excellent solution. The rectus abdominis muscle can be easily rotated into the groin and proximal portion of the thigh by using its inferior epigastric blood supply. Maximum rotation is achieved by skeletonizing the pedicle and then dividing the inguinal ligament, which allows transfer almost to the knee. Extensive vascular skeletonization of the iliofemoral system may result in division of the deep inferior epigastric artery (DIEA), and the reconstructive surgeon often begins the procedure with exploration of this vessel before the muscle is harvested. Laterally, the tensor fasciae latae muscle with its fascial extension is excellent for reconstruction of the lower abdominal wall and proximal part of the thigh, either anteriorly or posteriorly. Although the muscle bulk is quite small, the fascial extension, which can be harvested to just above the knee, is an autogenous fascial substitute for the lower abdominal wall when synthetic materials are contraindicated. Morbidity from this flap involves lateral knee destabilization and should be candidly discussed preoperatively.

The rectus femoris muscle is a bulky member of the quadriceps group and can be rotated on its pedicle, which is located approximately 10 cm below the inguinal ligament. It will effectively cover the groin and can be advanced under the inguinal ligament almost to the aortic bifurcation for covering exposed vascular prostheses. The quadriceps mechanism will be weakened, but morbidity is minimized by approximating the vastus medialis and vastus lateralis insertions to reconstruct the quadriceps tendon centrally in the distal anterior portion of the thigh. The gracilis muscle, the most superficial member of the adductor group, enjoys almost no functional donor site morbidity. Although the muscle is usually too small for significant thigh defects, it is popular as a free tissue transfer when a small amount of muscle is required. The vastus lateralis and vastus medialis can both be rotated in the anterior of the thigh, and a distally based vastus lateralis flap for knee reconstruction has been described. Both flaps require extensive dissection in the quadriceps mechanism and have limited arcs of rotation.

In contrast to the proximal aspect of the thigh, the knee and proximal third of the leg contain superficial bony structures in a tight fasciocutaneous envelope. Flap coverage is often required for traumatic soft-tissue defects as well as orthopedic wound breakdowns. These wounds often contain hardware as well as exposed bone. The gastrocnemius muscle, as an example of type I muscle circulation, is most effectively utilized in this area. Either head of the gastrocnemius muscle can be harvested independently on a single proximal vascular pedicle and reach from the top of the patella to the junction of the upper and middle thirds of the tibia. The medial head is larger than the lateral head, but flap choice is based on the position of the defect. The muscle rotation can be maximized by dividing both the origin and insertion of the muscle, and the length of the flap is maximized by scoring the deep fascia on the muscle. The circulation also allows for longitudinally splitting the distal aspect of the muscle to accommodate complex wound contours. The morbidity of the transfer of a single head of the gastrocnemius muscle is minimal, and skin-grafting the muscle surface provides excellent surface contour. On

TABLE 32–4.
Reconstructive Muscle and Myocutaneous Flaps of the Lower Extremity

Flap	Origin	Insertion	Muscle Type	Blood Supply	Motor Nerve	Skin Paddle	Morbidity
Proximal third of the thigh							
Rectus abdominis	Anterior chest wall	Pubis	3	Sup. & Inf. epigastric	Segmental	+ + +	Hernia
Tensor fasciae latae	Ant. Sup. iliac spine, greater trochanter	Lateral knee	1	Lateral femoral circumflex Br.	Inferior gluteal	+	Lateral knee destabilization
Rectus femoris	Ant. inf. iliac spine, acetabulum	Patellar tendon	1	Lateral femoral circumflex Br.	Femoral	+ +	Weakened knee extension
Gracilis	Pubis	Pes anserinus	2	Br. of profunda femoris, minor pedicles	Obturator	+/−	Minimal
Knee/proximal third of the leg							
Gastrocnemius medial head	Femoral condyle	Achilles tendon	1	Sural	Popliteal	+ +	Minimal
Gastrocnemius lateral head	Femoral condyle	Achilles tendon	1	Sural	Popliteal	+	Minimal
Middle third of the leg							
Soleus	Proximal tibia & fibula	Achilles tendon	2	Popliteal Br. (proximal) Segmental (distal)	Tibial	−	Minimal for hemisoleus
Distal third of the leg*							
Latissimus dorsi	Thoracolumbar fascia, iliac crest	Intertubercular groove of the humerus	5	Thoracodorsal, paraspinous perforators	Thoracodorsal	+ + +	Weakening of upper extremity "push off"
Serratus anterior	Ribs 7–10	Apex of the scapula	3	Thoracodorsal br., lateral thoracic	Long thoracic	+	Minimal if upper 4–5 slips preserved
Foot							
Abductor hallucis	Medial calcaneous	Great toe, proximal phalynx	2	Medial plantar	Medial plantar	−	Minimal
Flexor digitorum brevis	Medial calcaneous	Middle phalanges	2	Medial & lateral plantar	Medial plantar	+ + +	Minimal

* Free tissue transfer: The rectus abdominis and gracilis muscles are also reliably transferred free flaps.

TABLE 32–5.
Fasciocutaneous Free Flaps

Flap	Artery	Vein	Cutaneous Nerve
Radial forearm	Radial	Cephalic; venae comitantes	Lateral antebrachial cutaneous
Ulnar forearm	Ulnar	Cephalic; venae comitantes	Medial antebrachial cutaneous
Lateral thigh	3rd perforator of profunda femoris	Venae comitantes	Lateral femoral cutaneous
Lateral arm	Posterior radial collateral	Venae comitantes	Posterior cutaneous nerve of the arm
Scapular	Circumflex scapular	Venae comitantes	None
Temporoparietal fascia	Superficial temporal	Venae comitantes	Auriculotemporal
Dorsalis pedis	Dorsalis pedis	Saphenous; venae comitantes	Superficial peroneal

the other hand, the musculocutaneous gastrocnemius flap can be harvested to within 6 to 8 cm of the malleolus but creates significant aesthetic deformity of the leg, which has led many surgeons to prefer a free tissue transfer under these circumstances.

In the middle third of the leg, the soleus muscle is most often used. The distal aspect of the muscle relies on circulation that is segmental, and therefore great care must be taken in elevating the muscle from its bed. Although the hemisoleus flap has a reasonable arc of rotation, it provides little bulk. The muscle is also intimately related to the tibia, and high-energy injuries to the leg can result in significant muscle tearing and bruising. In such injuries, a free tissue transfer supplying a much larger volume of tissue from outside the zone of injury may be indicated.

The distal third of the leg and the ankle represent injury sites frequently requiring free tissue transfer. Early coverage is required with extensive soft-tissue loss; unstable cutaneous coverage and osteomyelitis may require free muscle transfer in the late postinjury period. External fixation can be helpful during soft-tissue reconstruction of the distal third of the leg and should be placed so that the frame is not obstructing the approach for microvascular free tissue transfer. Bone and soft-tissue debridement must be meticulous prior to free tissue transfer so that healing can occur per primum. Dead space is most difficult to handle when segmental bone loss has occurred. Local fasciocutaneous flaps handle this problem poorly because of their inability to be contoured and are relatively contraindicated with significant bone deformity. Free muscle transfer can fill the bony gap and effectively collapses the dead space. At the time of flap reelevation for bone grafting, however, a bloody and difficult dissection can be expected. An alternative involves antibiotic-impregnated methyl methacrylate beads utilized as a bone spacer placed under the free muscle transfer. The beads are removed at the time of bone grafting to not only preserve space for the graft but also make the dissection easier.

The harvest site for free muscle transfer to the distal third of the leg requires consideration of the size of the defect. The gracilis muscle provides a limited amount of tissue, while the lower four slips of the serratus anterior provide a broad, thin layer of muscle for coverage. The rectus abdominis muscle is the next largest muscle commonly utilized and has the advantage of excellent pedicle length and the ability to harvest the flap in the supine position. The latissimus dorsi alone or in conjunction with the serratus anterior muscle will provide the maximum amount of muscle coverage for a severely traumatized lower extremity. This flap can also be utilized in conjunction with the medial or lateral head of the gastrocnemius muscle to cover the entire leg from the knee to the ankle. Contour is best when a muscle transfer is skin-grafted because myocutaneous flaps create significant bulk and aesthetic deformity.

Several generalizations can be made about microvascular transfers in the lower extremity.

The microvascular anastomoses must be performed outside the zone of injury. Usually a proximal site where vessel diameter is maximal is chosen. End-to-side anastomoses tend to eliminate problems with size mismatch and preserve the distal circulation. Strict lower extremity elevation is required postoperatively to prevent significant venous congestion of the flap as well as problems with skin graft survival.

A traumatized foot provides a significant reconstructive challenge. Dorsally, coverage of extensor tendons can utilize techniques previously listed in the reconstructive ladder. On the plantar surface, however, tissue replacement is difficult because of the specialized nature of the plantar skin with its dense ligamentous attachments to bone. Additionally, any change in the skeletal architecture of the foot will alter the weight-bearing characteristics and create new areas of potential pressure damage. Sensation, to deep pressure, is considered essential for weight bearing, ambulation, and long-term durability.

Two small local foot muscles have been utilized for minimal defects. The abductor hallucis and flexor digitorum brevis can both be rotated into small, punched-out plantar defects. Additionally, fasciocutaneous flaps based on the medial plantar artery can transfer specialized plantar skin from non–weight-bearing areas in the arch of the foot to weight-bearing areas of the heel. The donor site is then skin-grafted. Again, this strategy is only effective for small defects.

Massive degloving injuries of the foot require serious consideration for amputation. Patients who select reconstruction must understand that it is an alternative to amputation and in no way will recreate a normal foot. Free tissue muscle transfer to the plantar surface with skin graft coverage can provide reasonable reconstruction, with most patients regaining ambulation. If the medial and lateral plantar nerves are intact, deep sensation is preserved in these patients, which accounts, in part, for the success of the procedure. Athletic and custom-made shoes have been useful in rehabilitation; the air inflatable athletic shoes that are widely available today can provide excellent foot protection at a reasonable cost.

Muscle flaps have several advantages for lower extremity reconstruction; limited, distal defects without infection, however, can often be closed with fasciocutaneous free flaps (see Table 32–5). Advantages of the fasciocutaneous flap include replacement with like tissue of defects over the foot dorsum, malleolus, and Achilles tendon. With small defects, the donor site for many fasciocutaneous flaps can be closed primarily. Alternatively, a meshed split-thickness skin graft will allow natural contraction of the donor site; the graft can be excised later. The vessels of many flaps are quite large, so microsurgery changes to macrovascular surgery. The temporoparietal fascia flap deserves special mention. It can be harvested with almost no donor site morbidity and provides a significant amount of ultrathin, highly vascularized soft tissue that has proved ideal for tendon glide as in the foot dorsum. When the flap is covered with a skin graft, contour has been excellent. Many fasciocutaneous flaps also contain sensory cutaneous nerves. The loose subcutaneous tissue of these flaps in the plantar position is, however, poor at resisting the shear forces in the foot. It is probably still preferable to use a muscle flap and skin graft in this location and rely on deep plantar sensation for protection from pressure necrosis.

In summary, the goals of soft-tissue reconstruction in the lower extremity include complete restoration of a musculocutaneous or fasciocutaneous envelope to achieve healing by primary intention following debridement. Reliable coverage for bone healing and bone reconstruction is essential. Significant disruption of veins and lymphatics secondary to trauma requires diligent postoperative care to prevent venous stasis breakdown as well as lymphedema. This may be accomplished by elastic bandage wraps in the initial ambulatory period and, in many cases, venous compression stockings on a chronic basis.

Nerves

Nerve reconstruction in a traumatized lower extremity may begin as early as the initial debridement. Dysfunctional nerves within the zone of injury are explored to confirm continuity. In the case of sharp trauma, transected nerves can be freshened and coapted acutely, provided that adequate soft-tissue coverage is available. Traction-type injuries outside the zone of immediate injury are generally observed for 3 months and then explored if recovery fails. Avulsion injuries and nerve gaps requiring nerve grafting, especially if greater than 8 cm, carry an unfavorable prognosis. In this type of injury, simultaneous tendon transfers should be considered. For example, a large gap in the common peroneal nerve might be treated with a nerve graft as well as transfer of the tibialis posterior tendon anteriorly and attaching it to the tibialis anterior tendon or (alternatively) to the middle cuneiform bone. Additionally, lower extremity orthoses and joint fusions may be utilized in the distal end of the lower extremity to compensate for nerve injuries with limited expectation of recovery. Transection of major cutaneous nerves should be repaired or the proximal end buried within the soft tissues to prevent painful neuromas. As with all peripheral nerve injuries, the prognosis is related to the mechanism of injury, the distance of regeneration necessary for motor end-plate reinnervation, the need for interposition nerve grafting, and the age of the patient.

Bones and Joints

Improvements in skeletal reconstruction have allowed aggressive bony debridement in high-energy comminuted fractures with a reduction in osteomyelitis. In general, nonvascularized bone grafting is successful in skeletal restoration when bone gaps are less than 6 to 8 cm. Although cortical bone provides some initial structural integrity, it is slow to heal by creeping substitution. Cancellous bone is the preferred graft material because of its fast revascularization through wide open bony channels. It is also an excellent source of osteoprogenitor cells for bone regeneration. The usual source of cancellous bone for grafting is the posterior iliac crest, which can supply a considerable amount of biological material with minimal morbidity. As with other free grafts, a well-vascularized, noninfected, nonscarred recipient bed gives the best result. Tibial gaps less than 8 cm from open fractures can be aggressively debrided and covered with a free muscle transfer and the bone gap maintained with antibiotic-impregnated methyl methacrylate. Six weeks after free tissue transfer, the flap can be elevated, the spacer removed, and the cavity irrigated and packed with cancellous bone graft. Stabilization of the bony skeleton is usually maintained with an external fixator. When complete soft-tissue healing is achieved following grafting, the patient can be placed in a cast. Alternatively, if pin site infections are a concern, a windowed cast can be substituted earlier. Serial x-ray examinations track bone healing prior to weight bearing. Nonunion requires regrafting and, if complicated by infection, may require an interim period before nonvascularized bone grafting can be reattempted. Alternatively, vascularized bone grafts or the Ilizarov technique may be substituted.

When bone gaps exceed 8 cm, or with scarred or irradiated recipient beds, vascularized bone grafts may be necessary for skeletal reconstruction. The fibula provides up to 24 cm of straight bone with excellent structural integrity. The graft is supplied by the peroneal arterial nutrient blood supply, which enters the bone in the middle third. Additionally, multiple segmental branches of the peroneal artery provide a significant periosteal blood supply. The fibula can be used ipsilaterally as a pedicle graft or as a free tissue transfer from the contralateral lower extremity. A skin paddle supplied by septocutaneous perforators penetrating the posterior leaflet of the lateral intermuscular septum can be reliably carried with the fibula and is an excellent sentinel for free tissue monitoring. The second choice for vascularized transfer is the iliac crest graft based on the deep circumflex iliac artery, a branch of the external iliac artery. A maximum of 10 cm of minimally curved bone can be harvested, with a skin paddle taken for microvascular monitoring. Vascularized bone grafts have the capacity for faster primary bone healing with immediate structural integrity. They do not rely on the slow creeping substitution of nonvascularized cortical bone grafts.

Gavriil Ilizarov, a Russian orthopedist, has

studied the tension-stress effect in long bones and has emphasized that axial traction in the extremity has a metabolic activating effect on bone and, when applied to a bony gap, results in distraction osteogenesis. Soft tissues including free tissue transfers appear to tolerate this procedure well, and the Ilizarov technique is rapidly becoming an effective therapeutic strategy for extensively damaged lower extremities. Principles of the Ilizarov technique provide for external fixation of the long bone and allow micromotion only parallel to the bone axis. A surgically created corticotomy is performed with repair of the periosteum and preservation of medullary tissues. A latent period of 5 to 7 days is followed by 1 mm/day distraction performed at four separate intervals across the bony gap. Simultaneously, the traumatic bony gap is closed. Following distraction, a period of neutral fixation approximately equal to the total distraction time allows ossification of the distracted bone gap (Table 32–6). Use of the extremity is permitted while the patient is in the Ilizarov apparatus. A steep learning curve has been noted (but one recent report documented 57 of 60 limbs successfully lengthened with 17 major and 10 minor complications).

In summary, vascular, soft-tissue, and bone reconstruction has improved significantly through advances in microvascular technique. Nerve injuries continue to be difficult to manage, with incomplete recovery frequent. Complex lower extremity reconstruction must be judged by the functional outcome measured against the time, cost, and morbidity of multiple procedures. Its ultimate success must also provide patient satisfaction with ambulation that is superior to amputation and use of a prosthetic device.

LEG ULCERS

The pathophysiology of cutaneous breakdown in the lower extremity varies significantly.

Ischemic Ulcers

Atherosclerotic arterial disease accounts for the majority of ischemic ulcerations in the lower extremity. The ulcers are characterized by superficial breakdown with a necrotic center, and the ulcers are characteristically extremely painful. They occur most often over bony prominences such as the malleolus. These ulcers usually begin with a traumatic cutaneous insult that may be minor. The occurrence of ischemic ulceration is enhanced by congestive heart failure and chronic venous insufficiency, which may occur concomitantly. Evaluation begins with a history and physical examination, with the circulatory status assessed by peripheral pulses, color, temperature, and capillary refill. Segmental Doppler examination with analysis of Doppler waveforms is next along with calculation of an ankle-brachial index by utilizing Doppler pressures, a reproducible and accurate indicator of ischemic etiology provided that the upper extremity circulation is relatively normal and that the vessels are not so heavily calcified as to be noncompressible. An ankle brachial index of less than 0.5 usually represents significant obstructive arterial disease, while an index less than 0.2 often indicates impending tissue loss in the lower extremity. Finally, arteriography helps to identify the anatomic sites of arterial obstruction.

Treatment of an ischemic peripheral ulcer involves local conservative measures including dressing changes, control of congestive heart failure, and elevation of the extremity to

TABLE 32–6.
Distraction Osteogenesis

Phase	Goals	Complications
Latency	7 days between corticotomy and distraction	–
Transport	Distraction: 0.25 mm 4 times daily	Failure of regeneration
Maturation	Increased mineral content of regenerated segment	Pin tract infection
Consolidation	Tubularization of cortical bone	Nonunion

reduce swelling along with conservative debridements until arterial reconstruction can be performed. Once this is accomplished, and there is no evidence for infection or heavy bacterial contamination skin grafting can often be successful if the ulcers fail to heal spontaneously. Free tissue transfer has also been successful. The morbidity of this procedure must be weighed against that of an amputation.

Neurotrophic Ulcers

Sensory changes create a common scenario for cutaneous breakdown. Most commonly, patients with diabetes mellitus complicated by a stocking/glove distribution of peripheral neuropathy with decreased response to pain frequently have neurotrophic ulceration. These are generally deep, painless ulcers with surrounding granulation tissue occurring at pressure points under the metatarsal heads or heel and are commonly known as malperforans ulcers. Additionally, because of intrinsic muscle dysfunction with peripheral neuropathy, there can be abnormal hyperextension of the metatarsophalangeal joints and compensatory flexion of the proximal interphalangeal joints with resultant increased pressure under the metatarsal heads. The Charcot joint that can occur in this setting also creates abnormal plantar pressure likely to lead to cutaneous ulceration.

Initial evaluation should document the peripheral neuropathy. In the case of diabetes mellitus, medial arterial wall calcification will often lead to noncompressible vessels with bounding peripheral pulses despite the contribution of ischemia to the lower extremity ulcerations. Doppler pressures will be abnormally high and may be unobtainable with severe calcific atherosclerosis. Digital pressures may be helpful, but it is likely that arteriography will be required to completely understand the macrovascular contributions to the etiology of the ulcer. Radiographs of the affected foot should be obtained because osteomyelitic changes are common. Extensive plantar abscesses, which may be very subtle from surface examination, can be suspected from air bubbles or soft-tissue swelling on radiographs. Cultures frequently yield multiple organisms, including gram-negatives, and antibiotic therapy should be appropriately directed.

In treating a neurotrophic ulcer, it is unlikely that the underlying pathophysiologic process will be altered. With osteomyelitis of the metatarsal head, the infected segment of bone must be resected, but the remaining metatarsal heads will bear increased weight and be subject to increasing forces for recurrent ulceration. Immobilization, leg elevation, debridement, and dressing changes along with antibiotics and glucose control are the mainstays of conservative treatment. Sepsis complicating a diabetic foot ulcer may require guillotine below-knee amputation with subsequent revision. When arterial reconstruction is indicated, bypass surgery often extends onto the foot. Limb salvage by arterial bypass, however, can be as successful as arterial reconstructions in nondiabetic atherosclerotic patients.

Venous Stasis Ulcers

Chronic venous insufficiency represents end-stage pathology of the valvular system within the veins of the lower extremity. Most often, this is a result of thrombosis and recanalization leading to valvular destruction. The pathophysiology of cutaneous breakdown with chronic venous insufficiency includes a high ambulatory venous pressure that is transmitted to the superficial venous plexus through perforating veins. This, in turn, leads to dilatation of capillary beds with an egress of large–molecular-weight proteins, including fibrinogen, into the intercellular interstitium. Fibrinogen in this extravascular location is converted to fibrin, which is only partially cleared. Fibrin and other deposited proteins are responsible for the disruption of nutrient flow to the skin, which becomes indurated, fragile, and finally ulcerated. Early in the pathophysiologic process, the skin is swollen and edematous, and visible varicosities lead to pigmented changes with erythema and stasis dermatitis. Finally, subcutaneous fibrosis occurs in the end stage of the disease.

This history is often positive for deep venous thrombosis, physical examination includes Trendelenburg's test, and duplex scanning is used to identify varicosities, deep venous obstruction, and recanalization channels. The color flow mode can document venous valve dysfunction. Phlebography is reserved for patients who may be candidates for valve transplantation.

The treatment of venous stasis disease remains similar to that described by Dr. Unna in 1883. The Unna boot is a compression dressing for lower extremity ulceration that is impregnated with zinc oxide, gelatin, and glycerin or calamine cream and is designed to locally treat cutaneous breakdown as well as counteract high ambulatory venous pressure. Although the majority of patients can be treated as outpatients, refractory ulcers require hospitalization for strict lower extremity elevation and dressing changes.

Only 10% of patients with venous stasis ulcers will require operative treatment. Surgery includes skin grafting after ulcer excision, which may be accompanied by ligation of subfascial perforating veins beneath regions of ulceration. Although not widely practiced, venous valve transplantation and valvuloplasty represent a direct assault on the pathophysiology of chronic venous insufficiency and have led to short-term success in several series.

LYMPHEDEMA

Lymphedema is an excess of interstitial fluid within tissues secondary to failure of lymphatic drainage. Lymphatic failure is caused either by congenital malformation and hypoplasia of the lymphatic system or by obstruction of major lymphatic channels secondary to excision, irradiation, infection, or tumor. Traditionally, lymphedema resulting from hypoplasia has been classified as primary lymphedema and seems to occur at three distinct ages. Congenital lymphedema is evident as limb swelling within several weeks of birth; lymphedema praecox, which accounts for 80% of the cases of primary lymphedema, is seen during puberty; and lymphedema tarda occurs after the age of 35 years. To date, no satisfactory pathophysiologic mechanism for presentation at these various stages has been proposed. Secondary lymphedema is synonymous with the acquired condition attributable to lymphatic obstruction.

Normally, lymph originating within the dermis collects in nonvalved dermal lymphatic channels and flows into the subdermal and subcutaneous plexus. Lymph collecting within the deeper tissues flows along intermuscular planes, and both systems parallel venous egress from the extremity. Communications exist at lymph node groups in the popliteal fossa and inguinal region. Although lymphovenous connections may exist, they are nonfunctional under normal physiologic conditions. Lymph flow is from a distal-to-proximal direction and is driven by the low hydrostatic pressure within the lymphatic system, permeability within the terminal lymphatic ducts, and valves within the system. Both lymphatic obstruction and lymphatic hypoplasia result in increased pressure eventually rendering valves incompetent and resulting in the buildup of interstitial fluid with a high protein content in the extremity. Clinically this is manifested as a brawny, nonpitting edema, with scaly skin changes designated as lymphostatic verrucosis. Lymphatic drainage beneath the deep muscle fascia seems to be somewhat less affected by obstructive processes secondary to the muscle pump mechanism. Extremities with lymphedema are very susceptible to infections that further increase fibrosis and damage to the obstructed lymphatic channels.

The diagnosis of lymphedema is essentially clinical. Contrast lymphography is contraindicated in lymphedema because of the damage it can cause to the remaining open lymphatic channels. Alternatively, lymphoscintigraphy utilizing technetium 99m combined with human serum albumin or dextran can provide static and dynamic studies of lymphedematous extremities. This study has been a significant advance in studying the physiologic effects of surgical intervention in lymphedema.

The treatment of the vast majority of patients with lymphedema is nonoperative. Prevention of infection or its early treatment are paramount. Elastic support garments are the mainstay of therapy, and sequential pneumatic compression devices are useful in conjunction with leg elevation in reducing uncontrolled lymphedema in the lower extremity.

The two basic formats for surgical intervention include excisional therapy and physiologic procedures. Various combinations of skin and subcutaneous tissue can be excised from massively edematous lower extremities with some improvement in contour and cosmesis. The Charles procedure, i.e., complete subcutaneous excision with skin grafting onto deep muscle fascia, is the most radical form of therapy but is fraught with significant and persistent skin symptoms as well as aesthetic contour deformity that is most obvious at the transition point about the knee. Staged subcutaneous excisions are now the usual ablative therapy and have superior aesthetic results.

For obstructive lymphedema, there have been several physiologic procedures proposed to bridge the damaged section of the lymphatic system. Lymphatic tracts in dermal grafts, muscle flaps, omentum, and bowel have all been transferred to the extremity with varying degrees of success. Additionally, lympholymphatic and lymphovenous anastomoses have been performed with short-term success. The durability of these procedures remains to be proved.

AESTHETIC DEFORMITY OF THE LOWER EXTREMITY

Thigh

By far, the most common aesthetic deformity of the lower extremity involves excessive adipose tissue in the hips, thighs, and buttocks. Sex variations in fat distribution make these deformities much more common in women. Recently, a greater understanding of the anatomy of the subcutaneous tissue in this region has been delineated. Two distinct layers, superficial and deep, have been histologically defined with the deep fat layer extending from the torso to the lateral proximal aspect of the thigh and gluteal region. It is this deep fat pocket that is most commonly targeted for removal.

Historically, body contouring in the lower extremity has been confined to direct excision. With this technique, skin and fat deformities are corrected. The major disadvantage is the significant scarring. The best candidates for dermal lipectomy include patients with massive weight loss who have redundant skin as well as remaining fat deposits.

Suction-assisted lipectomy is most often utilized for adipose deformity in the lower extremity. The technique removes deep subcutaneous fat through limited incisions placed in natural skin creases so that they are almost camouflaged. The final contour is determined by the fat remaining. Technical aspects of the procedure vary, but there is uniform agreement that a compression garment should be worn for at least 7 to 10 days after the procedure. Additionally, the very small access incisions can be left open or only loosely closed to allow drainage to minimize ecchymosis and hematoma formation. Appropriate fluid resuscitation is essential. In general, a 1% drop in the hematocrit can be expected for each 150 cc of fat suctioned, and intravenous replacement fluids should be administered in a ratio of three to one to the material removed. Autologous blood transfusion should be considered for suction lipectomy procedures exceeding 1,500 cc.

Ideal treatment of many aesthetic deformities of the thigh requires a procedure combining excision with suction lipectomy (Table 32–7). Effective treatment of crural excess can be achieved with a lenticular dermal lipectomy in the groin crease combined with suction-assisted lipectomy of the medial part of the thigh. Recurrence of the deformity has been successfully prevented by anchoring the inferior skin flap at the level of the excision to Colles' fascia. Another useful strategy involves lenticular incision in the buttock region with deepithelialization of the skin island over which the skin margins are closed to correct gluteal recess deformity, significant asymmetries, and iatrogenic deformities resulting from previous dermal lipectomy.

Calf

The subcutaneous tissue in the calf is a single layer, and contour deformities are most

TABLE 32–7.
Aesthetic Treatment of Hip/Thigh Deformities*

Deformity	Treatment
Crural excess	Medial thigh-plasty or SAL† and skin resection
Trochanteric excess ("saddle bag")	SAL
Gluteal recess	SAL
Composite trochanteric excess and gluteal recess	SAL and island deepithelialization of gluteal recess
Obesity—generalized	SAL
Asymmetry/trauma	SAL or SAL and island deepithelialization
Aging/atrophy	Skin reduction

* Adapted from Grazer FM: Suction-assisted lipectomy—Its indications, contraindications, and complications, in Habal M (ed): *Advances in Plastic and Reconstructive Surgery*. St Louis, Mosby–Year Book, 1984. Used by permission.
† SAL = suction-assisted lipectomy.

often attributable to the underlying muscle. Calf dysplasias secondary to poliomyelitis, trauma, or congenital deformities can result in significant aesthetic deformities. The gastrocnemius muscle is responsible for the calf silhouette described medially as a peak and laterally as a sweep. The deeper soleus muscle accounts for the overall size of the calf. Deformities in this region can be corrected with solid implants of silicone elastomer. The insertion technique involves an approach through a limited incision in the popliteal fossa that spares the cutaneous nerves. A subfascial pocket is created medially and laterally as needed, with implant placement creating the desired contour. Compression dressings are routinely worn in the postoperative period. The morbidity of this procedure has been acceptably low.

In summary, aesthetic surgery of the lower extremity most often involves reduction in its proximal aspect and augmentation distally, although suction-assisted lipectomy is, at times, performed in the calf/ankle region. Recent advances have allowed limited exposures to minimize scarring in the correction of aesthetic deformities of the lower extremity.

RECONSTRUCTION OF CONGENITAL DEFORMITY OF THE LOWER EXTREMITY

Congenital anomalies of the lower extremity are as diverse as those of the upper extremity. Skeletal anomalies are a frequent part of lower extremity anomalies. The incidence of congenital limb deformity in the lower extremity is approximately 0.3%. Genetic as well as environmental factors are believed to be etiologic, and classification is based on the embryologic failure leading to the deformity (Table 32–8).

Constriction Band Syndrome

The constriction band syndrome is believed to be an example of in utero mechanical disruption of limb development. The syndrome consists of a lower extremity constriction band with accompanying circulatory, lymphatic, and sensorineural disruption that varies in severity from a simple dermal groove to disruption affecting all layers of the limb and leading to congenital amputation. The syndrome is often accompanied by acrosyndactyly.

Treatment of the cutaneous aspects of the syndrome involve multiple, staged Z-plasty procedures. Severe manifestations of the constriction band syndrome may require amputation for an unsalvageable distal extremity.

TABLE 32–8.
Embryologic Classificaton of Lower Extremity Deformity

Failure of formation
Transverse
Longitudinal
Failure of differentiation
Duplication
Overgrowth
Constriction bands
Skeletal deformity

Syndactylism

As in the upper extremity, syndactylism is a failure of differentiation of the distal end of the extremity. Up to 20% of the cases are manifested as acrosyndactyly wherein the distal aspect of the digits are fused. A family history positive for syndactyly is present in 40% of cases, thus reflecting, at least in part, a genetic component. Functional manifestations of lower extremity syndactyly are usually minimal, and correction with Z-plasty and skin graft procedures is indicated primarily for aesthetic reasons.

SUGGESTED READING

Byrd HS, Spicer TE, Cierny G III: Management of open tibial fractures. *Plast Reconstr Surg* 1985; 76:719.

Courtiss EH: Suction lipectomy: A retrospective analysis of 100 patients. *Plast Reconstr Surg* 1984; 73:780.

Gelberman RH (ed): *Operative Nerve Repair and Reconstruction.* Philadelphia, JB Lippincott, 1991.

Gloviczki P: Treatment of secondary lymphedema, in Ernst CV, Stanley JC (eds): *Current Therapy in Vascular Surgery,* ed 2. Philadelphia, BC Decker, 1991.

Godina M: Early microsurgical reconstruction of complex trauma of the extremity. *Plast Reconstr Surg* 1986; 78:285.

Grazer FM: Suction-assisted lipectomy—Its indications, contraindications, and complications, in Habal M (ed): *Advances in Plastic and Reconstructive Surgery.* St Louis, Mosby–Year Book, 1984.

Gustilo RB, Anderson JT: Prevention of infection in the treatment of one thousand and twenty-five open fractures of long bones: Retrospective and prospective analysis. *J Bone Joint Surg [Am]* 1976; 58:453.

Ilizarov GA: Clinical application of the tension-stress effect for limb lengthening. *Clin Orthop* 1990; 250:8.

May JW Jr, Halls MJ, Simons SR: Free microvascular muscle flaps with skin graft reconstruction of extensive defects of the foot: A clinical and gait analysis study. *Plast Reconstr Surg* 1985; 75:621.

Nahai F, Stahl RS: Congenital deformities of the lower extremity, in Serafin D, Georgiade NG (eds): *Pediatric Plastic Surgery,* St Louis, Mosby–Year Book, 1984.

O'Donnell TF: Management of primary lymphadema, in Ernst CB, Stanley JC (eds): *Current Therapy in Vascular Surgery,* ed 2. Philadelphia, BC Decker, 1991.

Russell WL, et al: Limb salvage versus traumatic amputation. *Ann Surg* 1991; 213:473.

Rutherford RB (ed): *Vascular Surgery,* ed 3. Philadelphia, WB Saunders, 1989.

Yaremchuk MJ, Burgess AR, Brumback RJ (eds): *Lower Extremity Salvage and Reconstruction.* New York, Elsevier, 1989.

PART VIII

Plastic Surgery of the Genitourinary System

Chapter 33

Anatomy/Embryology

Charles E. Horton, Sr., M.D.
Charles E. Horton, Jr., M.D.
Michael E. Hill, M.d., Ph.D.

CONTENTS

NOTE: The material in this chapter may be covered during the prerequisite training period of many plastic surgery residents. This chapter should serve as a valuable review of important material in such cases.

CHAPTER OBJECTIVES

At the end of this chapter the resident knows the anatomy and embryology of the genitourinary system and applies this information in the plastic surgical management of a variety of genitourinary problems.

LEARNER OBJECTIVES

On completion of this chapter the resident

1. Has acquired knowledge of the embryologic development of both the male and female genitourinary systems.
2. Is familiar with the anatomy of the genitourinary system as it relates to genitourinary reconstruction.
3. Can explain the genesis of common congenital anomalies of the genitourinary system based on interrelated embryology and anatomy.

CLINICAL PRACTICE ACTIVITIES

During the course of the training program, the resident

1. Applies the fundamental knowledge of genitourinary embryology, anatomy, and pathology in the treatment of plastic surgical problems of the genitourinary system, including congenital disorders, trauma, and reconstruction.

ANATOMY OF THE MALE AND FEMALE GENITOURINARY SYSTEM

The knowledge of normal genitourinary development is key to understanding its pathology. The essentials of the normal anatomy of both sexes are best illustrated with detailed anatomic drawings. The majority of more detailed anatomy will be discussed in the embryology section (Fig 33–1).

EMBRYOLOGY OF THE GENITOURINARY SYSTEM

During the fourth week of embryogenesis, the premature kidney (pronephric system)

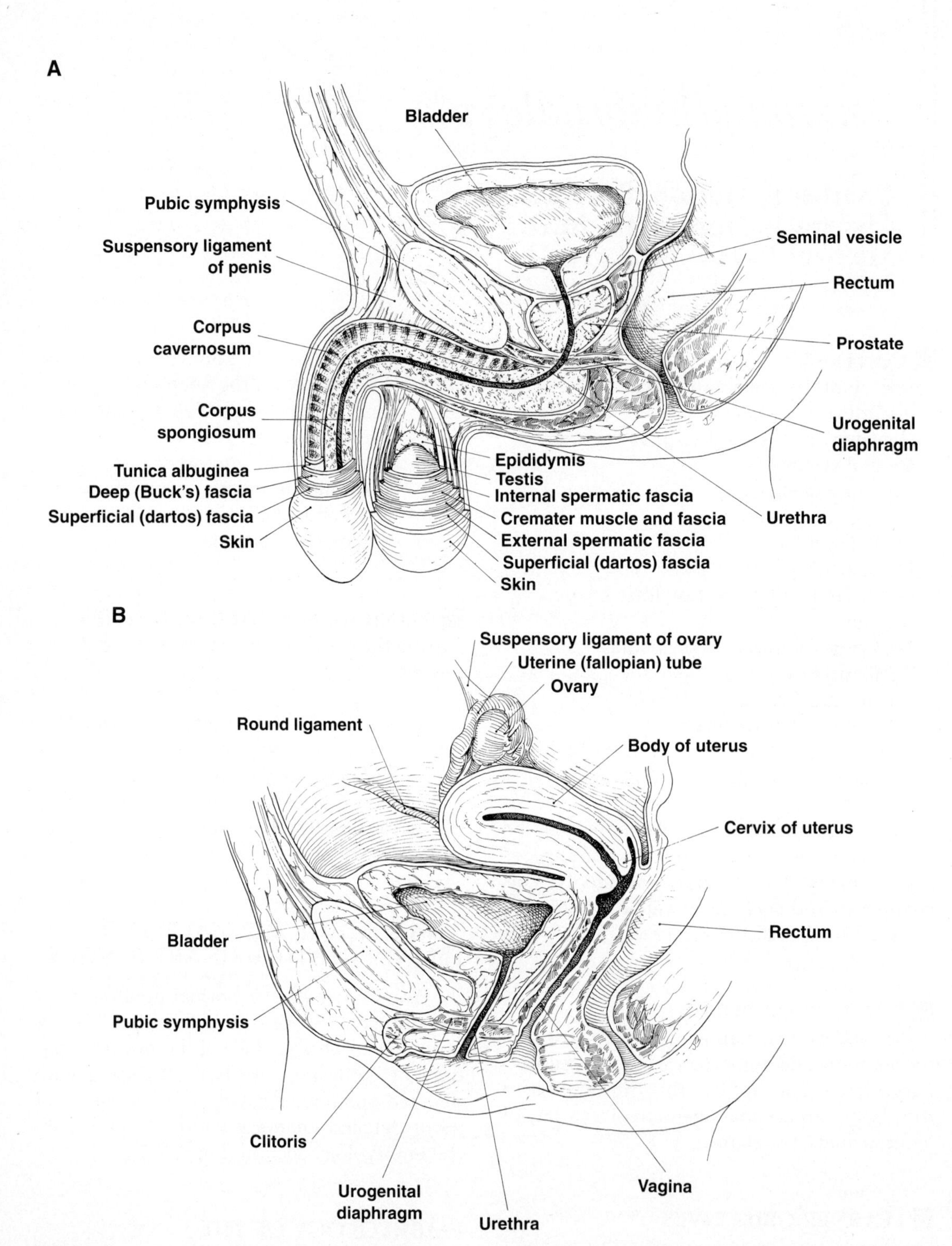

FIG 33–1.
A, normal male genital anatomy. **B,** normal female genital anatomy.

begins to develop in the cervical region of the embryo. This system quickly regresses as the mesonephric duct (wolffian duct) differentiates. Around the sixth week gonadal development begins on the medial aspect of the mesonephros, and this complex becomes known as the urogenital ridge. Under hormonal influence the mesonephric duct will persist in the male and degenerate in the female.

The definitive or permanent kidney arises from the third component of renal development, the metanephric system. The ureteric bud sprouts off of the caudal end of the mesonephric duct near the cloaca and grows into mesoderm, which forms the metanephric blastema. It is the ureteric bud that gives rise to the ureter, renal pelvis, and major and minor calyces. The renal parachyma evolves from the metanephric blastema.

Between the fourth and seventh weeks a urorectal septum will develop and divide the cloaca into a posterior anorectal canal and an anterior urogenital sinus. Two external membranes cover each respective cavity: (1) the anal membrane and (2) the urogenital membrane.

Further differentiation of the urogenital sinus gives rise to the urinary bladder, which communicates with the allantois via the urachus (median umbilical ligament in adults).

The pelvic segment of the urogenital sinus will develop into the prostatic and membranous urethra of the male.

As the genital tubercle is stimulated by androgens it elongates, and by the third month the urethral folds fuse over the urethral plate to form the penile urethra. The distal end of the urethra (fossa navicularis) is formed from an ingrowth of ectoderm that will eventually develop a lumen.

Genital System

The genetic sex of a child is determined at the time of fertilization by the presence of an "X" or "Y" chromosome of the sperm. Morphologic recognition of the sex is not determined until approximately the seventh week of development. Prior to this time, a period of indifferent gonadal development exists.

Proliferation of the coelomic epithelium and mesenchyme gives rise to the genital ridge, which is medial to the mesonephros. Primordial germ cells seed this ridge in a migratory fashion from the yolk sac via the dorsal mesentery. If the primordial cells do not reach the ridge, there will be an arrest in the development of the gonads.

In the male, the testis itself forms testicular cords consisting of germ cells and sustentacular cells of Sertoli. Between these cords are interstitial cells of Leydig. The Y chromosome triggers a cascade of events that leads to normal testicular development. A substance referred to as testis-determining factor (TDF) in concert with müllerian inhibiting factor (MIF) and androgens allow for the following events to occur: (1) the inductive effect of these substances stimulates the mesonephros to differentiate into the vas deferens and epididymis, while the paramesonephric duct is suppressed. The external genitalia are stimulated to differentiate into the penis and scrotum. The penis is derived from the genital tubercle and the scrotum from the labial-scrotal swelling. (2) Female morphology requires an XX chromosome pattern. Both chromosomes need to be present for normal development of the female. In the absence of MIF and androgens, the oviducts, uterus, and upper portion of the vagina develop from the müllerian ducts, and external genitalia take on the female phenotype.

Anatomy of the Penis

The penis is composed of three separate components, two corpora cavernosa and the corpus spongiosum. The corpora cavernosa are the erectile bodies of the penis that engorge with blood during an erection. The corpora cavernosa are covered by a strong and elastic tissue known as tunica albuginea. Between the two corpora cavernosa is an incomplete partition that morphologically has the appearance of teeth of a comb. The corpus spongiosum contains the urethra, which terminates at the urethral meatus located at the tip of the glans. The glans penis is derived from the corpus spongiosum and is separate from the two corpora cavernosa. All three corpora are enclosed by a layer known as Buck's fascia. The dorsal neurovascular bundle is located between the tunica albuginea and Buck's fascia. This neurovascular bundle is composed of two or more dorsal nerves that provide sensation to the glans penis, paired dorsal arteries, and a superficial and deep dorsal vein. The dorsal nerves are derived from internal pudendal nerves (located in Alcock's canal), and the dorsal vessels are the terminal branches of the pudendal artery and vein. The arterial flow is from the internal pudendal artery. As the artery enters the urogenital diaphragm, it gives off a bulbar branch, a dorsal branch that terminates in the glans, and the cavernosal branch that enters the corpora and terminates as the helicine arteries. The erectile function of the penis derives from the cavernosal nerves, which are branches from the pelvic parasympathetic plexus that when stimulated, relax the smooth muscle within the corpora and allow the inflow of blood to produce tumescence. Simultaneously there is a collapse of venous outflow until termination of the erect state occurs. Additional sensory nerves to the penis include the genitofemoral and sensory nerves.

In the genetic female, the effects of ovarian material and placental estrogens stimulate the paramesonephric duct (müllerian) to differentiate into the oviducts, uterus, and upper third of the vagina. Externally the labia, clitoris, and vaginal vault take on the morphology of the female.

PATHOLOGY AND PATHOLOGIC ANATOMY OF THE GENITAL SYSTEM

Hypospadias

An abnormal opening of the urethral meatus on the ventral surface is secondary to abnormal or incomplete fusion of the urethral folds. The prepuce develops as a hood and is deficient ventrally. The presence of ventral fibrous bands causes chordee. Some form of hypospadias occurs in 1 in 350 live male births in the United States. Of these, 90% occur in the distal end of the shaft or glans. Figure 33–2 depicts the locations that have been reported.

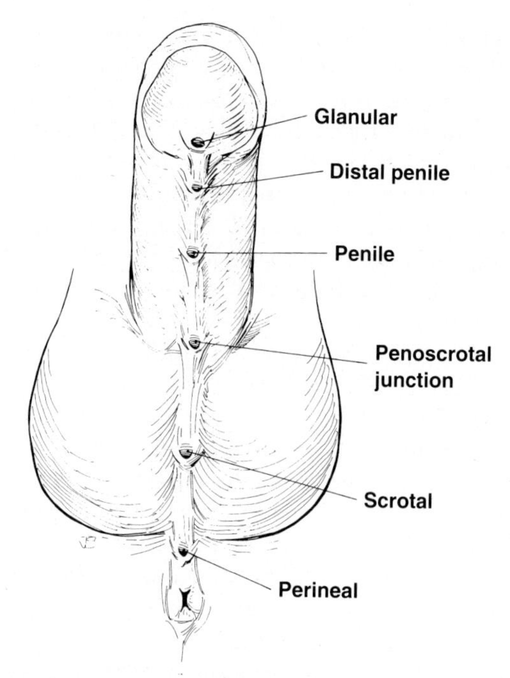

FIG 33–2.
Hypospadias variants, based on the position of the urethral meatus.

Chordee, or downward bending, of the penis can occur without hypospadias.

Good preoperative evaluation of these patients is critical. "Preurethroplasty" circumcision should never be performed on patients with hypospadias because the prepuce may be needed for subsequent reconstruction.

The authors believe that one-stage repairs are preferable to multiple-stage repairs. Multiple-stage repairs were performed in the past because many surgeons felt that chordee resulted from growing tissue and could recur. It is now known that chordee is static and fibrous; once corrected, it does not recur.

For historical reasons, four multiple-stage techniques are of significance. Prior to modern surgical techniques the four most popular reconstructive techniques were the Duplay, Denis Browne, Cecil-Culp, and Nové-Josserand and McIndoe techniques.

In 1955, Horton began a series of one-stage hypospadias repairs using full-thickness skin grafts from the prepuce. With this technique surgeons were able to correct chordee and reconstruct the urethra with good success and low morbidity.

Repairs performed from 1955 through the 1960s were one-stage repairs. In the 1980s the vascularized preputial flap became popular. For defects of the proximal or mid portions of the shaft, skin grafts or vascularized preputial flaps are ideal. For a distal defect, the meatal advancement glansplasty incision (MAGPI), urethral advancement, or flip-flap techniques can be utilized. (For additional discussion of surgical methods, see Chapter 34.)

Other Congenital Abnormalities of the Penis

Chordee Without Hypospadias

This is defined as an abnormal curvature of the penis with the urethral meatus located in its normal position at the tip of the glans. It has also been referred to in the literature as hypospadias without hypospadias and congenital short urethra; however, this last term is felt to be a misnomer because it is very rare for a short urethra to cause penile curvature. Chordee without hypospadias results from a deficiency of either the corpus spongiosum, Buck's fascia, or dartos fascia, which are replaced by dense fibrous tissue lying adjacent to or beneath the urethra. It can usually be corrected by resecting abnormal tethering tissue; alternatively, wedge resection of the tunica albuginea opposite the area of maximum curvature with primary closure can be used to correct this deformity.

Micropenis

Micropenis refers to a normally formed phallus with the median raphe, foreskin, glans, and meatus all normally developed; however, the phallus has a stretched length less than 2.5 SD from the mean for the child's age. This term should not be confused with the term microphallus, which refers to a small, ambiguous-appearing structure that is not clearly penile looking, such as that found in case of congenital adrenal hyperplasia. Micropenis is felt to result from inadequate virilization of an XY individual because of unresponsiveness to androgens or inadequate androgen production. This can be a very difficult problem to treat. If a male karyotype is confirmed and the phallus is borderline in size, a trial of testosterone therapy in combination with human chorionic gonadotropin (HCG) stimulation can be given for 6 weeks and the penis subsequently assessed for growth. If the phallus fails to respond to hormonal stimulation, gender reassignment should be considered. A more recent treatment option has emerged with the development of free tissue transfer techniques and total phallic reconstruction; consideration can now be given to raising these otherwise normal XY individuals in the male gender with the intent of performing total phallic reconstruction at around 6 years of age. This is a very complex and controversial issue.

Concealed Penis

Concealed penis refers to a phallus that is of normal size for the child's age but appears too diminutive because of concealment by surrounding scrotal and lower abdominal tissue. This is caused by dysgenetic tissue continuous with Scarpa's fascia that binds the penile shaft below the prepubic fat pad. The hidden penis can be released by resection of these abnormal bands together with mobilization of the corporal bodies and prepubic lipectomy.

There is a group of miscellaneous penile abnormalities that are all very rare. These include aphallia, diphallia, and penile torsion. All of these are felt to result from some abnormalities in development of the genital tubercle.

Scrotum Abnormalities

All abnormalities of the scrotum are rare and are often only a part of more extensive deformity of the genitalia. Scrotal abnormalities include the prepenile scrotum, which refers to a normally developed penis lying behind an essentially well formed normal scrotum. In a webbed scrotum a tethering band extends between the penis and the scrotum, as is usually seen in cases of intersex. There have been isolated reports of ectopic scrotum occurring and located on the inner aspect of the thigh, near the external inguinal ring, or on the anterior abdominal wall. Scrotal hypoplasia refers to a flat and discoid appearance of the scrotum and is associated with anorchia or cryptorchidism.

Epispadias and Exstrophy of the Bladder

The epispadias-exstrophy complex refers to failure of normal development of the dorsal surface of the penis, the abdomen, and the anterior bladder wall. The most common variant is exstrophy with complete epispadias, which occurs in 1 in 30,000 births and is three to four times more common in males. Isolated epispadias without bladder exstrophy is much more rare and occurs in approximately 1 in 250,000 births. In epispadias, the urethral mucosal groove is dorsally placed on the penis and creates a depression between two loosely attached corpora cavernosa. As with hypospadias, the epispadiac urethral meatus can be located distally on the penile shaft, midshaft, or more proximally in the penopubic area. The more proximal the urethral meatus, the more likely the abnormality is to be associated with urinary incontinence. The penis is usually short because of tethering of the corpora to widely separated pubic bones. Corpus spongiosum is rudimentary or absent. The prepuce is redundant ventrally. Erectile ability is unimpaired. Usually there is severe dorsal chordee.

The embryology of epispadias is controversial. The most widely accepted hypothesis states that persistence of the cloacal membrane prohibits migration of adjacent somatic mesoderm, which would ultimately have formed the anterior abdominal wall and dorsum of the urethra. When associated with bladder exstrophy, the treatment of epispadias is usually undertaken at a later stage following earlier bladder closure. Epispadias repairs are similar to techniques used for hypospadias: combinations of free grafts and vascularized flaps for urethroplasty. Critical to successful epispadias repair is adequate correction of dorsal chordee and penile lengthening.

Abnormalities of the Female Genitalia

Congenital absence of the vagina is also known as Mayer-Rokitansky syndrome. Congenital absence of the vagina often goes undetected until puberty, when the patient may be seen because of an abdominal mass associated with pain that is caused by accumulation of menses within the uterus. Absence of the vagina is often associated with renal problems, and these patients should have screening ultrasonography of their urinary tracts. Reconstruction of the vagina should be performed in these cases and can be done with either skin graft techniques or by utilizing various bowel segments to form a neovagina. Vaginal reconstruction is best deferred until after completion of puberty.

The adrenogenital syndrome, also known as congenital adrenal hyperplasia, occurs in both males and females but presents more of a clinical problem in female children. The female external genitalia exhibit a spectrum of masculinization from mild to complete, with fusion of the labia scrotal swellings and massive clitoral hypertrophy resembling a fully formed phallus. This syndrome results from an adrenal enzymatic deficiency impeding the formation of cortisol; a buildup of androgens proximal to the enzymatic block results in masculinization of the genitalia and can also be associated with significant electrolyte abnormalities that can be a life-threatening situation in neonates and must be diagnosed and treated early. Physical examination of these girls will uncover virilized genitalia with pigmentation of their genitals and scrotum as well as their nipples. Most importantly, there are no gonads palpable within what appears to be the scrotum. These children should always be sex-assigned females because they are otherwise completely normal and can indeed subsequently bear children. Immediate treatment involves hydrocortisone and mineralocorticoid supplementation with subsequent reconstructive surgery as needed. Reconstructive surgery in these cases involves clitoral recession and mobilization of the high vagina and can be successfully performed between 1 and 2 years of age.

SUGGESTED READING

Abbé R: New method of creating a vagina in a case of congenital absence. *Med Res* 1989; 54:836.

Devine CJ Jr, Blackley SK, Horton CE, et al: The surgical treatment of chordee without hypospadias in men. *J Urol* 1991; 146:325–329.

Devine PC, Winslow BH, Jordan GH, et al: Reconstructive phallic surgery, in Libertino JA (ed): *Pediatric and Adult Reconstructive Urologic Surgery,* ed 2. Baltimore, Williams & Wilkins, 1987, p 553.

Duckett JW Jr: Hypospadias. *Pediatr Rev* 1989; 11:37–42.

Gilbert DA, Horton CE, Terzis JK, et al: New concepts in phallic reconstruction. *Ann Plast Surg* 1987; 18:128.

Horton CE, McCraw JB, Devine CJ Jr, et al: Secondary reconstruction of the genital area. *Urol Clin North Am* 1977; 4:133.

McCarthy JG: *Plastic Surgery,* ed 6. Philadelphia, WB Saunders, 1990, pp 4153–4245.

Sadler TW: *Langman's Medical Embryology,* ed 6. Baltimore, Williams & Wilkins, 1990, pp 260–295.

Chapter 34

Trauma/Reconstruction/Functional Disorders

Lawrence J. Gottlieb, M.D.
Daniel P. Greenwald, M.D.
Laurence A. Levine, M.D.

CONTENTS

CHAPTER OBJECTIVE

At the end of this chapter the resident understands the principles of management of congenital, acquired, and functional disorders of the genitourinary system and undertakes comprehensive surgical management of such problems.

LEARNER OBJECTIVES

On completion of this chapter the resident

1. Understands the etiology and diagnosis of developmental abnormalities of the vagina.
2. Knows the principles and techniques of vaginal reconstruction.
3. Knows the principles and techniques of reconstruction of the male urethra and repair of hypospadias.
4. Knows the principles and techniques of reconstruction of the penis.
5. Recognizes the role of urologists and/or gynecologists in the collaborative management of selected cases.
6. *Knows how to evaluate ambiguous genitalia.*
7. *Understands the principles of diagnosis and treatment of transsexualism and is familiar with the techniques of male-to-female and female-to-male gender reassignment surgery.*

CLINICAL PRACTICE ACTIVITIES

During the course of the training program, the resident

1. Performs vaginal construction and/or reconstruction.
2. Participates in urethral construction and reconstruction in collaboration with the urologist.
3. Performs penile construction and/or reconstruction.

4. *Participates in the care (including surgical management) of transsexuals.*
5. *Evaluates and treats patients with vaginal, penile, urethral, and/or ambiguous genitalia disorders.*

While the urinary and genital systems are functionally different, they are anatomically and embryologically related. Both develop from a common mesodermal ridge, and both communicate during development with the cloaca. The differentiation of indifferent anlagen is under hormonal control and results in either the male or female phenotype. Interruptions or misdirections in ontogeny lead to abnormal development of gonads, ducts, and genitalia. Embryology provides the key to understanding these abnormalities. (For a detailed discussion of genitourinary embryology, see Chapter 33.)

SYNDROMES

Gonadal Dysgenesis

Patients can be 44-XY or 44-XX. Gonads do not differentiate (the etiology is unknown), and phenotypic development is female. Patients maintain infantile secondary sexual characteristics because of a lack of endogenous estrogen. Patients have primary amenorrhea.

Turner's Syndrome

Patients are female, 43-XO. Presentation is identical to gonadal dysgenesis with the addition of a webbed neck, a wide chest with broadly spaced nipples, and short stature. Its incidence is 2 in 3,000.

Klinefelter's Syndrome

Patients are male, 44-XXY. They are sterile and have testicular atrophy and gynecomastia. The incidence is 1 in 500 in the normal population and 1 in 100 among mentally retarded males. Evaluation of any male with gynecomastia should involve examination of the testicles and, where indicated, a sex chromatin determination. Therapy is hormonal and surgical (for gynecomastia). The sterility is irreversible.

Testicular Feminization

The incidence is reported as 1 in 20,000 to 64,000. Patients are 44-XY. Target tissues are unresponsive to normal levels of fetal androgen because of absent or dysfunctional receptors. Phenotypic development is female, and the outward appearance is unremarkable with the exception of scant axillary and pubic hair. Paramesonephric ducts are inhibited by normal levels of suppressor substance, so the vagina is short and ends blindly, and the uterus and fallopian tubes do not develop. Testes are small and typically located in the inguinal canal. As undescended testes, they are at risk for malignant degeneration and should be removed or placed into the scrotum (to facilitate surveillance) soon after the diagnosis is made. Presentation is primary amenorrhea.

Female Pseudohermaphroditism (ambiguous genitalia)

The most common cause is adrenogenital syndrome. Patients are 44-XX but have excess production of adrenal androgens because of abnormal steroid metabolism in fetal adrenal glands. Masculinization occurs and ranges from clitoral hypertrophy to almost male genitalia. Early gender identification is important so that appropriate hormonal and surgical intervention can be planned. Ductal development is normal, and normal female development can be expected with proper treatment.

Male Pseudohermaphrodites (ambiguous genitalia)

Patients are 44-XY with variable internal and external sex characteristics. This syndrome is thought to be due to inadequate androgen production or to production not in concert with target tissue sensitivity. Early gender identification is important so that appropriate surgical intervention can be planned.

HYPOSPADIAS

Hypospadias results from a failure of completion of development of the male external genitalia. The external urinary meatus is located on the ventral surface of the penis, between the perineum and the ventral aspect of the glans, depending on the severity of the condition. Hypospadias is a relatively common abnormality present in 3 to 5 per 1,000 live-born males. Eighty-five percent of patients have the urethral meatus located on the distal end of the penile shaft.

The penis and penile urethra form by a complex sequence of foldings and invaginations that generally progress proximally to distally. Hypospadias results from arrest of distal development of the ventral penile tissues. The urethral meatus is located along the ventral penile shaft. The location is variable and is described (in increasing order of severity) as glanular, distal penile, penile, scrotal, or perineal. The urethral groove persists from the hypospadiac meatus to the groove in the glans penis. In this groove the mesenchymal anlagen of corpus spongiosum, Buck's fascia, and dartos fascia fail to differentiate. This is characterized by a fan-shaped fibrous band from the meatus to the ventral glans, which may result in a ventral curvature or chordee with erection. In addition, there is a deficit of ventral preputial skin.

Other congenital abnormalities are commonly found with hypospadias. Full evaluation is necessary to rule out undescended testes, kidney abnormalities, and hernias. Cystoscopy is used to look for urethral valves or diverticula that can impede catheterization and/or voiding.

Preoperatively, it is important to assign an accurate gender. Circumcision before urethroplasty is contraindicated. Obstructive uropathy must be addressed immediately. Corrective surgery should be performed before the patient enters school.

The goal of surgery is an aesthetic and functional penis. This requires relocation of the urethral meatus to the tip of the penis and resection of the fibrous chordee. Techniques for reconstruction are chosen according to the severity of the defect and the availability of tissues. Preputial skin from the dorsum can be used for ventral coverage. It can be tubed and transferred to form a neourethra as a proximally based flap. To verify the adequacy of chordee release, saline is injected into the corpora to create an artificial erection (Gittes' maneuver).

The modern approach to hypospadias strives for one-stage corrective surgery. This is usually possible with one of four basic reconstructive techniques, each of which can be modified to suit a particular situation. These include the meatal advancement glansplasty incision (MAGPI), flip-flaps, full-thickness flaps, and preputial flaps.

The MAGPI approach is indicated for glanular hypospadias. A circumcision incision is combined with a dorsal longitudinal incision to place the meatus in the normal position. Repair should be accomplished by the age of 2 years.

The flip-flap technique is used for distal shaft hypospadias. This procedure is modified as needed in the presence of chordee. Complete release of chordee requires resection of all subcutaneous tissue located between the meatus and the glans.

If the skin over the urethra is too short to reach as a flip-flap, skin grafting is required. Dorsal or ventral proximally based preputial flaps as well as bladder mucosal flaps can be used as tubed neourethras. Combinations of flip-flaps, grafts, flaps, and MAGPI are used depending on the deficiency to be corrected.

EPISPADIAS

Epispadias, bladder exstrophy, and cloacal deformity are variants of the epispadias/exstrophy syndrome. These deformities of unknown etiology are complex, and correction is usually undertaken in a systematic and staged fashion. Simple epispadias involving only the glans occurs in 1 per 120,000 live male births. A more severe presentation is usually seen as part of the epispadias-exstrophy complex (1 per 30,000). Females are seen with bladder exstrophy and a bifid clitoris (the same frequency as in males).

This class of defects results from a failure of somatic mesoderm to form the lower abdominal wall. This is thought to be due to an overly prominent cloacal membrane that holds the lateral processes of somatic mesoderm apart. The anatomic presentation is variable, from a minimally abnormal dorsal meatus to complete exstrophy. In severe (proximal) cases there is no umbilicus, and the rectus abdominis muscles diverge inferiorly. Midline abdominal fascia may be absent. In these cases, the pubic ramus is split, and there is lateral segment rotation. This causes lateral hip displacement and anterior rotation of the anus. The bladder is open and exposed on the abdomen. The bladder neck may be formed, but the sphincter is usually cleft. The corpora are separated, and the dorsal neurovascular bundles are laterally located. The penis is short and tethered dorsally to the lower part of the abdomen. Many patients require several surgeries and often come to the plastic or urologic surgeon with a long surgical history and significant scar tissue.

In patients with epispadias, cystoscopy is used to look for valves or diverticula that can hinder catheterization and/or voiding. Renal workup is indicated when exstrophy is present. Patients with the more severe variants of epispadias are plagued with chronic and recurrent pyelonephritis, sometimes accompanied by hydroureter.

Surgical therapy must release the penis, correct the chordee, and repair or reconstruct the urethra, abdominal wall, and anterior of the bladder. Surgery is multistaged and designed to repair the bladder, sphincter, and external genitalia. Release of the penis is accomplished with various abdominal and groin skin flaps. These are used for dorsal coverage and can be used for urethroplasty. Urethroplasty is accomplished as for hypospadias, only on the dorsum of the penis and usually with a greater degree of difficulty. Bladder reconstruction proceeds by mobilizing the everted bladder edges and approximating them in the midline. The abdominal wall is reconstituted with rectus muscle and/or fascia flaps. Fibers of the cleft urinary sphincter are imbricated around the bladder neck in an attempt to restore continence.

Complications of the procedure include frequent urinary infections as a result of obstruction and incomplete emptying. The goal of therapy is to protect the upper urinary tract from progressive deterioration. Females have a better chance for continence, but males can expect improvement during prostatic growth at puberty. Sexual counseling for males is often indicated.

Repair of epispadias/cloacal deformity is complex and should not be undertaken by surgeons who are not routinely involved in the care of these patients.

PEYRONIE'S DISEASE

Peyronie's disease most commonly occurs in 40- to 60-year-old men and is characterized by a curvature of the erect penis. Ten percent of affected patients also have Dupuytren's palmar fasciitis. Its etiology is unknown but thought to be related to epigenetic factors (i.e., mechanical stress) superimposed upon a genetically or age-related predisposition to fibrous scarring of the tunica albuginea. Its incidence is approximately 1%.

The curvature is caused by localized scarring of the tunica albuginea, a tough fibrous layer of tissue that envelops the corpora cavernosa. The etiology is unclear, but it appears to be a disease of abnormal wound healing stimulated by epigenetic factors. A familial predisposition has been reported. The disease may progress, remain stable, or resolve spontaneously (approximately 10%).

Therapy is indicated when there is interference with intercourse or in the presence of penile pain. Vitamin E has been tried with minimal success, and surgery remains the mainstay of treatment. The operative technique is to gain exposure to the plaque through circumferential degloving incisions. Buck's fascia is elevated with the neurovascular bundle. The phallus may then be straightened by excising ellipses of tunica from the longer, convex side (Nesbitt procedure) or by excision of the plaque with grafting of the tunica defect. Complete scar removal is essential. Plaque excision is complete when the erect penis is straight. The tunica may be patched with a deepithelialized dermal graft, tunica vaginalis, or synthetic material. Intercourse is avoided for at least 6 weeks. Satisfaction, as judged by patient interview, is approximately 85%. Placement of a penile prosthesis may be necessary if preoperative erectile rigidity is suboptimal. Recurrence after surgery is unusual.

TRAUMA/INFECTION

Extensive loss of soft tissue can result from infections or trauma in men and women. The basic principles of management are as for any vital body part. For genital injuries, knowledge of anatomy is critical.

Infection

Infections can destroy genital tissue in men and women. Treatment is as for infections in other body sites: incisure and drainage where indicated, antibiotics, rest, and avoidance of prolonged dependency. More severe infections can occur with quite dramatic presentations, rapidly destroy tissue, and even threaten life. These are usually clostridial or mixed anaerobic infections that produce gas, necrosis, and sepsis.

Fournier's gangrene is a severe, rapidly spreading, destructive infection of the perineum caused by mixed aerobic and anaerobic organisms. This rapidly progressive condition usually affects debilitated or immunocompromised individuals and is sometimes the initial symptom of patients with occult cancer of the gastrointestinal tract. Other risk factors include poor hygiene, anal-rectal infection, diabetes, and urinary incontinence. Early recognition and treatment are mandatory because this can be life-threatening. Reconstruction follows removal of nonviable tissues and the attainment of a quantitative bacterial balance in the wound; grafts, local-regional flaps, and free tissue transfer are employed as needed.

Trauma

Most civilian injuries to the genitalia result from motor vehicle accidents or accidents involving industrial or farm machinery. Males are many more times afflicted than females. As with any type of trauma, the severity and type dictate the treatment. Patterns of injury are in part determined by local anatomy. Fascial planes determine patterns of spread or containment of extravasated urine, blood, and infection. In males, important fascial layers include the dartos fascia of the penis and scrotum, Buck's fascia of the penis, and Colles' fascia as it reflects over the deep urethra and genitourinary diaphragm. Dartos and Colles' fasciae are in continuity over the perineum and continue over the lower part of the abdomen as Scarpa's fascia. Subdartos layer collections are kept from involving the testes and cord structures by the external spermatic fascia.

Lymphedema

Lymph normally flows from the penis and scrotum (labia majora) to the medial superficial inguinal nodes. Testicular drainage is direct to the lumbar nodes, bypassing the inguinal basins. Lymphedema has been classified by Bulkley as primary or secondary. Secondary lymphedema is much more common than primary and results from scarring of normal lymph channels and/or blockage of lymph drainage. Primary edema results from aplastic, hyperplastic (tarda group), or hypoplastic lymph channels and is divided into three types: (1) congenital (Milroy's), (2) lymphedema praecox (pubertal), and (3) lymphedema tarda (manifested after the age of 35 years). Secondary lymphedema is classified on the basis of obstructive etiology (filariasis, lymphogranuloma, tuberculosis, syphilis, leprosy). Secondary lymphedema is also seen after elective lymph node dissection and in patients with carcinoma, postradiation destruction of lymphatics, cardiac and renal failure, venous thrombosis, and hypoproteinemia. Treatment depends on the etiology. The mainstay of therapy for refractory genital edema is surgery. Replacing edematous skin with uninvolved skin recruited from local flaps offers a good chance for relief. Complete skin excision with skin grafting is efficacious and usually successful. If the penile or scrotal skin is normal, it should be harvested and used as an isotropic full-thickness graft after resection of subcutaneous tissues. Lymphangioplasty has met with variable results, as has lymphaticovenous shunting. Wicking procedures using threads are no longer recommended. Omental flaps can offer early relief, but late scarring in the groin leads to the reformation of edema. Edema from filariasis is almost impossible to treat, and surgery is contraindicated because of increased scarring and worsening of the condition.

PHALLIC RECONSTRUCTION

Modern techniques have made possible the construction of an aesthetically pleasing, functional penis. The goals of reconstructive/constructive phallic surgery are the same regardless of the surgical indication (acquired, developmental, transsexualism). Ideally, the reconstructed phallus should fulfill several criteria to be functionally and psychologically satisfying. Any technique should provide reliable one-stage reconstruction that allows standing in order to micturate, intromission, protective sensation, erogenous sensation, and acceptable appearance. The radial forearm fasciocutaneous free flap fulfills most of these criteria. The "tube within a tube" design provides for a vascularized urethra. Neurorrhaphy between the flap's antebrachial cutaneous nerves and the pudendal nerves provides both protective and erogenous sensation. The development of protective sensation is crucial for long-term prosthesis retention.

Some patients may not be candidates for radial forearm flap penile reconstruction. Most alternative methods have the major limitation of lack of sensation and may have limitations of inadequate urethral reconstructions. These other reconstructive options include other free flaps, bilateral gracilis muscle flaps, rectus muscle flaps, and the standard groin flap or other tubed pedicle flaps. Subsequent muscle atrophy is a significant limitation of muscle flap reconstructions.

VAGINAL AGENESIS

Vaginal agenesis occurs in 1 in 4,000 to 80,000 women. Its etiology is unknown, but it is associated with abnormalities/malformations of the uterus and urinary tract. Ovaries are normal, and secondary sexual characteristics develop normally.

The diagnosis of vaginal agenesis is frequently missed at birth. Patients are initially seen because of primary amenorrhea, occasionally with an abdominal mass secondary to hematometra. Genitourinary workup generally includes intravenous pyelography, retrograde urethrography, ultrasound, and cystoscopy. Karyotyping may be necessary to distinguish vaginal agenesis from testicular feminization in infants.

VAGINAL RECONSTRUCTION

The goal of vaginal reconstruction is to provide a neovaginal tube with stable epithelial lining. It should be psychologically satisfying and of an adequate length and width to permit sexual intercourse. Candidates for this procedure include patients with congenital vaginal absence or maldevelopment, loss of the vagina because of tumor ablation or trauma, and male-to-female transsexuals.

Options for neovaginal epithelial lining include grafts (cultured epithelium, split thickness or full thickness) or flaps (fasciocutaneous, musculocutaneous, bowel or penile inversion—in transsexuals). There are advocates of each of these options. The advantages and disadvantages of each of these options are related to their relative technical complexity and the potential morbidity of the surgery, the donor site, the quality of the lining epithelium, and requirements for long-term stenting.

Incomplete vaginas can be treated with continued pressure in the perineal dimple to gradually deepen the vaginal canal (Frank procedure), but this is primarily of historical interest. Graduated obturators are used to maintain the introitus, and vaginal stenting is required forever.

Split-thickness grafts can be applied by stent to line a pocket dissected in the perineum between the bladder and rectum. This technique (McIndoe, 1938) requires permanent stenting to minimize progressive contraction of this epithelial-lined tube. In addition, there is the added morbidity of the donor site. Vaginal constructions with full-thickness grafts contract less, thus obviating the need for permanent stents. Full-thickness grafts offer the added dimension of growing proportionally with the patient. Complications of grafts include stenosis, loss of grafts, and fistulas. Transplanted squamous cell carcinoma has been reported. Grafting procedures generally require strict bed rest for 7 to 10 days.

Regional fasciocutaneous flaps are advocated for their simplicity and reliability. There is little need for long-term stenting, and the donor sites are frequently well hidden in the groin crease. There is some concern as to whether or not adequate length is provided by these flaps.

Regional musculocutaneous flaps are generally recommended for adult vaginal reconstruction. The gracilis musculocutaneous flap was the first to be described for vaginal reconstruction. Because of a high incidence of partial cutaneous loss, the need for bilateral flaps, unsightly donor site scars, and difficulty in reconstructions when the distal end of the native vagina was preserved, the rectus abdominis musculocutaneous flap was developed for vaginal reconstruction. It is robust, relatively straightforward to elevate, and requires no stenting.

Intestinal rectosigmoid flaps have been used in an effort to provide the most natural substitute for vaginal tissue. These obviate the need for stents and provide a mucosally lined introitus. The major drawback of this approach is the need for laparotomy with its inherent morbidity. In addition, they may manifest excess mucus secretion.

The penile inversion technique is an alternative technique in the gender dysphoric population. Its main advantage is in the use of healthy tissue that would otherwise be discarded.

Techniques that use skin as vaginal lining lack natural lubrication and tend to have an odor from desquamation. Circumferential introitus suture lines should be interrupted with Z-plasties or some sort of skin interdigitation to avoid stenosis.

SUGGESTED READING

Carson CC III, Barwick WJ: Penoscrotal lymphedema, in Georgiade NG, Georgiade GS, Riefkohl R, et al (eds): *Essentials of Plastic, Maxillofacial, and Reconstructive Surgery.* Baltimore, Williams & Wilkins, 1987, pp 809–815.

Chang KN, Mathes SJ: Reconstruction of genitalia, in Jurkiewicz MJ, Krizek TJ, Mathes SJ, et al (eds): *Plastic Surgery: Principles and Practice.* St Louis, Mosby–Year Book, 1990, pp 1255–1280.

Edgerton MT, Kenney JG, Langman MW: Gender reassignment surgery, in Georgiade NG, Georgiade GS, Riefkohl R, et al (eds): *Essentials of Plastic, Maxillofacial, and Reconstructive Surgery.* Baltimore, Williams & Wilkins, 1987, pp 780–796.

Gottlieb LJ, Saunders J: Burns of the perineum, in Achauer BM (ed): *Burn Reconstruction.* New York, Theime Publishers, 1991.

Horton CE, Sadove RC, Devine CJ: Reconstruction of male genital defects: Congenital, in McCarthy JG (ed): *Plastic Surgery.* Philadelphia, WB Saunders, 1990, pp 4153–4179.

Horton CE, Sadove RC, McCraw JB: Reconstruction of female genital defects, in McCarthy JG (ed): *Plastic Surgery.* Philadelphia, WB Saunders, 1990, pp 4203–4212.

Horton CE, Sadove RC, Spindel MR: Reconstruction of male genital defects: Acquired, in McCarthy JG (ed): *Plastic Surgery.* Philadelphia, WB Saunders, 1990, pp 4180–4202.

Horton CE, Stecker JF, Jordan GH: Management of erectile dysfunction, genital reconstruction following trauma, and transsexualism, in McCarthy JG (ed): *Plastic Surgery.* Philadelphia, WB Saunders, 1990, pp 4213–4245.

Hurwitz D: Congenital deformities of the female genitalia, in Georgiade NG, Georgiade GS, Riefkohl R, et al (eds): *Essentials of Plastic, Maxillofacial, and Reconstructive Surgery.* Baltimore, Williams & Wilkins, 1987, pp 774–779.

King L: Anomalies of the male genitalia, in Georgiade NG, Georgiade GS, Riefkohl R, et al (eds): *Essentials of Plastic, Maxillofacial, and Reconstructive Surgery.* Baltimore, Williams & Wilkins, 1987, pp 754–773.

Langman J: *Medical Embryology.* Baltimore, Williams & Wilkins, 1981, pp 234–268.

Laub DR, Wisnicki JL, Laub DR II, et al: Penoscrotal trauma and reconstruction, in Georgiade NG, Georgiade GS, Riefkohl R, et al (eds): *Essentials of Plastic, Maxillofacial, and Reconstructive Surgery.* Baltimore, Williams & Wilkins, 1987, pp 797–808.

Manstein CH, Manstein ME: Embryology of genitalia, in Georgiade NG, Georgiade GS, Riefkohl R, et al (eds): *Essentials of Plastic, Maxillofacial, and Reconstructive Surgery.* Baltimore, Williams & Wilkins, 1987, pp 747–753.

McCraw JB, Horton CE, Horton CE Jr: Basic techniques in genital reconstructive surgery, in McCarthy JG (ed): *Plastic Surgery.* Philadelphia, WB Saunders, 1990, pp 4125–4152.

PART IX

The Practice of Plastic Surgery

Chapter 35

Patient Management/Office Management

Ronald B. Berggren, M.D.

CONTENTS

CHAPTER OBJECTIVE

At the end of this chapter the resident is familiar with patient evaluation, ICD-9 and CPT terminology, and office operating room management.

LEARNER OBJECTIVES

On completion of this chapter the resident

1. **Understands how to interview and evaluate patients, especially the aesthetic surgery candidate.**
2. Knows the coding of diagnoses by the ICD-9-CM system.
3. Knows the coding of procedures by the CPT system.
4. Understands how to take standardized medical photographs.
5. Is thoroughly familiar with the principles of risk management.
6. *Knows the basic principles of how to equip and organize an office operating suite to comply with AAAAPSF standards.*

CLINICAL PRACTICE ACTIVITIES

During the course of the training program, the resident

1. **Participates in outpatient management, including both clinic experience in which the resident has independent responsibility and observation of faculty managing private patients, including initial consultation and management of complications.**
2. Codes diagnoses by the ICD-9-CM system.
3. Codes procedures by the CPT system.
4. Photographs his own patients with a standardized format.
5. Attends risk management seminar or studies risk management techniques and discusses principles with faculty; applies these principles in the daily practice of plastic surgery.

EVALUATION OF THE PATIENT

The most important person in the practice of plastic surgery is the patient. All activities of surgeons and their staff should focus on delivering the best care and service to the patient. This begins at the time of the first contact, which is usually with a member of the office staff. The staff should be friendly and professional in the greeting, in making the appointment, and in determining its purpose. This first contact often establishes the relationship between the patient and the surgeon and the surgeon's office staff. Since it is difficult for the surgeon to evaluate how this function is performed, there is merit in having someone call the office for the surgeon from time to time to evaluate the quality of the first contact.

A patient's time is valuable, and the patient should not expect to wait too long from the time of the appointment. When the surgeon is unavoidably detained, patients who are waiting should be informed of this fact and the reason for the delay. An offer should be made to make a new appointment for those who cannot wait. This change in appointment should not be a repetitive procedure.

When meeting the surgeon, the patient should expect to have sufficient time devoted to the visit to receive enough information to make an informed decision about the proposed treatment. When scheduling patients it is wise to leave a period in the middle of office hours free of appointments to allow the surgeon to get back on schedule if a patient requires an unusually long interview or examination. When on schedule this time can be used to make phone calls and catch up on other responsibilities.

The surgeon must begin the evaluation of the patient at the time of their first meeting. The initial contact is best carried out in the comfortable setting of the office rather than in an examining room. When the patient is fully clothed, in a comfortable seat, and relaxed, the probability is that there will be a better exchange of information. The preoperative and postoperative discussions should be carried out honestly and with demonstrable respect for the patient. While the language should not be too complex, it should not be too simplistic either.

The preoperative evaluation is particularly important for the patient seeking aesthetic surgery. While the primary indication for aesthetic surgery is a visible deformity for which correction is desired and improvement is possible, contraindications may be physical or emotional. The latter are the harder to uncover and evaluate. There are, however, certain patients who should raise concern on the part of the surgeon. Many times the only indication is that the surgeon feels uncomfortable with the patient. In this case and perhaps in many cases, additional visits should be required before undertaking a surgical procedure on the patient. In some cases the wisest course is to refuse to undertake the procedure at any time. In this instance the patient may challenge the surgeon with the question, "Don't you think you can do the operation?" The best answers are "No" or "Not to satisfy your expectations."

There are more specific warning signs: A patient who is indecisive or secretive about the requested treatment should be eschewed. If the patient has undergone a recent emotional event (e.g., divorce, bereavement), it might be best to wait until the patient has worked through the stress before undertaking the treatment. Since the surgery is designed to make the patient happier, family disapproval could lead to postoperative criticism and negate any gain that the patient may have accrued. This could lead to significant dissatisfaction and legal action against the surgeon. The surgeon may come to rue the day that an operation was performed upon a patient who was too demanding or who had a history of multiple procedures. These patients are frequently never satisfied and become very difficult.

Surgery should not be done in haste. There must be sufficient time for the patient to consider the procedure and its risks and consequences. In many cases, two or more preoperative appointments are appropriate. The use of printed educational material for the patient is very helpful.

RISK MANAGEMENT

Every surgeon will have results that do not please the patient. How these results are handled and the relationship developed by the surgeon will determine whether the issue is settled in court or in the surgeon's office. The surgeon should be sensitive to the signs of dissatisfaction. The first indication will be the concerns voiced by the patient in the postoperative period. This is even more important when the patient is accompanied by a member of the family or a friend when visiting the office. If the patient fails to keep follow-up appointments or expresses disproportionate distress, the surgeon should be wary.

The groundwork for the management of unsatisfactory results or complications is laid during the preoperative visits. Information for consent for surgery should include the following:

1. Description and explanation of the problem and the proposed treatment.
2. Description and explanation of the risks involved and the incidence of each.
3. Common side effects of the treatment (e.g., swelling, ecchymosis, scars, etc.).
4. A statement that a guarantee of complete satisfaction is not available. (This does not abrogate the responsibility to procede within the standard of care.)
5. Questions by the patient should be encouraged.
6. There should be acknowledgment that the consent can be withdrawn at any time.
7. The patient should realize that a second opinion may be obtained if desired.

The consent form itself should attest that these issues have been covered. A signed form should be obtained from every patient before surgery and included in the chart. There are many types of forms, and many have been successful in addressing the above issues. Advice on the best form can be obtained from an attorney knowledgeable in this area or from a representative of the professional liability insurance carrier.

During the preoperative discussion there should be a discussion of the manner in which unsatisfactory results or complications will be handled and *the cost.* If a fee is normally charged for a secondary procedure and it is not in a particular case, this may be construed as evidence that the surgeon erred.

The surgeon should listen to the concerns of the patient and be ready to help the patient resolve the problem. Frequent visits and close follow-up give the patient needed support during this difficult time. Written complaints should be answered in writing. There should be a policy established for the office staff in managing these situations. The staff must show as much concern as the surgeon. Second opinions should be encouraged, and these consultations should be offered at the surgeon's expense.

The surgeon must be prepared to handle patients who seek consultation because they are unhappy with the care received from another surgeon. The consultant should accept the patient's version of the incident cautiously. Written authorization for release of the medical records should be obtained and the records reviewed before an opinion is rendered. It is unwise to accept a patient who refuses to identify the physician. The discussion should be focused on the plan to remedy the problem, and there should be no discussion of liability or fault. The primary goal is to correct the deficit and satisfy the patient.

Some patients will seek legal remedies in spite of the careful attention given to them by the surgeon. Medical malpractice can be demonstrated only when a doctor/patient relationship has been formed. The patient must have sustained an injury that is the result of the surgeon's action or lack of action that was shown to be a deviation from the standard of care. This standard is usually determined by expert witnesses obtained by the patient's attorney and the surgeon's attorney. When there is conflict in the definition of the standard, the jury must decide between the options.

The best prevention for a charge of malpractice is to adhere to the standard of care in every situation. Allergies should be noted prominently on the charts to avoid administration of inappropriate medications. Patients should be advised of the effect of smoking on the outcome of surgery, and in some cases surgery should not be done if the patient does not stop smoking for a reasonable time before and after the operation.

Efforts to collect upaid fees are often the precipitating factor in the filing of a suit. Fees and other cost of secondary procedures should be discussed before surgery. Preoperative decisions should be obtained from insurance carriers if the patient expects to have the procedure paid for by the carrier. When a determination of prior approval is requested from the group responsible for the payment of the medical bills, the appropriate codes from the *International Classification of Diseases-9—Clinical Modification (ICD-9-CM)* and the *Current Procedural Terminology (CPT)* should be included. An unexpected bill can make the outcome of surgery look much less acceptable.

The medical record is the surgeon's best friend and worst enemy. When the records are complete and accurate, they will be a support if legal action is taken. Sloppy and incomplete records can lose the case before it gets to trial. When the patient seeks the advice of an attorney, the medical record is the first document reviewed, and it is upon this review that the decision to take the case may be made. Experts will use the record to determine whether the surgeon has deviated from the standard of care, and it will be the facts in the record upon which the jury bases its verdict.

Abbreviations and illegible entries in the record may lead to confusion and misinterpretation and should be avoided. Missed appointments should be documented because that may lay the foundation for the conclusion that the patient is partially responsible for the outcome. The content, time, and date of telephone calls should be entered into the record. All entries should be signed or initialed. If they have not been read, that should be indicated. When an error is detected, it should be crossed out but not obliterated. The correction should be initialed and dated. A record should never be altered to avoid liability after a claim or suit has been filed. When there is evidence such as this that impugns the honesty of the surgeon, he may be dropped by the insurance carrier from whom he has purchased liability insurance.

The professional liability insurance carrier should be notified promptly if there is an indication that a claim or suit will be filed. Policies have a requirement concerning this notification, and stipulations of the policy should be determined as soon as possible so that the surgeon will not be deemed out of compliance with the policy when notification is necessary.

Professional liability insurance comes in two basic forms. The first is an occurrence policy. This is becoming less common. This type of insurance covers the policyholder for any suit filed for an act that occurred during the term of the policy. For example, a suit filed 10 years after the policy was terminated regarding an act that occurred during the duration of the policy would be covered by the policy.

The second form is a claims made policy. Under this policy all claims made during the term of the policy are covered regardless of the time of the occurrence of the act causing the claim. This leaves the policyholder vulnerable after the termination of the policy unless a policy to cover the "tail" is purchased. This latter policy will cover claims made after the termination of the claims made coverage. Such termination may occur at the time of the retirement of the physician.

PHOTOGRAPHY

Photographs may be used to educate the patient in preparation for surgery. The surgeon must be careful that the photographs are not used to "sell" the surgery. Including fair and poor results along with good results will blunt the salesmanship. It may be useful to show patients the common side effects of the surgery (e.g., swelling, ecchymosis, or crusting following a chemical peel or dermabrasion).

There are other reasons to take good photographs. They will become an important part of the patient's record. Most patients will appreciate the opportunity to see before and after pictures of themselves. When the change is not fully appreciated, viewing of the preoperative photographs will demonstrate the change more clearly. The surgeon can also evaluate the results and appreciate his progress in doing the procedure. There is also the opportunity to see how the procedure might be done better in the future.

Pictures are frequently helpful or necessary to convince the payer of the significance of a problem and of the appropriateness of the request for payment. They are helpful in court for personal injury cases or medical malpractice cases.

Photographs must be taken carefully and as accurately as medical records if they are to be of optimal use. The equipment necessary does not have to be complex or expensive. The procedures should be standardized and the results reproducible. A 35-mm single-lens reflex camera with an attached electronic flash is the most versatile. Photographs of the limited regions of the body can best be taken with a

90-mm, 100-mm, or 105-mm macro lens. Half- or full-body photographs will require a greater camera-to-subject distance if these lenses are used, and a 50-mm or 35-mm macro lens may be preferable. The use of an extension tube on any of these lenses will allow close-ups to be taken. Zoom lenses should be avoided for general clinical photography since the results are not as uniform.

A separate photography room is the most desirable arrangement. If this is not feasible, the examining rooms can be arranged to allow for photographs. A distance of about 8 ft is enough unless full-body photographs are to be taken with a long–focal length lens. The background should be uncluttered and in a color that will allow contrast and easy viewing. Light blues, grays, or black may be used. Black may not give adequate contrast for patients with dark skin tones. The background can be made from rolls of colored paper produced for this purpose or a colored window shade. The advantage of these methods is that the background material can be pulled down onto the floor to provide a continuous background for photographs of the feet and lower part of the legs. The background can also be created by painting a section of the wall expressly for this purpose.

The best lighting is a two-light system to effect good modeling of the subject. This is more difficult to establish unless there is a dedicated photography room. The poorest lighting is probably produced with a ring light because it tends to subdue contours. A flash on the camera will serve the average surgeon well. Standardization of the methods and careful preparation of the subject are essential, as is avoidance of shadows.

There are some excellent materials available covering clinical photography. *Photographic Standards in Plastic Surgery* is a system prepared on a laminated card by the Plastic Surgery Educational Foundation Clinical Photography Committee in 1991 and is a good basis for building a system.

It is important to be consistent. This can be done by establishing the lens, lens opening (f-stop), camera-to-subject distance, shutter speed, and subject position for all the common regions that are photographed in the office. This can be recorded, and members of the staff may be taught to take many of the routine photographs.

The primary goal of subject preparation is to clearly demonstrate the areas of interest and produce a clinical picture. Glasses should be removed in most instances. Makeup should be minimal or nonexistent. There should be a similar amount of it in the preoperative and postoperative pictures. Jewelry should be removed or placed out of the picture. Long hair should be behind the shoulders in photographs of the breasts. Clothing should not be left partially on so that it is visible in the picture. In most cases a clinical photographic garment can be used to prevent embarrassment to the patient.

There are many systems for storing photographs. In most cases they are in the form of 35-mm transparencies. These are easily stored in racks or plastic loose-leaf pages. There are advantages and disadvantages to all repositories for these photographs. If they are kept in the patient's chart, they are always available when the patient is seen. However, they are not as readily available for teaching and other presentations. A solution to this dilemma is to duplicate all slides that will be used for presentation and leave the originals in the patient's chart. Be certain that all photographs that identify the patient are covered by a release signed by the patient. This can be included in the consent form.

The availability of a slide viewer in the office makes it easier for the patient to view the slides. Prints of the slides can be made for patient education or for the payer when they are determining approval for payment. There are inexpensive units that will make instant prints in the office.

CODING

The introduction of computers into the health care system has made the identification of patients, physicians, hospitals, diseases, and procedures increasingly dependent upon numbers. The use of these numbers to identify diseases and procedures has increased the need for the practicing surgeon to understand the system. Improper coding not only affects the amount of remuneration received but could also open the surgeon to accusations of fraud and abuse of the system. The disease is designated by a code from the ICD-9-CM. This listing is modified every 10 years. The procedures are identified in the CPT. This listing is produced by the American Medical Association and is updated annually. There are courses given regularly by specialty societies (including the American Society of Plastic and Reconstructive Surgeons), health insurance companies, state medical societies, and various government agencies. It is worthwhile for surgeons and their staff to attend certain of these instructional courses to remain current on this important subject.

The Surgeons should not leave the function of assigning codes to the various procedures to staff members. The surest method for the surgeon to learn the system is for the surgeon to do the coding. If there is an experienced staff person who can do the routine coding, the responsibility can be transferred. In this instance the surgeon regularly reviews samples of the coding and the surgeon does the unusual coding.

The ICD-9-CM code must be compatible with the CPT code. CPT codes must not represent a level of care or complexity of care that exceeds what was delivered ("upcoding," "code creep"). Multiple codes must not be used ("unbundling") if there is a single code to cover the procedure.

SUMMARY

Patient selection is an art that must be developed over time. It requires patience, discipline, and the courage to tell patients that the surgeon will not operate upon them at that time or ever. Risk management is based on respecting the patient and the trust that she is placing in the surgeon. This trust is repaid by practicing within the standard of care and within the surgeon's range of knowledge and ability. Good practice management requires the same attention to detail that is required in the operating room. Record keeping, photography, and coding are not as challenging as surgery. They will bring other rewards and protect the surgeon from embarrassment or worse.

SUGGESTED READING

Goin JM, Goin MK: *Changing the Body; Psychological Effects of Plastic Surgery.* Baltimore, Williams & Wilkens, 1981.

Goldwyn RM: *The Patient and the Plastic Surgeon,* ed 2. Boston, Little, Brown, 1991.

Goldwyn RM (ed): *The Unfavorable Results of Plastic Surgery, Avoidance and Treatment,* ed 2. Boston, Little, Brown, 1984, pp 3–46.

Zupko KA (ed): *Office and Practice Management Notebook.* Chicago, American Society of Plastic and Reconstructive Surgeons, 1992.

Index

B

C

E

H

M

S

T

V

W